# Public Health and Community Medicine

## 2nd edition

# Public Health and Community Medicine for the allied medical professions

## 2nd edition

**LLOYD EDWARD BURTON, M.S., Ph.D.**
Professor, College of Pharmacy
University of Arizona

**HUGH HOLLINGSWORTH SMITH, M.D., M.P.H.**
Research Professor, Department of Microbiology and Medical Technology
University of Arizona
Formerly: Associate Director, Division of Medicine and Public Health
The Rockefeller Foundation, New York

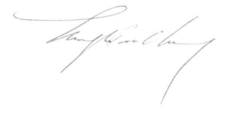

The Williams & Wilkins Company
Baltimore

Copyright ©, 1975
The Williams & Wilkins Company
428 E. Preston Street
Baltimore, Maryland 21202

*Made in the United States of America*

**Library of Congress Cataloging in Publication
Data**

Burton, Lloyd Edward, 1922–
Public Health and community medicine for the
allied medical professions.

   Includes bibliographies.
   1. Hygiene, Public. 2. Medical care – United
States.   I.   Smith,   Hugh   Hollingsworth,
1902–      joint author. II. Title. RA425.B83
1975     362.1'0973   74-13225   ISBN
0-683-01235-5

First edition, 1970
Reprinted 1971, 1972, 1973

Composed and Printed at
The Waverly Press, Inc.
Mt. Royal and Guilford Avenues
Baltimore, Maryland 21202

*With appreciation and affection*
*to our respective wives,*

CHIO  BURTON  and  MARY  ROYHL  SMITH

# Preface to the second edition

In the five years since our book first appeared, events have moved rapidly on many fronts in the health care field. The scope and rate of change are seen more prominently in health care legislation as Congress is seeking ways to bridge existing gaps. In revising this textbook, we have attempted to review the highlights of the recent changes in health care policies and to discuss proposed measures for improving the distribution of services to all people on an equitable basis. In addition, as we move more into the preventive aspects of health care, there is an increasing, gnawing suggestion that perhaps we should place more emphasis on the causes of health rather than on the causes of disease.

In our view, public health is a function of government and voluntary agencies to promote and protect the health of the community. In addition to health professionals, there are many civic leaders, public officials, and interested citizens who are deeply concerned with the success of this "systemized social action." The tools of public health are such "population based disciplines" as epidemiology, statistics, sociology, and demography.

Our concept of community medicine is that it is concerned with problems relating to the health of the people, falling between the private practice of medicine in the office, clinic, or hospital and the services provided by public health agencies.

Community medicine involves both preventive and curative procedures. Its approach is to families or groups of the population not adequately served by other available agencies. Problems relating to social and occupational situations that affect the people's health are of special concern. Initiation of programs in community medicine may be sponsored by medical colleges, community hospitals, medical societies and other professional organizations, or by other agencies in the community interested in conducting studies or in operating health care programs in this field. We have tried to keep this concept in mind in our description of the current scene of human health and in the discussion of specific disease entities.

Advances in biomedical research continue to flow from the great number of university laboratories and from research institutes of the world. Indeed new scientific and technological information is received at a far higher rate than it can be assimilated and put into effective use. The intensification of investigations on many fronts brings hope for the prevention or cure of several types of malignant tumors and for more secure protection against the infectious diseases.

In the preparation of this revised edition, the authors have made particular use of the following publications for which they wish to express sincere appreciation:

1. Report of the Committee on Infectious Diseases of the American Academy of Pediatrics; 17th Ed., 1974.
2. The Report by the Carnegie Commission on Higher Education, "Higher Education and the Nation's Health," 1970.
3. Anne R. Somers, "Health Care in Transition—Directions for the Future," published by Hospital Research and Educational Trust, Chicago, 1971.
4. Rosemary Stevens, "American Medicine and the Public Interest," Yale University Press, 1971.

The authors also would like to record their gratitude to Dr. George A. Bender, noted authority on the art and science of pharmacy. Dr. Bender has kindly reviewed our first chapter suggesting a number of valuable contributions on pharmaceutical history and on the mutual relationships of the professions of pharmacy and medicine.

A special acknowledgment goes to Richard A. Seggel, Senior Professional Associate, Institute of Medicine, National Academy of Sciences, in gratitude for his considerable help. Thanks to Mr. Seggel, we were able to obtain last minute changes in structure and function of the Public Health Service which, in turn, provides the reader with a more current text.

Appreciation is also due to Ms. Susan Horowitz, Public Health Service, Bureau of Health Resources Development, Office of Special Programs, for most helpful assistance in obtaining current data on health programs in her area of jurisdiction.

It is a pleasure, too, to acknowledge our debt to the World Health Organization, and to the Indian Health Service, Desert Willow Training Center, Tucson, Arizona, who have generously provided us with photographs of some aspects of public health programs in their areas of operation.

L. E. Burton
H. H. Smith

# Preface to the first edition

At this exciting point in 20th century society, there has emerged the philosophy that good health and the availability of adequate medical services should be included in the rights of citizenship. National attention has been focused upon this new obligation and increasingly larger percentages of the tax dollar are being appropriated to fund this rapidly enlarging endeavor. The constant demands for improved quality of medical care, combined with greater numbers of people seeking health services from public supported programs, require a more comprehensive definition of the words "public health."

Health is associated more and more with community hygiene, whether it be in the field of mental health, chronic illnesses, communicable diseases, accidents, or environmental pollution. Also, the dividing line between public health and private medicine is becoming more diffuse. Therefore, it has become urgent for those who are to enter the allied medical fields to obtain a good understanding of the circumstances impinging upon the various health professions as they struggle to cope with the problems of their communities. In addition, experience has demonstrated that the active participation of all educated members of the community is required to overcome the inertia of traditional attitudes that have obstructed progress toward many desirable goals.

One recognizes that there is already a considerable list of excellent books on public health and preventive medicine. Why then have the authors undertaken to launch another book which treats these topics? To paraphrase one of Thomas Jefferson's ringing phrases—"a decent respect to the opinions of mankind requires that they should declare the causes which impel them to"—write this book. Some years of teaching public health and preventive medicine to groups of university students of widely divergent backgrounds, whose future plans were as varied as their past experiences, have furnished the time to observe the trends in public health and to evaluate teaching methods and materials. Our students included premedical students, students planning to enter the field of public administration, and those being educated for pharmacy, nursing, and medical technology. There are textbooks on public health of superior quality for use in graduate schools and for medical students, and there are good books prepared in simpler terms for those who are satisfied by a superficial review of the subject matter, but the authors felt that there was no text suitable for undergraduates with a keen interest in health careers. Our objective in undertaking the book now being presented is to adjust the discussion to a level of appeal for those being trained in the health field—pharmacists, nurses, medical technologists, medical social workers, and the many other highly important members of the allied medical professions.

Our effort has been to describe the converging interests of public health and private medicine—to emphasize the closely knit relationship and interdependencies of all community activities, to promote, to restore, and to maintain the health of the people at the highest possible level. It is generally recognized that the numerous barriers to health care and the obstacles that prevent optimal medical services could be removed if all concerned pulled together in the right direction. Action on the political scene has made strides toward removing financial barriers and in providing greatly increased physical facilities for care. Under Federal guidance, first steps toward comprehensive health planning are being taken in many states. Other programs for regional medical care are in process of organization in all sections of the United States. The pot is really boiling! It remains for professional members of the medical health community to be made aware of the significant parts they can perform in making community medicine and public health a reality in the next decade.

As an acute observer, Robert Burton, (1577-1640), pointed out long ago, "They lard their lean books with the fat of others' works." The authors must plead guilty to this indictment. Without the works of others, one could not prepare such a textbook. Special appreciation is due the varied and numerous publications of the United States Public Health Service, and of its dependencies, the National Communicable Disease Center and the National Center for Health Statistics. No one can discuss public health during recent times without frequent reference to their valuable works. We are also grateful to the National Academy of Sciences of the National Research Council and to the National Commission on Community Health Services for much important source material.

In discussing the prevention of communicable disease, the authoritative reports of the Committee on Communicable Disease Control, of the American Public Health Association, and of the Committee on the Control of Infectious Diseases of the American Academy of Pediatrics are indispensable. The authors gratefully acknowledge their frequent references to these works.

The historical introduction is based solidly upon the great work of Fielding H. Garrison, of whom Dr. Henry R. Viets of Boston has said, "It was Garrison's task in life to take a narrower path and climb it higher than any of the others—the rocky path of the history of medicine."

Another important source of concepts, information, and views of the future that we are pleased to acknowledge is the recent book *Man Adapting* by René Dubos, New Haven, Yale University Press, 1965. This book should be read by every educated person. It is a splendid source of wisdom and of well-considered comments on the trends in health sciences in our current society.

Considerable reliance has been placed on two well-known books for guidance in the general principles of public health and preventive medicine. These are: (1) Rosenau-Maxcy, *Public Health and Preventive Medicine,* edited by P. E. Sartwell, New York: Appleton-Century-Crofts, 1965; and (2) *Preventive Medicine,* edited by D. W. Clark and B. MacMahon, Boston: Little, Brown, and Company, 1967. In the account of representative diseases of man, we relied, to a considerable extent, on the excellent *Cecil-Loeb Textbook of Medicine* for clinical data. These volumes, now in their 12th edition, are edited by Paul Beeson and Walsh McDermott and are published by W. B. Saunders Company. All of these professional treatises can be recommended without reserve, and the authors acknowledge their indebtedness with great appreciation to both the publishers and authors of these works.

The World Health Organization kindly supplied the photograph of its headquarters building in Geneva and a series of fascinating photographs illustrating several facets of their far flung health programs. The Pan American Health Organization generously provided the photograph of its imposing new headquarters building in Washington, D.C.

Special appreciation to Dr. Roger D. Baker is due for his kind permission to make use of a number of his excellent photographs reproduced from his textbook *Essential Pathology* published by the Williams and Wilkins Company.

Finally, thanks are due the Honorable Morris K. Udall, Representative from Arizona in the Congress of the United States, for obtaining the up-to-date information set forth in Chapter III on the activities of the medical departments of the Armed Forces of the Unites States and of the Veterans Bureau.

An attempt has been made to acknowledge the many additional debts to the works of others in the lists of references cited at the end of each chapter and in the notes on the sources of the many borrowed figures, tables, and photographs. Our thanks are extended to all of these upon whose works we have built and to those who have generously allowed us to borrow their thoughts in the form of quoted material. Indeed, our task has been largely that of compilation, synthetization, and interpretation of the work done or described by others.

Lloyd E. Burton
Hugh H. Smith

# Contents

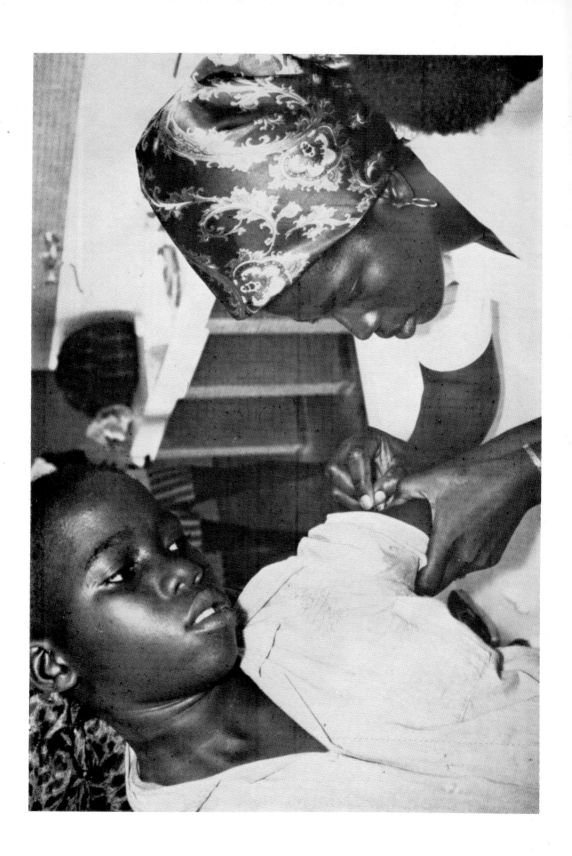

# 1

# *Historical introduction*

Nothing is lost in history: Sooner or later every creative idea finds opportunity and development, and adds its color to the flame of life.

WILL DURANT

But I am no historian and my hope is rather to make you feel the general circumstances, the sweep and movement of medicine, its interest and its fiery vitality.

ALAN GREGG

The successes of medicine and the medical sciences have not been lightly won; from a multitude of failures they are the survivals, the fortunate productions of the best or the most-favored men among an endless succession of skillful physicians.

LAWRENCE J. HENDERSON

To wrest from nature the secrets which have perplexed philosophers in all ages, to track to their sources the causes of disease, to correlate the vast stores of knowledge, that they may be quickly available for the prevention and cure of disease—these are our ambitions.

SIR WILLIAM OSLER

But on that account, I say, we ought not to reject the ancient Art, as if it were not, and had not been properly founded, because it did not attain accuracy in all things, but rather, since it is capable of reaching to the greatest exactitude by reasoning, to receive it and admire its discoveries, made from a state of great ignorance, and as having been well and properly made, and not from change.

HIPPOCRATES, *On Ancient Medicine*

---

## PRIMITIVE MEDICINE

From the beginning, man was faced with the fearful hazards of sickness, wounds, childbirth, and premature death. To soften the blows of these fierce aspects of nature, man has endeavored from the earliest times to discover remedies for his ailments and preventives to ward off ill health. Some notion of the evolution of such skills has been gained by studying the few remaining primitive peoples on the earth, but perhaps more has been learned by those who have attempted to reconstruct all aspects of the lives of prehistoric man from the surviving artifacts.

The common meeting point of all medical folklore appears to be animism, *i.e.*, the idea that the world swarms with invisible spirits which are frequently the cause of disease and death.[1] It must be understood that attempts to explain and treat illnesses were only one phase of a set of magic or mystic processes designed to promote the welfare of the group. Such matters as averting the wrath of angered gods or evil spirits, fire making, rain making, purifying streams or habitations, improving sexual potency, preventing crop failures, and warding off epidemic diseases were all functions of one person, be he god, king, sorcerer, priest, or medicine man. These important affairs all formed the savage's concept of "making medicine."

In religion, primitive man was essentially a pantheist. He worshipped the sun, the moon, the stars, trees, rivers, fire, springs, and even animals. Winds, storms, clouds, earthquakes, or other unusual experiences in nature were to him outward and visible signs of malevolent gods, demons, spirits, or other supernatural powers. Disease came to be regarded as the work of an evil spirit, and, as such, the spirit had to be placated or driven out. Primitives also believed that disease may be produced by a human enemy possessing supernatural powers. These he strove to ward off by appropriate spells and sorcery, similar to those employed by the enemy himself.

Another way of looking at disease was that it resulted from the actions of offended spirits of the dead, whether of man or animals. As these concepts developed, there came the advent of the medicine man or witch doctor, who assumed a supervisory relation to the cure of disease not unlike that of the priest to religion. He did his best to frighten away the demons of disease by assuming a terrifying aspect, covering himself with the skins of animals, shouting, slapping his hands, shaking a rattle, or pretending to suck away the demon through a hollow tube. The patient was provided a special fetish to be worn or carried to prevent future attacks by the same demon. These methods are not essentially different from faith-healing of our own day.

Primitive medicine fits in midway between magic and religion, by protecting against ill health through propitiation of the gods, by warding off evil influences, or through control of supernatural processes. As primitive man advanced in knowledge gained from experience, some improvement in the art of medicine was made. A special talent was developed for herb-doctoring, bone-setting, and rude surgery. One finds that savages in widely separated regions get to know the most fatal arrow poisons—curare, ouabain, among others—as well as the value of some plant derivatives as opium, hashish, coca, cinchona, tobacco, jalap, and numerous other herbs. North American Indians knew that arbutus was useful in treating rheumatism, lobelia for coughs, wild sage tea for fevers, wild ginger and ginseng for digestive disorders. The Iroquois around Quebec introduced Jacques Cartier to the use of an infusion of the bark and leaves of the hemlock spruce for the successful treatment of scurvy among his crew.

Primitive surgery made use of sharpened flints or obsidian knives and fishes' teeth. Blood was let, abscesses were opened, skulls were trephined, and ritual operations like circumcision were carried out. Wounds were dressed with moss or fresh leaves, ashes or natural balsams.

The midwife is one of the most ancient of medical figures. To assist women in childbirth, there was a universal tendency among primitives to adopt measures to aid or hasten delivery. The obstetric chair appears to be of great antiquity and is still used by some peoples of the Far East.

Primitive people learned from long experience the need for burying or burning refuse and human and animal excreta and for protecting water supplies from pollution. The dead were buried or placed in trees at places kept apart from the habitations of the group. The primitive man's reasons for such customs were based on magic. He buried his excrement so that something which had been a part of himself could not be employed by his enemies to cause him harm; he refrained from throwing refuse into the water so as not to offend the spirit of the river. The ceremonial of the burial rites was intended to propitiate the powerful ancestral spirits.

Although tribal customs arose mainly from superstition, many effective methods of disease prevention have been handed down from the past. They believed that evil spirits could affect everything belonging to the sick person: his clothing, his possessions, anything that he had touched. Fear of these spirits led to keeping the sick apart from the healthy. Many savages were prepared to burn down the infected hut and its contents. Other peoples unable to cope with a spreading infection by the usual incantations and charms burnt the entire village and moved to a new location.

William Osler,[2] the great medical teacher, reminds us that, "Civilization is but the filmy fringe on the history of man." Is it surprising that some concepts of our primitive background remain with us today?

## OLD WORLD (OR ANCIENT) MEDICINE

When prehistoric man discovered that wild wheat and barley could be cultivated, he gave up his nomadic existence. As man became settled in favorable circumstances, he soon unearthed copper and tin (the combination of which produced a harder and more useful product, bronze). So men began to develop complex urban civilizations concentrated in the great river valleys of the East: along the Nile, the Tigris and Euphrates, the Indus, and the great Yellow River of China. Among each of these civilized peoples, medicine became a systemized professional discipline based, at least to some extent, upon the primitive medicine employed from the earliest times.

The Sumerians of Mesopotamia (about 4000–3000 B.C.) laid the foundations of modern civilation by the invention of pictorial writing and the development of astronomy. In all of the early civilizations, we find astronomy applied to the practical affairs of life as astrology. Wars, epidemics, famines, and other matters of public or private interest were closely studied in relation to equinoxes, eclipses, comets, and changes of the moon and stars. For the most part, the Babylonian physicians regarded disease as the work of demons which swarmed in the earth, air, and water and against which long litanies or incantations were invoked.[3]

The oldest pharmaceutical document which has been translated is a clay tablet (now in the University of Pennsylvania Museum) written by an unknown Sumerian about 2100 B.C. The hand-sized slab of baked clay presents, in cuneiform characters, a number of formulas (or prescriptions) composed of recognizable drugs and vehicles. It was one of thousands of tablets dug up at Nippur.[4]

More is known of early Egyptian medicine because of the remarkable preservation of records in the tombs buried in the desert sands along the Nile Valley. Archaeological excavations of sites of the Old Kingdom (3400-2400 B.C.) to the New Empire (1580-1200 B.C.) reveal the continuous development of a highly specialized society. In addition to pictorial records found in the tombs, the main source of knowledge of Egyptian medicine is the papyri that have been carefully translated. These paperlike sheets made from the papyrus reed were covered with a closely written cursive script. Also, the Egyptian custom of embalming the dead has provided an unusual opportunity to investigate the kinds of diseases that flourished in that time.

The Egyptians believed that astrological events had a great influence on health and disease. The various Egyptian gods when displeased frequently punished the people with plagues and illnesses. In the case of severe sickness, the physician or sorcerer was called in, and the treatment consisted of spells, incantations, and other magic or religious rites. By such means, the gods might be placated. The physician also understood the value of a sound diet and of personal hygiene. The Egyptians believed that exhalation of decomposing bodies produced pestilence. This notion passed into rational medicine in the miasmic theory of disease causation.

It is probable that the Egyptians never carried surgery to the extent of opening the body,

although circumcisions and possibly surgery of the neck and limbs were undertaken. Splints to hold fractured bones in position have often been found on mummies. Egyptian knowledge of anatomy and physiology was of the most rudimentary character.

Egyptians classified over 260 diseases. The causes of these were mostly unknown. Stereotyped instructions for the recognition and treatment of these were handed down without change from one generation to another. A rich variety of drugs was available in Egyptian medicine: tonics, emetics, enemas, and so on. The Ebers Papyrus, a scroll some 20 meters long, written about 1500 B.C., and a compilation from many earlier documents, throws considerable light on pharmaceutical knowledge in ancient Egypt. More than 700 drugs are included in over 800 prescriptions recorded in the scroll. Botanical drugs predominate, but others derived from the animal and mineral sources.[5]

The main interest of Egyptian medicine lies in its great influence on the development of Greek medicine. Doubtless, the ancient Greeks learned as much of medicine as of chemistry from the civilized people of the Nile. Their first visits to Egypt began in the 12th to 13th centuries, B.C. By the 7th century B.C., there was frequent contact between the Greeks and the Egyptians.

Among the Semitic peoples, the concept of disease as punishment for sin was generally accepted. Even in Babylonian medicine, which was primarily built on demonology, the thought of disease as associated with bodily impurity or sin appears. In the Old Testament this concept comes to full flower. The overwhelming mass of references to disease in the Old Testament involves the concept of punishment for sin and the gospel of punishment for sin and the gospel of righteousness as its only remedy. "If ye walk contrary unto me, and will not hearken unto me; I will bring seven times more plagues upon you according to your sins" (Leviticus 26:21). "So the Lord sent a pestilence upon Israel from the morning even to the time appointed: and there died of the people from Dan even to Beersheba seventy thousand men" (II Samuel 24:15). After David had made appropriate burnt offerings and peace offerings, the "Lord was intreated for the land, and the plague was stayed from Israel" (II Samuel 24:25).

In China, the early history of medicine is

purely legendary. As far back as 2737 B.C. the Emperor is said to have experimented with poisons and classified medicinal plants. Emperor Shen Nung (ca 2000 B.C.) is credited with having sought out and investigated the medicinal values of several hundred herbs, some of which he tested upon himself. He also is credited with authorship of the first "Pen T'sao" or native herbal, the base from which Chinese pharmacy sprang.[6] Aside from a considerable skill with drugs, Chinese medicine was based on a theory of Taoist philosophy that life is an interplay between two forces: Yang (light, heat, and life) and Yin (darkness, cold, and death). A proper balance in the body of these two forces meant harmony and health. If either force became predominant, disharmony and disease appeared. The treatment for this imbalance was acupuncture. This method, used for 4000 to 5000 years in China, consists of sticking fine needles into the body at carefully selected places. The theory assumed that the life force flows through certain channels, and that these are related to points on the skin. The acupuncture needles were inserted for 2 to 3 mm. through the skin at the appropriate points, acting as a stimulus. Yang and Yin were restored to harmony.

In recent years the Chinese have experimented with considerable success with acupuncture as a method of providing anesthesia for surgical procedures. With the improvement of relations between China and the United States there have been several exchanges of visits between physician groups of the two countries. This has resulted in a marked increase of interest in acupuncture among physicians and laymen in the United States. Some states permit the use of acupuncture in medical practice; others limit its use to research groups which are seeking to learn what may be the scientific basis, if any, for acupuncture.

The Chinese were adept at massage. They were early acquainted with identification of individuals by fingerprints. Ancient Chinese knew of preventive inoculation against smallpox, which practice was probably gotten from India.

In India, the ancient Hindus became skillful in surgery. About 120 different surgical instruments including scalpels, lancets, saws, needles, hooks, probes, trocars, catheters, and so on were described in early records. The Hindus apparently knew every important operative

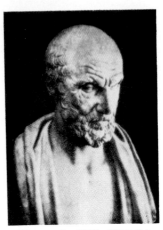

Hippocrates (460–370 B.C.)
Source: Garrison, F. H. *An Introduction to the History of Medicine,* Ed. 4. Philadelphia: W. B. Saunders Co., 1929, p. 93

procedure except the use of the ligature. They amputated limbs, checking hemorrhage by cauterization. At the time of Alexander's expedition (327 B.C.), Indian physicians enjoyed a high reputation for superior knowledge and skill.

In summary, medicine advanced considerably among the early Eastern Civilizations. According to Garrison[7] "The Babylonians had some intuition of the nature and prevention of communicable diseases; the Jews originated medical jurisprudence and public hygiene, and ordained a weekly day of rest; the Chinese introduced anthropometry, fingerprints, massage (osteopathy), acupuncture, and many drugs, and the Hindus demonstrated skill in operative surgery."

## GREEK MEDICINE

The philosophical and scientific revolution (6th century B.C.) in Greece had its antecedent inheritance not only in prescientific beliefs, myths, and cosmogonies of the Greeks themselves, but also in treasures of Babylonian and Egyptian thought of 2000 years. Knowledge of stellar movements, approximate determination of the cycles of solar and lunar eclipses, the Egyptian calendar, the achievements in algebra and geometry, the superb Egyptian technology in metallurgy, mining, and building gave rise by coalescence with Greek thought to Grecian triumphs. Their almost total lack of an experimental method and dependence on empirical observation led to a general approach to the understanding of natural phenomena.[8] From Egypt came many drugs as well as the basis of medical ethics. Some Egyptian surgical instruments were copied.

The role of the gods in medicine clearly persisted. By the 5th century B.C., however, it had been discarded by the Greek intellectual leaders in favor of a philosophy which marked, in the words of Winslow,[9] "perhaps the most important turningpoint in the whole history of human thought." The concept that the universe is a rational system working by discoverable laws seems to have first appeared as a definite belief among the Greeks. If disease is postulated as caused by gods or demons, scientific progress is impossible. The concept of natural causation was the first essential step.

Hippocrates (460–370 B.C.), often called the Father of Medicine, gave to Greek medicine its scientific spirit and its ethical ideals. All that a man of genius could do for medicine, with no other instrument of precision than his own open mind and keen senses, he accomplished. Hippocrates virtually founded the bedside method which has been the distinctive technique of all true clinicians up to our own day.

The Greek concept from Hippocrates onward attributes all disease to disorders of the fluids of the body. Some 100 papers from members of the Hippocratic school have survived. It is impossible to know which of these were actually written by Hippocrates himself. They are obviously written by physicians of great intellectual power and experience.

The achievements of the Hippocratic school cleared the air as never before of the fog of superstition and fear surrounding human illness. However, in the understanding of disease, Greek physicians were handicapped by their ignorance of anatomy, physiology, and pathology. They conceived that arteries were full of air, since they were found empty at death. They imagined that arteries came from the heart and veins from the liver; for 2000 years this error was perpetuated.

It was the Greeks who gave to the world the profound and sensible belief in the healing power of nature. The physician assisted the patient's natural powers of resistance by simple remedies such as rest, good food, fresh air, massage, and hydrotherapy.

Excellent treatises on "Fractures, Dislocations, and Wounds of the Head," "Nutriment," "Epidemic Diseases," and "Regimen in Acute Diseases" were produced by Hippocrates or by his associates. "Airs, Waters, and Places" was perhaps the greatest of the Hippocratic writings. It is essentially a treatise on epidemic diseases to give the basic Greek theory of the controlling influence of climate, weather, water, and physiogeography on the occurrence of epidemics. The author recognized that there were always certain diseases present in a population. These he called endemic. Other diseases at certain times became excessively frequent. These were termed epidemic. The harmful effects of swamps in the causation of summer fevers (malaria) were well recognized.

The greatest scientific name after Hippocrates is that of Aristotle (384–322 B.C.), who gave to medicine the beginnings of botany, zoology, comparative anatomy, embryology, and physiology. He taught anatomy by dissection of animals. He was, in fact, the greatest biologist who appeared for some 2000 years. For more than 2000 years the philosophy and medical thought of Aristotle constituted the principal source of intellectual stimulus of mankind. Without the contributions of Aristotle to biology, the development of rational medicine might have followed a different course.

Soon after the death of Aristotle about 300 B.C., a great medical school was founded in Egypt at Alexandria. Greek physicians formed the teaching faculty of this school. Among these was Herophilus, who may be regarded as the founder of anatomy, and Erasistratus, who conducted important studies in physiology. Dissections of human cadavers were permitted in public, probably for the first time.

After the first generation or two, the high quality of the Alexandrian school began to wane. The school continued on a reduced basis for centuries. Thus, Greek science and culture were firmly implanted in the ancient Egyptian civilization and served to spread Greek doctrine to the East.

## ROMAN MEDICINE

After Corinth was destroyed in 146 B.C., Greek medicine to a large extent migrated to Italy. Before that time, Romans had relied mainly on medicinal herbs, superstitious rites, and sacrifices to the gods. As Rome conquered the Mediterranean World and took over the legacy of Greek culture, she acquired Greek knowledge of medicine and hygiene. As usual, the Romans stamped Greek ideas with their own peculiar character and altered them to suit their own purposes. In medicine, the Romans were strictly imitators, but, as engineers and administrators, as builders of baths and sewer systems, as providers of aqueducts for water supplies, they set the world a great example.

Frontinus (40–104 A.D.)[10], Water Commissioner of Rome for some years, published an account of the aqueducts of Rome. This report is the first full account of an important branch of public administration. According to Frontinus, the inhabitants of Rome from the earliest days obtained water from the Tiber River and from wells. By the time of the death of Frontinus, 13 large aqueducts were required to supply the city, delivering an estimated 222 million gallons a day. Because of its purity, water from some aqueducts was reserved for drinking purposes. The more polluted waters were used for gardens. The general supply was to fountains, baths, and other public facilities. Supply to private houses was only by an imperial grant.

Throughout the Empire, the Romans provided their cities with similar water supplies on a smaller scale. Many of the Roman cities also had sewerage systems carrying off surface water and sewage from the streets.

The earliest scientific medical work in Latin is the *De Re Medica* by A. Cornelius Celsus, prepared about 30 A.D. Celsus, a gentleman of culture but not a physician, compiled from Greek authors the available medical knowledge of his day. His work proved durable and was one of the first medical books to be printed (1478 A.D.), afterward passing through many more separate editions than almost any other scientific treatise. *De Re Medica* was a compendium of existing knowledge. Good accounts are given of the malarial fevers of Italy and their treatment, of gout, and of the treatment of different forms of insanity. Celsus was also the first important writer on medical history.

Pharmacy in the areas controlled by Rome was raised from magic and legend to a more scientific position by the works of Pedanios Dioscorides, a Greek who accompanied the Roman legions to most parts of the world known in the 1st century A.D. Dioscorides described drugs, their sources, their collection and preservation, and their supposed medicinal virtues.[11]

The ancient period closes with the name of the greatest Greek physician after Hippocrates, Galen (131–201 A.D.). A native of Pergamum in Asia Minor, Galen studied at Smyrna and at Alexandria. He traveled widely and practiced medicine in many cities of the Empire. At Rome, beginning practice in 164 A.D., he soon attained the leadership of his profession, but retired early to devote himself to study, travel, and teaching. Galen, with remarkable facility, substituted theorizing for plain observation and interpretation of facts as taught by Hippocrates. He developed a theoretical scheme to explain disease which remained in vogue until the 17th century. It supposes three types of so-called spirits associated with three types of the activity of living things. There were the natural spirits formed in the liver and distributed by the veins, the vital spirits formed in the heart and distributed by the arteries, and the animal spirits formed in the brain and distributed by the nerves. The animal spirits were especially associated with the higher functions of sensation and motion. The scheme presupposed minute pores in the system of the heart, through which the venous blood charged with natural spirits passed from the right ventricle into the left where it became charged with vital spirits. Arterial blood charged with vital spirits became converted to animal spirits in the brain and was thence distributed by the nerves.

Galen was the most voluminous writer of his times. His works are a huge compilation of current knowledge including nine books on anatomy, 17 on physiology, six on pathology, 16 essays on the pulse, 14 on therapeutics, 30 on pharmacy, and one on the method of medical practice. Galen also operated the equivalent of a pharmacy in Rome. He de-

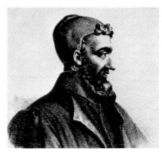

Galen (131–201 A.D.)
Source: National Library of Medicine, Bethesda, Maryland, Neg. No. 67-1028

veloped many methods of mixing, extracting, refining, and combining drugs. These ideas carried over into the late 18th century, and have come down to us today in that class of preparations known as galenicals.

After Galen's death, his writings on anatomy, physiology, and disease were regarded as the final authority. By modern standards, this medicine was severely limited, but it gave acceptable answers which were applied for 1500 years, and provided the correct impetus and direction for the rise of modern medicine.

Another important contribution of Rome is the hospital for the care of the sick or wounded. These began as valetudinaria, or infirmaries, for slaves. Public hospitals for civilians were paralleled by military institutions located at strategic areas of the Empire. Eventually, under the influence of Christianity, hospitals were created as benevolent acts of charity. The first of this kind was established in Rome in the fourth century.

Roman medicine was best in its practical aspects: in public health, the advance of surgery, and the creation of a hospital system. It surpassed all previous developments. It suffered as had the previous systems from limited knowledge of the sciences basic to medicine. Their hygienic achievements, such as cremation, town planning, well-ventilated, heated houses, public baths, paved streets, and so on were of more consequence than their other medical advances.

## MEDICINE IN THE MIDDLE AGES

Following the collapse of Rome, the problem in Europe was to weld together the culture of the barbarian invaders with the classical heritage of the fallen Empire and with the belief and teachings of the Christian religion. The Church became the repository of knowledge, not only of medicine but of learning in general. In this unfavorable medium for its growth, science was disregarded, not in any hostile spirit but as unnecessary. Under the edicts of the Church, supernatural origins of disease were revived. According to the teaching of St. Augustine, in the fifth century, all diseases could be ascribed to demons, sent to torment the human spirit. For almost eight centuries the study of medicine in the West was nearly static.

During the Middle Ages, when successions of invaders destroyed many libraries and museums, remnants of Western knowledge of pharmacy and medicine were rescued and preserved by religious orders in some of the monasteries. Manuscripts from many lands were laboriously copied by monks and the knowledge obtained from these manuscripts was taught in the cloisters to monk-practitioners. Disease was treated by the monks through prayers, laying on of hands, penances, and the exhibition of holy relics. The extent of such practices became so great that finally Pope Innocent III in 1139 A.D. barred priests from the practice of medicine.

The Eastern Roman, or Byzantine Empire, with its capital in Constantinople, continued to foster the Greco-Roman cultural legacy. Between the third century and the fall of Constantinople in 1453 A.D. the tradition of Greek medicine was kept alive as a flickering light. This source of enlightenment was returned to Europe through the escape of many Greek scholars bringing precious manuscripts when Constantinople capitulated.

Another and more important enrichment of medical science arose from the East. By the seventh century the Christian world had extended far eastward, almost to China. Most of these eastern Christians were Nestorians, who had been driven from their churches and homes because of alleged heretical beliefs. In Edessa, Asia Minor, and Persia, the Nestorians established schools, libraries, hospitals, and centers of learning which attracted hundreds of Christian, Hebrew, Syrian, Greek, and Persian scholars. The physicians of these schools became famous, having adopted the scientific methods of other peoples and added to them by their own discoveries.

In the 7th century there began a phenomenal change in human affairs. The followers of Mohammed arose to conquer vast areas formerly belonging to the Byzantine Empire and within a century had swept over Egypt, North Africa, and Spain in the West. As the primitive desert Arabs came into contact with the more enlightened peoples in their conquests, their leaders began to recognize their own backwardness and to appreciate the value of all that was best in Greco-Roman civilization, especially in the fields of medicine and of science. The existing centers of learning were preserved. Moslem students began to learn Greek or Syriac and soon translations were made into Arabic.

The cultivation of medicine was encouraged

by the Arabs. Before the end of the 9th century they were in possession of all of the science of the Greeks; they had produced from their own people scholars of the first order. From this time they showed an aptitude for the exact sciences.

It was the Arabs who first separated the arts of the apothecary and physician. In Baghdad's bazaars, late in the 8th century, they established the first privately owned apothecary shops. To the Greco-Roman wisdom obtained by translating original manuscripts into Arabic, the Arabs added their own innovations, such as syrups, confections, conserves, and products of distillation such as waters, elixirs, and alcoholic liquids.

The first outstanding physician of the Arab world was Abu Bekr Muhammad al-Razi (844-926), known in Europe as Rhazes.

Having studied chemistry and medicine in Baghdad, Rhazes made careful observations on disease. To him is owed the first accurate description of smallpox, which he differentiated from measles. Rhazes, writing in Arabic, produced some 131 books, half of which were on medicine. His two chief works were *Kitah al-Hawi (The Comprehensive Book)* and *Kitah al-Mansuri (Book for Mansur,* the Prince to whom it was addressed). These books were surveys of all medical knowledge of his time. They were immensely popular and later served in their Latin translations as textbooks in European medical schools for several centuries.

Rhazes introduced new remedies such as mercurial ointment and the use of animal gut for sutures.

One of the greatest names in the history of medicine was Abu Ali al-Husein ibn Sina (980–1037), known in Europe as Avicenna or The Prince. Born in Bokhara in Persia, Avicenna was something of an infant prodigy. Having studied medicine on his own with the aid of tutors, he served as court physician to a number of the Persian rulers. He is the author of the most famous medical textbook ever written; *Qanun-fi-l-Tibb (The Canon of Medicine)* is a gigantic survey of physiology, hygiene, and therapy. Avicenna wrote not only about medicine; two of the five books in the *Canon* contained much material about pharmacy and the preparation of substances for use in medicine. His teachings, pharmaceutical as well as medical, were accepted as authority in the

West until the 17th century, and for another 200 years in the Orient. Innumerable manuscripts of *The Canon* exist. A Latin version was printed in 1472 and repeated editions appeared, the last in 1663.

In Spain, the western Arabs attained their brightest prosperity. Remarkable schools of medicine were founded in Seville, Toledo, and Cordova.

Surgery among the Arabs had fallen to a low state. This was mainly due to religious objections to touching a dead body, which prohibited autopsies and anatomical dissection. The only textbook on surgery by the Arabs was written by Abul Oasim Abulcasis (1013–1106) of Cordova. This man recognized the decadence of surgery in his country and was determined to restore surgical science to life. His book is especially valuable because of the many illustrations of surgical instruments. The cautery iron was a favorite instrument recommended by Abulcasis. His book was an important element in the revival of surgery in Italy and France.

An important physician in this period of Moslem medicine was Abu Marwan ibn Zuhr (1091–1162) of Seville, known to Europeans as Avenzoar. His ability lay in accurate clinical descriptions; he provided clear pictures of mediastinal tumors, pericarditis, intestinal tuberculosis, and pharyngeal paralysis. His best known book, *Kitah al-Tasir (Book of Simplication on Therapeutics and Diet),* translated into Hebrew and Latin, greatly influenced European scholars.

Averroës, Abu al Wahd Muhammad ibn Rushd (1126–1198), is better known as a philosopher than as a physician. Albeit, Averroës was a great physician. He was the first to explain the function of the retina and to recognize that an attack of smallpox confers immunity. His encyclopedia of medicine was translated to Latin and widely used as a textbook.

Abu Muhammad ibn Baitar (1190–1248), of Malaga, gathered all Islamic botany into a vast work of extraordinary learning. This book remained the standard of botanical authority until the 16th century, and marked him as the greatest botanist and pharmacist of the Middle Ages. In his volume, Baitar lists 1400 plants, 300 of which were said to be new.

Arabian medicine was based on Greek science. No contributions were made to anatomy, as dissection was prohibited, nor to physiology, and the pathology was that of Galen. Several new and important diseases were described; a number of new drugs were introduced, chiefly from the plant kingdom. Arabian hospitals were well organized and became famous. It was in the field of chemistry that the Arabs made the greatest advances. Probably Arabian chemistry was based largely on the earlier knowledge of the Egyptians.[2]

In the words of Will Durant[12] "for five centuries, from 700–1200 A.D., Islam led the world in power, order and extent of government, in refinement of manners, in standards of living, in humane legislation and religious toleration, in literature, scholarship, science, medicine and philosophy."

Medicine in the 11th and 12th centuries in Europe was elevated to a higher plane by the medical school founded at Salerno, a little seaside town on the coast near Naples. This southern area of Italy was still under strong Greek influence. The teachings of this famous center, the first independent medical school of the time, brought an invigorating freshness into the dreary stagnation of the Dark Ages. Anatomy was still based on dissection of animals. The Galenic theories still prevailed. Observations of patients and study of disease was undertaken with keenness and vigor. The most important source of this knowledge was Spain, particularly Toledo, where from the middle of the 12th until the middle of the 13th century, an extraordinary number of Arabic works in medicine, philosophy, mathematics, and astronomy were translated into Latin. Many of the ablest translators of this period were Jewish scholars. The teachers at Salerno were the first medieval physicians to cultivate medicine as an independent branch of science. Salerno was the first European university to bestow a medical degree.

During this period several great medieval universities were founded: Paris, 1110; Bologna, 1113; Oxford, 1167; Montpellier, 1181; Padua, 1222; and Naples, 1224. Although such schools flourished and medicine was highly respected, its scientific study did not progress. Generally speaking, human dissection was not allowed. In this respect, the rest of Europe was far behind Italy. Here the importance of anatomical study was recognized. Such universities as those at Padua, Venice, Florence, and Bologna began the dissection of the bodies of executed criminals handed over by the

authorities for this purpose. This break with tradition was essential for progress of medicine and surgery.

Hospital construction and maintenance were characteristic developments in medieval Europe. Arising from the experience of military hospitals of the Romans and from their valetudinaria for the sick poor, the Christian church fostered the creation of Hotel Dieu, a place for God's hospitality, in many cities. This movement was greatly stimulated by the human miseries resulting from the Crusades. Several religious orders such as that of St. John of Jerusalem, St. Elizabeth of Hungary, and the Teutonic Knights were initiated and devoted their energies to the care of the sick poor.

In 1198, Pope Innocent III launched a great campaign for hospital building. This church influence led to the completion of many fine hospitals in European cities during the later years of the Middle Ages.

As the 13th century dawned, the lower segment of Italy was joined with its neighboring island to form the Kingdom of the Two Sicilies, ruled by Frederick II, who also was Emperior of Germany. His capitol, Palermo, was the crossroads of three dominant cultures—Moslem, Jewish, and Christian. Frederick's talent for reform and organization brought about a change of great significance both to medicine and pharmacy. About 1240, Frederick issued an edict separating pharmacy and medicine into two distinct professions, with rules and limitations concerning practice. This event is considered to mark the beginning of pharmacy as a separate profession, distinct from medicine.

## MAJOR EPIDEMICS OF THE MIDDLE AGES

Leprosy was the first widespread epidemic disease to threaten Europe during the Middle Ages. It was a result of the Crusades that leprosy was brought back by the military expeditions returning from the Near East. A charitable order, the Knights of Saint Lazarus of Jerusalem, introduced leper hospitals, named "lazarettos" from the order, all over Europe. It has been estimated that as many as 19,000 lazarettos existed in Europe. In England, the first leper hospital was founded in 1096, the last in 1472.

Leadership was assumed by the Church, as medicine had little to offer. Based on the concepts of contagion in the Old Testament, lepers were strictly isolated from the healthy community. Lepers were compelled to wear a characteristic costume and to sound a bell or clapper to warn of their approach. As these measures of isolation took effect, leprosy began to recede and gradually almost disappeared from Europe. This represents perhaps the first great success in combating a widespread contagious disease.

The most dreadful calamity ever to visit the human race occurred in the middle of the 14th century when an epidemic of bubonic plague was introduced from Asia to Europe by way of Constantinople. By 1350, the whole continent from Russia to Scandinavia was in the grip of the plague. One-half of the population of England perished and probably at least one-fourth of the entire European population succumbed to plague. The social disturbance resulting from the Black Death was profound. The power of the Church and of Civil authorities was diminished. Commerce was dislocated. This great event marked the end of the Middle Ages and cleared the way for a new advance of European civilization built upon the relics of the old.

It was the Black Death that finally demonstrated the contagiousness of disease. The idea of infection had not been universally accepted in Greek medicine. Winslow names the Black Death as "the great teacher" in this field. Leprosy had offered a preliminary course of instruction, and, at the end of the 15th century, a postgraduate course was offered by syphilis which swept over Europe in a highly virulent epidemic form.

Knowledge of the contagiousness of plague led to the initiation of another public health measure. As a result of experience with leprosy, strict regulations were set up to combat plague. Every house containing a plague victim was put under a ban. All who came in contact with the sick were placed in isolation. When a plague victim died, his home was aired and fumigated, and his effects were burned.

The City of Venice in 1348 was the first to introduce quarantine as a protective measure. Based on the belief that plague was brought into the city through infected goods carried by ships, the incoming ships and their crews were isolated at an island in the harbor for a period of 40 days, hence the term "quarantine" (meaning, 40 in Italian). This system was adopted in Italy, southern France, and neighboring areas to combat contagious disease and is to some extent useful in the practice of modern public health.

The third great epidemic scourge of the Middle Ages was syphilis. This outbreak is supposed to have appeared first in 1495 in Naples, which at that time was under siege by the French. In the opinion of some, syphilis had recently been introduced to Spain upon the return of Columbus's sailors from the West Indies. Certainly, the disease behaved like a newly imported infection in that a rapidly spreading, malignant form of syphilis became widely prevalent in Europe. Many died of the acute effects of the disease. Mercury ointment became a routine drug for the treatment of syphilis. Guaiac from the bark of a West Indian tree was also a favorite remedy.

## THE PERIOD OF THE RENAISSANCE

Many forces aided in the transition of civilized mankind from medieval to modern conditions. Among these was the invention of gunpowder and the printing press. These served to free man from the bonds of feudalism and to provide him with the means of acquiring knowledge. The voyages of the great explorers uncovering the wonders of the New World established the astronomical ideas of Copernicus. The events of the Reformation allowed free thought to come into its own. Critical spirits began to flourish. Byzantine-Greek scholars came to Italy in large numbers following the

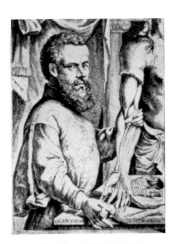

Vesalius (1514–1564)

Source: Garrison, F. H. *An Introduction to the History of Medicine,* Ed. 4. Philadelphia: W. B. Saunders Co., 1929, p. 217

fall of Constantinople to the Turks in 1453, bringing with them the written records of Greek thought and restoring the inquiring intellects of Plato and Hippocrates to favor.

The increase of world trade created by exploration and colonization of new lands brought prosperity to the Old World and provided capital for scientific and educational advances.

In the 15th century, an enthusiasm for classical study arose. Knowledge of Greek became general among scholars and accurate translations of the Greek works of Galen began to appear. The printing press made these improved translations of the ancient scientific treatises available to students and led to a new interest in medicine as a scientific study.

It was at the end of the 15th century, too, that medicine and pharmacy, separated as professions some 160 years, were found coming together again in a cooperative interprofessional endeavor in the Italian city-state of Florence. In 1498, the Florentine Guild of Apothecaries and the Medical Society collaborated in writing and printing the *Nuovo Receptario*, or New Formulary, with the authority of the Florentine government as represented by the monk, Savanarola. This small book of standards, written in the Italian vernacular instead of classical Latin, is probably the first pharmacopeia to have been produced with governmental approval and authority.

Fresh impetus to a study of the human body was given by a school of artists in Florence, the most noted of whom was Leonardo da Vinci. Even though opportunities for dissection were still limited, a number of first-rate anatomists made distinguished studies. Sylvius at Paris, Vesalius, Fallopius, Fabricius, and Eustachius of Italy were all teachers of anatomy who left their names with us as discovers of anatomical structures. Of these, Vesalius (1514–1564) was the master spirit of the science. Working in Padua, he published his great work, *De Fabrica Humani Corporis*. This work marks a definite breaking with past tradition and struck a fatal blow at the dead hand of Galen.

Three strong men of aggressive temperament in the medical world of the 16th century, Paracelsus, Vesalius, and Ambroise Paré, by shouldering past men of traditional views, literally "blazed the way" for a general advance in medicine and for a liberalization of thought. Paracelsus (1493–1541), physician, chemist,

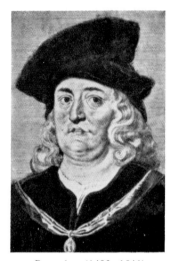

Paracelsus (1493–1541)
Source: Garrison, F. H. *An Introduction to the History of Medicine,* Ed. 4. Philadelphia: W. B. Saunders Co., 1929, p. 204

teacher, traveler, reformer, was born in Switzerland. He publicly burned the works of Galen and the Arabians and advocated observation and experimentation as a basis for knowledge. No medical writer did more to break the shackles of classical dogmas.

Ambroise Paré (1510–1590), of Paris, strove mightily to rescue surgery from the neglect and degradation to which it had fallen in the Dark Ages. He rejected the use of boiling oil for treatment of gunshot wounds and amputations in 1536. Later he reintroduced the use of ligatures to control hemorrhage (1552). The ligature had been used in ancient medicine, but had been replaced through Arab influence by the cautery iron to control bleeding. Before Paré, amputations were rarely performed with success. The procedure became common thereafter. Paré was especially successful in the treatment of gunshot wounds. His faith in the healing power of nature is summed up in the famous inscription on his statue: "I treated him, God cured him."

Another man of genius of this period is Fracastorius (1478–1553). Born in Verona, he studied in Padua. A many-sided man, he was at once a physician, geologist, and astronomer, and shares with da Vinci the true interpretation of fossil remains. His medical fame rests on authorship of the celebrated poem, *Syphilis sive Morbus Gallicus* (Venice, 1530). It was this poem that gave the disease its name. His greatest

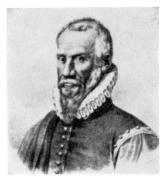

Ambroise Paré (1510–1590)
Source: Garrison, F. H. *An Introduction to the History of Medicine,* Ed. 4. Philadelphia: W. B. Saunders Co., 1929, p. 225

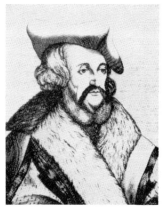

Fracastorius (1478–1553)
Source: National Library of Medicine, Bethesda, Maryland, Neg. No. 65-396

tain peak in the history of disease causation.

## THE SEVENTEENTH CENTURY

The 17th, like the 16th century, was a brilliant period of human history. In the field of medicine, the discovery of the circulation of the blood by William Harvey initiated the modern science of physiology. Harvey (1578–1657), an Englishman, studied in Padua. The doctrine of Galen that the blood ebbs and flows in closed arterial and venous systems still prevailed.

Harvey, by experimental vivisection, ligation, and perfusion, established that the heart acts as a muscular pump to propel the blood through the circulatory vessels and that the motion of the blood is continuous and in a cycle or circle. Harvey applied mathematical measurements for the first time in a biological experiment to prove that the blood must return to the heart by way of the veins. Although Harvey lectured to the students in London on his experiments, he was hesitant to publish so revolutionary a concept. He waited for 15 years to put his studies before the public in a famous book, *De Motu Cordis,* 1628. Harvey's trepidation was justified. His colleagues and contemporaries ridiculed him and his theories.

Aristotle had taught that the heart is the center of life, the mind, and the soul. Harvey demonstrated that the blood is of prime importance, while the heart is only a pump to keep it in motion. Harvey did not, however, solve the function of respiration of air, but adhered to

work, *De Contagione* (1546), proposed germs (*contagium animatum*) as the cause of a wide variety of diseases. He theorized about three types of contagion: (1) those which infect by direct contact only, (2) those which may also be spread by fomites, such as excreta or clothing contaminated by the patient, and (3) those which may be spread at a distance.

There has been some difference of opinion as to just what germ or contagium animatum meant to Fracastorius, but Winslow states[9]:

It is precisely the glory of Fracastorius that, by close observation and clear thinking, he worked out a clear and essentially accurate analysis of the way in which living "germs" operate, without ever suspecting that they were living.

Each disease is specific and has its specific "germ." It is the first really intelligent statement of the contagiousness of disease—a moun-

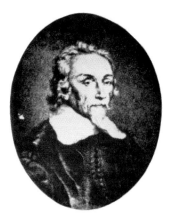

William Harvey (1578–1657)
Source: Garrison, F. H. *An Introduction to the History of Medicine,* Ed. 4. Philadelphia: W. B. Saunders Co., 1929, p. 246

the old doctrine that breathing in air served only to cool the hot blood.

It was early in the 17th century, too, that another step forward was taken in the development of pharmacy as a profession. Opening of trade routes to the East Indies had developed a lucrative trade in drugs and spices, which in the British Isles was monopolized by the Guild of Grocers. This Guild also had jurisdiction over the apothecaries. The apothecaries found allies among court physicians and in the philosopher-politician, Francis Bacon, who persuaded King James I of England to grant a charter in 1617 which formed a separate company known as the "Master, Wardens and Society of the Art and Mystery of the Apothecaries of the City of London"—the first organization of pharmacists in the Anglo-Saxon world.

Athanasius Kircher (1602–1680) was probably the first to use the microscope to investigate the causes of disease. In his publication, *Scrutinium Pestis* (Rome, 1658), Kircher describes experiments upon the nature of putrefaction, demonstrating that maggots are developed in the decaying matter. His primitive microscope magnified only to 32-power, so it is unlikely that he actually saw bacteria. Robert Hooke (1635–1703), a mechanical genius of England, also made use of an early microscope. In his book, *Micrographia* (1665), there are many fine plates illustrating vegetable structures. He refers to the "little boxes or cells, distinct from one another." This is the first use of the term "cell" in a biological sense.

The greatest of the early microscopists was Antonj van Leeuwenhoek of Delft (1632–1723). Among his accomplishments, Leeuwenhoek became an expert lens grinder. He produced some 247 microscopes with 419 lenses. His energy in studying microscopic preparations was amazing. He was the first to describe the spermatozoa, gave the first good account of red blood cells, was the first to see protozoa, and described bacteria, bacilli, and spirillae from material taken from his own mouth. Some 375 scientific communications were sent to the Royal Society of London. These appeared in the Society's transactions.

Soon the great Italian, Marcello M. Malpighi (1628–1694), using the microscope (an instrument not available to Harvey), discovered the existence of the capillary system connecting the small arteries and veins, and made Harvey's discovery a certainty. Malpighi was professor of anatomy at Bologna, Pisa, and Messina. He is credited as being the founder of microscopic anatomy or histology. His descriptions of the capillary bed and bronchial tree in the lungs gave a basis for the studies on respiration soon to come.

Two other great Italian scientists made contributions of importance. Francesco Redi (1626–1697) dealt a hard blow to the old doctrine of spontaneous generation. It was widely held that maggots and grub worms appear spontaneously in decaying organic matter. Redi exposed meat in jars, some uncovered and others covered with gauze. Maggots appeared on the uncovered meat, but not in the meat protected from flies.

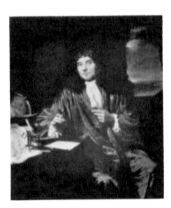

Athanasius Kircher (1602–1680)
Source: Garrison, F. H. *An Introduction to the History of Medicine,* Ed. 4. Philadelphia: W. B. Saunders Co., 1929, p. 253

Antonj van Leeuwenhoek (1632–1723)
Source: Burnett, G. W., and Scherp, H. W. *Oral Microbiology and Infectious Disease,* Ed. 3. Baltimore: The Williams and Wilkins Co., 1968, p. 4

The other celebrated professor was Santorio Santorio (1561–1636) of Padua, called Sanctorius. This man was a clever inventor of precision instruments, including a crude clinical thermometer and a pulse timer which were promptly forgotten for 100 years. His chief fame is as the founder of physiological metabolism through his experiments on himself. Having carefully constructed a chair balanced on a sensitive weighing machine, he conducted studies on his weight changes before, during, and after taking food.

In the latter half of the century, the distinguished chemist, Robert Boyle (1627–1691), carried out experiments with animals *in vacuo* proving that air is necessary for life as well as for combustion. Robert Hooke (1635–1703) demonstrated that artificial respiration can preserve life in dogs with an opened thorax. John Mayow (1643–1679) experimented on exposing dark venous blood to certain gases. He fully grasped that the function of respiration is to cause an interchange of gases between the air and the blood. It took another 100 years until oxygen was finally discovered.

Perhaps the greatest physician of the century was Thomas Sydenham (1624–1689), educated at Oxford and Montpellier. His career as a London practitioner was one of continued success. An intelligent, keen observer, he reintroduced the bedside study of disease as employed in the ancient days of Hippocrates. Sydenham made no single great contribution to medicine but did describe many new diseases, such as chorea, scarlatina, gout, and hysteria. His concept of disease was a developmental process, running a regular course, each with its peculiar natural history. He thought that certain diseases have "epidemic constitutions" and are influenced by cosmic or atmospheric forces. Sydenham's studies on the effects of geography and meteorology on epidemic diseases and the rhythmic periodicity of their recurrence qualify him as one of the founders of the science of epidemiology.

The bearing of children continued to be a fearful hazard, but toward the end of the century there appeared several books setting forth new ideas on midwifery. Francois Mauriceau (1637–1709), of Paris, was in some respects the leading obstetrician of his time. His book gives a good account of the conduct of normal labor. He corrected the ancient view that pelvic bones separated during delivery.

Hendrik van Deventer (1651–1724), a native of Holland, has been called "the father of modern midwifery." His book accurately describes the common pelvic deformities and explained how labor is complicated by such abnormal birth canals. The use of men as obstetricians began to come into fashion in France and England.

Blood letting as a therapeutic measure continued to be heroically practiced. The patient was given large quantities of water to drink before the bleeding, the theory being that the process was a kind of blood washing to rid the body of poisonous substances. The famous surgeon, Guy Patin, bled his wife 12 times for a chest complaint, his son 20 times for a long continued fever, and himself seven times for a cold in his head.

The materia medica in common use during the period is characterized by absurdity. Among the remedies listed are lozenges of dried vipers, foxes' lungs, oil of ants, crabs' eyes, oil of spiders and earthworms. There was an increasing number of proprietary preparations for which wild claims were made and large sums collected.

In public health, probably the outstanding contribution was in the field of biostatistics. William Petty (1623–1687), physician and economist, urged the collection of figures on population, diseases, revenue, and other related topics. While Petty knew the importance of quantitative studies of health, the best contribution to such studies came from his friend, John Graunt (1620–1674), whose important book, *Natural and Political Observations upon the Bills of Mortality,* appeared in 1662. Studying the figures on death that were available to him, Graunt noted the excess of male over female deaths, the excess of the urban over the rural death rate, and the variation of death rates by seasons. His work contains the beginnings of statistical methods of analysis of vital data.

It is clear that this seventeenth century was one of extreme activity in medical science, and that far greater advances were made in its various branches than in any preceeding hundred years.[13]

Yet the level of medical practice for the public at large improved very little.

## THE EIGHTEENTH CENTURY

The 18th century was a time of emancipation of human thought. The craving for liberty (political, spiritual, and intellectual), begun with the Reformation, could now flourish with little restraint. The age was one of theorists and system makers. Hermann Boerhaave (1668–1738), of Leyden, was the leading physician and teacher in the early decades of the century. He taught chemistry, physics, and botany as well as bedside medicine. His lectures were famous throughout Europe. His books were enormously influental and served to bring a more rational view of clinical medicine.

Another physician whose influence was enormous was the great Swedish doctor, Carl von Linne, better known as Linnaeus (1707–1778), who gave incentive to classification of diseases by his lifetime devotion to identification and arrangement of plants into a systematic schemata. All known plants were separated by genus and species—a monumental task. The sexual parts of plants were used as the basis of differentiation. Linnaeus believed in the fixity of species with no allowance for evolutionary changes.

One of the great chemists of the 1700's was the German pharmacist Andreas S. Marggraf (1709 1782). He differentiated between potassium and sodium compounds, identified magnesium, was the first to prepare potassium cyanide, and introduced many reagents. His most important discovery, reported in 1747, was development of methods to extract sugar from sugarbeets.[14]

A pharmaceutical "dynasty" was begun in Philadelphia in 1729 when Irish immigrant Christopher Marshall established his apothecary shop. It became a leading retail store; a practical training school for apprentices; the base for large-scale chemical manufacturing; and an important supply depot for drugs during the Revolutionary War, when Marshall became known as the "fighting Quaker." His sons, Charles and Christopher, Jr., earned individual fame in pharmacy and manufacturing; and Christopher's granddaughter, Elizabeth, who took over the shop in 1804, probably was the first woman pharmacist in the United States.[15]

Hospital pharmacy was introduced to the Colonial American scene in 1752. The Pennsylvania Hospital had been established the year before in a rented house in Philadelphia, prime movers being physician Thomas Bond and Benjamin Franklin. When the hospital received a large shipment of drugs from London, it was decided to place an apothecary in charge of them. First apothecary was Jonathan Roberts. In 1755, he was replaced by John Morgan, a pupil of Dr. John Redman.[15]

Perhaps greatest of the pharmacist-chemists was Karl Wilhelm Scheele. As a young apprentice in Swedish pharmacies, under the understanding eyes of his preceptors, Scheele began a life-long series of chemical experiments. Although he operated his own pharmacy in Köping, and always considered himself a pharmacist, in his short 43 years of life (died in 1786) Scheele reported one discovery after another. Among his contributions were chlorine, basis of bleaching and laundry industries; fruit acids, of high importance to the food and beverage industries; tungsten and molybdenum, indispensable to the steel industry; and glycerin, which enters into countless commodities as well as explosives. Scheele also is credited with independent discovery of oxygen.[15]

From a small laboratory in his pharmacy, German pharmacist Martin H. Klaproth (1743–1817) brought forth many chemical discoveries, some of which have a profound effect on our world today. Among the several elements he discovered was, in 1789, uranium, the key to the atomic bomb which initiated our atomic age, which began some 150 years after Klaproth's time. Also, he is considered the father of modern analytical chemistry.[16]

One of the early triumphs of preventive medicine in Europe was the introduction from the East of inoculation against smallpox. This disease had become epidemic throughout Europe in the 16th and 17th centuries. Voltaire states that

in an hundred persons that come into the world, at least sixty contract smallpox; of these sixty, twenty die—and twenty more keep very disagreeable marks of this cruel disorder as long as they live.[17]

The use of inoculation of smallpox matter from a mild case to immunize children by inducing a light infection had been practiced in India and China for hundreds of years. The first introduction of this method to Europe came through a communication of two Greek physicians to the Royal Society of London around 1713 to 1716. Lady Mary Wortley Montague, wife of the English Ambassador to Turkey, had her 3-year-old son inoculated in Constantinople in 1718 and soon afterward brought the method into use in London. During a severe smallpox epidemic in Boston in 1721, Dr. Zabdiel Boylston (1679–1766) inoculated his own son, thus introducing this preventive measure to America.

The use of inoculation against smallpox became widespread and many improvements in technique were developed. Edward Jenner (1749–1823) made inoculation obsolete, however, by his discovery published in 1798 that cowpox virus applied to human skin produced an inocuous pustule that gave solid immunity to smallpox. This method, called vaccination, was safer than inoculation. It was rapidly adopted throughout the civilized world and must be considered the first and certainly one of the most effective of all measures of disease prevention.

Surgery received a forward impetus in France in 1686 when the royal surgeon, Charles-Francois Felix successfully cured a *fistulo in ano* on the person of Louis XIV. Both Felix and his successor, Georges Mareschal (1658–1736), were made royal surgeons. In 1724, Mareschal persuaded Louis XV to create five chairs of surgical instruction. The Academy of Surgery was founded in 1731. Louis XV soon after ordered that no one could practice surgery without a degree in the arts. Paris soon became the surgical center of the world.

In England, the surgeons were separated from the barbers in 1745, but it was not until 1800 that George III gave its charter to the Royal College of Surgeons of London.

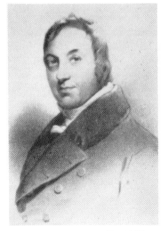

Edward Jenner (1749–1823)
Source: Burnett, G. W., and Scherp, H. W. *Oral Microbiology and Infectious Disease,* Ed. 3. Baltimore: The Williams and Wilkins Co., 1968, p. 33

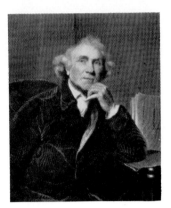

John Hunter (1728–1793)
Source: National Library of Medicine, Bethesda, Maryland, Neg. No. 66-485

John Hunter (1728–1793), the great Scottish anatomist, put surgery on a scientific basis. Coming to London in 1748, his work was many sided. He created a valuable museum of anatomical and pathological specimens. As a pioneer in experimental and surgical anatomy, he made many contributions. As a surgical pathologist, he described shock, phlebitis, and gunshot wounds and studied inflammation. As Garrison says, "it is no exaggeration to repeat that Hunter found surgery a mechanical art and left it an experimental science."[18]

The surgery of the eye was advanced by Jacques Daviel (1696–1762), of Paris, who was the originator of the treatment of cataract by extraction of the lens (1752). By 1756, he had recorded 434 lens extractions with only 50 failures.

During the 18th century, care of women in childbirth began to pass from the midwife to the trained male obstetrician. This led to a growth in knowledge. William Smellie (1697–1763) learned his obstetrics in Paris and settled in London to practice. Smellie's book in 1752 laid down for the first time safe rules for the use of forceps in delivery. He taught methods for pelvic measurements to discover contracted pelves that would render delivery difficult.

The Manchester surgeon, Charles White (1728–1813), emphasized the vital need for surgical cleanliness in obstetrics. He stands out as a pioneer in aseptic childbirth, preceding Oliver Wendell Holmes and Semmelweis of the next century.

Two great movements shook the world in the latter part of the period: (1) the American and

French Revolutions, and (2) the Industrial Revolution. The political overturns in America and France broke down many old barriers to progress and freed the energies of these peoples for great advances in the period ahead.

Many factors combined to promote industrial development. Wars created a greater demand for production and distribution of goods. Growth of population provided increased markets. Wood had been the major source of fuel, but forests were being rapidly depleted. Coal was needed. Mining of coal was still a primitive process. The problem of lifting water from the mines called for better pumps and led to the steam pumps of Savery and Newcomen. Production of coal mounted so that by 1750 coal burning was already darkening the London skies. By this time, London was the largest city on the globe with a population of 725,000.

Coal and coke had been used early in the century for smelting iron, but by 1740 high-grade steel was produced, making it possible to produce the machinery required in the Industrial Revolution.

After the invention of the flying shuttle and the spinning machine, textile factories began to spring up in England, bringing thousands of rural people to add to the already overcrowded, unsanitary urban areas. Without adequate water supplies and with no sewerage systems, the conditions of life deteriorated until relief was provided by the public health movement of the Victorian Age.

Many new hospitals were built in the 18th century, but, from the point of view of cleanliness and administration, they were at a very low level. In 1788, Jacobus–Rene Tenon published a description of the old Hotel Dieu of Paris. There were some 1220 beds, most of which held from four to six patients. In the halls were sick lying miserably on filthy heaps of straw. Ventilation was so faulty that attendants could not enter in the morning without a sponge wet with vinegar held to their faces. Conditions were no better in many other large European hospitals.

Treatment of insane persons was even worse. They were chained or put in cages like animals in a zoo. The public for a small fee, could come to view them.

The French physician, Philippe Pinel (1745–1826), early in the 1790's ordered chains and fetters removed from insane women and men in Parisian hospitals. Despite political opposition, Pinel replaced cruelty and inhumanity with kindness, understanding, and rational therapy. He is considered to be the Father of Psychiatry. In the United States, Dr. Benjamin Rush of Philadelphia wrote the first text on psychiatry, "Medical Inquiries and Observations Upon Diseases of the Mind," published in 1812.[19]

Two men of strong character arose in England to devote themselves to the betterment of their fellow man. John Howard (1726–1790) became interested in the welfare of prisoners, hospital inmates, and other unfortunates. He found the jails to be endemic fever nests. His recommendations were for flushing floors, daily baths, ovens for baking clothing, white washing of cell walls, and attendance of a physician. William Wilberforce (1759–1833), a member of Parliament, devoted himself to a campaign against slavery and to the cause of political reform.

In 1761, there appeared in Venice a book by a distinguished Italian physician, Giovanni Battista Morgagni (1682–1771), *De Sedibus et Causis Morborum* (*On the Seat and Causes of Disease*). This work contains the lifetime studies of Morgagni, who observed his patients carefully and carried out detailed dissections on those who died, a true foundation of modern pathology. Many diseases were described accurately by Morgagni for the first time.

An important advance in preventive medicine came from the Scottish physician, James Lind (1716–1794), who was a surgeon in the Royal Navy. Scurvy was a formidable problem among all sailors, especially in the naval service. The British fleet had 2400 cases of scurvy after a 10–week cruise in the Channel in 1779. Knowing that the Dutch had used orange and lemon juice to treat scurvy in the 16th century, Lind conducted a series of clinical experiments that definitely proved citrus fruits and their juices would cure scurvy. Using six pairs of sailors suffering from scurvy, Lind gave a different alleged remedy to each pair—cider, vinegar, elixir of vitriol, sea water, spices, and citrus fruits. After six days, those given citrus fruits were fit for duty; at the end of two weeks the others showed no appreciable improvement. As a result of Lind's persuasion, the admiralty ordered that preserved lemon juice be carried on all naval ships and regularly be issued to the men.[20,21] After this order finally took effect, scurvy disappeared like magic from the Navy.

Lind was also the founder of naval hygiene in England. He introduced regular uniforms, bathing, and delousing, and even devised a method of distilling sea water for drinking purposes.

Public health was advanced on other fronts. Bernardino Ramazzini (1633–1714) opened up an entirely new field of medicine—trade diseases and industrial hygiene. His book, *De Morbis Artificum Diatriba (Discourse in the Diseases of Workers)*, published in 1700, gave to occupational hygiene what Vesalius gave to anatomy and Morgagni to pathology. Ramazzini called attention to tuberculosis among stonecutters and miners, eye troubles of printers, and various other disorders related to occupation.

From Germany, Johann Peter Frank (1745–1820) issued six volumes entitled, *A Complete System of Medical Polity*. A great physician and teacher, Frank's treatise laid the foundation of all modern public hygiene. Covering the whole of a man's life "from womb to tomb," he discussed water supply, sewerage, sex hygiene, and school hygiene, indeed all measures to be taken by government for the protection of the health of the public. Frank's philosophy had an important effect in shaping governmental action on health matters during the next century.

Outbreaks of epidemic disease were more scattered and isolated than in previous centuries. Plague and syphilis had subsided to a great extent. Malarial fevers, influenza, scarlet fever, and diphtheria were often prevalent. Smallpox appeared, but methods for control had now become available. Typhus and intestinal fevers were a scourge of the military during the wars. Yellow fever had become a threat to the port cities of America and Europe, having been frequently introduced by sailing ships from the American tropics.

At its best, medical practice by the end of the 18th century had greatly improved and was based to a considerable degree upon careful studies in the fields of physiology and anatomy. Leading physicians enjoyed social and cultural advantages of a high order. The fashionable London physician wore a powdered wig, a red satin or brocade waistcoat, short breeches, buckled shoes, and a three-cornered hat, and carried a cane.

Treatment of patients was still often heroic. Purging and bleeding were frequently employed.

For the most part, the general public received little medical care and that was of the poorest quality. The novelists of the period paint a sorry picture of the average practitioner. Quackery in many forms flourished and patent medicines enjoyed a ready sale.

## THE ADVANCE TO MODERN MEDICINE

In the evolution of modern medicine three factors seem of especial importance: (1) the great industrial or social democratic movement of civilized mankind, following close upon the political revolutions in America and France, intensified the demand for intellectual and economic liberty and upheld the new idea of the dignity of man; (2) the publication of such works as Helmholtz's *Conservation of Energy* (1847) and Darwin's *Origin of Species* (1859) did away forever with many silly concepts of man as the center of the universe; and (3) physics, chemistry, and biology came to be studied as objective laboratory sciences, disassociated with previous attempts to keep them as applied disciplines secondary to the practical needs of man.[22] Medicine also owes much to the great mathematicians and physicists of the preceding times who developed the theory of vision and a knowledge of the respiratory process.

Relief of pain for suffering patients, and introduction of a new class of medicinal agents, came from experiments conducted by the young German apothecary, Frederich W.A. Sertürner. In 1816, Sertürner confirmed his earlier isolation of morphine from opium; demonstrated its effectiveness by bold clinical trials in his apothecary shop in Einbeck; and declared the importance of a new class of organic plant constituents, the alkaloids.

Taking their cue from Sertürner's alkaloidal experiments, Pierre-Joseph Pelletier and Joseph-Bienaime Caventou isolated emetine, strychnine, and brucine in their laboratory in the back of their Parisian apothecary shop. Then they tackled the baffling problem of the Peruvian barks that were so useful, if not consistently reliable, against malaria. In 1820, they announced methods for separation of quinine and cinchonine from the cinchona barks.[23]

The modern scientific movement did not attain full stride until well after the midpoint of the 19th century. The progress of medicine in the decades preceding continued at the slow pace characterizing the beginning of the century. It took a long time to demonstrate that the development of medicine as a science could only come through the performance of a vast amount of chemical, physical, and biological research by thousands of eager investigators.

Many nations have contributed significantly to the advance of medicine. The center of progress does not remain long with one people, but shifts periodically to other lands. France was the leader in the advancement of clinical medicine in the early 19th century. Students from America and European countries were attracted to the clinics and hospitals of Paris. The great names of Pierre-Charles-Alexander Louis (1787–1872), Rene-Theophile Hyacinthe Laënnec (1781–1826), and Gaspart-Laurent Bayle (1774–1816) were built on their studies of tuberculosis. Laënnec introduced the stethoscope and wrote a classic work on its usefulness in the study of chest diseases—*Traite de l'Auscultation Mediate*. Pierre Bretonneau (1778–1862) accurately described diphtheria, giving it its present name. He performed the first successful tracheotomy to save life in croup. Philippe Pinel (1745–1826) stands high in medical history as the first to institute humane treatment of the insane.

Purging and blood letting continued to be the major measures of treatment of most diseases by most physicians. Some carried blood letting to absurd degrees. Gabriel Andral (1797–1876) joined with Pierre Louis in protesting such vigorous and generally useless procedures. Andral was the first to advocate chemical examination of the blood as a diagnostic procedure (1843).

In the United States, in 1820, came the development and publication of the first United States Pharmacopoeia by physicians representing medical organizations—the first book of standards for medicines that had been prepared entirely by professional persons.

In 1821, the first professional organization of pharmacists was launched—the Philadelphia College of Pharmacy. Concerned with professional problems, ethics, purity of drugs, and pharmaceutical competence, the organization also founded pharmacy's first educational institution, which is still in existence under the name of the Philadelphia College of Pharmacy and Science.[23,24]

In the middle years of the 19th century, the physicians of the British Islands produced a number of brilliant clinicians: John Cheyne (1777–1836), Abraham Colles (1773–1843), Robert Adams (1791–1875), Robert James Graves (1796–1853), and William Stokes (1804–1878), of the Irish School in Dublin. All gave excellent descriptions of disease phenomena. The English clinicians, Richard Bright (1789–1858), Thomas Addison (1793–1860), Thomas Hodgkin (1798–1866), and James Parkinson (1755–1824), are all well known to medical students. Their names have been applied to important disease entities that they so ably differentiated.

In Germany, the scientific movement had been delayed somewhat by the devastating effects of the Napoleonic Wars. In Germany, Johannes Müller (1801–1858) is given the title of "Founder of Scientific Medicine." He was equally eminent in biology, comparative anatomy, pathology, physiology, and chemistry. As a teacher, Müller produced many brilliant investigations. His handbook, *Handbuch der Physiologie des Menschen* (1834–1840), and his journal, *Archiv für Anatomie, Physiologie, und Wissenschaftliche Medizin* (1834), exerted a profound influence among students of medicine during the 19th century.

Jacob Henle (1809–1885), building on the prior studies of Schleiden and Schwann, became the leading German histologist and one of the greatest anatomists for all time. He recognized the cell as the basic structural and functional unit in all living organisms. Apart from his anatomical contributions, Henle wrote an essay on "On Miasmas and Contagia" (1840) in which is given the first clear statement of living agents of disease.

In chemistry, Justus von Liebig (1803–1873) was the originator of laboratory teaching. His laboratory in Giessen established in 1826 was the first of its kind connected with a university. Here, Liebig began the chemistry of carbon compounds. He and his associate, Friedrich Wöhler (1800–1882), were the creators of modern chemistry of metabolism.

Three names dominate the science of physiology during the second half of the 19th century: (1) Hermann von Helmholtz (1821–1894) established that all modes of energy, heat, light, electricity, and all chemical phenomena are capable of transformation from one to the other, but are otherwise inde-structable and impossible of creation. His invention of the ophthalmoscope made oph-thalmology an exact science. His great *Hand-book of Physiological Optics* (1856–1862) remains a permanent classic. (2) Claude Bernard (1813–1878), the greatest physiologist of mo-dern France, is the founder of experimental medicine. He discovered that cane sugar in-jected in the veins appears in the urine, but not if treated previously with gastric juice. This led to his discovery of the glycogenic function of the liver. Equally important were his studies on the pancreatic juice. His third great accomp-lishment was his demonstration of the vaso-motor mechanism by which the nervous impulses regulate the blood flow in the small arterioles. (3) Carl Ludwig (1816–1895), the founder of the Physiological Institute at Leipzig, is regarded as perhaps the greatest teacher of physiology who ever lived. He did little writing. Most of his important discoveries were reported under the names of his pupils. Ludwig's principal contributions were on the regulatory mechanisms of blood circulation, the physiology of urinary excretion, and the de-velopment of techniques for laboratory studies.

Another great German who contributed greatly to the rise of modern medicine is Rudolf Virchow (1821–1902), the founder of cellular pathology. Professor and director of the Pathological Institute in Berlin, Virchow became known as a man of wide culture. As an anatomist, pathologist, epidemiologist, sani-tarian, anthropologist, archaeologist, editor, and teacher, Virchow became easily the most influential medical personality of Berlin. "In pathology, he had only Morgagni as a possible competitor before him and no one after him."[25]

Virchow defines disease as a conflict among the cells of the body brought about by the action of external forces. He was the first to observe and define leukocytosis. He separated pyemia from septicemia and demonstrated the importance of embolism in arterial disease. Perhaps Virchow's demand that all unproved hypotheses be subjected to searching inquiry and that no authoritarian voices be accepted without questioning is his most valuable impetus to advancing the modern spirit of medicine.

French medicine produced another out-

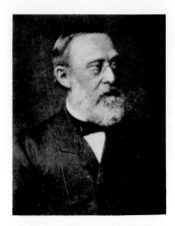

Rudolf Virchow (1821–1902)
Source: Garrison, F. H. *An Introduction to the History of Medicine,* Ed. 4. Philadelphia: W. B. Saunders Co., 1929, p. 569

standing clinician in this period in the person of Jean-Martin Charcot (1825–1893). In 1862, he became physician to the great hospital of the Salpetriere in Paris. Here, over the years he created a neurological clinic which attracted students from all over the world. Not only did Charcot make numerous contributions to neu-rology, but he shed light on many chronic diseases and senile disabilities. His studies in diseases of the nervous system are summarized in five volumes, but much of his work, as with Ludwig, appeared in the publications of his students.

The professional status of pharmacy was strengthened with the formation of the American Pharmaceutical Association in 1852. Chief architect of the organization was William Proctor, Jr., professor at Philadelphia College of Pharmacy, who became the APhA's first secre-tary, and also edited the nation's first pharma-ceutical journal.[26]

### Technological Achievements

One of the most significant accomplishments that has made modern surgery possible was the discovery of anesthetic agents. Since primitive medicine, various drugs—hashish, opium, alcohol, among others—had been used to reduce the suffering of those undergoing surgical manipulation. In 1842, a country doctor in Georgia, Crawford W. Long (1815–1878), used ether for a number of minor operations. Long published no results of his experience and had no influence on subsequent development of anesthetics. Sir Humphrey Davy (1788–1829) had suggested that the gas, nitrous oxide, might serve to control pain in certain types of surgery. It was not until 1844 that Horace Wells (1815–1848), a dentist in Hartford, Connecticut, began to use nitrous oxide in tooth extractions. William T.G. Morton (1819–1868), a partner of Wells, carried on, using ether as the anesthesia. He accomplished tooth extractions without pain. Morton persuaded surgeons at the Massachusetts General Hospital to try out ether in operative procedures in November, 1846. The success of these experiments led to the announcement of the great discovery to the world. The prestige of the Massachusetts General Hospital surgeons gave credibility to the good news. Oliver Wendell Holmes suggested the terms anesthesia and anesthetic.

Shortly afterward, 1847, Sir James Y. Simpson (1811–1870), of Edinburgh, introduced chloroform into obstetrical practice. This was opposed by some religious groups on the ground that God had condemned woman to bring forth children in pain. Queen Victoria put an end to most such objections by asking for the new anesthetic in the delivery of her younger children.

Another great technical advance was the introduction of accurate thermometry into medical practice. Knowledge of fever as a prominent component of many illnesses was as old as medicine. Few attempts to measure body temperatures accurately had been made and indeed no instrument well adapted to such studies had been available. A brilliant German professor at Leipzig, Carl R.A. Wunderlich (1815–1877), set himself the task of investigating animal heat in health and sickness. His book on clinical thermometry in 1868 made a study of the temperature a recognized feature in the diagnoses of the nature of all illnesses. "He found fever a disease and left it a symptom."[27]

The thermometer and hypodermic syringe played no significant part in the care of sick and wounded during the American Civil War. By 1868, a convenient pocket-sized clinical thermometer had been designed and its use became general within a few years. The hypodermic syringe came into general use about the same time.

Another step forward in administration of medicine by the hypodermic route was the invention of the ampoule in 1886 by Stanislas Limousin, a French pharmacist. This made possible sterile preservation of injectable medicines until time for use.[28]

With all of these great forward steps toward the establishment of a real scientific basis for medicine, it is doubtful that the average individual going to the average physician received better care in the middle of the 19th century than he might have received 100 years previously. One must then examine the developments that have led to the great medical proficiency that is available in many parts of the world today.

## Medical Education

The aim of medical education is to produce the kinds of practitioners, teachers, and research workers required currently or that will be required in the years ahead. As the problems to be met by medical graduates have changed so rapidly and so radically, it has proved difficult to keep medical faculties in tune with the requirements. This is, and will continue to be, one of the main obstacles to the raising of standards of medical practice.

To a considerable extent, medicine in the United States followed the pattern of the British system. The special feature of English clinical instruction, the hospital school, had its beginnings in such institutions as Guy's Hospital (1723), the Edinburgh Hospital (1736), the London Hospital (1785), and St. Bartholomew's (1790). To supplement the teaching of these schools, many notable practitioners gave private instruction.

Until after the Revolution, there was little advance in American medicine. In the Colonial period, all leading physicians and surgeons had received their training in Europe. The remainder were trained by these men under the apprentice system. The first medical school in North America was founded at the University of Pennsylvania in Philadelphia in 1765; the next at King's College, New York, 1767; Harvard University (1782) founded the third school. Soon, Dartmouth College launched a medical course in 1798. As the new lands to the West came to be settled, medical colleges appeared in Ohio, Kentucky, and the southern states.

In the earlier American schools, teaching was completely didactic, based on books that changed little from one generation to another. Most schools lacked good facilities for bedside teaching and hospital work was only provided for a small number of graduates who were chosen as interns. The more fortunate or well-to-do graduates went to Europe for post-graduate courses. At first, 1800 to 1840, Paris was the preferred center for training, then Vienna, England, or Scotland, and, during the last decades of the 19th century, the German universities provided the greatest attraction to American students.

As the population of the United States increased and moved westward, the demand for medical practitioners passed the supply. Private proprietary schools sprang up in all parts of the country and many became what were later termed "diploma mills." By 1869, there were 72 medical colleges in the United States.

The first real reform in American medical education was introduced by President Eliot of Harvard in 1871. He raised the entrance requirements of the Harvard Medical School, lengthened the course to 3 years, and provided better facilities for clinical and laboratory instruction. This general pattern was adopted by the Universities of Pennsylvania, Syracuse, and Michigan shortly afterward.

It is generally conceded that the founding of the Johns Hopkins Hospital (1884) and Medical School (1893) with funds provided by the Baltimore philanthropist gave the needed impetus to the forward movement of American medicine. Patterned on the excellent German university schools that had grown up after mid-19th century, Johns Hopkins required a bachelor's degree for entrance. Students were required to serve as clinical clerks on the wards as was done in the English hospital schools. Research in all departments of the School became a dominating feature. Graduates all spent several years as interns and residents in hospital wards. Such highly trained men were in great demand as teachers in other schools, so the influence of the Johns Hopkins institutions immediately became widespread.

In 1909 to 1911, Abraham Flexner, financed by the Carnegie Foundation for the Advancement of Teaching, made a comprehensive study of the status of medical education in the United States and abroad. The authoritative report prepared by Flexner laid bare the sad picture that there were many inferior schools incapable of providing an acceptable level of medical education. There were, for example, 39 schools in Illinois, 42 in Missouri, and 43 in New York. After the appearance of the Flexner report, many of these low grade schools closed their doors. The Council on Medical Education of the American Medical Association has continued over the years to set standards for high-class schools and to endeavor to promote better training for new physicians.

In recent years, American medical education has reached new peaks of excellence. Numerous large medical centers in all parts of the country provide first-class facilities for research, for teaching, and for the care of patients. As the expense of such facilities has increased, more and more of the financing has to come from tax funds.

Pharmaceutical education in the United States was gradually turned from apprentice-oriented training to college-based lecture and laboratory education due to the work of Dr. Albert B. Prescott, dean of the College of Pharmacy of the University of Michigan.

As the 1820 U.S. Pharmacopoeia had become out of date, a group from the American Pharmaceutical Association joined with the physician-manufacturer, Edward R. Squibb, in a revision of the compendium. The new Pharmacopoeia appeared in 1882. Since then this book has been recognized as the nation's leading reference on drug standards.[29]

## Medical Research

The cost of early investigations was borne to a large extent by the researcher from private funds. Outstanding scientists in the 19th century received encouragement and support from their respective governments. Laboratories or institutes were provided for Liebig at Giessen (1825), for Virchow in Berlin (1856), for Pasteur in Paris (1888), and for Koch in Berlin (1891). Special institutions devoted to medical research began to multiply, such as the Imperial Institute for Experimental Medicine at Petrograd (1890), the Lister Institute for Preventive Medicine in London (1891), Oswaldo Cruz Institute, Rio de Janeiro (1901), and, in the United States, the Wistar Institute of Anatomy and Biology, Philadelphia (1892), and The Rockefeller Institute for Medical Research in New York (1901). These institutes continue to turn out valuable research products, and now every university medical school and indeed many hospitals are devoting attention to the advancement of new knowledge in the health field. During and subsequent to World War II, the Federal Government has provided through congressional appropriations, huge sums to foster research, especially in medicine and medically related fields. This increased emphasis on the quest for new knowledge is producing results at a more rapid rate than can be assimilated. Indeed, so great is the current flow of new information from the research laboratories that it has been said that the past decade has produced more research data than did all of the years before added together.

In Figure 1 the tremendous growth of research funds in the medical field is shown with projected estimates for continued increase in funds in the years ahead. In 1966, more than $2 billion were invested in medical and health-related research in the United States. By 1972, the total of research funds in the medical field had risen to $3.3 billion, of which the Federal Government provided 63 per cent.

In Figure 2 is shown the astronomical growth of scientific publications beginning with a rapid increase in the late 18th century. As scientific publications grew, the need for abstract journals became apparent. The press of new information has now become so burdensome that computerized systems for the recall of specific data have come into frequent use.

The tremendous advance in pharmaceutical research and manufacturing in the United States and world-wide, especially since World War II, has contributed many outstanding medicinal products and devices. Pharmaceutical manufacturing, described as "a child of wars," and research grew rapidly under stimulus of shortgages of medicines during World War I. With the advent of World War II, limitations in supply again became acute, and methods of developing new products to fill shortages (such as quinine, needed for malaria) stimulated intensive research. Development of new chemotherapeutic agents and antibiotics taxed both manpower and manufacturing equipment. Only in recent years, has this flow been constricted by regulations of the Federal Food and Drug Administration.[30]

It is impossible even to list the important discoveries that have affected medical thought and practice during the past hundred years. A few significant additions to knowledge are cited only to point up the directions that medicine has taken.

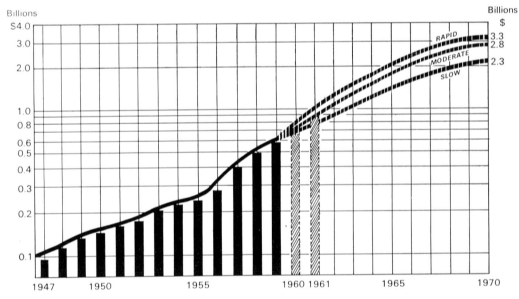

Fig. 1.1. National Expenditures for Medical Research, 1947 to 1959 and alternative projections, 1960 to 1970. Source: National Institutes of Health, Resources for Medical Research, Report 3, January, 1963. United States Public Health Service Publication 1001.

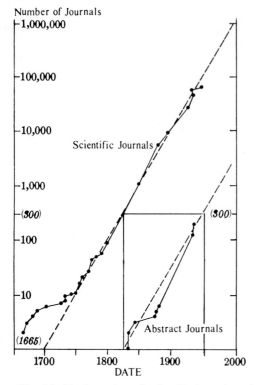

Fig. 1.2. Total number of scientific journals and abstract journals founded, as a function of date. Source: de Solla Price, D. J. *Science since Babylon.* New Haven: Yale University Press, 1961.

The founders of bacteriology were Louis Pasteur (1822—1895) and Robert Koch (1843—1910). Pasteur, a chemist, did brilliant work on the different forms of tartaric acid. This led to studies on fermentation. His studies on bacteria suggested experiments to refute spontaneous generation of life. His work on fermentation brought a request that he investigate the problems of the wine and beer industry in France. The research on wine resulted in the method of control by "pasteurization" or partial heat sterilization. The silkworm industry was threatened by a disease of the worms. After 5 years of patient study, Pasteur learned that there were two distinct diseases killing the silk-worms. Methods for control were introduced.

The idea that fermentation was due to microorganisms convinced Pasteur that some communicable diseases might be also. Working with anthrax, he demonstrated that cultures of the *Bacillus* would produce the disease in sheep, but germ-free filtrates of the cultures would not do so.

Pasteur discovered vaccines for three separate diseases: one for anthrax produced by growing the organism at high temperatures; one for chicken cholera by leaving cultures of the organism at room temperatures for prolonged periods; and one for rabies by transferring of the virus in rabbits for a long series of passages. He used the name "vaccine" in honor of Edward Jenner, the discoverer of cowpox vaccination against smallpox (*vaccus,* in Latin, means cow).

Pasteur trained many colleagues in the methods of bacteriology, and they continued his life's work in the Institute Pasteur in Paris.

One of the first important by-products of the germ theory was the discovery of antiseptic surgery by Joseph Lister (1827—1912), of Glasgow. Using dilute preparations of carbolic acid to control infections, Lister got far better results with his patients than could be obtained by previous methods. Aseptic surgery was soon introduced and prevails today.

Robert Koch, a physician, was great as an innovator and teacher. He introduced such well-known methods for the study of bacteria as fixing and drying preparations on glass slides, staining them with analin dyes, and obtaining pure cultures of organisms by distributing colonies on plated media. Koch discovered the bacillus of tuberculosis and later prepared tuberculin from its cultures, discovered the cholera agent, enunciated "Koch's postulates" for the establishing of the etiological role of a microorganism, and, with Merke, perfected

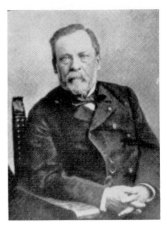

Louis Pasteur (1822—1895)
Source: Burnett, G. W., and Scherp, H. W. *Oral Microbiology and Infectious Diseases,* Ed. 3. Baltimore: The Williams and Wilkins Co., 1968, p. 10

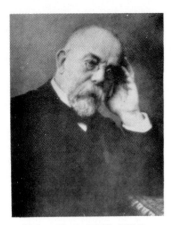

Robert Koch (1843–1910)
Source: Burnett, G. W., and Scherp, H. W. *Oral Microbiology and Infectious Disease*, Ed. 3. Baltimore: The Williams and Wilkins Co., 1968, p. 24

methods of steam sterilization.

Pasteur and Koch were the great architects of microbiology. Many others have filled in the bricks and mortar. One of Koch's pupils, Friedrich Loeffler (1852–1915), and Edwin Klebs (1834–1913) discovered the diphtheria bacillus. A few years later, colleagues of Pasteur, Emile Roux (1853–1933) and Alexandre Yersin (1863–1943), demonstrated that the deadly effects of the diphtheria bacilli were caused by a powerful toxin secreted by the organisms in the infected tissues. This finding quickly led to another fundamental method of preventive medicine. Emil von Behring (1854–1917) discovered that the serum of animals immunized by small doses of diphtheria toxin protects other animals against the usually fatal doses of the toxin. Thus were developed the methods of treatment of diphtheria and later of immunization of children against the disease.

Production of diphtheria antitoxin began in 1896; early crude products soon were refined and concentrated. Within five years, deaths from diphtheria were reduced from 45 to 5 per 100 cases. Further research developed antitoxins for other infections, and soon these were followed by successful vaccines for prevention of the major contagious diseases.[31]

Another of Koch's assistants rose to great prominence. Paul Ehrlich (1854–1915) became director of the Institut für Experimentelle Therapie at Frankfurt on the Main. He became a pioneer in experimental intracellular chemistry, such as the microchemical reaction of tissues to stains. Ehrlich came to the belief that protozoan diseases must be treated by drugs that can sterilize the patient's body of the parasites without injuring the body's tissues. His most effective drug discovery was "606," or Salvarsan, for the treatment of syphilis. Later, Neosalvarsan, equally effective but less toxic than Salvarsan, was produced.

Contemporary with Ehrlich was French pharmacist Ernest F.A. Fourneau, another of the successful researchers who helped give birth to the age of chemotherapy. For 30 years, Fourneau headed the research laboratories of the Pasteur Institute in Paris. Early in his work he introduced organic bismuth salts for syphilis which proved less toxic than the arsenicals. He paved the way for discovery of the life-saving sulfonamide compounds, and from his laboratories came the first group of chemicals having recognized antihistaminic properties.[31]

The concepts of Ehrlich have guided subsequent workers. It was not until after 1935 that Prontosil and the sulfanilamides became available, and, shortly thereafter, through the investigations of Dubos, Fleming, Florey, Chain, Waksman, and many others, the era of antibiotics came along with their great usefulness in the treatment of almost all infectious diseases. Penicillin became available during World War II followed by streptomycin, erythromycin, the tetracyclines, and many other powerful antibacterial agents. Amphotericin B and griseofulvin soon were produced to combat fungal infections and so the list continues to expand.

The modes of spreading some infectious diseases were readily apparent. Smallpox and measles were obviously contracted by direct contact with individuals ill with these diseases in the infectious stages. Rabies was well known to be spread by the bites of rabid animals. There was strong evidence that cholera and typhoid fever were water-borne. Other diseases presented puzzling features. Sir Patrick Manson (1844–1922), working on the China Coast, provided the first clue by demonstrating in 1878 that culex mosquitoes transmitted the filaria causing elephantiasis. Shortly after, Theobald Smith (1859–1934) and F.L. Kilborne proved that a tick is the carrier of the parasite of Texas fever in cattle. Then came the brilliant studies of Sir Ronald Ross (1857–1923) and the Italian workers, Amico

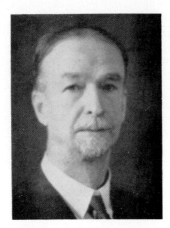

Theobald Smith (1859–1934)
Source: Burnett, G. W., and Scherp, H. W. *Oral Microbiology and Infectious Disease,* Ed. 3. Baltimore: The Williams and Wilkins Co., 1968, p. 36.

Bignami (1862–1929), Guiseppe Bastianelli (1862–1959), and Giovanni Battista Grassi (1854–1925), who clearly showed that the *Anopheles* mosquito is the carrier of malaria to man. Thus, mosquito control could offer a method for preventing this ancient scourge of man. In 1901, Walter Reed (1851–1902), head of the U.S. Army Commission in Havana, conducted experiments on a common mosquito long proposed by Dr. Carlos Finlay (1833–1915) as the vector of yellow fever. Beyond a shadow of doubt, the *Aedes aegypti* mosquito was convicted as the carrier of urban epidemic yellow fever. This information was quickly put into use by William C. Gorgas (1854–1920) in effecting the control of yellow fever in Cuba and Panama.

Another important discovery of the Reed Commission was the proof that yellow fever is caused by a filter-passing agent smaller than all known bacteria. This is the first proven virus disease of man.

Shortly thereafter, the roles of the flea in the transmission of plague and that of the tick in typhus fever were demonstrated. It is now wellknown that arthropods are transmitters of a number of other important diseases of man, especially those caused by viruses.

Wilhelm Konrad Röntgen (1845–1922), professor of physics in several German universities, discovered a new ray that passed through most substances. In reporting his discovery to the Würzburg Society in 1895, Rontgen predicted that the new rays (which he called X rays)

would be useful in medicine. With amazing rapidity, X rays, or Röntgen rays, were put to many uses in the medical field. Indeed, modern medicine could not have developed to the precision in diagnosis that has been attained were it not for this valuable aid.

Among the greatest achievements of research are those in the field of nutrition. The starting point of recent knowledge of vitamins was the experiments of Eijkman and Grijns of the Dutch East Indies, who, over a period of years (1897–1906), conducted studies on the production of beriberi (polyneuritis) in chickens by a limited diet. Their discovery of an antineuritic substance in rice husks and beans led eventually to the identification of Vitamin B1 (or thiamin). In 1913 to 1916, McCollum, Davis, and Kennedy demonstrated a growth-producing factor in butter fat and eggs. This proved to be what is now known as Vitamin A. Water-soluble Vitamin C was finally demonstrated in citrus fruits. It had long been known empirically that citrus juice prevented scurvy. Although it had been shown that cod liver oil could prevent rickets, the active principle, Vitamin D, was not extracted until 1917 by Windaus. Joseph Goldberger (1874–1929), in a remarkable series of dietetic experiments, demonstrated that pellagra was the result of an inadequate diet. In 1937, it was shown that niacin (or nicotinic acid) was the factor in the

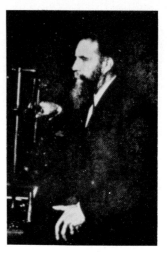

Wilhelm Konrad Röntgen (1845–1922)
Source: Garrison, F. H. *An Introduction to the History of Medicine,* Ed. 4. Philadelphia: W. B. Saunders Co., 1929, p. 721.

diet that protects against pellagra. It was soon demonstrated that Vitamin B12 has an important role in the formation of new red blood cells. Vitamin K for the hemorrhagic conditions and other accessory food factors have also come to light as a result of recent research.

Thus, effective preventive measures were now available for such troublesome human ailments as beriberi, scurvy, rickets, pellagra, and pernicious anemia.

The importance in nutrition of certain minerals has been clearly demonstrated. Iron is known to be essential in the formation of hemoglobin. If the diet is deficient in iron, anemia results. This can be controlled by dietary supplements. Calcium and phosphorus were shown to be important in the young for growth and development of the bones.

Iodine is essential for thyroid hormone production in the body. In old glacial regions, the soil and water are low in iodine compounds. A high incidence of endemic goiter frequently results. Research has provided a preventive measure for this condition by recommending the general use of iodized table salt in low iodine areas. More recently, it has been demonstrated that fluorides in the drinking water will reduce the incidence of dental caries by about one-third among children who consume the treated water. Also, topical application of fluorides has proved effective in lowering tooth decay. Many communities have provided for an addition of fluorides to their water supply as such a preventive measure.

Equally fascinating have been studies on the glands of internal secretion. The discovery of insulin in 1923 by Frederick Banting and Charles Best has prolonged life for millions of diabetic patients. Intensive research has greatly enlarged our knowledge of the functions of the pituitary gland, thyroid, parathyroid, and adrenal glands bringing better understanding and methods of treatment for many human disorders. Studies on sex hormones have been highly interesting. These control reproduction, sexual maturity, lactation, and other body functions. Important discoveries are still to be expected by continuing research in this field.

No field of medical science is more fascinating than immunology. An understanding of the immunological relationship of human blood groups provided by the studies of Karl Landsteiner (1868–1943) and many others has led to the extensive use of whole blood and

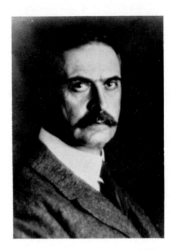

Karl Landsteiner (1868–1943)
Source: National Library of Medicine, Bethesda, Maryland, Neg. No. 10511.

blood fractions in medicine. Blood transfusions are saving thousands of lives each year. During the past 10 years, the transplantation of vital organs from one individual to another has offered promise of another important lifesaving measure. Available knowledge of the basic immunological concepts that will make such transplantations generally acceptable is still much too scanty. Many interesting leads are being vigorously pursued by research workers. Early success in this quest seems assured.

In the area of clinical psychology, Sigmund Freud (1856–1935), of Vienna, made great contributions. Collaborating with another Viennese physician, Joseph Breuer (1842–1925), a method was discovered of treating hysteria by getting the patient to recollect in a state of hypnosis the circumstances of early life that had led to the symptoms. This "cathartic" method of treatment was the initial step in the development of what was later called psychoanalysis. In 1894, Freud replaced hypnotism as a means of recalling hidden memories by a method of "free association" which is the heart of psychoanalysis. Freud studied a variety of psychoneurotics, as well as some individuals with apparently normal minds. His major discoveries were: (1) the existence of the unconscious and its influence on the conscious state, (2) the importance of repression in burying certain mental experiences, and (3) the importance of infantile sexuality.

With a number of colleagues, a series of International Congresses on Psychoanalysis was initiated. The first was held in 1908.

Although many of Freud's concepts are not generally accepted, his theories have had a wide impact not only on psychiatrists and psychologists, but also have strongly influenced anthropologists, educators, artists, and writers.

In the years following Freud, tremendous progress has been achieved in the understanding and treatment of mental diseases. In a preventive way the introduction of effective drugs in the treatment of syphilis has greatly reduced the incidence of general paresis. Likewise, the improvement of nutrition and the introduction of niacin has prevented thousands of cases of insanity due to pellagra. Lithium compounds are proving valuable in the control of depressive states. The psychopharmacological products are a boon in the management of many emotional disturbances. It appears that a new day is dawning in psychiatry.

One of the fastest moving fields in medicine is virology. Apart from the studies on yellow fever by the Reed Commission in Havana and the isolation of the virus of poliomyelitis in 1908, little progress was made in the study of viruses for many years. The gradual development of techniques and the discovery of convenient laboratory animals has recently brought rapid results. Effective vaccines against yellow fever and influenza were produced. With the introduction of continuous cell lines and by the use of human cell cultures, a great impetus was given to virus research. Perhaps the most notable triumphs have been the production of efficient vaccines to combat poliomyelitis, measles, and mumps. Another hopeful aspect of recent virological research is the demonstration that viruses may be directly related to some malignant tumors in the human. This may offer means to combat successfully some types of cancer.

The availability of adequate blood supplies for transfusion and the control of infections through antibiotics have made advances in radical surgical procedures possible. Operations to remove a lobe or even a whole lung that is diseased are now commonplace. Repairs of heart valves and replacement of segments of large blood vessels are carried out with considerable frequency.

One of the most fascinating advances in human medicine has been the development of the transplantation of organs from one individual to another. Beginning with kidney transplants about 20 years ago, surgeons have progressed to the transfer of hearts, bone marrow, lungs, livers, and thymus glands. Reports have been collected on over 3000 kidney transplants, over 130 heart transfers, and a lesser number of transplantations of other organs.[32],[33]

In the course of studying the immunological phenomenon involved in the body's efforts to reject the newly transplanted organ, scientists have made great advances in the field of immunology. The use of antilymphocyte serum (ALS) to diminish the donor's intolerance for the new tissues has become highly important. This serum appears to be much more satisfactory than the immunosuppressive agents previously employed.

While transplantation of organs must still be regarded as in an early stage of evolution, it would appear that this approach to human disease may have real potentiality for the future.

These fundamental advances in medical education and in research activities give promise for revolutionary progress in medical practice. The public is becoming better informed through modern communication media of the possibilities of medical science in the preservation and restoration of the health of the individual. The demand for medical service expands continuously. New methods of distributing medical care are becoming necessary. Experiments in this direction are being undertaken on all sides.

## The Rise of Public Health

The rapid rise in population of the industrial urban areas in Britain in the early 19th century led to intolerable sanitary and housing conditions. The spark that finally led to reform was set by Edwin Chadwick (1800–1890) with his report in 1842 on the "Sanitary Condition of the Labouring Population of Great Britain."[34] The publication of this report stimulated Parliament to formulate the Public Health Act of 1848. A General Board of Health was created. This Board is credited with persuading Parliament to legislate acts to control housing conditions, to establish sewerage systems and proper water supplies, and to provide for medical officers of health. The City of London was fortunate in its selection of Sir John Simon (1816–1904) as its first health director. He proved to be an outstanding public health leader in England for the second half of the century.

Another stimulus to sanitary reform was provided by the repeated waves of Asiatic cholera that swept across Europe and America during the 19th century. Britain was hard hit by the cholera epidemics of 1831 to 1832, 1848 to 1849, and 1853 to 1854. Chadwick's concept of communicable disease was based on the belief that such diseases were bred in filth and that the air polluted by foul odors arising from decaying organic matter was the means of transmitting contagion. Chadwick's explanation is not accepted today, but the close association of filth and disease is now generally admitted.

Two remarkable Englishmen, John Snow (1813–1858) and William Budd (1811–1880), demonstrated the germ theory of disease before Pasteur and Koch had brought their big guns to bear on the problem. Snow in 1849 in a pamphlet, "On the Mode of Communication of Cholera," and in subsequent papers developed his theories of contagion. During the London cholera epidemic in 1854, he put his theories to the test. Snow stated:

Diseases that are communicated from person to person are caused by some material which passes from the sick to the healthy, and which has the property of increasing and multiplying in the system of the person it attacks.

He proceeded to carry out a careful study of an outbreak of cholera centering around Broad Street in the London district of Soho. Almost immediately he suspected the Broad Street pump as being the source of infection. He persuaded the authorities to remove the handle of the pump and the epidemic quickly subsided.[35]

William Budd came to similar conclusions in his study of typhoid fever. Beginning his studies in 1839, Budd published a paper in 1856 entitled, "On Intestinal Fever; Its Mode of Propagation." Budd imagined the agent of typhoid to be "so low in the scale of created things that the mildew which springs up on decaying wood must be considered high in comparison." Budd carried out a most convincing study of a typhoid outbreak in the village of North Tawton, of which he was the sole physician. He concluded that "the tainted hands of those who wait upon the sick," bed linen, and other clothing of the sick (citing the high prevalence of the disease among washer-women) are frequent sources of infection. The principal way, he considered, is by contamination of drinking water by the excreta of the sick.[36]

In Massachusetts, Lemuel Shattuck (1793–1859), a book dealer serving in the State Assembly, complained so frequently of a lack of progress in sanitation that he was appointed chairman of a legislative committee for the study of health and sanitary problems of the State. The report for which Shattuck was largely responsible appeared in 1850, "Report of the Sanitary Commission of Massachusetts," and is a remarkable one.[37] Although the report attracted little attention at the time, one of its recommendations was put into effect. In 1869, the Commonwealth of Massachusetts set up a state board of health made up of physicians and laymen. Although Louisiana had set up a board or commission to deal with yellow fever epidemics as early as 1855, it is not generally considered to have created the first state board of health in terms of the general functions of such boards.

Other states organized state boards of health in quick succession: California, 1871; Virginia, 1871; Minnesota, 1872; and Michigan, 1873. The American Public Health Association was launched in 1872 and has since served as a standard bearer in all public health campaigns. The United States Public Health Service (as it is now called) took over quarantine functions in ports from 1878, having evolved from the old United States Marine Hospital Service founded in 1798 for the medical care of seamen.

Dr. C.-E.A. Winslow (1877–1957)[38] has outlined the development of public health during his long career:

When I entered in the late nineties, public health consisted only of two lines of attack. It included sanitation, the control of filth as advocated by Chadwick, and the beginning of the control of contagious diseases by the use of serums and vaccines. In 1900, we had a pretty good basis for sanitation and we had a preview of the tremendous possibilities of the application of bacteriologic methods to the diagnosis, treatment, and prevention of disease. Those two phases then comprised the whole of public health; it was nothing but sanitation and the control of communicable disease.

By 1910, control of typhoid, cholera, and diphtheria had progressed successfully. The leading cause of death was tuberculosis. Thirty-five years before, Edward Trudeau (1848–1915) had established the first sanitorium for tuberculosis in this country at Saranac Lake, New York. Public health leaders knew that there were two ways to fight tuberculosis: to check the spread of infection and to build up the patient's vital resistance.

An important new phase of public health was introduced. Education in personal hygiene became the third major health program. The principles of personal hygiene were applied in the second decade of the century to the control of infant mortality, to improvement of the health of school children, and finally to mental hygiene. Education to change people's habits of life based on knowledge of physiological hygiene has become a major objective of public health.

This phase of public health was greatly fostered by the development of the public health nurse. This movement began in New York City starting for the purpose of teaching good health practices in the homes of the poor. In 1902, Lillian Wald (1867–1940) organized the first school nursing program in New York, setting up a pattern which was rapidly followed throughout the country.

The need for local health departments to bring health knowledge to the people soon became apparent. Yakima County, Washington, and Guilford County, North Carolina, created the first such departments in 1911. This led the way to the organization of similar health departments across the nation.

The growth of state and local departments of health created a demand for trained personnel. Beginning with 1912, a program of study was organized at the Massachusetts Institute of Technology by William T. Sedgewick. Later, MIT joined with Harvard University to offer a broader program. Dr. Milton J. Rosenau was a member of this faculty. His book, *Preventive Medicine and Hygiene,* appearing first in 1913 and continuing to appear in new editions written by new men from time to time until the present day, has done as much to advance public health as any other single factor.

The Rockefeller Foundation of New York, organized in 1913, adopted public health as one of its basic fields of interest. Through financial aid and through strong leadership, this Foundation assisted in the establishment of schools of public health both in the United States and abroad. Johns Hopkins University School of Public Health opened its doors for teaching and research in 1919. The reorganized School of Public Health at Harvard University came into being in 1923. At present there are 18 such schools in this country devoted to preparing leaders in public health administration, public health nursing, sanitary engineering, biostatistics, and laboratory and research fields. It is through the leadership of these schools that the basic disciplines of public health (biostatistics and epidemiology) have been brought to their current state of development.

In 1949, Winslow[39] offered the following definition:

Public health is the science and art of preventing disease, prolonging life, and promoting physical and mental health and efficiency through organized community efforts, for the sanitation of the environment, the control of community infections, the education of the individual in the principles of personal hygiene, the organization of medical and nursing service for the early diagnosis and treatment of disease, and the development of the social machinery which will ensure to every individual in the community a standard of living adequate for the maintenance of health.

As public health gained in maturity, astounding results were achieved. The average length of human life was greatly extended, infant and maternal mortality were greatly reduced, and the burden of communicable disease has been diminshed to a low level. The life expectancy of man in the western world has been greatly extended. On the other hand, a whole new set of problems has arisen: cardiovascular disease, cancer, and accidents are now major factors in our death rates. Extension of conventional health department activities to areas not previously served is now required. This is especially true in the field of medical care. It is essential that the practicing physicians, the hospitals, health departments, and all other health agencies work together in close symphaty to extend a good quality of medical care to the whole community.

Certainly the most significant development of the 20th century in medicine has been the increasing concern of governments at all levels for the health of the people. Traditionally, governments have assumed some responsibility for the medical care of their indigent citizens.

In general, this care has been limited in scope, of poor quality, and rather grudgingly administered. As medical science has progressed, it has become clear to all that far more can now be done than formerly to preserve and restore health and to prolong the period of useful living. In recent decades, government has gradually extended its coverage for medical care to larger numbers of the population.

Under the 1965 Amendments to the Social Security Act, almost all persons over 65 years of age are eligible for coverage under a basic plan that provides payment for a large proportion of hospital and nursing home costs through Social Security taxes. A voluntary supplementary insurance plan financed by monthly payments by each enrollee, matched by payments by the Federal Government, covers most physicians' charges and cost of certain medical services not included under the basic plan.

In addition, the Federal Government will supply financial aid to states to provide medical assistance for medically indigent aged, for blind and disabled persons, and for poverty-stricken families with dependent children. Each state decides for itself whether it wishes to adopt this program. The state determines what people will be included, the services that they are entitled to, and the manner in which the program will operate. Although each state will determine the speed and pattern of its program growth, by 1975 all state medical assistance programs are expected to provide medical care for substantially all the people who cannot pay for it themselves.

Other federally sponsored programs are certain to have an effect on the evolving American health care system. The Comprehensive Health Planning Act of 1966 and the Health Maintenance Organization Act of 1973 are among the significant recent developments.

What the effects of these far-reaching programs will be on the future of medicine and its allied professions cannot now be foreseen. It is clear that the impact will be profound. The "winds of change are blowing across the land." Medical practice will be different in the years ahead.

## The Emergence of the Nursing Profession

Organized nursing arose under the auspices of the Catholic Church during the Middle Ages to meet the needs that developed from the great crusades against the Moslems in the East. The guiding principle of nursing in those times was charity. Three nursing orders became outstanding: (1) the Knights of St. John, (2) the Teutonic Knights, and (3) the Knights of Lazarus. Corresponding with these orders were three orders for women who cared for female patients in special hospitals. Many other nursing orders were established as the number of hospitals grew, for example, the Augustinian Sisters at the Hotel Dieu in Paris. Within the limitations of the state of medical knowledge, these hospitals performed a great service to the poor classes.

Nursing sank to a very low level in those European countries in which the Church organizations were overthrown by the Reformation. The heads of such governments closed monasteries, churches, and hospitals. The religious nursing orders were forced to cease their services. Only women from the lowest classes undertook nursing as a career. In countries still loyal to the Catholic Church nursing remained more or less static, but continued to provide devoted service.

Indeed, the period between the latter part of the 17th century up to the middle of the 19th was the "dark age" of nursing. Not only did the status of nurses sink miserably, but the condition of hospitals also sank during the 18th century to the lowest level ever. Hospitals continued to be notoriously filthy until well into the last century.

A number of factors contributed to the emergence of nursing as a profession. The emancipation of women can be traced to the trend toward personal freedom arising from the Industrial Revolution and other movements for social reform. Without the emancipation of women, the evolution of nursing would surely have taken a far different course.

In the British Isles, efforts to improve nursing were made in Ireland by the Sisters of Charity and the Sisters of Mercy. Starting in 1812 and 1830, respectively, these orders are significant as the first modern nursing organizations in Great Britain. They were Catholic and based on the tradition and experience of the French orders.

The need for better nursing was recognized in Germany. Theodor Fliedner (1800–1864), Protestant pastor at Kaiserswerth, near Düsseldorf, and his wife opened a training school for deaconesses and a small hospital. The girls who attended were taught ethics and religious principles, practical nursing of the sick, and some knowledge of pharmacy. For the first time in history, there was available a school with most of the essential elements for the training of nurses. When Fliedner died in 1864, branches of his institution had already been established in the Near East and in London, Pittsburgh, and Milwaukee. Some 1600 women had been trained as deaconesses.

Florence Nightingale (1820–1910), a lady of the British upper classes, became deeply interested in social betterment. Impressed by the highly unsatisfactory status of patient care in hospitals, Miss Nightingale made a thorough study of all aspects of the situation. She studied institutions in several European cities and visited the Kaiserswerth Hospital and School for Deaconesses repeatedly.

When the horrible conditions of the British sick and wounded in the Crimean War became known in London, Florence Nightingale volunteered to recruit a group of women to go out to give what assistance they could. The brilliant results achieved by these nurses under Miss Nightingale's leadership are known to all. The grateful public raised, by popular subscription, a sum of $220,000 for the "Nightingale Fund" to be used for the establishment of the first British School of Nursing at St. Thomas's Hospital. With the opening of the School in 1860, the demand for the "new style" nurses greatly exceeded the supply. Soon other hospitals opened similar schools which led to a rapid growth of English nursing. Miss Nightingale's books, *Notes on Hospitals* and *Notes on Nursing,* had a tremendous influence on all sides.

Close association between leaders in the United States and Florence Nightingale made sure that her concepts would strongly influence American schools that were founded in the years after the Civil War. In 1873, the Bellevue Hospital School of Nursing began in New York. In Boston, two schools were of importance: The New England Hospital, modeled on the Kaiserswerth plan, opened in 1872, and the Massachusetts General Hospital beginning in 1873. In Connecticut, the New Haven Hospital, following Miss Nightingale's principles, organized its school as a unit independent of the hospital. It also admitted the first students in 1873.

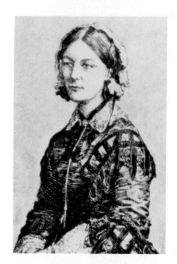

Florence Nightingale (1820–1910)
Source: William H. Welch Medical Library, Johns Hopkins University, Baltimore, Maryland

During the next 25 years, steady progress was made. The number of nursing schools increased. The growth was closely related to the development of scientific medicine and surgery. Originally, 1 year was set for the training of a nurse. As more knowledge and skill became necessary, the period of training had to be extended. The founding of the Johns Hopkins Hospital School of Nursing in 1889 gave a great impetus to nursing. Thus, during this period, the advance of nursing was characterized by a rapid increase in the number of schools, by improvement and extension of the courses, by the provision of better equipment, and by appropriate textbooks. Perhaps more important was the appearance as leaders of nursing of a remarkably able group of women, who were to initiate the next significant steps toward the creation of a profession.

The first of these steps was the organization of nursing schools by universities. Miss Adelaide Nutting (1858–1948), a Canadian by birth, graduate in the first class in nursing at the Johns Hopkins Hospital and afterward principal of that school, became the first nurse ever to be made a university professor. She took the chair at Teachers College, Columbia University, in 1907 and made a splendid contribution toward the creation and development of the Department of Nursing and Health in that institution. The University of Minnesota, in 1909, created the first school of nursing organized as an integral part of a university. Since that time,

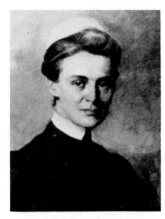

Adelaide Nutting (1858–1948)
Source: William H. Welch Medical Library, Johns Hopkins University, Baltimore, Maryland

dozens of university schools of nursing education both for undergraduates and graduate students have been organized throughout the United States.

Another great step forward in the growth of nursing as a profession was the formation of professional associations and the establishment of professional journals. The American Nurses Association founded in 1911 grew out of alumnae associations of the early schools of nursing. The National League of Nursing Education and the National Organization for Public Health Nursing have also played important roles in setting standards of education and of practice that have progressively raised the influence of nurses in the health field.

A movement of deep significance for public health is generally credited to Miss Lillian Wald (1867–1940). She became interested in the great need for nursing service among the poor of New York City. She was instrumental in founding the Henry Street Settlement in 1893. This settlement became the field training area for nurses and social workers from Columbia University and gave strong impetus to the creation of public health nursing which is the mainstay of all health work among the people. In 1902, Miss Wald organized the first nursing program for school children in New York City, creating a pattern that has rapidly spread across the country.

Thus, by the end of the first decade of the present century, all of the steps which were required to place the nursing profession on the way to its current high peak of performance had been taken. Without these developments, medical care and public health could not have advanced to their current levels of excellence.[40]

## REFERENCES

1. Garrison, F.H. *An Introduction to the History of Medicine,* Ed. 4. Philadelphia: W. B. Saunders Co., 1929, p. 20.
2. Osler, W. *The Evolution of Modern Medicine.* New Haven: Yale University Press, 1921.
3. Garrison, F.H. *An Introduction to the History of Medicine,* Ed. 4. Philadelphia: W. B. Saunders Co., 1929, p. 61.
4. Kremers, E. *Kremers and Urdang's History of Pharmacy,* Revised by Glenn Sonnedecker, Ed.3. Philadelphia: Lippincott, 1963, p. 5.
5. Kremers, E. *Kremers and Urdang's History of Pharmacy, Revised by Glenn Sonnedecker, Ed. 3. Philadelphia: Lippincott, 1963, p. 7.*
6. *Bender, G. A. Great Moments in Pharmacy,* Detroit: Northwood Institute Press, 1966, p. 17
7. Garrison, F.H. *An Introduction to the History of Medicine,* Ed. 4. Philadelphia: W. B. Saunders Co., 1929, p. 78.
8. Saunders, J. B. de C. *Transitions from Ancient Egyptian to Greek Medicine.* Lawrence, Kansas: University of Kansas Press, 1963.
9. Winslow, C.-E. A. *The Conquest of Epidemic Disease.* Princeton, New Jersey: Princeton University Press, 1943.
10. Rosen, G. *A History of Public Health.* New York: M. D. Publications, Inc., 1958.
11. Bender, G. A. *Great Moments In Pharmacy.* Detroit: Northwood Institute Press, 1966, pp. 36–38.
12. Durant, W. *The Story of Civilization. IV. The Age of Faith.* New York: Simon and Schuster, 1950.
13. Dana, C. L. *The Peaks of Medical History.* New York: Paul B. Hoeber, Inc., 1926.
14. Kremers, E. *Kremers and Urdang's History of Pharmacy.* Revised by Glenn Sonnedecker, Ed. 3. Philadelphia: Lippincott, 1963, pp. 316, 423.
15. Bender, George A., *Great Moments in Pharmacy.* Detroit: Northwood Institute Press, 1966, pp. 80–91.
16. Kremers, E. *Kremers and Urdang's History of Pharmacy.* Revised by Glenn Sonnedecker, Ed. 3. Philadelphia: Lippincott, 1963, p. 419.
17. Durant, W., and Durant, A. *The Story of Civilization. IX. The Age of Voltaire.* New York: Simon and Schuster, 1965, p. 590.
18. Garrison, F.H. *An Introduction to the History of Medicine,* Ed. 4. Philadelphia: W. B. Saunders Co., 1929, p. 347.
19. Bender G. A., *Great Moments in Pharmacy.* Detroit: Northwood Institute Press, 1966, pp. 152–168.
20. Bender, G. A., *Great Moments in Pharmacy.* Detroit: Northwood Institute Press, 1966, pp. 124–130.

21. Roddis, L. H., *James Lind*. London: Heinemann, 1951, pp. 52–62.
22. Garrison, F. H. *An Introduction to the History of Medicine,* Ed. 4. Philadelphia: W. B. Saunders Co., 1929, p. 407.
23. Bender, G. A., *Great Moments in Pharmacy*. Detroit: Northwood Institute Press, 1966, pp. 96–110.
24. Kremers, E. *Kremers and Urdang's History of Pharmacy,* Revised by Glenn Sonnedecker, Ed. 3. Philadelphia: Lippincott, 1963, pp. 171–173.
25. Garrison, F. H. *An Introduction to the History of Medicine.* Ed. 4. Philadelphia: W. B. Saunders Co., 1929, p. 570.
26. Bender, G. A., *Great Moments in Pharmacy*. Detroit: Northwood Institute Press, 1966, pp. 118–136.
27. Garrison, F. H. *An Introduction to the History of Medicine,* Ed. 4. Philadelphia: W.B. Saunders Co., 1929, p. 431.
28. Bender, G. A. *Great Moments in Pharmacy*. Detroit: Northwood Institute Press, 1966, pp. 166–170.
29. Bender G. A. *Great Moments in Pharmacy*. Detroit: Northwood Institute Press, 1966, pp. 138–151.
30. Bender, G. A. *Great Moments in Pharmacy*. Detroit: Northwood Institute Press, 1966, pp. 186–205.
31. Bender G. A. *Great Moments in Pharmacy*. Detroit: Northwood Institute Press, 1966, pp. 172–184.
32. Moore, F. D. *Transplant–the Give and Take of Tissue Transplantation* (Revised Edition). New York: Simon and Schuster, 1972.
33. *Research Advances in Human Transplantation.* Department of Health, Education, and Welfare

Publication No. (NIH), 73–108. U. S. Government Printing Office, 1973.
34. Chadwick, E. *Report on an Inquiry into the Sanitary Condition of the Labouring Population of Great Britain, Poor Law Commissioners.* London: W. Clowes for Her Majesty's Stationery Office, 1842.
35. Snow, J. *On Cholera.* New York: reprinted by The Commonwealth Fund, 1936.
36. Budd, W. *Typhoid Fever, Its Nature, Mode of Spreading and Prevention.* New York: reprinted by The Commonwealth Fund, 1931.
37. Shattuck, L. *The Report of the Sanitary Commission of Massachusetts, 1850.* Cambridge: reprinted by Harvard University Press, 1948.
38. Winslow, C.-E. A. *The Evolution and Significance of the Modern Public Health Campaign.* New Haven: Yale University Press, 1923.
39. Winslow, C.-E. A. The evolution of public health and its objectives. In *Public Health in the World Today,* edited by J. S. Simmons. Cambridge: Harvard University Press, 1949.
40. Griffen, J. J., and Griffen, H. J. K. *Jensen's History and Trends of Professional Nursing,* Ed. 5. St. Louis: The C. V. Mosby Co., 1965.

## ADDITIONAL SUGGESTED READING

1. Scarborough, J., *Roman Medicine*. Ithaca, New York: Cornell University Press, 1969.
2. Singer, C., and Underwood, E. A. *A Short History of Medicine,* Ed. 2. New York: Oxford University Press, 1962.
3. Dubos, R. J. *Louis Pasteur: Free Lance of Science.* Boston: Little, Brown and Co., 1952.
4. Sigerist, H. E. *American Medicine.* New York: W. W. Norton and Co., 1934.

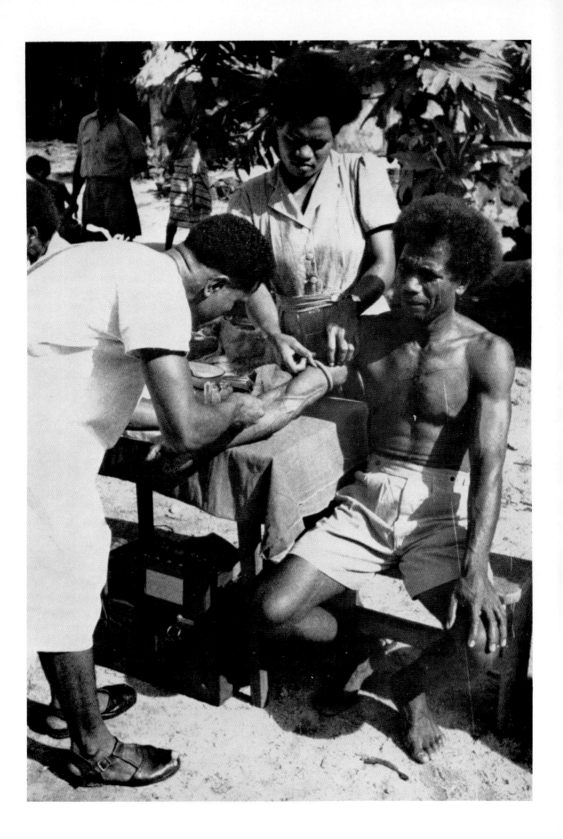

# 2

# Organization and administration of health agencies

The dogmas of the quiet past are inadequate to
the stormy present. . . . As our case is new, so
we must think anew and act anew. We must
disenthrall ourselves.

ABRAHAM LINCOLN
*Message to Congress,* December 1, 1862

Everywhere the old order changeth and happy
are those who can change with it.

WILLIAM OSLER

## INTERNATIONAL HEALTH ORGANIZATIONS

### Introduction

International public health had its origin over
a century ago in the International Sanitary
Conference held in Paris in 1851. The motivating force for this meeting was the continued
threat of Asiatic cholera to European nations.
The recent introduction of steam as a source of
power for railways and ships had laid the
foundation for international trade on an unprecedented scale and had increased speed of
transportation.

The object of the first International Sanitary
Conference was to attempt to reach agreement
among the 12 nations represented on quarantine regulations to prevent the spread of
cholera. Although the delegates labored man-
fully for six months, in the end, the conference
must be reckoned a failure, as governments
were unwilling to put its recommendations into
effect.[1]

This was not an isolated example of interest
in international co-operation. During the first
half of the 19th century, many bilateral
conventions had been concluded between individual countries on technical matters. For
example, agreements to control postal communications were arranged. These limited conventions gave way in the second half of the century
to international conferences to enable

nations to reach agreement on numerous
technical subjects. Among such subjects were
postal and telegraphic communications, weights
and measures, patents, trademarks, copyrights,
navigation safeguards, the slave trade, and labor
legislation.

During the next 50 years, at least nine other
international sanitary conferences were convened to consider the mutual problems presented by cholera and other epidemic diseases
such as plague and yellow fever. In retrospect,
it must be admitted that progress in the
promotion of international public health was
very slow during this period.[2] It could hardly
have been otherwise in the prevailing state of
medical science. National authorities strongly
disagreed on the elementary aspects of causes
and modes of spread of the epidemic diseases.
The next century brought a flood of technical
information upon which effective international
action could be based.

### Pan American Health Organization

To the Americas goes the honor of having
established the first permanent international
health organization. It was created by an
International Conference of American States
held in Mexico City in 1902. The participating
governments were mainly concerned to protect
against the interruption of regular commerce
and trade caused by epidemic disease.

The new health agency, with headquarters in
Washington, D.C., was designated the International Health Bureau. It was assigned a single
room in the Pan American Union building and
was given an annual budget of $5000. The staff
consisted of six part-time officials and two
clerks. For the first two decades of its life, the
Bureau was largely a clearing house to collect
and distribute information on disease, to call
periodic conferences of health officials, and to
aid participating governments to better sanitary
conditions of seaports.

In 1924, a Pan American Sanitary Code was adopted and the name of the agency was changed to the Pan American Sanitary Bureau. At that time, the United States Public Health Service agreed to lend to the Bureau two of its medical officers as field workers. Under the Code, which was eventually signed by all of the American governments, a wide range of functions was assigned to the Bureau and it was designated as the central co-ordinating agency for health in the Americas. A director was appointed in 1920. Dr. Hugh S. Cummings, former Surgeon-General of the USPHS, was selected and held the directorship until 1947, when he was replaced by Dr. Fred L. Soper. The current director, Dr. Abraham Horwitz of Chile, replaced Soper in 1959.

In 1947, an overall organization, the Pan American Sanitary Organization, was established, with the Bureau designated as its operating arm or general secretariat. Finally, in 1958, a new name was adopted for the basic organization, the Pan American Health Organization.

As of 1973, there are 26 member governments in PAHO with three participating governments representing colonial areas in the region.

In 1949, PAHO signed an agreement with the World Health Organization through which the Bureau assumed the functions of WHO Regional Office for the Americas. Thus, serving both PAHO and WHO, the Bureau has programs along several main lines: control or eradication of communicable diseases; strengthening of national and local health services; education and training of professional health personnel; and research. Principal campaigns have been directed against malaria, yellow fever, and smallpox. Another major program has been the development of safe community water supplies. PAHO and WHO now employ more than 1400 persons and administer funds that totaled more than $40 million in 1972 for over 700 health projects in the Americas.[3]

In 1965, a new building for permanent headquarters was opened in Washington, D.C. (Fig. 2.1). This building was made possible by a grant of the landsite by the United States

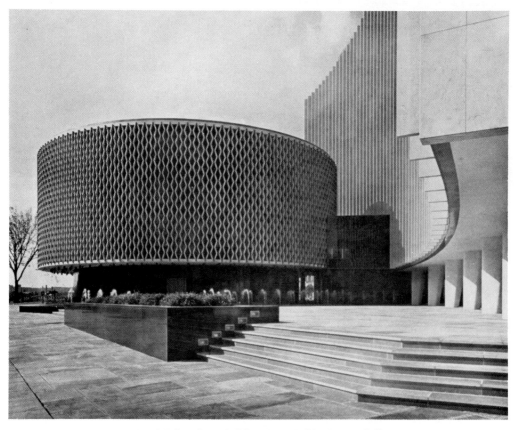

Fig. 2.1. PAHO and WHO building in Washington, D.C.

Government and by a loan of $5.5 million by the Kellogg Foundation for construction costs. This money was repaid by the American republics on an annual basis, but the funds repaid went for education, training, and water programs in the areas where this assistance is required.[3] In 1972, the Ministers of Health for the Americas meeting in Santiago, Chile, drew up an ambitious 10-year plan for the improvement of health services throughout the region.[4]

## Office International d'Hygiene Publique

As governments realized that knowledge of epidemic diseases was rapidly increasing, the need for a permanent office or center to deal with such matters became recognized. In 1907, delegates from 12 nations signed, in Rome, an agreement for the creation of an international office of public health—the Office International d'Hygiene Publique, to be located in Paris. The new Office was to be under the authority and control of a committee of technical delegates of member governments. Its main function was to disseminate to member states information of public health interest, especially that relating to the major epidemic diseases, as well as measures to combat these diseases; its secondary objective, derived from the first, was to ensure that the international sanitary conventions were kept up to date. The third function of the Office was to act as an arbitrating agency in international sanitary matters. Finally, the Office was to function as a kind of post office, facilitating prompt interchange of information without the cumbersome machinery of diplomatic exchange.

The staff and facilities of the Office were established in Paris in 1909. It operated fairly well until the advent of World War I. During the war, work of the Office ceased, except for publication of the monthly bulletin.

Attempts were made to absorb the Office into the Health Organization of the League of Nations, when that body began to function in 1920. This move was resisted by some of the participating governments and the Office continued to operate as a separate body until the outbreak of World War II in 1939. At the World Health Conference held in July, 1946, in New York, the delegates of 60 states signed a protocol agreeing that the Office be absorbed by the newly created World Health Organization. This transfer was completed by the end of 1950.

The Paris Office was a remarkably effective agency for its limited purpose, which was chiefly the prevention of the international spread of epidemic diseases.[1]

## The Health Organization of the League of Nations

The covenant of the League of Nations, coming into force in January, 1920, contained a mandate to the League to take action in international health. Acting on this directive, the Council of the League took steps to create an effective health organization. In addition to a general advisory health council, the Health Organization consisted of a standing Health Committee and a secretariat.

The activities of the Health Organization can be broadly grouped into the following:

1. Epidemiology, including the epidemic information service. At the end of World War I, vast epidemics of typhus and other diseases were afflicting Poland, Russia, and the Balkan States. An international epidemic commission was created to combat these outbreaks. The combined efforts of all concerned proved successful in reducing the ravages of these major epidemics.

An Epidemiological Intelligence Bureau was set up in Singapore and later another in Sydney, Australia, to collect information on disease occurrence and to disseminate it to interested governments. The weekly "Epidemiological Record," begun in 1925, served to supply health officers with recent data on epidemic diseases and quarantine measures. Data were broadcast by radio to ships at sea and to port authorities to inform them of recent outbreaks of disease.

2. Technical studies were carried out mainly by expert committees. A number of such committees were directed to study specific disease problems, e.g., malaria, plague, syphilis, tuberculosis, and cancer. Perhaps the most valuable contribution was in the field of international standardization of drugs, sera, hormones, and other important biologicals.

3. Technical assistance was provided to governments requesting aid. Nutrition, housing, and medical education were fields of special interest.

As the international political situation worsened from 1936 onward, the capability of the Health Organization to perform useful work diminished. Valiant efforts to maintain the basic activities of the Organization during World War II met with partial success. The weekly "Epidemiological Record" never ceased publication, although reports were incomplete. Work on biological standardization was continued in London and Copenhagen.[1]

## United Nations' Relief and Rehabilitation Administration

As World War II proceeded, health workers, mindful of the awful conditions which prevailed between 1918 and 1920, urged that plans be concerted on an international scale for relief and rehabilitation of war-torn countries. After some preliminary committee work in London, an agreement was signed in November, 1943, by 43 allied and associated nations, establishing a United Nations' Relief and Rehabilitation Administration (UNRRA). The functions of the Health Division were:

1. Assistance to national health authorities for the prevention of epidemics resulting from the war; the restoration of national health departments; the loan of technical personnel; the estimation of medical and sanitary supplies required; assistance in their procurement.

2. Revision and administration of international sanitary conventions for maritime and aerial quarantine.

3. Health protection of persons displaced by the war.

4. Training and rehabilitation of professional health and medical personnel.

UNRRA was, by definition, a temporary organization to handle emergency conditions resulting from the great war. In spite of difficulties resulting from the rapid organization of the program and from the recruitment of staff in the confusion prevailing at the termination of the world conflict, it performed a highly useful and necessary role. Indeed, it carried out by far the largest international health program ever executed.

UNRRA was dissolved by action of the participating governments in August, 1946. Its remaining funds were transferred to the Interim Commission of the World Health Organization, with the recommendation that the technical assistance program be continued to those countries requesting aid.[1]

## World Health Organization

The charter of the United Nations adopted at the international conference meeting in San Francisco in 1945, contained an article calling for the establishment of a specialized health agency with wide powers. After considerable preparatory planning, the World Health Conference was convened in New York in June, 1946. Delegates were present from all 51 members of the United Nations, while observers representing a number of non-member states were also present.

The Conference succeeded in producing the constitution of the World Health Organization. It also arranged for an Interim Commission to prepare for the first World Health Assembly and to carry on, without interruption, the surviving activities of the League of Nations' Health Organization and those of the Office International d'Hygiene Publique and of UNRRA.[5]

It had been expected that the Interim Commission would come to an end in a matter of months, but delays in ratification of the WHO constitution prolonged its existence for nearly two years. It was not until September 1, 1948, that the World Health Organization finally came into being. Headquarters were established in the Palais des Nations, in Geneva, Switzerland (Fig. 2.2).

Membership in WHO is open to all states. Each state desiring to enter WHO must ratify the constitution and receive a majority vote of the Health Assembly.

The administration of WHO is through a director-general and five assistant director-generals each of which is in charge of three divisions of the program. The staff, excluding that of PAHO, numbered 3758 as of November 1972.[6]

The work of WHO is carried out by:

1. The World Health Assembly, composed of delegates representing members. This Assembly meets in regular annual session and in such special sessions as may be necessary.

2. The Executive Board, consisting of 24 persons designated by as many members. These members are selected by the Health Assembly. The member so selected shall appoint a person qualified in the field of health. The first Director-General of WHO was Dr. Brock Chisholm of Canada who served from 1946 to 1952; Dr. M. G. Candau of Brazil succeeded Dr. Chisholm and served from 1953 to 1973; Dr. Halfdan Mahler of Denmark has recently taken over the post from Dr. Candau.

The principal functions of the World Health

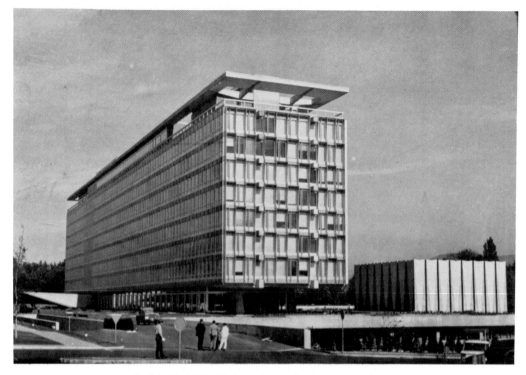

Fig. 2.2. World Health Organization headquarters in Geneva

Organization as outlined in the Constitution are:

1. To act as the directing and coordinating authority on international health work.

2. To establish and maintain effective collaboration with the United Nations, specialized agencies, governmental health administrations, professional groups, and such other organizations as may be deemed appropriate.

3. To assist governments, upon request, in strengthening health services.

4. To furnish appropriate technical assistance and, in emergencies, necessary aid upon the request or acceptance of governments.

5. To provide or assist in providing, upon the request of the United Nations, health services and facilities to special groups, such as the peoples of trust territories.

6. To establish and maintain such administrative and technical services as may be required, including epidemiological and statistical services.

7. To stimulate and advance work to eradicate epidemic, endemic, and other diseases.

8. To promote, in cooperation with other specialized agencies where necessary, the prevention of accidental injuries.

9. To promote, in cooperation with other specialized agencies where necessary, the improvement of nutrition, housing, sanitation, recreation, economic or working conditions and other aspects of environmental hygiene.

10. To promote cooperation among scientific and professional groups which contribute to the advancement of health.

11. To propose conventions, agreements, and regulations, and make recommendations with respect to international health matters and to perform such duties as may be assigned thereby to the Organization and are consistent with its objective.

12. To promote maternal and child health and welfare and to foster the ability to live harmoniously in a changing total environment.

13. To foster activities in the field of mental health, especially those affecting the harmony of human relations.

14. To promote and conduct research in the field of health.

15. To promote improved standards of teaching and training in the health, medical, and related professions.

16. To study and report on, in cooperation with other specialized agencies where necessary,

administrative and social techniques affecting public health and medical care from preventive and curative points of view, including hospital services and social security.

17. To provide information, counsel, and assistance in the field of health.

18. To assist in developing an informed public opinion among all peoples on matters of health.

19. To establish and revise as necessary international nomenclatures of diseases, of causes of death, and of public health practices.

20. To standardize diagnostic procedures as necessary.

21. To develop, establish, and promote international standards with respect to food, biological, pharmaceutical, and similar products.

22. Generally to take all necessary action to attain the objective of the organization.

The Constitution of WHO provided for the establishment of regional offices to function within the framework of the parent organization to meet the special regional needs. The first World Health Assembly meeting, in 1948, tackled the complex task of delineation of the regional areas. Within a period of some three and a half years, six regions came into being. These areas are: (1) Eastern Mediterranean area, with headquarters in Alexandria; (2) Southeast Asia, with headquarters in New Delhi; (3) the Americas (the Pan American Sanitary Organization), with headquarters in Washington, D.C.; (4) Africa, with headquarters in Brazzaville; (5) the Western Pacific, with headquarters in Manila; and (6) a regional office for Europe, with headquarters in Copenhagen.

WHO avoids the error of overcentralization by providing for six regional committees comprised of representatives of the member states of each region. These regional committees establish policies and oversee the activities of the regional offices.

In addition to its regular functions, WHO is carrying out an extensive program in co-operation with member nations to combat selected epidemic diseases. Campaigns to eradicate smallpox and malaria are being pushed vigorously.

In 1967, smallpox was reported in 42 countries, 30 of which were considered endemic for the disease. The actual number of cases was estimated at 2.5 million. By the end of 1972, only 19 countries reported cases of smallpox and of these, only in seven countries was the disease considered endemic. The estimated number of cases of smallpox for 1972 was under 200,000. The success of this campaign was attributed to the use of a potent and stable freeze-dried vaccine. Brazil—the last stronghold of the disease in the Americas—has eradicated smallpox. The eradication program there began in the late 1960's. As recently as 1969, there were 7407 cases in Brazil, but the total dipped to 19 in 1971. In 1973-74, smallpox flared up in Bangladesh, India, and Pakistan. WHO teams were sent to assist the official agencies in control campaigns.

More difficulty has been encountered with malaria. In embarking on a world-wide campaign in 1956, WHO relied on the interruption of malaria transmission by the use of residual insecticides. This campaign has met with some success. By 1972, it was estimated that 721 million people living in previously malarious areas had been freed from the threat of the disease, and another 631 million are now protected either by spraying operations or by drugs regularly administered. Some 480 million people are living in areas where eradication programs are not yet in operation, but many of these are benefiting from limited control measures.[6]

Tuberculosis continues to be one of the priority health problems in four of the six regions of WHO. Immunization with BCG vaccine on a large scale and the widespread application of chemotherapy are the main measures used for combating tuberculosis. Many years will be required in the less developed countries before this disease can be brought under control.

A constant vigil is kept on influenza to provide early notice of the appearance of new strains requiring modification of the current vaccines. Control programs to reduce the toll of venereal diseases and of tropical yaws are progressing well. Studies on other important diseases such as cholera and schistosomiasis have been initiated. Altogether, the program of WHO is a many faceted undertaking.

According to its constitution, the Health Assembly must approve budget estimates and apportion the expenses among the members in accordance with a scale to be fixed by the Health Assembly. WHO also receives special contributions from active member nations and from the United Nations' Technical Assistance Board.

For the first year after establishment of WHO (1949), the budget was $5 million. By 1961, the budget had grown to $21,114,348. The effective working budget for 1972 was $86,034,290; for 1973, the effective working budget was $93,847,000; and for 1974, at $100,250,000. A portion of the budget increases has resulted from the decline of the U. S. dollar on the world monetary market.[6]

In the framework of WHO, a number of countries have entered a cooperative program called the International Agency for Research on Cancer. In 1965, the participating countries (West Germany, France, the United Kingdom, Italy, and the U. S. A.) established this agency to be located in Lyons, France. The 1970 budget for research was $1,925,000.

Other important intergovernmental agencies concerned with health are the International Labor Organization, United Nations Educational, Scientific and Cultural Organization, and Food and Agriculture Organization of the United Nations. These agencies have cooperative arrangements with WHO.[6]

Prospects appear bright for the future success of WHO. Fortunately its mandate is broad, so that it can serve the emerging nations to strengthen and develop their total health services. The World Health Organization is set up as an independent agency, with its own constitution, membership, and financial sources. It is, of course, closely related to the United Nations, but is not dependent upon that agency. Unless major wars come to upset international cooperation, WHO should go on to greater and more significant accomplishments.

## United Nations' International Children's Emergency Fund

When the functions of UNRRA were terminated in 1946, the UNRRA Council recommended that a portion of its available funds be allocated to set up an International Children's Fund to continue relief and rehabilitation activities in countries that had been victims of aggression. The United Nations accepted this suggestion and created the Fund, requesting governments to make voluntary contributions for its support. The governing body is an executive board of representatives of 25 countries, originally nominated by the United Nations' General Assembly.

During its first three years of operation, this organization was allocated $418 million, in large part through appropriations made by 43 governments. The original program of the United Nations' International Children's Emergency Fund was limited to supplementary feeding of children in war areas. The organization extended its program, stressing child health and maternal and infant care. Through an agreement, WHO provides medical and technical personnel and supervises the implementation of programs in the field. The more important health programs have been directed to the control of tuberculosis, syphilis, trachoma, and malaria and to the improvement of maternal and child health.

Organized originally as a temporary emergency agency, it has filled such a need and obtained such financial support that, in 1953, it was made a permanent organization. Its name was changed to the United Nations' Children Fund.[6] In 1972, allocations of $46,200,000 were made by the Executive Board of UNICEF for its programs in the less developed countries.[6]

## Bilateral International Health Activities

One of the early developments of this nature was the Institute of Interamerican Affairs, established in 1942 by the United States to give assistance to several Latin American countries. The betterment of health was one of the major aims of this program. Technical assistance and financial aid to assist in the development of more adequate public health facilities and services were the main accomplishments.

Similar programs have been undertaken by the U. S. government on a wider scale since World War II. Aid has been given in special programs such as malaria eradication, yaws control, medical education, and so forth. The organizations administering this program have changed titles from time to time, but the objectives have been pursued continuously. Since 1967, the Agency for International Development, a dependency of the Department of State, has had responsibility for the program. Its predecessors, the International Cooperation Administration and the Economic Cooperation Administration, carried on similar programs.

The primary object of United States economic assistance is to help developing nations achieve improvement of agriculture, industries, educational and health services. While United States economic assistance programs have leveled off for the past few years, other western nations have increased their contributions. In 1963, the United States contributed about 63 per cent of the economic aid going to less developed countries; in 1973, the United States percentage had dropped to 38 per cent of the total bilateral and multilateral programs. The total United States AID program for fiscal year 1974 is proposed as $3.5 billion.[7]

At the request of President John F. Kennedy, Congress established the Peace Corps. Under this program, carefully selected young Americans, after a period of training, are sent to countries requesting such aid to assist people at a grass roots level to solve their problems. These individuals, on a people-to-people-basis, have met remarkable success in aiding people to improve their housing, their water supplies, and their agricultural practices. In some instances, health programs such as immunizations have been fostered. As of 1973, there were about 8000 volunteers in 58 countries. Of these countries, only 27 receive other kinds of bilateral aid from the United States. $77 million is proposed to Congress for FY 1974 for the support of the Peace Corps program.[7]

The Colombo Plan for Cooperative Economic Development in South and South-East Asia was formulated by British Commonwealth Ministers at Colombo, Ceylon, in 1950. It was designed as a cooperative effort in which Asian countries themselves, helped by countries outside the region, would develop their economies and raise the living standards of their people. There are now 24 member countries including the United States. The agreement set the duration of the Colombo Plan at six years. It has subsequently been extended three times and is currently set to expire in 1976. The total flow of external assistance in recent years is at a rate of approximately $2,400,000. The United States provides by far the largest contribution. The main thrust of the Plan has been improvement of agriculture, industrial development, production of power and minerals, extension of transport and communications, and the improvement of social services including education and health.[8]

## Voluntary Agencies

A large number of voluntary agencies have contributed to the improvement of health on an international basis. Perhaps the most significant programs have been conducted by such philanthropic agencies as The Rockefeller Foundation, the Ford Foundation, the Kellogg Foundation, the Wellcome Trust, and the Nuffield Foundation. Such programs include disease control, e.g., malaria, yellow fever, and hookworm, improvement of agriculture and nutrition, development of schools and institutes of public health, and the training of health personnel as teachers and leaders, as well as the financing of research programs. Recently the Robert Wood Johnson Foundation with a huge endowment has initiated support to activities aimed at improvement of health care services.

## FEDERAL HEALTH AGENCIES

### Introduction

The health system of the United States is as large and as complex as the country itself. Involved in this system are hospitals, nursing homes, university-related medical centers and biomedical research laboratories, producers of medicines and medical supplies, allied medical personnel, voluntary health agencies, and government health agencies at the Federal Government, particularly in recent years, has been increasingly active in supporting and augmenting the efforts of these partners within the health system.

The health-related activity of the Federal Government is widely distributed throughout the various departments, bureaus, and agencies. For example, the enforcement of narcotics and drug abuse laws is the responsibility of the Department of Justice; control of biologicals for animal use and problems of nutrition are assigned to the Department of Agriculture; provisions for industrial health standards and care are set and maintained in the Department of the Interior, the Bureau of Mines maintains an effective Health and Safety Division; the Atomic Energy Commission has a research and training program in biology and medicine; very large expenditures for health-related research and service are made annually by the Veterans Administration and the Department of Defense. Actually, every major department of the Federal Government has responsibility for and jurisdiction over some type of health activity, despite the fact that the word "health" is not found in the U. S. Constitution.

The major health activities for the nation, however, are centered in the Department of Health, Education, and Welfare (HEW). This department, formed in 1953 from the Federal Security Agency, incorporates the Public Health Service, Office of Education, Social Security Administration, Office of Human Development, and the Social and Rehabilitation Service (see Fig. 2.3). With the advent of Titles 18 and 19 to the Social Security Act and subsequent legislation preparing for national health insurance, other agencies of HEW (the Social Security Administration and the Social Rehabilitation Service) are assuming prominent administrative positions in health care, particularly for the elderly, the indigent, and the medically indigent. The direct involvement in extensive and comprehensive health-related research and service for the United States, however, is administered through the Office of the Assistant Secretary for Health of HEW and remains largely a function of the Public Health Service.

*Historical Background*

The U. S. Public Health Service had its inception in the Marine Hospital Service, established as a division of the Treasury Department in 1798 during the administration of President John Adams. The Secretary of the Treasury at that time, Alexander Hamilton, sponsored the Congressional Act, which provided hospitals for the relief of sick and disabled seamen. This service was financed initially by monthly deductions of $0.20 from the wages of each seaman and represented the first prepaid medical insurance program in the country. Castle Island, in Boston Harbor, was the site of the first hospital. Additional hospitals were established at principal ports and waterways during the next few years, continually extending westward until the establishment of a Marine Service Hospital in San Francisco in 1853. The Service was reorganized in 1870, with the formation of a commissioned officer corps having rank designations similar to those of the U. S. Navy.

With continued expansion of the nation and increasing health problems accompanying this expansion, it became obvious that a national public health organization was necessary. In 1912, the Marine Hospital Service was incorporated into the more comprehensive U. S. Public Health Service. This new organization was given the responsibility to co-ordinate and administer the major governmental health programs, including national hospitals. The Public Health Service was authorized to enforce quarantine laws, to co-operate with states and communities in the control of communicable disease epidemics, and to study and regulate the growing health problems of urbanization such as hygiene, sanitation, and water pollution. A laboratory was established in the Staten Island Hospital and from this humble beginning can be traced the National Institutes of Health.

Federal legislation continued to assign additional health duties to the Public Health Service. Noteworthy among these were the Social Security Act of 1935, which systemized assistance to the states for health manpower development, disease control programs, and limited health care; and the National Cancer Act of 1936, which established the National Cancer Institute. After World War II, Congress assigned increasing responsibility to the Public Health Service and continued to pass more health legislation, particularly after the Public Health Service was incorporated into HEW. The trend of Congress to promote social and health programs on an expanded scale has prompted even more health legislation. Within recent years, major new laws have been enacted that increase HEW's authority, responsibility, and appropriations in the fields of health care, protection, knowledge, and manpower. Each year additional bills are introduced which further expand such activity. The health programs coordinated or directed through the Office of the Assistant Secretary for Health involve more than 44,000 employees and $4.8 billion in annual expenditures. The Public Health Service, as the major direct health arm of HEW, is the agency which performs most of these functions.

The Public Health Service Commissioned Corps no longer represents a management structure but has become one of the two personnel systems on which HEW depends for the recruitment of health professionals, the civil service system being the other. At present, the great majority of the top officials and all other personnel of HEW's health programs are not in the Corps.

## ORGANIZATION OF THE PUBLIC HEALTH SERVICE

The past few years have seen a series of major

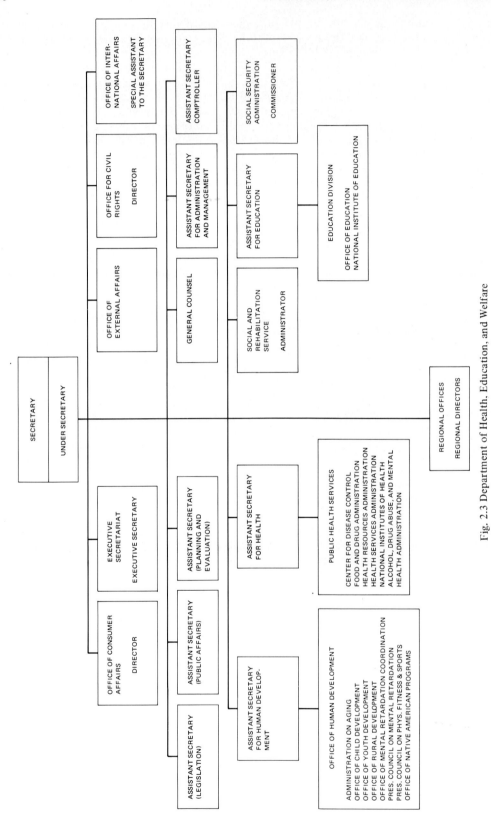

Fig. 2.3 Department of Health, Education, and Welfare

reorganizations of the Public Health Service. These changes, although designed to accommodate new and expanding programs and to provide for a more efficient and economical system of administration, have been somewhat confusing. Both observers and participants find difficulty in keeping track of reassignments, realignments, administration of new programs, and the death, burial, resurrection, modification, and relocation of old programs. Additional changes can be anticipated as the Federal government becomes even more involved in the various aspects of health planning, research, and delivery systems.

The present organization of the Public Health Service consists of the Office of the Assistant Secretary and his administrative assistants; a group of offices concerned with particular health related problems such as population, drug abuse prevention, nursing homes, international health, and professional standards review; intermediate coordinating offices; and six separate health divisions or agencies (see Fig. 2.4).

The six divisions are grouped according to special tasks and responsibilities. Because of the unique character and specific functions of the Center for Disease Control and the Food and Drug Administration, each of these agencies was raised to a separate division. The direct health service of the Federal government is assigned to the Health Services Administration and the support services such as statistics and evaluation are a function of the Health Resources Administration. The National Institutes of Health serve as the main health research arm of the Federal government and still remain as a separate agency. The newest division of the Public Health Service, at the time of this writing, is the Alcohol, Drug Abuse, and Mental Health Administration.

## Center for Disease Control

Wartime efforts to control malaria served as an originating base for the Center for Disease Control. Although the name has changed several times from the original Communicable Disease Control, the agency has always retained its initials (CDC) for identity purposes. CDC now has the responsibility for administering the Lead Paint and Rat Control programs, Occupational Safety and Health, and the Clearinghouse for Smoking and Health as well as those programs historically identified with CDC such as disease surveillance, smallpox eradication,

tropical disease, venereal disease, and epidemiology. The annual budget for CDC is approximately $138 million, and 3600 workers are employed.

## Food and Drug Administration

Regulatory agencies, generally, have not been associated with the health component of HEW. Most of these types of activity have been assumed by other Federal agencies or by the individual states. The Food and Drug Administration (FDA) is a notable exception. The FDA assumes a commanding position as a regulatory agency in the production and dissemination of drugs and medical devices, as well as the labeling which accompanies such products. One of their recent activities has been the review of non-prescription drugs to determine efficacy. Much of this type of review is conducted by advisory committees composed of experts plus non-voting industry and consumer representatives. Although the FDA prefers to encourage self-regulation and cooperative endeavors with industry, it has the power to issue sharp reprisals against those who transcend government regulations.

Reflecting its increasing responsibility and activity, the FDA added still another bureau in February, 1974, the Bureau of Medical Devices and Diagnostic Products. This Bureau is separated into four divisions: Diagnostic Product Standards and Research, Medical Device Standards and Research, Compliance, and Classification and Scientific Evaluation.[9]

Other responsibilities of FDA are the regulatory control of radiological products and the administration of the National Center for Toxicological Research. There are 6300 employees in FDA and the annual budget for health related activities is $135 million. Another $65 million is designated for its regulatory activity in the food industry.

## Health Resources Administration

This newly formed agency was created to help planning, staffing, and research in Federal health resources. These important functions have been brought together into three bureaus under one administrative umbrella in the first stage of a two-stage reorganization. The Health Resources Administration employs 2000 people and had a 1975 operating budget of $574 million. Significantly, this figure is $552 million

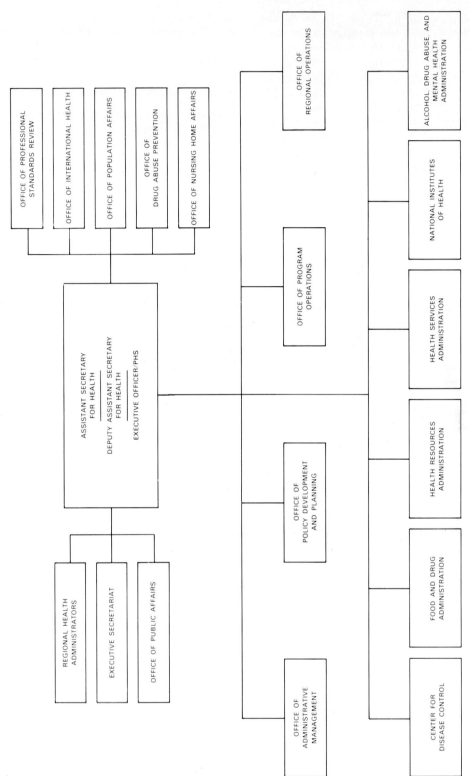

Fig. 2.4 Public Health Service

less than the $1126 million approved for 1974 and reflects the projected loss of funds for health planning, regional medical programs, and health facilities construction, as well as significant reductions in funds allocated for health manpower instruction and assistance.

### National Center for Health Statistics

This Center is the agency responsible for the collection, analysis, and dissemination of data on vital events and health, including the physical, mental, and physiological characteristics of the population. Their periodic publications on the various health indexes have proven to be invaluable for the voluntary and governmental health agencies in helping to prepare specific health programs. All national baseline health data systems maintained by the Federal government are brought together in this agency. In addition, the National Center for Health Statistics has the responsibility for research and development of the newer data systems and statistical methods in this field.

### Bureau of Health Services Research and Evaluation

The primary functions of this Bureau are to conduct research and analyses on the organizing, delivery, and financing of health services. Also, it supports the development and testing of new approaches to improvement of the distribution, utilization, and cost effectiveness of health resources and services. The Bureau has overall responsibility for the development of health services research and strategy for the Department of HEW and coordinates all such research activities throughout the various Federal health agencies.

### Bureau of Health Resources Development

This Bureau focuses on production, utilization, distribution, and rationalization of human physical resources in the health services field. Of particular interest to those in the allied medical professions, the Bureau of Health Resources Development has the responsibility for essentially all of the health manpower education programs. Examples of these programs are student assistance for loans and scholarships, continuing education, programs to increase the number of minority health professionals, physician assistant training, programs to

place former military medical corpsmen into health occupations, and financial assistance for health education institutions. Another effort of this Bureau is to help solve the problem of geographic maldistribution of physicians and a reordering of physician specialties. The Bureau of Health Resources and Development is organized into Divisions of Allied Health Manpower, Dental Health, Manpower Intelligence, Nursing, and Physician and Health Professions Education.

## Health Services Administration

Historically, the Federal government has provided direct health care for special groups, including the American Indians, Alaskan natives, merchant seamen, and certain Federal employees. Also, the government has assumed responsibility for providing direct health care for the Coast Guard, the Peace Corps, the Bureau of Prisons, VISTA, and the Health Service Corps. In addition to direct services Congress has passed legislation which provides indirect health services to the states and their political subdivisions. Examples of these indirect services include major financial assistance for establishing and staffing community health centers, maternity and child health projects, health maintenance organizations, and programs for family planning and migrant health.

The agency responsible for co-ordinating and administering all of these direct and indirect health-related functions is the Health Services Administration (HSA). In terms of numbers of people employed (15,380), HSA is the largest of the six agencies. Its budget of $1.18 billion is the second largest, exceeded only by the budget of the National Institutes of Health. HSA is divided into four large operating divisions: the Indian Health Service, Bureau of Community Health Services, Federal Health Programs Service, and the Bureau of Quality Assurance.

## National Institutes of Health

Research is essential to all progress in the health sciences and continues to be a major concern of the Federal government. The principal biomedical research arm of the Public Health Service, the National Institutes of Health (NIH) supports more than one-third of all medical research in the United States. A significant portion is conducted in the laboratories of the Institutes, but the major portion is done in universities and research centers. Each year NIH awards literally thousands of research grants and fellowships.

NIH is composed of ten institutes, two divisions, a clinical center, an international center, and the National Library of Medicine. The ten National Institutes are concerned principally with research into the health conditions that still present major problems and are separated into Cancer; Heart and Lung; Allergy and Infectious Diseases; Arthritis, Metabolism and Digestive Diseases; Child Health and Human Development; Dental Research; Eye; Neurological Diseases and Stroke; Environmental Health Sciences; and General Medical Science. There are 10,500 people employed in NIH, including the highest percentage of research scientists and health professionals. The budget of $1.83 billion is the highest of all the Public Health Service divisions. However, approximately one-third of this total amount, $600 million, is assigned to the National Cancer Institute and another $309 million to the National Heart and Lung Institute, accounting for about half of the total NIH budget.

*National Library of Medicine*

The central resource of medical literature for the United States is the National Library of Medicine. This Library is reputed to contain the largest and finest collection of medical literature in the world with well over one million books, journals, theses, pamphlets, and prints. The services extend through thousands of other libraries which receive millions of pages of material every year, largely in the form of photocopy and microfilm. The work of the National Library of Medicine is aided by MEDLARS, a computerized system which can conduct approximately 100 searches of medical literature simultaneously and answer specific requests on almost any medical subject. The use of computers has been pioneered in this Library, offering one of the answers to the storage and recall of rapidly mounting quantities of information. One of the recent innovations has been the development of MEDLINE (MEDLARS on-line) to provide health professionals with rapid access to current medical literature. Covering the basic and clinical sciences, the MEDLINE data base consists of approximately 400,000 citations to articles from 1200 journals published throughout the world. Although many of these services are provided on a cost-sharing basis, the Federal government assumes the major financial responsibility. This is reflected in the $28 million budget of the National Library of Medicine.

## Alcohol, Drug Abuse, and Mental Health Administration

Currently, the newest of the agencies to be formed, the Alcohol, Drug Abuse, and Mental Health Administration is a reflection of the administrative concern over drug abuse, the recognition that alcohol is our most heavily abused drug, and the extent of mental illness in the United States. As discussed in Chapter 8 of this textbook, mental illness ranks among the highest of the national health problems, taking a devastating toll in human suffering and filling one-third of the hospital beds. The abuse of alcohol and other drugs has reached such staggering proportions that programs to work effectively with these growing tragedies must be expanded accordingly. Therefore, separate agency status, enhanced budgets, and enlarged staffs have been assigned to supply needed support and coordination. Common to each of the three divisions in this agency are programs of research to determine cause, prevention, and cure, and programs for training both present staff and new personnel. The Drug Abuse and Alcoholism divisions feature project grants and contracts for community health agencies and institutions as well as grants to States to help finance local programs. The Mental Health division supports much of the staffing expense for the growing numbers of Community Mental Health Centers throughout the United States.

The Alcohol, Drug Abuse, and Mental Health Administration employs 5600 people and the combined budget is $735 million. Approximately one-half of this amount is assigned to the Mental Health division, $217 million to Drug Abuse, and $100 million to Alcoholism. Significantly, the budget for this combined agency has been reduced $150 million in the past three years, evidently with the expectation that the individual states and their political subdivisions will assume more of the financial responsibility in administering these programs on the local level.

The gradual evolution of the organization of the Public Health Service raises some interesting speculations. It is the opinion of numerous observers that the present structure is merely a holding pattern for even more profound changes. As more effective methods are devised to attract physicians and dentists into government service it is projected that the Public Health Service Uniformed Corps eventually will be absorbed into the civil service system. Even the title, "Public Health Service," has been challenged as to its appropriateness in designating the health related functions of the Federal Government. Also, there is considerable agitation for the creation of a separate Department of Health headed by a cabinet level Secretary.

It can be readily seen, then, that the Federal Government is a full partner in virtually all fields of health. The range of programs extends from the realm of disease prevention and research through the various methods of disease control and the delivery of health services, and even provides help in furnishing medical manpower to deliver these services. These are additional evidences that the United States is moving toward a program of total, high quality care for all people, regardless of their ability to pay, and reflects the growing philosophy that health is not a privilege but a right.

## STATE HEALTH ACTIVITIES

State constitutions usually define in broad terms the responsibility of state governments for the protection of the general health and welfare of its citizens. State legislatures have defined, by their various acts, the organizations in each state responsible for health activities. Such laws differ greatly in the 50 states. A few states have detailed public health laws, codified and classified to form a clear legal basis for health activities. In others, only broad principles are laid down and occasional laws are enacted to meet specific situations. In all 50 states, there is a provision for some kind of supervisory board of health. The functions of this board are usually advisory and quasi-legislative. In general, the majority of membership of boards of health is from the medical profession. The size of boards range from five to 19 members. The average is nine. Sixteen states have combined departments of health with at least one other agency, and, in four instances, have established large agencies combining

health, social services, and other functions such as vocational rehabilitation and mental health.

Powers and duties of state health boards vary considerably from state to state. In 37 states, the boards have responsibility for formulating codes and rules relating to health. In 15 states, the director of health is appointed by the board, and in three states, the board must approve the appointment, usually made by the governor. Eleven boards have supervisory powers over local boards of health. Sixteen state boards have the power to conduct health studies and investigations. Generally, courts have upheld the actions of health officers or boards of health, provided these actions seemed reasonable, and were clearly in the public interest.

Members of state boards of health are appointed by action of the governor, by the state legislature, and sometimes by professional societies of the state. In 45 states, the governor makes the appointments, but his selections must be confirmed in 25 states by the legislature. The terms of office of board members range from two to nine years, and the appointments are usually staggered to ensure continuity. Health professionals usually predominate on the boards, although 26 states have consumers on their boards of health.[10]

In past years, politics played too great a role in the affairs of health departments, but those years are passing. Public health has become a specialized form of medical practice, requiring years of special experience to equip personnel for their complex duties. In 1949, the Council on Medical Education and Hospitals of the American Medical Association authorized the formation of a specialty board, the American Board of Preventive Medicine and Public Health, to examine and certify qualified physicians. The American Public Health Association has also studied continuously, since 1928, education and training of all classes of public health personnel. The standards thus set are generally accepted by states as guides for selection of health personnel.

In the evolution of state government, recognition of responsibility for the public health was slow. The first permanent state health organization was not established until 1869, in Massachusetts. By 1900, some 38 states had developed some form of state health organization; by 1913, every state and territory in the Union had one. Control of epidemics and communicable disease was the first objective of these state organizations. This required the development of sanitary science and of laws and regulations to control water supplies, stream pollution, and sewage disposal. The establishment of laboratory service to assist in the diagnosis and control of communicable disease was also necessary.

Most state health departments are organized on a basis of divisions of bureaus to provide certain standard services. (See Fig. 2.4 for plan of organization of the Maryland State Department of Health and Mental Hygiene.) The usual divisions are:

1. Communicable disease control.
2. Vital statistics.
3. Environmental sanitation.
4. Maternal and child health.
5. Public health laboratory service.
6. Public health nursing.
7. Health education.
8. Local health services.
9. Mental hygiene.
10. Industrial hygiene.
11. Administration.

The American Public Health Association has defined the minimum functions of a state health department as:[11]

1. The study of state health problems and planning for their solution.
2. Coordination and technical supervision of local health activities.
3. Financial aid to local health departments.
4. The enactment of sanitary regulations applicable in local health programs.
5. The establishment of minimal standards for local health work.
6. The maintenance of central and branch laboratory services, including diagnostic, sanitary, chemical, biological, and research activities.
7. The collection, tabulation, and analysis of vital statistics.
8. The collection and distribution of information concerning preventable disease.
9. The maintenance of safe quality of water and the control of waste disposal.
10. Establishment and maintenance of minimal standards of milk sanitation.
11. Provision of services to aid industry in the control of occupational hazards.
12. The establishment of qualifications for health personnel.
13. Formulation of plans in cooperation

with other organizations for meeting all health needs.

As new health problems make themselves felt, the state health departments alter their organizational patterns to meet them. Such a problem is drug abuse practices among the younger population.

More recently, state health departments have become responsible in many states, in conjunction with Federal Agencies, for programs of hospital planning and licensure and for some phases of medical care to indigent and medically indigent individuals.

The state health officer is the administrative head of the organization. He is sometimes termed the Commissioner or Director of Health. His line of authority is generally from the governor, with the state board of health serving mainly as an advisory body.

A confusing factor in trying to understand a state health organization is that more than one agency has responsibility for activities in this field. According to studies made by the public health service, a total of 60 different types of state agencies contribute, in some way, to state health programs. With this fractionation of responsibility, it is easy to understand the difficulties encountered in developing uniform standards of performance and achieving common goals. Since the enactment of the Comprehensive Health Planning Act of 1966, states have created agencies for reviewing or producing plans for health programs on a statewide basis. A substantial proportion of federal funds is transmitted to the states for distribution by these Health Planning Agencies. At the present time, the role of state health departments vis-a-vis other state agencies with an interest in the health field is in a position of uncertainty.

In most states, direct personal services are not usually performed by the state health department. Its staff is limited largely to specialized personnel who visit local health departments as consultants. Some states do maintain mobile equipment and staff to serve local areas which request such aid. Mobile chest X-ray units or dental clinics are examples. Really, it might be said that the chief aims of a state health department are the promotion of local health agencies throughout the state and the assistance of such departments to carry out their functions in a satisfactory manner. Indeed the objectives of public health today should be to take responsibility for the development and

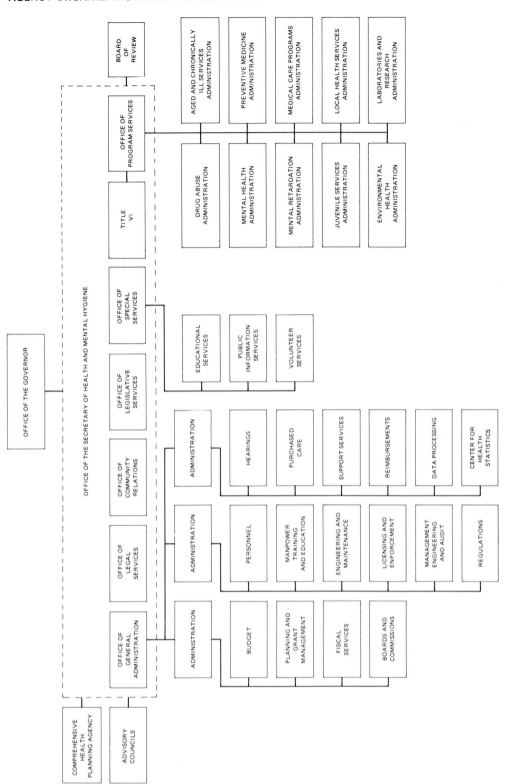

Fig. 2.5. Organization of Maryland State Department of Health, effective July 1, 1967

maintenance of political and social machinery, that will make possible the prevention of disease, the treatment of illness, the reduction of disability, the promotion of physical and mental health, and the protection and improvement of the quality of the environment.

## LOCAL HEALTH DEPARTMENTS

In every state, it is provided by law that some responsibility for health matters must rest with local agencies, with such authority resting in township, city, or county governments. As the need for public health services has grown, many states have encouraged local governmental units to combine for more economical and effective administration of health activities. As of 1971, there are about 1600 fulltime local health departments of one type or another serving about 2500 counties including more than 300 cities. They protect the health of a combined population of almost 180 million people.[12] Many of these local health programs are limited as to quality and number of services rendered.

In areas not covered by local health departments, services are frequently provided by personnel from the state health organization. In sparsely populated areas, the state sometimes sets up health districts which either may be served by local district staff or by staff from the state health department.

The patterns of local health organization vary from one region of the United States to another, depending largely upon the governmental systems. In the northeastern area, the city, town, or municipality is the type of local health jurisdiction most favored. In the South, single county health departments and multicounty health units are more frequently encountered. (See Fig. 2.5 for organizational plan of the Maricopa County Health Department, Arizona.)

In general, local health departments operate under the authority of the local governing body: mayor and council in cities and board of supervisors in the counties. Usually, a board of health is appointed by the governing authorities. This board, most frequently having five or seven members, represents community interest in health activities. It serves to adopt policies, rules and regulations, and sanitary codes and to conduct necessary hearings. The board should have the authority to appoint or recommend the appointment of the director of health.

The local director of health should be a full-time officer with adequate training and experience in public health practice. The size of his staff will vary with the population to be served and the resources available for health services. Probably, minimal requirements of staff for effective service are: one medical officer of health per 50,000 of the population, one trained public health nurse for each 5,000 population, supervisory nursing personnel, one for each six to eight staff nurses, one sanitarian to every 10,000 to 15,000, sufficient part-time physicians to assist in the operation of the various health department clinics, and office personnel, one per 15,000 population.[12]

Programs of local health departments have expanded rather rapidly during the past 25 years. The following activities are considered to be basic:

1. Collection of vital statistics.
2. Control of the sanitary conditions.
3. Control of communicable diseases.
4. Provision of laboratory services.
5. Protection of the health of mothers and infants.
6. Education of the public on health matters.

The local health department should participate in state or regional planning in a number of ways, such as:

1. Providing local health data.
2. Supplying details of health program activities and achievements.
3. Giving staff support which includes professional judgments and interpretations of problem areas.
4. Engaging in studies and surveys which will assist the planning agency to better understand and define issues.
5. Providing the state and regional planning agencies with health information that will assist them in keeping their plans current.

Many health departments are active in diagnosis of chronic diseases and rehabilitation of sufferers from long-term illnesses. The importance of mental illness has become ever more apparent and more attention is given to diagnostic and treatment facilities.

"Its fundamental responsibility," according to the 1963 Policy Statement of the American Public Health Association, "is to determine the health status and health needs of the people within its jurisdiction, to determine to what extent these needs are being met by effective measures currently available, and to take steps

RICOPA COUNTY DEPARTMENT OF HEALTH SERVICES

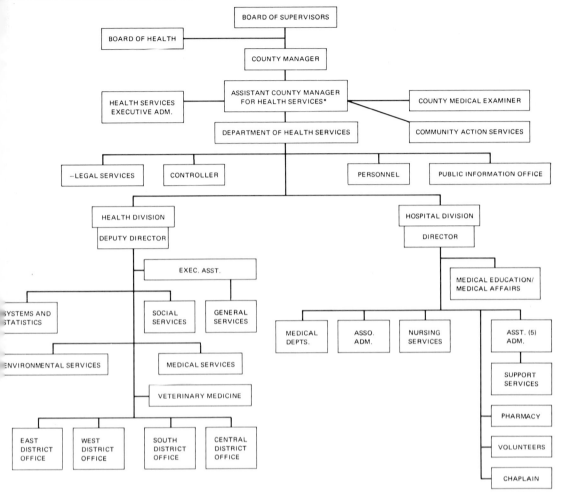

* DIRECTOR, HEALTH SERVICES
  DIRECTOR, HEALTH DEPARTMENT

Fig. 2.6. Organization plan of a county health department. Maricopa County, Arizona

to see that the unmet needs are satisfied."[13]

Since July 1, 1966, when Medicare came into effect, many local health departments have become involved in administration of home care programs for patients recently discharged from hospitals.

The finances necessary for the local health department come from the state, from the local government, and sometimes from grants from Federal agencies. Frequently, voluntary health agencies join with the official health department to finance specific health projects. There is no minimum cost figure that can be cited for satisfactory local health services. An expenditure of $3.50 to even $5.00 *per capita* prevails in some service areas. The cost will depend upon the quality and quantity of the services provided.

## PHILANTHROPIC FOUNDATIONS

One of the most remarkable phenomena of recent times has been the growth of philanthropic foundations. This has been made possible, of course, by the tremendous increase of wealth, resulting from the industrial and technological revolutions of the 19th and 20th centuries. More recently, the disposition of governments to increase income and inheritance taxes has also influenced many individuals to create tax exempt trusts.

According to the Foundation Directory, by the beginning of the twentieth century, some 18 philanthropic foundations had been created in the United States. Between 1901 and 1909, 16 new ones appeared; between 1910 and 1919, some 75 foundations were added; between 1920 and 1929, there were 157; between 1930 and 1939, came 259; between 1940 and 1949, the number skyrocketed to 1134; and between 1950 and 1959, the huge number of 2546 was established. By 1969, the number of American foundations was approximately 5454 and there was no let-up in the movement. (This figure does not include foundations with assets of less than $500,000 or those making grants of less than $25,000 per year).[14]

Of course, many of these trusts were relatively small and had limited objectives. A few possessed huge financial resources with broad programs of service. For example, The Rockefeller Foundation has granted many hundreds of millions of dollars "to promote the well-being of mankind throughout the world."

Education, welfare, international activities, research, and health have been the areas of most interest to those directing the expenditure of foundation funds. While the total amount of funds expended by all foundations is small in proportion to the money provided by governments for the same purposes, it has had a profound influence. "To prime the pump" is the expression frequently applied to initial foundation grants. The skillful foundation officer finds situations of potential importance that are ready to move if given a little impetus.

In the field of health, the philanthropies of the Rockefeller family have taken a high place. Mr. John D. Rockefeller founded The Rockefeller Institute (now Rockefeller University) for Medical Research in New York City in 1901. This Institute served to train more teachers of medicine and medical research workers during its early decades than any other center in the United States. In 1909, Mr. Rockefeller set up the Rockefeller Sanitary Commission to control hookworm disease in the southern states. This campaign, while successful in itself, demonstrated the need for stable state and local health departments. The General Education Board (1903) and The Rockefeller Foundation (1913) undertook the work of strengthening health departments, of building up medical schools, and later of creating schools of public health in the United States and abroad to prepare the thousands of trained health workers to carry on the newly created health services.

In control of specific diseases, aside from the hookwork campaign, The Rockefeller Foundation undertook widespread programs to study and control malaria, yellow fever, and other epidemic diseases on an international basis.[15]

Other foundations such as the Carnegie Boards, the Commonwealth Fund, the Milbank Fund, the W. K. Kellogg Foundation, the Nuffield Trusts, the Wellcome Trusts, and, recently, the Ford Foundation have also made great contributions in advancing medical science, medical, dental, and nursing education, and, the whole area of public health. The Robert Wood Johnson Foundation, in 1971 with assets valued at more than $1.4 billion, has recently announced its chief program interest is to be in a broad spectrum of health care programs, experiments, and studies.[16]

As a result of the general betterment of health and the preservation of life in wide areas of the world, the growth of the human population has been fantastic. A number of the foundations have, in the past two decades, devoted more of their resources to programs devoted to research on birth control methods and projects designed to foster family planning. A great deal of foundation money is also being devoted to improvement of agricultural practices and the development of better food crops for those regions of the world where the populations are poorly nourished.

## RED CROSS

### Introduction

The American National Red Cross is in a category all its own; it is neither a governmental agency nor can it be classified as a strictly private, voluntary organization. It is, therefore, more commonly referred to as a quasi-governmental agency. The honorary chairman of the American National Red Cross is the President of the United States and the honorary counselor and treasurer, respectively, are the Attorney General and the Secretary of the Treasury. The Red Cross is, however, essentially a volunteer organization. Annually, approximately 1.6 million Americans give their services voluntarily in 3177 local community chapters.

The beginning of the Red Cross movement was due largely to the interests and activities of a young man from Switzerland, Henri Dunant. In 1859, Mr. Dunant, more by chance than by previous intent, was present at the Battle of Solferino in Italy, where he attempted to care for wounded and dying men. He was so appalled at the conditions and the apparent disregard for suffering humanity that he crusaded for governments of various nations to authorize a neutral voluntary agency which would give help to wounded military men. Years of toil, with gathering support and approval, proved to be worthwhile. In 1863, a committee of Swiss businessmen met with Mr. Dunant in Geneva, Switzerland, to lay groundwork for an international organization to aid the suffering. The following year, delegates from 16 nations attended the Geneva Convention and signed the pact which provided for the establishment of the International Red Cross. The organization was to be governed by 25 Swiss citizens and the emblem adopted was the Swiss flag, with the colors reversed; in Moslem countries, the red crescent replaces the red cross. It was agreed that wounded soldiers should be treated humanely and that medical personnel should be non-combatants authorized to wear the Red Cross emblem. Additional provisions of the Geneva Convention extended the same type of neutral protection to voluntary aid societies recognized by their governments as relief agencies. Sea warfare later came under the same protection and standards were established for the treatment of war prisoners. Years later, international recognition was given to the Red Cross as a disaster relief agency during peacetime as well.

The headquarters of the International Red Cross are in Geneva, Switzerland, and continue to be governed by Swiss citizens. Much of the co-ordination of world-wide activities and administration of humane services in areas of conflict are conducted from these offices. In addition, there is a League of Red Cross Societies with offices in Paris. This League is composed of the Red Cross organizations of the various countries which have ratified the conventions. The promotion of mutually desirable programs, encouragement of international goodwill and understanding, exchange of personnel and ideas between national organizations, close co-operation with the Geneva office, and strengthening common bonds are only a few of the activities of this League.

The International Red Cross is representative of peoples' concern for people and governments' concern for their citizens. Countries that may differ rather significantly in many respects will readily participate in this humanitarian endeavor where they can meet on a common ground. Meetings of the International Congress of the Red Cross bring together Red Cross societies and governments from around the world to discuss and plan protection for victims of war, aid to refugees and disaster victims, and development of new Red Cross societies. Repeatedly demonstrated is the fact that in times of international confrontation and unrest when faith between nations is suspect, the one organization that retains the faith and confidence of both opposing factions is the Red Cross. Today, the Red Cross and its affiliated societies have spread to virtually all countries, representing about 99 per cent of the world's population. Each year, on May 8, commemorating the birthday of Henri Dunant, more than 200 million Red Cross workers around the world observe Red Cross Day.

The United States ratified the Geneva Convention of the International Red Cross in 1882, largely through the prolonged and determined efforts of Clara Barton, who then became the first president of the American society. Congress granted a charter to the American National Red Cross in 1900 and greatly enlarged and extended this charter in 1905. The Red Cross was specifically charged with service to military families and the obligation to carry on a system of national and international relief.[17]

The mission of the American Red Cross is officially stated as follows:

The American Red Cross is the instrument chosen by the Congress to help carry out the obligations assumed by the United States under certain international treaties known as the Geneva or Red Cross Conventions. Specifically, its Congressional charter imposes on the American Red Cross the duties to act as the medium of voluntary relief and communication between the American people and their armed forces, and to carry on a system of national and international relief to prevent and mitigate suffering caused by disasters. All the activities of the American Red Cross and its chapters support these duties. Nationally and locally the American Red Cross is governed by volunteers, most of its duties are performed by volunteers and it is financed by voluntary contributions.

The following statement, quoted from an opinion of the Honorable John W. Davis when he was Solicitor General of the United States, describes in broad terms the duty and obligation of the American Red Cross to carry out the requirements of its Congressional charter:

When any question arises as to the scope and activities of the American Red Cross, it must always be remembered that its Charter is not only a grant of power but an imposition of duties. The American Red Cross is a quasi-governmental organization, operating under Congressional Charter officered in part, at least, by government appointment, disbursing its funds under the security of a governmental audit, and designated by Presidential Order for the fulfillment of certain treaty obligations into which the Government has entered. It owes, therefore, to the Government which it serves the distinct duty of discharging all those functions for which it was created. Not only is it constrained by these considerations growing out of its organic character, but there is also a moral obligation resting upon it to its membership and to the American people who have so freely and generously contributed to its support.

Some of the services of the Red Cross deserve special mention.

### Services to the Armed Forces and Veterans

The experience of the American Red Cross in carrying out its congressional charter mission to assist U. S. servicemen, veterans, and their families on a world-wide basis enables its volunteer and career staff to respond promptly and effectively to the needs created by the United States' commitments throughout the world. Recreation centers and clubmobile units are established in the field and servicemen with urgent personal and family problems are assisted at military installations in the United States and foreign countries. Red Cross chapter workers aid military families when they are faced with problems resulting from family separations, involuntary extensions of enlistments, interruptions in pay or allotments, and emergencies in the home. Veterans are also helped in hospitals, in filing government claims, and in providing other personal and family services.

### Disaster Services

Hurricanes, floods, tornadoes, and other disasters marshal the forces of the local chapters in and near the involved area. Within a very short period of time, organized reinforcements begin arriving from regional, area, and national offices. Through the co-operation of other groups, the Red Cross helps to provide food, shelter, medical and nursing services, transportation, communication, and clothing to disaster victims. Rehabilitation services are rendered during the postdisaster period. No charges are made for these services or supplies.

### Blood Program

In 59 regional blood programs operating through 1700 chapters, the Red Cross collects approximately 4 million units of blood each year. This represents over 60 per cent of the voluntary blood donations in the nation, excluding those made to hospital blood banks. Most of the blood collected is furnished to approximately 4300 hospitals and blood banks. The remainder is used in the manufacture of products for blood component therapy and for research. A significant portion of the fractionated blood is used by the military.

There is no charge for use of blood collected in the Red Cross program. There is, however, an assessment as a partial reimbursement for the cost involved in collecting, processing, storing, and distributing the blood; most hospitals and blood banks pass this assessment on to the patient. Even with this partial reimbursement received from participating hospitals, the blood program is an expensive endeavor. In a recent year, the net cost of the program exceeded $11 million.[18]

### Safety Programs

One of the aims of the Red Cross is to conserve human life through programs of first aid and water safety. Well over 1.9 million first aid certificates and 2.6 million small craft and water safety certificates are issued annually to people who successfully pass courses of instruction. These courses are taught, for the most part, by volunteer lay instructors and are conducted in schools, churches, private and community swimming pools, industrial plants, military bases, labor halls, and local chapter buildings and facilities. The Red Cross also provides the American people with informal instruction by means of film showings and public demonstrations of safety techniques. In addition, approximately 14,000 highway stations, mobile units, and detachments provide first aid on the highways and at community events.

### Nursing Program

The Red Cross continues to develop and conduct nursing programs to provide health information to the American people and to expand nursing and health resources in the United States and various other countries. The nursing program began in Ohio, in 1912, in answer to an urgent need for nursing services, particularly in rural areas. The policy, set forth at the beginning, was to promote and assist in the development of local public health nursing programs. Also, the aim was to help establish full-time local health departments, to which it eventually turned over most of its work. Through these Activities, the American Red Cross has played a prominent role in the promotion of public health nursing units in state health departments.

Programs in nursing services are changing with the changing times. Attention is now directed more toward giving home nursing training to persons performing homemaker services, encouraging home health practices, and training nursing aides in nursing homes. Communities are thus provided with auxiliary nursing forces prepared to help meet every-day illness and accident situations and to give service in disasters or other major emergencies. Home nursing instruction has also been adapted to meet the special needs of such groups as the economically underprivileged, children who help take care of their younger brothers and sisters, and Spanish-speaking people living in the United States. Teaching home nursing courses has been facilitated by the development of programmed instruction books.

In addition, 62,000 professional nurses are voluntarily enrolled with the Red Cross to serve in chapter and community health programs. They are active in disaster relief operations and in the Blood Program. They also help to teach home nursing classes, and provide nursing and health services at clinics, first aid stations, and hospitals.

### Red Cross Youth

The Red Cross early recognized that the perpetuation of a strong and effective society depended upon the investments made in youth. The importance of youth, now and in the years ahead, is reflected in continuing efforts in the Red Cross to help young people gain greater understanding of the meaning of service. Junior Red Cross members fill approximately 57,500 friendship boxes annually for children in other countries; high school Red Cross members participate in community activities such as joining in beautification projects, helping retarded children learn to swim, tutoring the educationally underprivileged, visiting hospitals, and aiding disaster relief. It was recently reported that students from 38,000 elementary and secondary schools served through Red Cross chapters in one year and that 312,000 young people under 18 years of age participated in some phase of chapter service.[18] College students lead on-campus blood drives and participate in such community-oriented programs as rehabilitation of posthospital mental patients, teaching homemaking skills to residents of economically distressed areas, and teaching essential family health practices to migrant laborers.

## VOLUNTARY HEALTH AGENCIES

### Introduction

Before the turn of the century, while public health agencies were still in developmental stages, there appeared a different type of health endeavor which was destined to have a major influence on the entire health system of the United States. This was the voluntary health agency. The first such agency, the Anti-Tuberculosis Society of Philadelphia, was established in 1892. The effectiveness and success of this local agency provided the stimulus to organize, in 1904, the National Association for the Study and Prevention of Tuberculosis, later to become the American Lung Association. Over 25,000 health agencies have been established since that time. Many of the national agencies have divisions in each of the 50 states, units organized to cover the 3130 counties in the nation, and branches established as geographic subdivisions of unit areas. The total number of national, state, and local voluntary health organizations in the United States has been estimated to be well in excess of 100,000.

Voluntary health agencies are non-profit organizations having no legal powers and are not subject to governmental control. They usually are governed by a self-perpetuating board of directors comprising a wide range of community leadership. The agencies can be divided according to their special interests. One type is composed of those groups which are primarily concerned with certain organs or structures of the body, such as the American Heart Association and the National Society for the Prevention of Blindness. Other agencies are concerned with particular phases of health and welfare, such as the National Safety Council and the Planned Parenthood Federation of America. In addition, there are those groups, such as the American Diabetes Association and American Cancer Society, which are concerned with specific diseases. A representative list of national voluntary health agencies, with mailing addresses, is found in the "Appendix."

## Desirable Characteristics

In these health organizations are found large numbers of civic-minded citizens from all walks of life who give of themselves without financial recompense and who are united in a determination to conquer specific diseases, treat particular infirmities, or provide care for certain health conditions. Much of the support comes from individuals who are interested in the work of the agency because of personal or family experiences.

These agencies are an expression of the spirit of democracy and of the belief that each individual has a responsibility to himself, his neighbor, his community, and his country. The usual voluntary agency, to a greater degree than the tax-supported agency, gives the individual citizen a direct opportunity to help shape an important aspect of the life of his community. Nowhere else in the world is this possible to the extent that it is in our society.

The majority of the voluntary health agencies fulfilled a vital need at the time of their inceptions. For example, the National Tuberculosis Association was organized at a time when tuberculosis caused one-tenth of all deaths and was responsible for widespread destitution. The American Cancer Society was established in 1913, when fear, fatalism, and ignorance characterized the approach to cancer.

Voluntary health organizations have often led the attacks on public health problems. They have provided medical care for the poor before public funds became available; they pioneered diptheria immunizations and financed the development and field trials of Salk polio vaccine. Through health education, they have provided for public acceptance of communicable disease control programs such as tuberculosis and venereal diseases. In addition, these agencies have set up research projects to ascertain needs and solutions and have sponsored new health services which were not otherwise available through public health channels.

## Financing

Each year, the voluntary health agencies collect approximately ½ billion dollars from the American people through special appeals, fund drives, bequests, and legacies. Most of this money is used for public and professional education, health services, and research, but a significant portion is used for administrative expenses, particularly the costs of the fund-raising campaign itself. Different methods for solicitation of funds have been devised, but the most successful have been those which present an emotional appeal, pose a personal challenge, promoted by well-known personalities, and then solicit relatively small contributions from a vast number of private citizens. Charity balls, telephone solicitation, and appeals through the mails are commonly used. The tuberculosis Christmas Seal, adopted from Denmark, was so spectacularly successful that several other agencies have resorted to the same technique. One example is the Easter Seal, inaugurated in 1934 by the National Society for Crippled Children.

The success or failure of a fund drive depends, in many instances, upon the efficiency of the fund raisers and upon emotional rather than intellectual appeal. For example, pictures of crippled victims and specific disease slogans which imply that "you or members of your family may be on the waiting list" have been far more successful than a straightforward presentation of the facts, accompanied by an appeal for financing general health needs. The cost of these campaigns has ranged from about $0.06 of every dollar collected to approximately $0.40.

Much of the successful work of the voluntary health agencies has been due to the interest, sympathy, and kindness of the American public, but there is now such a multiplicity of fund drives and appeals that criticism and resentment have been stirred up. The public is deluged on the streets and through various communication media for contributions. Sometimes mild pressure and embarrassment are included, such as passing collection boxes in lighted theaters and using neighbors for door-to-door solicitation. There have been so many "weeks" and "months" set aside by proclamation, with accompanying appeals for funds, that it has resulted in confusion and misunderstanding among the public and conflict among some agencies.

A partial answer to this problem of multiplicity of fund drives has been the formation of the United Way, Community Campaign, or a similar federation of agencies which represents the voluntary health and welfare interests of the community. Prior to the annual fund drive, each representative agency submits and must justify a proposed budget for the forthcoming year. These budgets are reviewed by an executive council and are then combined to set a realistic goal for the annual community-wide solicitation of funds. The pledged and collected money is distributed among the agencies according to a previously approved and equitable system. If the federated drive does not achieve its goal, the reduction in allocations is also equitably distributed.

Federated fund drives have been largely successful in that they have furnished a workable method for community support without duplication of effort and expense. There are some agencies, however, that will not join the federated drives or will reserve the right to conduct supplementary campaigns if budget requirements are not met. Reasons given for this position are that the individual agency will be in danger of losing its identity and that publicity, education, and appeal concerning a particular disease or health need will be lost. In addition, fund raisers contend that people will give more money if they are asked for multiple small donations throughout the year rather than one large donation to be given annually.

Not infrequently, pharmacists, nurses, and other members of the allied medical professions are asked for opinions regarding voluntary health agencies which are deserving of public support. These opinions should not be given lightly. Most agencies welcome inspections and investigations and many of them publish annual reports including money collected and disbursed. Much information can be learned from these investigations. Facts concerning local and national affiliations, stated activities and goals, use of volunteers and paid staff, quality of management, percentage of collected money remaining in the community, quantity and quality of services performed, and community need of these services are all valuable guides upon which to base opinions. An important consideration is the percentage of the budget required for administration and financing. Reports are still received concerning some agencies that spend as much as 68 per cent of their income for office maintenance and fund raising.

In response to a need for screening agencies prior to fund drives, many community councils have established fund-raising review boards. Agencies anticipating fund drives in the community submit to the Board detailed reports concerning purposes, objectives, and operating expenses. After careful review, the Board may endorse the fund drive or withhold its endorsement. Since the Board does not have legal powers of enforcement, it cannot prevent the agency from conducting fund drives, but, if endorsement is withheld, there is usually enough publicity given to this action so that the fund drive will not succeed. Understandably, then, the endorsement of the fund-raising review board is highly desired and a significant number of agencies have modified their administrative procedures and have reduced operating costs in order to qualify for endorsement.

## Undesirable Features

The time has come when the public, with some justification, has begun to inquire into not just the financial integrity of an agency, but also the question of whether or not its program is effectively linked to those of other public and private agencies in the community. It is not too unusual for voluntary agencies to bring such pressure to bear on an official health department that the public health program may be thrown out of balance. This pressure may be exerted in two different ways. The voluntary organization, interested in a particular disease or health need, may strongly urge the health department to overemphasize this particular aspect of the total program. Conversely, the voluntary organization may feel that its speciality should be reserved for its own agency activities and may, therefore, exert pressure on the health department to under-emphasize this portion of the public health program.

With such a very large number of voluntary health agencies, it is inevitable that duplication of services will occur. A unique feature of voluntary health organizations is that they seldom die. Significant numbers of such agencies have been established for the purpose of developing a specific health program until that project could be taken over by an official agency, yet, upon reaching this predetermined stage of development, the voluntary agency is reluctant to give up its involvement. Not infrequently, these agencies will expand their horizons to include related diseases and health needs. The result is an even greater degree of overlapping and duplication, not only of health services, but also duplication of administrative costs and fund-raising activities. Reference has been made previously to the growing confusion of the public. This confusion results not only from the multiplicity of funds drives, but from overlapping of functions as well. The National Commission on Community Health Services, very much aware of these complications, has commented on this problem.

It may be both inevitable and desirable that there should be a number of separate health agencies at any one time; but it is entirely fair and necessary to question whether it is in any way appropriate for all of them to continue indefinitely as completely separate units, especially in view of the tremendous need to develop a well-integrated community program. There may well be a point in the study and interpretation of a single disease or condition at which the characteristics peculiar to it have been sufficiently analyzed, recorded, and publicized so that its further pursuit may be related to or combined with other similar efforts without loss of identity or support. Members of the professions have as yet shown few signs of working toward this kind of synthesis, despite complaints of contributors about the multiplicity of appeals.[19]

There is another related duplication of services which has come under close scrutiny. With individual and corporate income taxes constantly on the increase, the public is expecting more health services from the government and each year Congress is appropriating more tax dollars for medical research and health related activities. Many of these areas of government-financed activity are identical with the special interests of voluntary health agencies and there is a growing concern about contributing to these organizations when tax funds are used for the same purpose.

These problems are not new, but they are becoming more acute and voluntary health agencies are faced with the difficult situation of what to do about such trends. The National Health Council, founded in 1920 by a group of leaders who anticipated a vast expansion in health activities, foresaw the inevitable chaos that would develop unless health agencies had a mechanism for working together. This Council, representing a membership of 70 national organizations, has been partially successful in helping to integrate and co-ordinate the activities of health agencies. The annual National Health Forum, sponsored by the Council, furnishes an opportunity for leaders of the various organizations to discuss methods by which the voluntary health agencies can best serve our changing society. In addition, some of the individual agencies have recognized the need for re-evaluation and appraisals of positions, particularly in regard to their relations with other official and non-official organizations.

Today, it is generally recognized that most functions originally ascribed exclusively to the voluntary agency can be carried by the public agency as well, although not always to the same degree nor with the same potential flexibility. Proposals for some rather drastic changes in functions and activities of voluntary health agencies have been introduced in recent years. It has been suggested that, since the Federal Government has assumed a major role in such areas as communicable diseases, cancer, mental health, heart disease, dental health, convalescent care, and rehabilitation, the voluntary health agencies should relinquish these activities. It has also been suggested that research, health manpower production, public assistance, and the usual community health services should be the sole responsibility of Federal and state governments.

## Extended Opportunities for Service

What significant service, then, can the voluntary agencies contribute to the comprehensive health program of the nation? While their present role is not as distinct and unique as it once was, there are strong traditional, philosophical, and practical reasons not only for the continuance of voluntary agencies, but also for them to play a far more dynamic role than most of them do now. A number of progressive agencies have already demonstrated the opportunities for expanded and meaningful health endeavors.

Historically, voluntary agencies have been characterized by their flexibility and capacity for innovation, demonstration, and pioneering in new aspects of service. These characteristics are needed in the conduction of studies to determine the need for new services, to establish demonstration projects, and to initiate the service until it is sufficiently established to be ultimately taken over by the official agency. Since it depends upon tax support, even a progressive government must frequently be conservative when experimenting with new ideas. The voluntary organization can perform experimentation very suitably and demonstrate effectiveness until an interested government agency can be convinced of the desirability of incorporating this plan into its official program.

Another very valuable service of voluntary health agencies is public education. The widespread community participation, on which these agencies depend, serves as valuable sources for promoting increased understanding of health needs and programs. The educational work is so important and has accomplished so very much in the health field that it cannot be overstressed. Regardless of legal authority, no health department can function properly without the support of an informed and interested public. Since government action in a democracy should not precede public opinion, the public must be educated in health matters. It should now be recognized that the educative efforts of the voluntary health agencies, particularly in recent years, have changed public attitudes and concerns about health and have influenced the elected representatives. This has helped to attract a substantial amount of the gross national product to health programs and facilities and has contributed to an impressive growth and elaboration of the health sciences.

Still another very important service to perform, and one already rendered by some agencies to a limited extent, is purposeful action within the controversial fields. For example, the American Cancer Society has taken a very positive position against cigarette smoking and has used printed materials, public-speakers, radio, and television in a vigorous campaign to discourage the use of cigarettes. They have been joined this effort by the American Lung Association, along with rather' limited support from the Federal government. Yet, cigarette consumption in the United States is increasing every year. The present figures from the U. S. Department of Agriculture list 580 billion cigarettes smoked in the United States in one year. This figure is 90 billion above the total in 1964 when the Surgeon General's warnings were made public. The same report stated that smoking among teenagers showed a substantial increase since the last survey was made.[20] Certainly, much more remains to be done in this controversy involving a practice which is deleterious to health, including a reassessment of the effectiveness of current campaigns.

Another field for opportunity and expanded service lies in the health problems which are not publicly popular. One example is alcoholism. It is a tragedy that there are well over 9 million alcoholics in the nation with approximately 200,000 new alcoholics developing each year. This is an area of activity by the Federal Government but the existing voluntary agencies primarily concerned with this problem still need considerable help in providing public education and in encouraging community support for referral and treatment centers.

Additional opportunities for extended service include endeavors to find the most effective uses of leisure time, conduction of studies into the various methods of co-operation with government, and exploration of the full potential of a creative partnership between voluntary and governmental services. Co-operation with public agencies in developing and maintaining standards to ensure high quality health care and the continued role of helping to formulate public policy with respect to health needs for the entire community are also functions which can be carried out by voluntary agencies.

Finally, most government agencies are pledged to provide only one standard of health service for all of the people. It is generally recognized, however, that there are geographic areas and segments of the population that require additional programs and supplemental services to meet health needs. Voluntary agencies can and do serve as valuable allies by rendering needed service in a community when such service is not covered adequately by the public agency.

It is important not to lose sight of the fact that total community health is the objective sought by all those who give of their time and energies for health-related endeavors. Duplication, fragmentation, and conflict can seriously interfere with the attainment of that objective. The demands of the future point clearly to the necessity for closer working relations among the various voluntary health agencies on one hand and between governmental and voluntary agencies on the other.

## PROFESSIONAL HEALTH ORGANIZATIONS

Health education and health care in the United States are among the best in the world and much of the success in setting and maintaining these high standards can be attributed to the professional health organizations. Essentially all of the separately identifiable health-related professions have their own societies. These societies were formed to promote the public health in general and, more specifically, to advance the standing of their particular discipline among their own colleagues, within the medical profession and among the public and governmental agencies. It has long been recognized that the quality of health care and services provided is in direct proportion to the competency of the persons who provide the care or service. The separate health professions are well aware of this fact and realize that only through constant upgrading of education and performance can their group maintain a position of respect and professional stature in this rapidly changing field. Through committees, conferences, and conventions, these organizations have raised the educational requirements. They have also promoted continuance of education beyond graduation by presentation of clinics, seminars, short courses, and symposia. To assure that standards are maintained, many groups have established accreditation committees to conduct periodic evaluations. The reports of these accreditation committees can be of major significance to the institution evaluated. For example, if an educational institution is not granted accreditation, the students graduating from that school may be prevented from taking licensing examinations for their chosen health profession.

Other functions of professional organizations are those of mutual protection and assistance. By banding together, they have been able to raise salaries, act as pressure groups in political issues, discourage unqualified competitors, lobby for desired legislation, and promote favorable public relations. Many of the rulings and standards initiated by the various professional groups have been incorporated into laws.

Similar to the situation found in voluntary health organizations, there are now so very many professional health groups that there is evidence of fragmentation, duplication, and conflict among some of the societies. Among groups having common goals, there is competition for membership, differing philosophies among leaders which result in divided loyalties, and failure to present a united front to the public and to the legislators. The resulting confusion and misunderstandings almost invariably work for the detriment of the profession and frequently are not in the best interests of public health. Efforts are presently being made among leaders of some of the leading professional organizations to determine ways in which these groups can meet on common grounds, combine talents and assets, and work together harmoniously. Certainly, no health profession is so strong or so self-sufficient that it can attempt to maintain itself without the strong organizational support of its members.

The following national groups are representative of the single field organization: American Dental Association, American Dietetic Association, American Nurses Association, American Pharmaceutical Association, American Hospital Association, American Medical Association, and National Association of Sanitarians. Most of these organizations are parent societies, having state and local divisions; in addition, there are academies, sections, and related organizations. For example, an annual convention of the parent American Pharmaceutical Association calls for ancillary meetings of the Academy of General Practice, Academy of Pharmaceutical Sciences, Military Section, and Student Section, and includes concurrent meetings of the American Society of Hospital Pharmacists, American College of Apothecaries, American Institute of History of Pharmacy, and Council of State Pharmaceutical Executives.[21]

There is one association in the United States which brings together all of the broad interests and disciplines of the community health professions. This is the American Public Health Association, founded in 1872. It is in the Public Health Association that all of the different professional groups meet to consider the various health problems that must be settled on a community-wide basis. As evidence of expanding interests in public health and in co-operative efforts to solve community health problems, annual conventions of the American Public Health Association are attracting increased numbers of representatives from related health professions. These representatives hold separate meetings to determine how their particular profession can best serve in the combined public health endeavor. At a recent convention, in addition to the 20 section meetings of the Association, 42 national associations and sections within associations conducted such programs and conferences.[22]

With such a multiplicity of professional health organizations and related societies, it is not unusual for a professional person to be urged to join at least three or four groups whose special interests relate to his area of activity. Of course, each of these organizations has membership dues, usually magazine subscriptions, and local, regional, and national meetings. For the young person entering his profession, it would be well to study and evaluate the various organizations and be selective about joining. With limitations on funds and available time, it would be far better to concentrate on doing a good job with one or two groups rather than to be so extended as to become ineffective. Certainly, the young professional is urged to join his parent organization, for only through organized effort can the prime purpose of his profession be realized.

## REFERENCES

1. Goodman, N. M. *International Health Organizations and Their Work,* Ed. 2. Baltimore: Williams and Wilkins Co., 1971.
2. Howard-Jones, N. Origins of international health work. *Brit. Med. J., 1:* 1032, 1950.
3. Pan American Health Organization–1972 Annual Report of the Director. Official Document No. 124, Washington, D. C., 1973.
4. Pan American Health Organization–Ten-Year Health Plan for the Americas. Official Document No. 118, Washington, D. C., 1973.
5. *The First Ten Years of the World Health Organization,* Geneva: World Health Organization, 1958.
6. The Work of WHO, 1972. Annual Report of the Director-General to the WHO Assembly and to the United Nations. Official Records of WHO, No. 205, Geneva: 1973.
7. Agency for International Development–Introduction to the FY 1974 Development Assistance Program Presentation to the Congress. Washington, D. C., 1973.
8. The Colombo Plan. British Information Services, Central Office of Information. London: 1971.
9. Pharmaceutical Manufacturers Assn. Newsletter, *16:*8, 1974.
10. Gossert, D. J. and Miller, C. A. State Boards of Health, their members and commitments. *Amer. J. Pub. Health, 63:* 486-493, 1973.
11. American Public Health Association. The state health department–services and responsibilities. *Amer. J. Pub. Health, 44:* 235, 1954, and *55:* 2011-2020, 1965.
12. Hanlon, J. J. and McHose, E. *Design for Health–School and Community. Philadelphia: Lea and Febiger, 1971.*
13. American Public Health Association. The local health department–services and responsibilities. *Amer. J. Pub. Health, 41:* 304, 1951, and *54:* 131–139, 1964.
14. *The Foundation Directory.* Prepared by the Foundation Center, Editor: M. O. Lewis, Ed. 4. New York: Columbia University Press, 1971.
15. Fosdick, R. B. *The Story of the Rockefeller Foundation.* New York: Harper and Brothers, 1952.
16. The Robert Woods Johnson Foundation. Wealthy Foundation seeks to affect care. *American Medical News,* September 10, 1973, pages 1 and 11-13.
17. Red Cross Charter. Public Law 4, 58th Congress, 3rd Session, January 5, 1905.
18. Annual Report, 1973. Washington, D. C.: American National Red Cross, 1973.
19. Report of Task Force on Organization of Community Health Services. National Commission on Community Health Services, Bethesda, Maryland 1965.
20. American Medical News, Nov. 19, 1973.
21. The 120th APhA Annual Meeting. *J. Amer. Pharmaceutical Assn. NS13:*9, 1973.
22. Program and Abstracts, 101st Annual Meeting, APHA and Related Organizations, 1973.

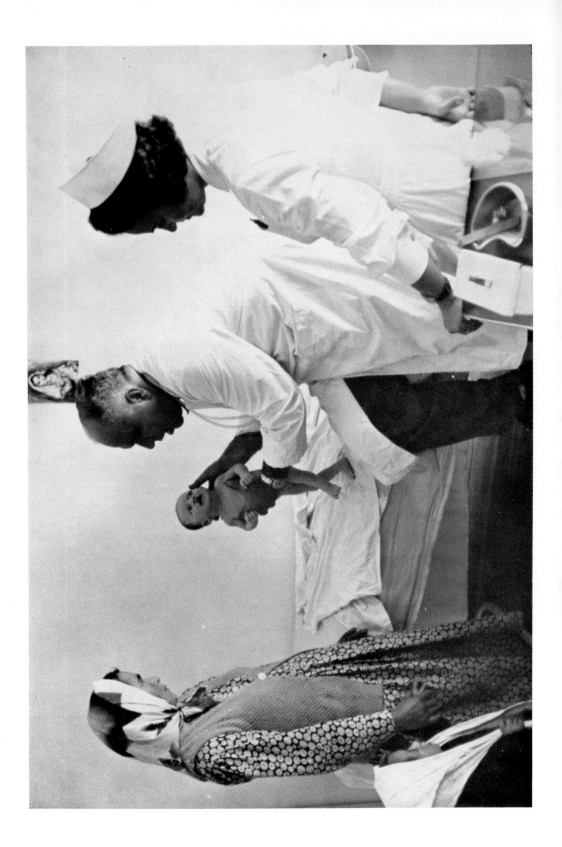

# 3

# Convergence of private medicine and public health

Change is the hallmark of our society. This is as true of medicine as it is of any institution on the American scene. The technology of medicine has been transformed within a generation; at the same time, contemporary social philosophy has defined health broadly and has asserted that good health is the right of all. These factors, in an era of limited manpower and rising costs, have conjoined to change the relationship between physician and patient in fundamental ways. The challenge to this medical generation is the designing of new institutional forms which will preserve the best medical traditions of service to those in need and of professional freedom for the physician.

LEON EISENBERG, "Change, Challenge and Choice"*

One reason for the rising demand to see the doctor is that the many minor ills which befall us all are no longer regarded as inevitable consequences of being alive. We all desire not simply life but abundant life, not an absence of disease but a feeling of mental and physical fitness. Modern life, with its struggle for existence, its frustration, and its unhappiness, imposes a strain which is too great for the unaided citizen. The doctor has become a symbol of society's need for support and consolation. Nor is there any sign that this is a temporary phase. Modern man, for all his technology, is a frightened creature as much in need of guidance and more in need of faith than his forefathers. He is likely to become increasingly dependent on medicine as knowledge advances.

C.H. STUART-HARRIS, "The Frontiers of Medicine"†

* From *Johns Hopkins Med. J., 122:* 1. © Johns Hopkins University Press, Baltimore, 1968.
† From *The Lancet, 2:* 429. © *The Lancet,* London, 1958.

## The Changing Medical Scene

The United States is in a period of drastic changes in the patterns of medical care. The concept that access to health services of good quality is a social right of every citizen is spreading among the people. Governments have felt the pressure for greater availability of modern medicine and are responding to the appeals of their citizens. James W. Haviland, M.D., speaking at the 1965 Health Conference of The New York Academy of Medicine,[1] gave the following statement as a reasonable goal for health workers of the United States: "To provide appropriate health care for all at an attainable cost." The attainment of this goal will require many readjustments in present methods of providing for the health needs of the population.

At the beginning of the 20th century, the practice of medicine was largely led by general practitioners. At best, however, the doctor's arsenal against disease was sadly limited. There were no crowded waiting rooms in those days. Medical practice took place mostly in the homes of the patients. Surgery was frequently undertaken on the kitchen table. There were few specialists, so that one physician usually took care of every medical need. The individual general practitioner of the old school required only casual assistance. Few laboratory procedures existed. Drugs with specific actions were hardly known. Office equipment consisted of a thermometer, a stethoscope, a prescription pad, a few surgical instruments, and chemicals to test urine for albumin and sugar. A few more advanced physicians owned microscopes.

As the century advanced, improvements in medical education became general. This led to advances of medical science with the use of new diagnostic and curative procedures. As examples of this progress, the introduction of X ray by Röntgen and of arsphenamine by Ehrlich for the treatment of syphilis may be cited. Re-

## TABLE 3.1

*Type of practice and primary specialty of active non-Federal and
Federal physicians: 1967 and 1971*

| Primary Specialty | Total active[1] | M D.'s (Dec. 31, 1971) | | | | D.O.'s (Dec. 31, 1967) |
| | | Patient care | | | Other profes-sional activity[2] | |
| | | Office-based practice | Hospital-based practice | | | |
| | | | Training programs | Full-time physician staff | | |
|---|---|---|---|---|---|---|
| Total | 318.699 | 197.764 | 52.840 | 36.644 | 31.451 | [3]11,381 |
| General practice[4] | 73,194 | 54,137 | 7,531 | 6,008 | 5,518 | [5]8,651 |
| Specialty practice | 245,505 | 143,627 | 45,309 | 30,636 | 25,933 | 1,416 |
| Medical specialties | 81,926 | 46,255 | 16,532 | 9,340 | 9,799 | 354 |
| Allergy | 1,641 | 1,376 | | 84 | 181 | 2 |
| Cardiovascular diseases | 6,016 | 4,026 | | 791 | 1,199 | 2 |
| Dermatology | 4,149 | 3,049 | 571 | 266 | 263 | 20 |
| Gastroenterology | 1,857 | 1,183 | | 234 | 440 | |
| Internal medicine | 46,202 | 24,245 | 11,917 | 4,973 | 5,067 | 266 |
| Pediatrics[6] | 19,918 | 11,508 | 4,044 | 2,278 | 2,088 | 64 |
| Pulmonary diseases | 2,143 | 868 | | 714 | 561 | |
| Surgical specialties | 101,336 | 69,221 | 18,224 | 9,115 | 4,776 | 841 |
| Anesthesiology | 11,557 | 7.775 | 1,619 | 1,412 | 751 | 180 |
| Colon and rectal surgery | 654 | 594 | 21 | 24 | 15 | 43 |
| General surgery | 30,897 | 18,806 | 7,564 | 3,106 | 1,421 | 273 |
| Neurological surgery | 2,721 | 1,765 | 537 | 255 | 164 | 5 |
| Obstetrics and gynecology | 19,770 | 14,299 | 2,914 | 1,513 | 1,044 | 80 |
| Ophthalmology | 10,252 | 7,903 | 1,402 | 545 | 402 | 133 |
| Orthopedic surgery | 10,121 | 6,971 | 1,882 | 948 | 320 | 73 |
| Otolaryngology | 5,592 | 4,088 | 844 | 439 | 221 | 23 |
| Plastic surgery | 1,688 | 1,266 | 233 | 123 | 66 | 1 |
| Thoracic surgery | 1,928 | 1,280 | 242 | 249 | 157 | 5 |
| Urology | 6,156 | 4,474 | 966 | 501 | 215 | 25 |
| Psychiatry and neurology | 27,767 | 13,436 | 4,630 | 5,741 | 3,960 | 31 |
| Child psychiatry | 2,171 | 1,182 | 248 | 348 | 393 | |
| Neurology | 3,317 | 1,347 | 771 | 523 | 676 | 3 |
| Psychiatry | 22,279 | 10.907 | 3,611 | 4,870 | 2,891 | 28 |
| Other specialties | 34,476 | 14,715 | 5,923 | 6,440 | 7,398 | 190 |
| Aerospace medicine | 1,046 | 321 | 69 | 230 | 426 | |
| General preventive medicine | 826 | 221 | 60 | 50 | 495 | |
| Occupational medicine | 2,624 | 1,851 | 14 | 72 | 687 | |
| Pathology[7] | 11,103 | 3,484 | 2,451 | 2,714 | 2,454 | 46 |
| Physical medicine and rehabilitation | 1,563 | 578 | 238 | 562 | 185 | 9 |
| Public health | 2,975 | 613 | 50 | 152 | 2,160 | |
| Radiology[8] | 14,339 | 7,647 | 3,041 | 2,660 | 991 | 132 |

[1] Excludes 3.207 M.D.'s with addresses unknown, and 3,529 unclassified M.D.'s.
[2] Includes medical teaching, administration, research, and other.

search received more generous support, especially to meet the demands for new knowledge generated by World War I. Patterns of health care began to change rapidly. The hospital began to replace the home as the preferred locale for patient care. Another facet of change was the rise of specialization in medicine. Of doctors in private practice in the United States in 1931, over 80 per cent were general practitioners, whereas by 1965 only 36 per cent of physicians were listed as being in general practice. In 1971, there were 318,699 medical doctors in active practice in the United States and 11,381 doctors of osteopathy. Of the medical doctors, approximately 23 per cent were general practitioners and 77 per cent were specialists[2] (see Table 3.1). A still larger proportion of those practicing in large cities are engaged in the practice of one or another of the 50-odd medical specialties.

In 1947, the American Academy of General Practice was formed with the objective of upgrading its members through graduate training programs. Members are required to undertake 150 hr. of accredited postgraduate study every 3 years. Although the activities of this Academy have been noteworthy, they have not stopped the overall decline in the number of general practitioners.

The number of offical and fully certified specialties is not fixed. New ones are continually evolving. Subspecializations within these fields develop as new knowledge and new techniques become available. Internal medicine is now subdivided into rheumatology, endocrinology, allergy, and others.

Medical students are taught almost exclusively by specialists. It is not common for the medical student to have extended contact with general practitioners of medicine. According to Magraw,

In the succeeding classes of medical students in the years since 1960, three factors appear to have entered into the choice of those who have planned to go into general practice: (1) indebtedness and the need for immediate income; (2) the student's personal characteristic of aggressive striving for independence summed up in the phrase "rugged individualist," and (3) commitment to an ideal of personal or family medical care still nurtured after four years of medical school. Of these, the first two appear the more frequent motivations.[3]

Specialization pervades American medicine and shows signs of increasing. This is largely because of the great expansion of scientific and technical knowledge since World War II. During the war, grants from the Federal Government to support medical research increased enormously. This program proved so popular with the public and with Congress that funds for research in medicine and medically related areas have continued to increase. In 1972, the nation spent an estimated $3.3 billion on medical research. The Federal Government provided about 65 per cent, industry supplied 27 per cent, and 8 per cent came from other sources.[4] (see Figure 3.1).

The public is well aware that medical science has produced amazing results. This public knowledge has led to greater expectations on the part of patients from their physicians. Antibiotics, tranquilizers, cardiac surgery, and effective vaccines to prevent poliomyelitis and

[3] Includes 1,314 D.O.'s (775 in training program, 181 in full-time hospital staff positions, 186 in other professional activities, and 172 Federal D.O.'s) for whom data are not available on specialties.
[4] Includes no specialty reported and other specialties not listed.
[5] Includes 827 with practice limited to manipulative therapy.
[6] Includes pediatric allergy and pediatric cardiology.
[7] Includes forensic pathology.
[8] Includes diagnostic roentgenology and therapeutic radiology.

Sources: AMA Center for Health Services Research and Development: *Distribution of Physicians in the United States, 1971, Regional, State, County, Metropolitan Areas.* G.A. Roback, Chicago, American Medical Association, 1972.

AOA Membership and Statistics Department: *A Statistical Study of the Osteopathic Profession, December 31, 1967.* Chicago, American Osteopathic Association, June 1968.

*Health Resources Statistics, 1972–73,* National Center for Health Statistics, Public Health Service. DHEW Publication No. (HSM) 73 - 1509, June, 1973

The Share of NIH Funds in the Nation's Medical
Research and Development (1972 estimate)

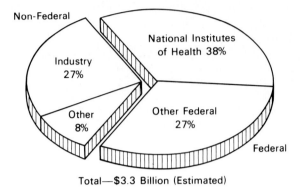

Total—$3.3 Billion (Estimated)

Funds Obligated for Medical Research and development
(Source: National Institutes of Health)

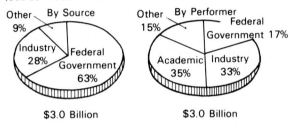

$3.0 Billion                              $3.0 Billion

Fig. 3.1. Source: American Medical Association Medical News: J.A.M.A., June 12, 1971.

measles are only a few of the new measures available to health workers.

As for selection of physicians, the public likes the idea of a personal physician. Those engaged in general practice have full offices and maintain heavy schedules of practice. As the number of generalists continues to decline, the public has been compelled to seek medical attention directly from specialists. To some degree, pediatricians and internists have undertaken the role of personal physician. Patients now directly seek specialists who in their judgment, can best diagnose and treat the current set of symptoms. This system results in piecemeal practice.

## COMPREHENSIVE HEALTH CARE

As pointed out above, the great complaint against medical practice at present is the disappearance of the personal physician. This has led to treatment of disease on an episodic basis rather than the long-term continuous care

of the individual as a whole being. The fragmentation of practice that has resulted from the great predominance of specialists leaves patients disturbed and dissatisfied. These defects in today's medical practice have been widely recognized and discussed. In 1962, the National Commission on Community Health Services was created by the American Public Health Association and the National Health Council. Six reports from this Commission have been published covering such topics as: (1) comprehensive personal health services; (2) environmental health; (3) health manpower; (4) health care facilities; (5) financing community health services and facilities; and (6) organization of community health services. A synthesis of these six reports has also been prepared entitled *Health is a Community Affair.*[5]

The American Medical Association is aware of the decrease in personal physicians, although the AMA prefers the term "family physician." A committee appointed by the Association in 1964 to consider all problems related to "Education for Family Practice" submitted its report in September, 1966.[6] The committee defined the family physician as

one who (1) serves as the physician of first contact with the patient and provides a means of entry into the health care system; (2) evaluates the patient's total health needs, provides personal medical care within one or more fields of medicine, and refers the patient when indicated to appropriate sources of care while preserving the continuity of his care; (3) assumes responsibility for the patient's comprehensive and continuous health care and acts as leader or coordinator of the team that provides health services; and (4) accepts responsibility for the patient's total health care within the context of his environment, including the community and the family or comparable social unit.

Interest is growing in the field of family practice. Forty-nine medical schools now are operating undergraduate programs in family medicine. Most of these were established since 1970. Another 11 schools have programs in the developmental stage. By mid-1973, there are 25 full departments of family practice. At the graduate level, the number of approved residencies has increased from 70 in 1971 to 172 in 1973. A total of 1771 residents were in training in 1973.

The American Medical Association recognized that these steps, although encouraging, were not sufficient to meet the need for primary care physicians. Efforts are to be increased toward persuading a much larger proportion of medical graduates to adopt family practice as their field of choice.[7]

## TYPES OF MEDICAL PRACTICE

### Solo Practice

Although no precise data are available on the proportion of physicians in the various forms of medical practice, it seems that over half of all practicing physicians have individual offices and conduct a "solo" practice. This has been the traditional method. The doctor completed medical school and then "hung out his shingle" to await the approach of his patients. Sometimes the wait was a long, dreary one. The physician, working only with the office assistants that he can afford, in an office that he

rents or purchases and equips with his own capital, and with patients who freely choose him as their doctor, represents professional independence or "personal autonomy."

The disadvantages of this form of practice for the physician are: (1) isolation from professional colleagues; (2) concern over financing his investment; (3) leanness of early and late stages of his career; (4) difficulty in controlling and regularizing work hours; and (5) difficulty in taking adequate time off for postgraduate education.

For the patient, solo practice does not provide much assurance of professional competence and integrity that generally results when physicians are working in groups under the surveillance of critical colleagues. Frequently, too, the patient is subjected to inconvenience and expense in having to seek laboratory tests, X-ray examinations, and consultation by specialists frequently at some distance from their own doctor's office.

### Combined Practice

Along with increasing technological and scientific complexity of medicine there seems to be a strong tendency for doctors to want to work in close association with other physicians. There has developed during the past few decades a broad range of formally organized group practices and a variety of other forms of combined practices. These include partnerships of many kinds, some with few, some with many doctors. Some combinations include general practitioners and various types of specialists. Others are made up of specialized physicians or of general practitioners only. There is a great variety of private clinics, industrial and labor union groups, hospital and medical school groups, and consumer-sponsored groups. Changes in forms of medical practice are occurring at a rapid rate, so that it is difficult to follow all developments precisely. In fact, many doctors engage in more than one form of practice.[8] The American Medical Association has published a booklet on group practice directed to physicians interested in joining or forming a group.[9]

There are at least three forms of combined practice evolving today. These represent stages of involvement and are characterized by: (1)

sharing physical facilities—this may imply only an arrangement between two physicians to reduce office expenses and to cover calls for one another in their hours of leisure, or it may involve a formal, cooperative agreement whereby physicians have their own patients and collect their own fees, but share expenses of office, equipment, assisting personnel, and other necessary items; and (2) sharing income—this form of practice usually means a partnership to share expenses as well as income. A legal agreement is drawn up between two physicians or more which provides for mutual responsibility to their patients and to each other. The partnership agreement should anticipate all foreseeable future problems that might confront the partners and provide procedure for handling them. Partnership arrangements may include two or more physicians.

## Group Practice

Group medical practice [as defined by the Council on Medical Service of the American Medical Association, October 3, 1964] is the application of medical service by three or more physicians formally organized to provide medical care, consultation, diagnosis, and/or treatment, through the joint use of equipment and personnel, and with income from medical practice distributed in accordance with methods previously determined by members of the group.[9]

The size and complexity of group practice units vary widely from small ones composed of a few general practitioners to such large well-known institutionas as the Mayo Clinic in Rochester, Minnesota, or the Lahey Clinic in Boston, Massachusetts.

After the sudden rise in growth following World War II, group practice has been growing slowly, but steadily, especially in some sections of the United States.

The American Medical Association's Department of Survey Research conducted a survey of all known medical groups in 1969.[9] Questionaires were sent to 7891 medical groups. Replies were received from 6371 groups meeting the AMA definition of group practice. This survey showed 40,093 physicians practicing in the 6371 groups. Of the total number of non-Federal physicians practicing in 1969 (227,758), approximately 17.6 per cent practiced in groups. Internes and residents were not included in this computation.

The average size of groups were slightly over six physicians. Of the 40,093 physicians practicing in groups, 91 per cent were full-time; the remaining 9 per cent were part-time group members.

There are in general three types of groups: (1) single specialty groups, which accounted for 3169 of the total groups and 13,053 physicians. Most of this group type consisted of three to five physicians. (2) Multispecialty groups composed of three or more physicians representing two or more fields: 2418 multispecialty groups with 24,349 physicians were listed in the 1969 survey. (3) General practice groups with three or more general practitioners. There were 784 of these groups with 2691 physicians.

Of the three group types, single specialty groups experienced the fastest growth rate between 1965 and 1969.

Most groups operate on a fee-for-service basis, but a number of important experiments have been undertaken with prepayment of fees by an insurance plan. Groups that have used this system include Ross-Loos, Kaiser Foundation Health plans in California, the Health Insurance Plan of New York, and several group cooperatives in other cities. In the 1969 survey of medical groups, only 85 groups reported that over 50 per cent of their income was derived from prepayment.

Many studies of group practice have been undertaken in recent years. The results of these investigations are well summarized by Fein in his recent book.[10] The view most generally held is that the advantages of group practice for both patients and participating physicians far outweigh the possible disadvantages of the system. Among the advantages usually cited are:

1. Higher productivity of physicians in a group setting as compared to those in solo practice.

2. Reduction of wasteful overhead costs by more efficient use of personnel and expensive equipment.

3. Less hospitalization of patients because of the emphasis on ambulatory diagnosis and treatment.

4. Better supervision of professional activities by group discipline.

5. Provision of more continuous and unified patient care.

6. Greater convenience for patients in obtaining consultation with specialists, laboratory tests, X-ray, and other special examinations.

7. Greater opportunity offered to physicians and other staff for postgraduate training.

8. Opportunity for physicians to have regular time off for relaxation and recreation.

9. More secure income for physicians, especially for the difficult periods at the beginning and termination of professional activity.

10. Retirement income for members of the group staff in accordance with their periods of service.

11. Relief for physicians to a large extent from administrative burdens for devotion of a larger share of energy to medical pursuits.

12. More complete and better unified patient record systems than in the offices of physicians in solo practice.

Practice in groups is not well-suited to all physicians. The strongly individualistic person is more adapted to a solo professional life not subjected to conformity to group discipline. Unquestionably a physician surrenders some independence when he joins a group. His group may at times be subject to criticism for actions of one or another of his group fellows. His actions are to a certain extent subject to review by his colleagues. Group members must abide by decisions of the majority, which may be displeasing to individual members. Excessive incomes by individual specialists are discouraged in group practice.

In October, 1966, the Secretary of Health, Education and Welfare called a National Conference to explore ways to stimulate the group practice of medicine in the United States. Some 150 conferees attended this conference which met at the University of Chicago.

A whole series of recommendations came from this 2-day discussion: (1) suggestions on how to overcome the legal barriers which exist in some states; (2) plans to expand the Hill-Burton program to encourage group practice; (3) provision of Federal subsidy for major prepayment group practice plans; and (4) other recommendations related to the use of manpower in group practice.[11]

A form of group practice, the "Health Maintenance Organization" (HMO) has recently received widespread national attention. Essentially, an HMO is an organization that provides complete health services to an enrolled population in return for a prepaid enrollment fee. Payment of the annual fee entitles the subscriber to all services (including hospitalization) that might be required during the year. The Nixon administration has advocated HMO's as the most effective delivery system of health care. Proponents of the HMO system of prepaid group practice maintain that (1) the quality of health care will be improved; (2) the scope of care would be broadened to include early detection of disease and preventive measures; and (3) the cost of health care would be reduced by eliminating over-utilization of hospital services. In October, 1972, Congress enacted H. R. 1 which permits Medicare beneficiaries to enroll in HMO's.

The HMO Act of 1973 provides $375 million over five years to aid in the establishment of HMO's across the country. To qualify for federal aid, HMO's must meet standards set by the government of minimal benefits offered, stay open for 24 hours a day, provide open enrollment, and conform to other requirements. The Act requires larger employers to offer workers an HMO option when existing health insurance contracts expire, provided an HMO is available in the community. This large-scale experiment will test consumer and provider acceptance of prepaid group care delivery. A period of rough sailing for the plan is anticipated as there appears to be little enthusiasm for the program either on the part of the public or of the medical profession.[12,13]

*Medical Care Foundations*

In response to the growth of prepaid group practice plans, a number of county and state medical societies have organized non-profit medical care foundations. Typically, such foundations are incorporated. Participating physicians maintain their separate and independent practice. Subscribers pay the foundation a prepaid fee to cover the cost of medical services.

The first such foundation was formed by the San Joaquin County Medical Society of California in 1954. The movement has extended rapidly in recent years. In 1971, the American Association of Foundations for Medical Care was formed. According to AAFMC as of November 1973, there were 71 foundations as members in 29 different states.[14,15]

The government appears to be keenly interested in the foundation approach and has expressed willingness to provide limited funds via HMO planning and developmental grants to several medical care foundations. To qualify as HMO's, physicians would have to subcontract with hospitals and other facilities to provide the necessary range of additional services which an HMO must offer.

Some physicians concerned over the encroachment of government in the regulation of medical practice have decided to form organizations to protect the interests of their members. In Massachusetts, the doctors call their organization a Federation of Physicians and in Florida, the American Physicians Guild. In Nevada and California, some twelve medical unions have been formed with membership of some 25,000 doctors and dentists. Plans are being discussed for a national union of physicians and dentists.[16]

Legal advisers have pointed out that as physicians are largely self-employed, there may be legal obstacles in having a union to represent them on the same basis as labor unions bargain for employee rights. Also, the American Medical Association's House of Delegates has expressed strong opposition to the movement to join unions.[17]

### The Growth of Allied Medical Professions

Medical specialism is making it necessary for physicians to develop cooperative arrangements with a wide range of allied medical professions. In these days, diagnosis depends on a battery of laboratory, X-ray, and other instrumental tests. In addition to the traditional medical team—physician, nurse, laboratory technician—there is clearly a great growth of other health workers essential to successful diagnosis, treatment, and rehabilitation of patients. In 1971, about 4.4 million persons were employed in the health professions and occupations in the United States. A total of more than 600 primary and alternate job titles have been identified and probably this inventory is incomplete.[2] The estimate is that by 1980 about 5.31 million people will be employed in the health field (See Table 3.2).

Until quite recently, the main thrust of the Federal Government in the health field was to increase the supply of basic resources rather than to improve the efficiency of their utilization. Under the terms of the Economic Opportunity Act of 1964, funds have been used to develop experimental neighborhood health centers to provide comprehensive health services in urban areas having high concentrations of poverty and a marked lack of health services. As of June, 1972, 129 such centers were in operation throughout the country.[2]

The chief characteristics of the neighborhood health center are:

1. It focuses on the needs of the poor.
2. Ready accessibility in terms of time and place in which a wide range of ambulatory health services are made available.
3. Involvement of the population to be served as policy makers and employees.
4. Integration with existing sources of services with formal referral channels to other institutions.
5. Assurance of high quality professional care.
6. A program of preventive medicine and health promotion.
7. Varied sponsorship, some being affiliated with private or teaching hospitals such as Montefiore in New York; some with medical schools; for example, the Tufts-Delta Health Center in Mississippi; and some by corporations created by groups of consumers and providers.

Although neighborhood health centers have met the needs of some population groups to some extent, they tend to prolong the separation of medical care into that designed for the better-off people and that arranged for the poor. No group of American citizens desires to be relegated to second-class status. The health services industry ranks third among all industries in the employment of personnel. Only in agriculture and construction are there greater numbers employed.[13]

Around 1900, the number of physicians in proportion to all the other professional health workers combined equalled about three to five. By 1950, the percentage of doctors dropped to 23 per cent. Today, approximately one in five of the professionally trained health personnel is a physician (See Fig. 3.2 and Table 3.2).

## OUTPATIENT CLINICS

For over 200 years, outpatient clinics have provided medical care for the ambulatory sick among the poor of the United States, especially in the larger cities. The first such clinic, or dispensary as it was then called, was established by the Pennsylvania Hospital in Philadelphia in 1752. Within a few years, similar dispensaries were opened in New York and Boston.

During the 19th century, the number of outpatient clinics increased slowly—most of those organized being attached to hospitals. By 1904, only 150 such clinics were available, nearly all located in the larger cities. Health

Persons (thousands)

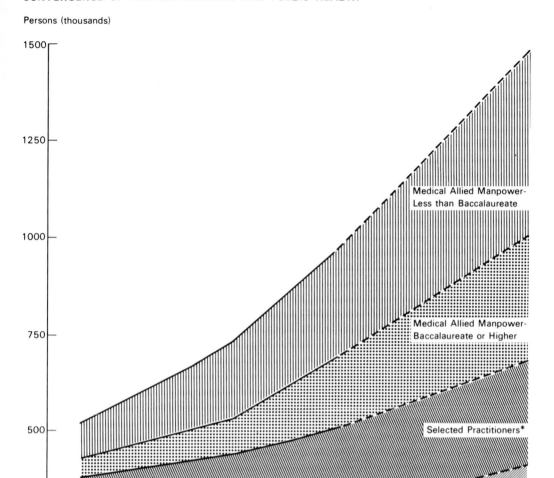

Fig. 3.2. Medicine and allied services Employment 1950–1980
* Selected Practitioners: Optometrists, pharmacists, podiatrists, clinical social workers, chiropractors and naturopaths, and lay midwives.
Source *Health Manpower Source Book* 21 Pennell, M. Y., and D. B. Hoover, Public Health Service-National Institutes of Health, Bureau of Health Professions Education and Manpower Training, Public Health Service Publication No. 263, Section 21, 1970.

departments began to operate clinics for the diagnosis and treatment of tuberculosis about that time. In 1910, there were some 450 outpatient clinics in the United States, and by 1952, a total of 3500. There has been a tendency for independent dispensaries to disappear, because hospitals have begun to operate ambulatory services and governmental agencies have begun to assume their responsibilities for providing medical care.

## TABLE 3.2

*Estimated employment in health occupations: 1967 and*
*projections to 1975 and 1980*

| Occupation within Group | 1967 | 1975 | 1980 |
|---|---|---|---|
| Total, all occupations | 3,515,000 | 4,634,500 | 5,316,300 |
| Other than "allied health" | 2,708,500 | 3,512,500 | 3,972,300 |
| "Allied health"—at least baccalaureate | 229,500 | 350,000 | 410,000 |
| "Allied health"—less than baccalaureate | 577,000 | 772,000 | 934,000 |
| Medicine and allied services, total | 956,800 | 1,281,500 | 1,477,300 |
| Physicians (M.D. and D.O.) | 305,500 | 361,500 | 407,300 |
| Selected practitioners[1] | 199,800 | 250,000 | 275,000 |
| "Allied health"—at least baccalaureate | 175,000 | 270,000 | 320,000 |
| "Allied health"—less than baccalaureate | 276,500 | 400,000 | 475,000 |
| Dentistry and allied services, total | 235,700 | 248,000 | 271,000 |
| Dentists | 98,700 | 109,000 | 120,000 |
| "Allied health"—less than baccalaureate | 137,000 | 139,000 | 151,000 |
| Nursing and related services, total | 1,754,000 | 2,362,000 | 2,720,000 |
| Registered nurses | 659,000 | 816,000 | 895,000 |
| Licensed practical nurses | 320,000 | 546,000 | 675,000 |
| Nursing aides, orderlies, and attendants | 775,000 | 1,000,000 | 1,150,000 |
| Environmental Health services, total | 218,000 | 313,000 | 398,000 |
| "Allied health"—at least baccalaureate | 54,500 | 80,000 | 90,000 |
| "Allied health"—less than baccalaureate | 163,500 | 233,000 | 308,000 |
| All other services, total | 350,500 | 430,000 | 450,000 |

[1] Optometrists, pharmacists, podiatrists, clinical psychologists, clinical social workers, chiropractors and naturopaths, and midwives.

Sources: 1967 estimates based on table 1 in "Measuring the Supply of Health Manpower" by M. Y Pennell. *Health Manpower, United States, 1965–1967.* Public Health Service Publication No. 1000, Series 14, No. 1. Washington, Government Printing Office, 1968. 1975 and 1980 projections by the Bureau of Health Professions Education and Manpower Training, Public Health Service.

*Health Resources Statistics,* 1972-73. National Center for Health Statistics, Washington, D.C. Public Health Service. DHEW Publication No. (HSM) 73-1509, June, 1973.

A survey conducted by the American Hospital Association in 1972, outpatient visits increased by 19.5 million for all hospitals reaching a total of 219.182 million. Since 1967, outpatient visits have increased by 47.9 per cent for all hospitals. Of the 6622 hospitals reporting, only 2038 or 30.8 per cent have organized outpatient departments, while 5023 or 75.9 per cent maintain emergency departments.[18]

To provide the comprehensive health care that is considered to be the goal of a modern health delivery service, some means must be found to increase the effective use of the physician's skills. This need has led to the development of "physician's extenders" which includes physician's assistants, nurse practitioners, and dental therapists. For many years, nurses following varying periods of special training have assumed such roles as nurse midwives, nurse anesthetists, nurse attendants in intensive care units, and public health nurses. In recent years, courses of training to fit nurses to be physician's associates, especially in the pediatric field, are being offered. It appears certain that nurses will wish to fit themselves for other important roles in the medical care field.

Physician's assistants are defined as those who by training and experience are prepared to work under the supervision of a licensed physician in carrying out his patient care responsibilities. The physician's assistant is prepared to take medical histories, carry out general physical examinations and routine laboratory tests, and to administer treatments as prescribed by the physician. The physician's assistant may be prepared and permitted to perform other technical or clinical tasks as determined by his training program and the supervising physician.

As of November, 1973, there are over 40 training programs for physician's assistants in about 30 states. The Federal Government has provided financial support to some 30 of these training centers to fulfill the mandate of the Comprehensive Health Manpower Training Act of 1971. By the end of 1973, a total of 637 physician's assistants will have received training; an additional 793 will have graduated by the end of 1974.[19],[20] One important shift in the use of hospital outpatient services is the rapid growth in popularity of the emergency room. Originally intended to provide care only in true cases of emergency, these departments now are major sources for medical care of the community (see Table 3.3 for the years 1962-71). In

a study conducted in Rochester, New York, in 1965, Kluge, Wegryn, and Lemley made the following observations on the increasing use by the public of hospital emergency rooms:

The reasons for this increase are many: (1) Patients are learning that physicians are available at the hospital emergency department 24 hours a day and that they can receive very adequate care there. (2) Whereas formerly transportation was more of a problem, patients can now get to a hospital some distance from their home in a short period of time and do not have to depend on the availability of their nearby family doctor. (3) The increased mobility of our population causes situations in which medical problems develop in families which have recently moved, before they learn of a family physician to whom they can turn for help. (4) Some patients do not want to bother their doctor for relatively minor complaints. This attitude of patients may be due to the feeling that the specialist who treated them a short time ago is not interested in their total health problems, or that he does not wish to accept the responsibility for patient care outside of his own field of interest. (5) In many areas the cost of hospital emergency care is lower than the cost of the same care given by their own physician. (6) Many insurance plans cover emergency department visits, whereas

TABLE 3.3

*Patient visits to emergency departments and organized outpatient departments: 1962 through 1971*

| Year | Number | | | Hospitals reporting patient visits | Patient Visits (in millions) | |
|------|--------|--|--|------|------|--|
| | Hospitals reporting | Emergency department | Organized outpatient departments | | Emergency departments | Organized outpatient departments |
| 1971 | 6622 | 5137 | 2132 | 5870 | 51 | 82 |
| 1970 | 6570 | 5519 | 2498 | 5223 | 45 | 63 |
| 1969 | 6651 | 4959 | 2475 | 5124 | 40 | 53 |
| 1968 | 6695 | 5415 | 3445 | 5113 | 36 | 58 |
| 1967 | 6783 | 5658 | 3713 | 5309 | 35 | 55 |
| 1966 | 6660 | 5554 | 3619 | 5233 | 33 | 58 |
| 1965 | 6422 | 5370 | 2941 | 4756 | 30 | |
| 1964 | 6665 | 5565 | 2950 | 4622 | 27 | 46 |
| 1963 | 6834 | 5654 | 3114 | 4771 | 25 | 48 |
| 1962 | 6814 | 5725 | 3165 | 4297 | 20 | 34 |

Sources: American Hospital Association: Hospital Guide Issue, Part 2. *J.A.M.A.* Chicago, August 1971. Also prior annual editions.

American Hospital Association: *Hospital Statistics, 1971,* Chicago, 1972.

*Health Resources Statistics,* 1972-73. National Center for Health Statistics. Public Health Service. DHEW Publication No. (HSM) 73-1509, June, 1973, Table # 278, p. 483.

they do not cover office visits or house calls. (7) More physicians now are becoming specialists and arrange office hours by appointment only, sometimes weeks in advance. This leaves little room and no encouragement for the patient with an unexpected problem to be seen in the office. (8) Many physicians refer patients to the emergency department of the hospital where multiple diagnostic facilities are readily available along with the personnel to do these services.[21]

Hospital outpatient services round out the role of hospitals as true focal points of community health, professional education, and service to man. They select cases requiring hospital care, permit follow-up of patients discharged from the hospital, and reduce the number of hospital admissions by providing ambulatory care.

In 1972, outpatient revenue per outpatient visit was $16.62, an increase of 13.3 per cent since 1971.[18]

Outpatient clinics have been found to be increasingly useful in the study and treatment of mental disorders. Mental health clinics are now being extensively developed by local health departments or by other public and private agencies. The minimal staff for such clinics is composed of a psychiatrist, a clinical psychologist, and a psychiatric social worker. The functions of mental health clinics are: (1) to help patients about to enter a mental hospital; (2) to help former mental hospital patients; (3) to treat those not requiring hospital care; (4) treatment of children with behavior problems.

With the cost of care in the various types of hospitals rising so precipitously, the use of the outpatient clinic services is bound to continue to increase rapidly. Many patients have been hospitalized needlessly for diagnostic studies that could have been performed as well and at a lower cost in a properly administered clinic for ambulatory patients.

## HOSPITALS

Hospitals are occupying a continuously more important role in the totality of community health care. More than 33 million Americans were admitted to general hospitals in 1972, and 47 per cent of them had surgical operations. There has been a steady increase in hospital utilization during the past half-century. Perhaps the principal reason for this is that hospitals have more to offer to the sick than in the past. Also, there is no other place where the complex skills and apparatus of medical science can be applied so effectively. The growth of prepaid insurance including Medicare and Medicaid has brought hospital care within reach of middle and low income groups of the population. The increase of older people in the population has added to the burden of chronic disease that often requires hospitalization. Finally, the modern home situation is not such as to provide extended sick care to elderly members of the family. Inpatient admissions to non-Federal, short-term general hospitals have increased from 126.8 per 1000 population in 1958 to 141.4 per 1000 in 1970 and to 160 per 1000 in 1972.[18] (See Table 3.4 for admissions data for years 1967, '71, and '72 and Table 3.6 for admissions data for 1971 and 1972.)

The past 30 years have seen great changes in hospital financing. The previous pattern of support by private donors became obsolete, while at the same time, proprietary hospitals were for the most part converted into non-profit community institutions. As a result, communities, to an increasing degree, have a voice in hospital policy and management. A second major change has been the advent of prepaid insurance and the increasing support of municipal, county, state, and Federal financial support for hospital care.

In the period since World War II, hospitals have continued to charge at an accelerating rate. Many factors contribute to these changes. Intensive care units, organ transplantation, and other recent technological advances have added greatly to the costs of hospital services.

From 1967 to 1972, hospital expenditures have increased by 99.2 per cent. From 1971 through 1972, hospital expenditures per resident increased from $140 to $157, a 12.1 per cent increase.

Although there was an increase of 13.3 per cent in admissions to all registered hospitals between 1967 and 1972, the average length of stay decreased from 16.4 days in 1971 to 15.5 days in 1972[18] (see Table 3.4).

During 1972, total expenditures for community hospitals increased by 13.7 per cent to $25.5 billion. This increase is lower than corresponding increases each year from 1967 (see Table 3.5). Hospital charges advanced far more rapidly than did the Consumer Price Index, physician's fees, the cost of drugs, and prescriptions (see Fig. 3.3 and Table 3.7).

TABLE 3.4

*Selected measures in all U. S. Hospitals, 1967, – 71, – 72*

| Measure | All U.S. Hospitals | | | | | Community Hospitals[1] | | | | |
|---|---|---|---|---|---|---|---|---|---|---|
| | | | | Per cent change | | | | | Per cent change | |
| | 1967 | 1971 | 1972 | 1967-72 | 1971-72 | 1967 | 1971 | 1972 | 1967-72 | 1971-72 |
| Hospitals | 7.172 | 7.097 | 7.061 | – 1.5 | – 0.5 | 5.850 | 5.865 | 5.746 | – 1.8 | – 2.0 |
| Beds (000s) | 1.671 | 1.556 | 1.550 | – 7.2 | – 0.4 | 788 | 867 | 879 | 11.5 | 1.4 |
| Average number beds per hospital | 233 | 219 | 220 | – 5.6 | 0.5 | 135 | 148 | 153 | 13.3 | 3.4 |
| Admissions (000s) | 29.361 | 32.664 | 33.265 | 13.3 | 1.8 | 26.988 | 30.142 | 30.709 | 13.8 | 1.9 |
| Average daily census (000s) | 1.380 | 1.237 | 1.209 | –12.4 | – 2.3 | 612 | 665 | 663 | 8.3 | – 0.3 |
| Average length of stay (days) | ² | 16.4 | 15.5 | ² | – 5.5 | 8.3 | 8.0 | 7.9 | – 4.8 | – 1.2 |
| Occupancy (per cent) | 82.6 | 79.5 | 78.0 | – 5.6 | – 1.9 | 77.6 | 76.7 | 75.4 | – 2.8 | – 1.7 |
| Outpatient visits (000s) | 148.229 | 199.725 | 219.182 | 47.9 | 9.7 | 109.987 | 148.423 | 162.668 | 47.9 | 9.6 |
| Average outpatient visits | 20.668 | 28.142 | 31.041 | 50.2 | 10.3 | 18.801 | 25.307 | 28.310 | 50.6 | 11.9 |

[1] Community hospitals include all nonfederal, short-term, general, and other special hospitals except psychiatric and tuberculosis hospitals.
[2] Comparable data not available.

Source: *Hospital Statistics, 1972*, American Hospital Association, Chicago, 1973.

## TABLE 3.5

*Expenditures of all U. S. hospitals, in millions of dollars*
*1970–72*

| | | | | Per Cent Change | |
| Category | 1970 | 1971 | 1972 | 1970-71 | 1971-72 |
|---|---|---|---|---|---|
| Total U. S. hospitals | $25,556 | $28,812 | $32,667 | 12.7 | 13.4 |
| Payroll | 15,706 | 17,635 | 19,530 | 12.3 | 10.7 |
| Non-payroll | 9,850 | 11,177 | 13,137 | 13,5 | 17.5 |
| Community hospitals | 19,560 | 22,400 | 25,462 | 14.5 | 13.7 |
| Payroll | 11,421 | 13,053 | 14,459 | 14.3 | 10.8 |
| Non-payroll | 8,139 | 9,347 | 11,003 | 14.8 | 17.7 |
| Noncommunity hospitals | 5,996 | 6,412 | 7,205 | 6.9 | 12.4 |
| Payroll | 4,285 | 4,582 | 5,071 | 6.9 | 10.7 |
| Non-payroll | 1,711 | 1,830 | 2,134 | 7.0 | 16.6 |

Source: *Hospital Statistics,* 1972, American Hospital Association, Chicago, 1973.

## TABLE 3.6

*Measures of inpatient utilization in all U. S. hospitals, 1971–72*

| | Total United States | | | Community Hospitals | | |
| Measure | 1971 | 1972 | Per cent change | 1971 | 1972 | Per cent change |
|---|---|---|---|---|---|---|
| Population[1] (000s) | 206,230[2] | 208,232[2] | 1.0 | 204,254[3] | 206,451[3] | 1.1 |
| Beds per 1000 population | 7.5 | 7.4 | −1.3 | 4.2 | 4.3 | 2.4 |
| Admissions per 1000 population | 158 | 160 | 1.3 | 148 | 149 | 0.7 |
| Patient days per 1000 population | 2,189 | 2,123 | −3.0 | 1,188 | 1,174 | −1.2 |

[1] Source: *Current Population Reports,* Series P-25, No. 497, March 1973.
[2] Total resident population.
[3] Civilian resident population.

Source: *Hospital Statistics,* 1972, American Hospital Association, Chicago, 1973.

The total number of hospitals registered by the American Hospital Association in 1972 was 7061 or 36 fewer than in 1971 and 111 fewer than in 1967. The number of beds set up and staffed was 1.6 million in 1972. This number is 121,000 less than in 1967. All decreases were in the non-community hospital group. The average number of beds in community hospitals has been consistently increasing. (see Table 3.4).

The Hill-Burton Act passed by Congress in 1946 placed upon United States Public Health Service the administrative responsibility for authorizing grants to states for surveying needs and developing state plans for construction and equipping needed public and voluntary non-profit general, mental, tuberculosis, and chronic disease hospitals and public health centers. Each year since 1947, the Congress has appropriated substantial funds for this purpose, the Federal contribution being matched by from one-third to two-thirds by state or local funds. From the inception of the program in 1946 through 1972, grants totaling $3.8 billion have been awarded to 10,939 projects costing $13.2 billon. These projects arose from nearly 3900 communities of the nation.[22]

From 1969 to 1972, there was a trend toward construction of ambulatory care facilities instead of more costly hospitals. In 1972, nearly half (47 per cent) of the 191 projects approved

TABLE 3.7

*National health expenditures, by type of expenditure and source of funds, fiscal years and 1972–73 (in millions)*

| Type of Expenditure | Total | Source of Funds | | | | | |
| --- | --- | --- | --- | --- | --- | --- | --- |
| | | Private | | | Public | | |
| | | Total | Consumers | Other | Total | Federal | State and local |
| | | | | 1972-73[1] | | | |
| Total | $94,070 | $56,516 | $51,925 | $4,591 | $37,554 | $24,620 | $12,934 |
| Health services and supplies | 87,562 | 53,553 | 51,925 | 1,628 | 34,009 | 22,005 | 12,004 |
| Hospital care | 36,200 | 16,951 | 16,483 | 468 | 19,249 | 12,609 | 6,640 |
| Physicians' service | 18,040 | 13,999 | 13,986 | 13 | 4,041 | 2,992 | 1,049 |
| Dentists' services | 5,385 | 5,097 | 5,097 | | 288 | 188 | 101 |
| Other professional services | 1,680 | 1,439 | 1,404 | 35 | 241 | 168 | 73 |
| Drugs and drug sundries | 8,780 | 8,110 | 8,110 | | 670 | 360 | 310 |
| Eyeglasses and appliances | 2,109 | 2,025 | 2,025 | | 84 | 48 | 37 |
| Nursing-home care | 3,735 | 1,512 | 1,485 | 27 | 2,223 | 1,350 | 873 |
| Expenses for prepayment and administration | 4,198 | 3,335 | 3,335 | | 863 | 685 | 178 |
| Government public health activities | 2,811 | | | | 2,811 | 1,215 | 1,596 |
| Other health services | 4,624 | 1,085 | | 1,085 | 3,539 | 2,392 | 1,147 |
| Research and medical-facilities construction | 6 508 | 2,963 | | 2,963 | 3,545 | 2,615 | 930 |
| Research | 2,277 | 220 | | 220 | 2,057 | 1,977 | 80 |
| Construction | 4,231 | 2,743 | | 2,743 | 1,488 | 638 | 850 |
| Publicly owned facilities | 971 | | | | 971 | 136 | 835 |
| Privately owned facilities | 3,260 | 2,743 | | 2,743 | 517 | 502 | 15 |

[1] Preliminary data.

**Source:** *National Health Expenditures,* FY 1973. Social Security Administration, Office of Research and Statistics. Research and Statistics Note # 24 - 1973.

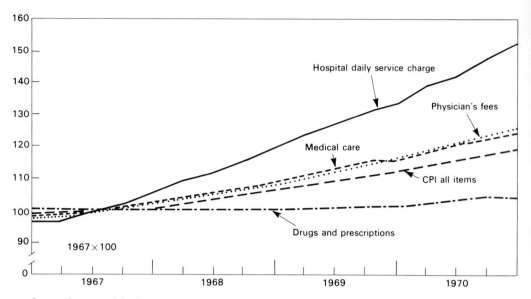

Source: Consumer Price Index, Bureau of Labor Statistics
Fig. 3.3. Quarterly index of consumer and medical care prices, 1967-1970
Source; *Medical Care Prices Fact Sheet,* 1966-70; Social Security Administration, Office of Research and Statistics, Note *2, 1971.*

for Hill-Burton grant funds were for construc-tion or modernization of public health centers, outpatient and rehabilitation facilities.[22]

In the period 1964 to 1969, new nursing home facilities with 5838 beds were constructed under the Hill-Burton program at a total cost of $86.8 million of which $30.3 million were Federal funds.

One hundred and thirty-one nursing homes were improved by additions, alterations, or replacements under the same program providing a total of 9754 beds. The cost of these operations was $157.3 million of which Federal funds amounted to $47.3 million.

During recent years under the Hill-Burton program Federal funds have been devoted to modernization of obsolete hospital beds. Over 272,000 beds were reported to be obsolete and the total cost for bringing these beds into modern condition was estimated to be $8.8 billion.

Although direct grants-in-aid will be continued, Congress has directed (1970) that far greater financial assistance will be provided through direct loans, and loan guarantees with interest subsidies. Regulations for the loan programs became effective in 1972.[22]

### The Hospital as a Center of Community Health

In some of the large cities, there is a movement to extend the functions of hospitals to that of a community health center. For some time, a few hospitals have served as the base for comprehensive prepaid medical service plans. According to Dr. George Baehr of New York City, the hospital of the future will be required to assume more responsibility to the community by extending its services extramurally so as to provide continuing medical care to low income families. Key staff members will be salaried internists and pediatricians serving as personal physicians for enrolled families. These physicians will be aided by a variety of allied medical personnel.[23]

Many physicians are finding it convenient to locate their offices either in hospitals or in medical office buildings in the immediate vicinity of hospitals. According to Dr. Rufus Rorem, already some 400 hospitals are renting space for offices to an estimated 15,000 physicians who are conducting their practices from hospitals.[24] The rationale of this location is to conserve the doctor's limited time and to provide convenient access to diagnostic facilities. The effect is to draw the doctor and the hospital into a more intimate association. Such arrangements will create in the public mind the concept of medical care which is hospital-based.

### Hospital-Physician Relationships

As hospitals have become more complex with larger and more diversified staffs, relationships with physicians have altered. The basic issue is whether hospitals will be responsible for providing care to patients or whether physicians shall retain their professional leadership.

The advent of the professional hospital administrator has done much to formalize hospital functions and to establish lines of authority. Graduates of university courses in hospital administration began to appear in numbers shortly after World War II. To them, the governing boards of hospitals devolve responsibility for the organizational and house-keeping functions of administration. To the medical staff is given responsibility for the quality of the medical care that the hospital patient receives. The medical staff, through appropriate committees set up to audit the professional practice of the staff, controls the quality of patient care.

Another important aspect of the physician's relation to the hospital is his attitude toward the other members of the medical care team. Nurses, social workers, dieticians, therapists, technologists, and psychologists represent only a partial list of the some 30 distinct specialties related to medicine. These medically related professions are striving for position in the social order of the medical institutions in which they work. Physicians are deeply involved in the problems, status, and identity of these groups. Most of these other professions now possess knowledge and skills that are essential to the practice of modern medicine. In good hospital practice, the tendency is for the addition of more and more special skills to assist with the treatment and rehabilitation of the patient.

## Progressive Medical Care

The principal objective of the concept of progressive care is to provide better care by organizing hospital services around the individual patient's needs. Specially planned and organized units are arranged to which patients are assigned in accordance with their degree of illness and need for care.

Progressive care applies not only to individual hospitals but should encourage the development of a coordinated system of services and facilities on a community basis. There is a growing tendency to establish on a common site a medical center that includes a hospital offering various levels of care, a nursing home, a home for the aged, a health service center containing offices for both official and volun-

tary health agencies, a building for physicians' offices, and a motel for ambulatory patients.

A number of elements go to make up progressive medical care. The *intensive care unit* offers maximal supervision to critically ill patients requiring constant nursing care and observation. All necessary emergency equipment, drugs, and supplies are immediately available.

Units for *intermediate care* are designed for persons requiring a moderate amount of nursing attention. Included in this group are patients partially able to care for themselves.

*Self-care units* are mainly for convalescent patients who are ambulatory but still require treatment or diagnostic services. Here the nurse instructs the patient in self-care within the limitations of his illness.

*Long-term care units* provide prolonged medical and nursing care. For these patients, emphasis is placed on rehabilitation, occupational therapy, and physiotherapy.

For those no longer needing institutional facilities, medical care may be adequately arranged at *home* through the extension of limited services from the hospital. Voluntary community services may be utilized in this program, but the hospital usually assumes responsibility for coordinating the patient's overall care.

*Outpatient care* may provide diagnostic, therapeutic, preventive, or rehabilitative services for ambulatory patients.

The basic philosophy of progressive patient care is not new, but its impact on hospital design only began to have extensive effect in the mid-1950's. Through this system, the patient receives the degree of attention suited to his needs. The time of skilled professional personnel is used to best advantage.[25]

## Institutions for Long-Term Care

The increasing incidence of chronic disabilities and long-term degenerative diseases which is accentuated by the growing number of older people in our population has presented health-planning agencies with an acute problem. On the basis of data in 1971, there were an estimated 22,558 institutions in the United States which provided nursing, personal, or hospital care to the aged or chronically ill.[2] In these facilities, there were some 1.235 million beds. They provided care at the time of the survey to 1.106 million residents or patients.

Many of the existing long-term care facilities are becoming rapidly obsolescent. This is partly because of advances in medical science which now make possible more effective approaches to treatment, care, and rehabilitation of long-term patients.

The type of institution best suited to a patient depends upon his individual needs. The sheltered care home provides to people who are essentially able to manage the usual activities of daily living such services as room, board, laundry, and general supervision with only occasional assistance. These services are found primarily in homes for the aged, foster homes, and other facilities for group care. (see Table 3.8 for number of nursing home beds in selected years 1963 through 1971 and the types of care available).

The nursing or convalescent home furnishes a wide range of services to chronically disabled persons. The chronic disease hospital is designed to supply all services. These homes for sheltered care, nursing homes, and chronic disease hospitals are frequently privately owned, but are inspected and licensed by state or local health departments.

In planning and providing services required by a community for the aged and chronically ill, it is highly important that a careful study be made of existing facilities and programs in terms of effectiveness of program, adequacy of staff, and suitability of structure and location. The Comprehensive Health Planning agencies are charged now in each state and community with responsibility for estimating the requirements for additional long-term care facilities.

The advent of Medicare and Medicaid has increased the demand for beds in long-term institutions. This demand has stimulated new construction.

## MEDICAL CARE PROVIDED BY FEDERAL AGENCIES

The role of the Federal Government in providing medical care has grown steadily during the past few decades. In addition to specific public programs for which it is directly responsible, the government subsidizes and stimulates medical care in other ways. Tax incentives are offered to employers who carry the costs of health insurance for their em-

TABLE 3.8

*Number and beds in nursing care and related homes: selected years 1963 through 1971*

| Type of Nursing Care and Related Homes | Number | | | Beds | | |
|---|---|---|---|---|---|---|
| | 1963 | 1969 | 1971 | 1963 | 1969 | 1971 |
| Total | 16,701 | 18,910 | [1] 22,558 | 568,560 | 943,876 | [1] 1,235,405 |
| Nursing care | 8,128 | 11,484 | 13,204 | 319,224 | 704,217 | 944,697 |
| Personal care homes with nursing | 4,958 | 3,514 | 3,645 | 188,306 | 174,874 | 196,955 |
| Personal care homes without nursing | 2,927 | 3,792 | 5,506 | 48,962 | 63,532 | 90,432 |
| Domiciliary care | 688 | 120 | 203 | 12,068 | 1,253 | 3,321 |

[1] Preliminary data.

Sources:    Unpublished data from the National Center for Health Statistics Master Facility Census.

       National Center for Health Statistics: *Development and Maintenance of a National Inventory of Hospitals and Institutions.* PHS Pub. 1000–Series 1–No. 3–Public Health Service, U.S. Department of Health, Education, and Welfare. Washington. U. S. Government Printing Office, February 1965.

       *Health Resources Statistics,* Health Manpower and Health Facilities, 1972-73, DHEW Publication No. (HSM) 73-1509.

ployees. Individuals are allowed tax exemptions for their personal and family medical expenses. Benefits prescribed by law, such as the workmen's compensation program, ensure medical attention to large numbers of individuals who might not otherwise be cared for. Federal participation in other programs is highly varied. Characterized by the kind and degree of public control, there are at least five general patterns:

1. Provision of services directly by the responsible agency, as in the Defense Department's care of servicemen and the Veterans Administration's hospitals.

2. Purchase of services from the vendors by the government agency, as in public assistance programs or the Veterans Administration "home town" programs.

3. Purchase by government of specified services through fiscal agents as in the program for dependents of armed forces personnel or in Medicare.

4. Government purchase of health insurance coverage from private plans or carriers as in the federal employee program.

5. Mandatory purchase by employers of insurance coverage as in workmen's compensation.[8]

The programs for provision of direct medical services by Federal agencies are briefly described below.

## United States Public Health Service

The USPHS provides medical and hospital care for certain groups of the population designated by Congress as eligible for such care. Among these are seamen of the American Merchant Marine, personnel of the United States Coast Guard, American Indians, and civilian employees of certain branches of the government. The Service assigned medical personnel for the ship and shore establishments of the United States Coast Guard and the Maritime Administration, for Federal prisons and reformatories, and for other governmental agencies.

As of 1970, the clinical facilities administered by the Public Health Service were 2482 general hospital beds and 357 beds at the leprosarium at Carville, Louisiana. The total population cared for was estimated at 1,744,502 persons. From this population, 36,894 were admitted to hospitals and 140 persons to the leprosarium. The total number of visits to outpatient facilities was 1,707,468.[26]

## Veterans Administration

As of July, 1973, there were 29,073,000 veterans of the Armed Services of the United States. It is estimated that over three million of these individuals avail themselves of regular or periodic care provided by the Veterans Administration.

From time to time, Congress has altered the eligibility requirements for veterans seeking medical care. Those now eligible for admission to a Veterans Hospital are:

1. Veterans with service-connected disability—unconditionally eligible.

2. Veterans with compensable disabilities, not service-connected—eligible, if a bed is available.

3. Veterans in need of hospitalization who state that they are unable to pay the necessary expenses thereof—eligible if a bed is available, irrespective of whether disability, disease, or defect were caused by military service.

As of April 30, 1973, the Veterans Administration controlled 170 hospitals with a total of 97,075 beds. It was estimated that 1,007,228 would be admitted to hospital in fiscal year 1973 and that there would be 11,632,000 visits to outpatient clinics (not including dental cases). Below is listed the number of professional personnel (figures expressed as full-time employee equivalents).[26]

Number of professional personnel divided by areas of professional competence: figures expressed as full-time employee equivalents*

| | |
|---|---|
| Consultants and attendants | 123 |
| Nurses | 20,111 |
| Dentists | 918 |
| Physicians | 9,154 |
| Clinical and counseling psychologists | 950 |
| Wage rate employment | 34,727 |
| Purchase and hire | 329 |
| Other personnel | 87,234 |
| Total | 153,546 |

* An employee equivalent is one 40-hour-week work slot. This work slot is not necessarily worked by one employee, therefore the above figures are the number of employees.

As the number of veterans grows and as the age of the veteran population increases, hospital requirements appear likely to expand.

In addition to hospital care, the VA conducts a large scale outpatient medical program in its various hospitals and regional office clinics.

Since 1945, treatment for veterans with service-connected disabilities has been made available in their home towns. The physician of his choice is paid for his services on a fee-for-service basis. Also an extensive program of dental care is conducted for veterans in the various outpatient clinics.

## Armed Forces

Complete medical care services are provided for members of the armed forces and for certain of their dependents. The following statements outline facilities available, personnel to man these facilities, and the numbers of services rendered during a recent fiscal period: *United States Army (Fiscal Year 1973)*[26]

Daily average of beds occupied:
Active duty army ................. .3876
All patients ....................... .8091
Total population cared for: 17,630,114
Number of hospital patients: 491,298
Number of outpatients visits: 17,138,816
Number of professional personnel divided by area of professional competence:
(as of June 30, 1973)
Medical corps officers ............... 3,392
Civilian medical doctors ............... .163
Army Nurses ...................... 2,495
Civilian nurses .................... 1,800
Other officers ...................... .210
Enlisted medical corps ............. 22,763
Other civilians ................... 18,933
(includes non-medical workers assigned to support medical facilities)

*United States Navy (1973)*[26]
Medical Personnel:
  Medical Officers ................. 2,382
  Dental Corps ..................... .156
Nurse Corps ...................... 1,920
Medical Service Corps ................. .651
All other officers .................... .93
Enlisted personnel ................. 9,684
Civilian ......................... 7,033
  Total ....................... 21,919
Number of hospital patients:        248,035
Number of outpatient visits:      14,819,756
Authorized beds:                     9,780
Population served: information not available.[27]

*United States Air Force*[26]
Number of hospital beds available (1972):8,378

Number of hospital admissions: 212 per average 1000 strength per year
Number of outpatient visits (1972: 16,533,685
Number of professional personnel divided by areas of professional competence: (1973)
  Medical corps ................... 3,707
  Dental ......................... 1,627
  Veterinary ..................... .343
  Medical services ................ 1,441
    Students ..................... .350
  Biomedical ..................... 1,313
  Nurses ........................ 3,801

  Total ....................... 12,050

From the accounts above, it will be seen that the Federal Government is obligated by statute to provide medical care in whole or part to a substantial proportion of the population of the United States. Of the 7061 registered hospitals in the United States in 1972, a total of 401 are owned and operated by the Federal Government. These Federal hospitals have 9.3 per cent of all hospital beds. Of the total hospital admissions, 5.3 per cent (1.769 million patients) entered Federal hospitals in 1972 and 46.09 million visits were paid to outpatient departments maintained by Federal hospitals. This number represents about 21 per cent of total hospital outpatient clinics.[18]

## THE LIAISON OF MEDICINE AND PUBLIC HEALTH

Modern public health may be said to have come to life in 1848 with the enactment of the Public Health Act by the British Parliament. In the United States the public health movement was initiated on a similar basis a few years later, as individual states began to organize boards of health. In its early years, the responsibilities of boards of health lay in the collection of vital statistics, the sanitation of the environment. and the control of epidemic disease. In disease control, isolation of infectious patients and quarantine were the principal methods available. One brilliant exception was the use of cowpox virus for smallpox immunization . With such well-defined objectives, there was no occasion for conflict between practicing physicians and those engaged in the field of public health. Physicians served those patients who chose to come to them on a fee-for-service basis. Health officers attempted to control communicable disease largely through measures provided for by legislation, based upon police power.

As is usual with human affairs, the situation did not remain static. Even the modest activities of public health departments resulted in a lowering of the death rates and a consequent sharp increase in the population. Social and economic conditions also improved with the increase in the general wealth. Scientific and technological advances brought new and effective methods to those engaged in medical practice and to public health agencies. The Age of Bacteriology, for example, gave a rational basis for purification of water, milk, and food-stuffs. Also the knowledge of specific agents of disease produced specific methods of prevention and treatment. Vaccines and immune sera became quickly available. Effective drugs made therapeutic prophylaxis possible. Knowledge that certain important diseases such as typhus fever, yellow fever, and malaria were borne by lice, fleas, or mosquitoes led to effective measures for reducing the danger of infection by these insects.

Public health officers became concerned with the diagnosis and treatment of diphtheria by antiserum. Laboratories became essential. Soon it became clear that women during pregnancy and in the postnatal period, at least among the poorer people, were not receiving adequate medical supervision. Clinics for prenatal and postnatal care and for well babies were organized by many health departments. The use of public health nurses for home visits and for clinics early in this century soon demonstrated how valuable such trained individuals could be in the education of families in health matters.

Tuberculosis, at the turn of the century, was by far the most important communicable disease. The value of special hospitals for the treatment of this disease had been demonstrated by such men as Dr. Edward L. Trudeau of Saranac Lake, New York. For such an expensive control program, the community turned to health departments to establish and operate the hundreds of tuberculosis sanitoria and clinics that were required throughout the country. Many cities, during the first decades of this century, discovered the need for municipal hospitals for the isolation and treatment of acute infectious diseases, such as scarlet fever, diphtheria, meningitis, and poliomyelitis. Frequently these "fever hospitals" were adminis-

tered and controlled by the official health agencies.

Responsibility for the prevention and treatment of venereal disease has largely been in the hands of health departments by common consent for many decades. Many physicians treat individuals with such infections with care and skill in their offices, but, of course, do not have the staff to trace contacts of patients nor do they have the legal power to force cases of infectious venereal diseases to undergo isolation or proper treatment in order to protect the public.

Since the years of the Great Depression, public health has felt an increasing sense of responsibility for the personal health of individuals who cannot afford to pay for private care. The narrow line between preventive and curative medicine has become even less well-defined with the tremendous progress of medical science. Society in many states has placed on public health an increasing obligation to assure that essential health services be more generally available. School health programs, health education, and detection of dental, visual, hearing, and other defects are becoming commonplace. More and more health departments are undertaking services designed to help control such chronic diseases as cancer, heart disease, diabetes, and arthritis.

In the face of increasing public pressure for better and more equitably distributed health care services, the Federal Government has during the past decade moved to provide funds for the construction of health facilities, for the training of health personnel, for aid toward the establishment of comprehensive health centers and for setting up comprehensive health planning agencies on state and local levels. At the present time, developments in the health care field are in a state of flux. No plan for national health services exists and yet well-informed individuals believe that Congress will enact some form of national health insurance coverage by 1976.

Both the public health agencies and the medical profession are vitally interested in such plans to provide an extension of medical care to people in the lower economic groups. In many urban areas, the departments of public health are now charged with operation of city or county hospitals and outpatient clinics. No doubt administration of various types of community health centers and health maintenance organizations will be added. As such plans develop, health departments can be relieved of the responsibility of operating separate clinics for maternal and child care, tuberculosis, and venereal disease. The coming decade will be marked by much experimentation designed to remove the gaps that have existed between public and private medicine.[28,29]

With the abatement of epidemic disease, public interest is turning toward the field of personal health care. Such care is likely to be delivered in neighborhood health centers, HMO's, in physician's offices, and in hospitals. In the future it seems likely that the role of health departments in the delivery of personal health care will be diminished. Health departments can assume the role of public defenders to ensure that the public receives the health care it needs. This is especially true in programs directed against specific diseases for which control programs on a mass basis have been devised. In this role, the health department can exercise the important function of educating the public in health matters. One thinks of such problems as drug abuse, lung cancer, cancer of the cervix, and other health entities about which the public is in need of accurate information.[30]

## GOVERNMENT INFLUENCES AND CONTROLS

### SOCIAL LEGISLATION

" . . .we have reaffirmed our adherence to the ecumenical and universal concept of health as a science and a philosophy at the service of man and the humanization of development."

Ministers of Health of the Americas[31]

As was mentioned previously, the term "health" is not found in the United States Constitution. Despite this, the Federal Government is assuming a continually more prominent position in the provision and dispensing of health care and services. This central body now plays such a major, dominant role in the field of health that some aspects of virtually all types of health care are controlled, regulated, or influenced by the Federal Government and, to a lesser degree, by state and local governments.

The concepts and philosophies associated with government provision of health care have modified within recent years and the rate of change is constantly increasing. Whereas in former generations it was generally accepted to be the responsibility of the individual to keep himself in good physical condition and free from disease, this responsibility is now shifting to government. Whether as a matter of economic necessity in a dictatorship to keep high production levels, or as a right in a democracy, people are looking to their governments for protection from illness and for assurance that they will receive adequate, high quality care when they become sick, regardless of ability to pay. As taxes increase the public expects more from their government in return, and high on this list of expectations is adequate health care. Leading politicians and social planners, reflecting the nation's increasing concern for the health and welfare of its people, have taken the position that the United States Government must assume the responsibility for providing three essential services for its citizens; they are defense, education, and health care.

The elected representatives have sensed this growing reliance upon the Federal Government and many of them have interpreted it as a mandate from the people. As a result, there is a continually increasing number of health-related bills which are introduced in each succeeding session of Congress. For example, over 200 bills involving health legislation have been introduced in the current session of Congress. Various aspects of national health insurance are the subject of 15 bills in the House of Representatives and 19 in the U.S. Senate.[32] Other bills pertain to subjects such as Medicare Prescriptions, Medical Devices, Emergency Medical Services, Expanded VA Health Care, Mental Health, Rural Health, and Dental Care for Children. A particularly interesting bill, H.R. 12053, entitled the National Health Policy and Health Development Act of 1974, proposes to make sweeping changes in health planning and to establish finally a formal Health Policy for the United States.[33] The bills are prepared and introduced largely by social-oriented legislators and usually not by men with a medical background. Although legislators frequently consult members of the medical profession, these elected representatives are far more concerned about the end results than methods of getting there. Working out the details, implementing the legislation, and preparing various groups within the medical profession to adjust to the growing list of qualifications, exclusions, requirements, coverages, stipulations, restrictions, and benefits are the obligation of other government workers and of professionals in the medical field.

To adopt a common phrase—this is a new ball game. Regardless of the term used to describe the social preoccupation with health and the increasing activities in this field, it is apparent that the nation is moving toward a program of total health care for all its people. Such a program, it appears, will be principally financed through tax funds and social security payments. It is incumbent upon the members of the various medical professions to recognize this trend, to learn of the emerging programs, and to become involved in community activities so that allied medical groups can have a more effective voice in public affairs. Equally important is the support of national professional organizations so that representatives of these professions can become more intimately involved in helping to write medical legislation and in formulating policy. It is unrealistic to sit back and wait for political groups, social planners, and health agencies to seek advice from the allied medical professions or to withhold participation until specifically invited. If the allied health professions do not offer cooperative assistance and do not assume prominent positions in the planning of expanding government medicine, it is altogether possible that the reticent profession will be assigned a minor role and will be given ample time and opportunity to suffer the consequences of its inactivity.

## Constitutional Bases of Participation

It must be remembered that the 13 original states were very cautious about relinquishing to the Federal Government any of their rights. Accordingly, the functions and authorities which were delegated to the Federal Government were very limited, with the strong implication that all of the other powers and activities which were not so delegated were retained by the states. Since the Constitution was written approximately 100 years before the germ theory of disease was established and about 75 years before the creation of the first state health department, it is understandable that the founders and leaders of the nation did not specifically include public health functions as a designated power of the Federal Government. The omission of these functions, however, has had a profound influence upon the development of public health in the United States and is largely responsible for the delay in establishing a uniform system of health care throughout the nation.

In delegating powers to the Federal Government the writers of the Constitution phrased the designated responsibilities and duties in terms sufficiently broad to allow liberal interpretations. It is through these interpretations that the Federal Government has assumed such a wide range of activity in these matters relating to health.

The following provisions of the U.S. Constitution have been broadly interpreted to provide the majority of the legal bases of government participation in the health field.

### Regulate Commerce with Foreign Nations

Under this provision the Federal Government assumes the authority of quarantine and of many of the health regulations pertaining to people and products which enter the United States from foreign nations. The U. S. Public Health Service presently assumes the major responsibility in international quarantine.

### Regulate Commerce among the Several States and with Indian Tribes

Through control of interstate commerce the Federal Government can exercise the power of quarantine and can regulate the passage of diseased persons from one state to another, as well as control interstate shipments of biologicals, food supplies, animals, and other similar articles that may involve public health. The Federal Government also controls the quality of containers as well as the labels on these containers. An important use of this power was the enactment of the Food and Drug Law. Vital statistics and direct responsibility for the health of the American Indians have also been assumed under this provision.

The control of interstate commerce has been extended to give authority over certain groups and practices within the boundaries of a single state. An example of this was the Federal suit against the Nothern California Pharmaceutical Association. In this action the Federal Government claimed authority to bring such a suit because pharmacists in the Association were handling products in interstate commerce.

*The Establishment of Post Offices and Post Roads*

This provision has led to the right of the Federal Government to prevent passage through the mails of materials deleterious to health. Legislators are presently taking a long look at mail-order prescriptions.

*The Power to Raise and Support Armies and to Provide and Maintain a Navy*

The authority to provide for the common defense also carries the power to do whatever is necessary to protect the health of the armed forces, even within state boundaries. This obligation, along with health expenditures in the Veterans Administration, represents one of the major annual financial outlays for health services.

*Promote the General Welfare*

This phrase appears in the Preamble to the Constitution and again in the body of the document. The generous, liberal interpretation of this has been the floodgate through which has flowed the vast majority of social legislation relating to health. The Department of Health, Education, and Welfare with its far-ranging programs of grants-in-aid, subsidization, and direct services owes its very existence to the intent which has been read into the "general welfare" clause. The same is true for many other programs and agencies of the Federal Government.

Because the Federal Government is a creation of the states, it was originally intended that this central power could exercise authority and control only in those areas which had been specifically granted by the states. Each state is sovereign unto itself except for the powers given to the central government. Theoretically, therefore, the United States government is restricted in its public health work within the states.

Actually, however, there is considerable Federal Government health activity in all of the 50 states. Through the process of grants-in-aid the national government sets specific requirements which must be met before the money is granted. In addition, it reserves the right of audit and of conducting periodic checks to assure that the promised work is being performed. This proffered money is attractive to the states and its political subdivisions since

there are rarely enough local tax funds to meet the existing needs. Counties usually receive the bulk of their operating expenses from taxes on real property, whereas most states levy a relatively small income tax to pay for their expenditures. It is the Federal Government with its broad tax base which collects and disburses the large majority of public funds. To qualify for increasing quantities of these funds the individual states are entering into cooperative agreements whereby the Federal Government exercises a far-reaching influence on state health administration.

Another reason for increased Federal Government influences and controls in the health field is the need to exercise authority over the public health hazards created by large urban populations which cross county and state boundaries. Of the 210 metropolitan areas identified by the Bureau of the Census, 79 are multicounty and 27 are interstate. The concept of a metropolis has now given way to that of the megalopolis, a supercity where numbers of metropolitan areas have become so extended and enlarged that they have joined together to form one large mass of urban living. The New Jersey-New York-Connecticut section of the eastern seabord, the Chicago complex, and portions of Southern California are representative of the megalopolis development in this country. These areas are confronted with problems that must be solved on a regional cooperative basis. An example is the Metropolitan Washington Council of Governments, a joint organization of the District of Columbia, five counties in bordering states, and six major cities in the National Capital area. Regardless of territorial lines these areas have common problems relating to sewage, garbage disposal, transportation, air and water pollution, and substandard housing conditions breeding filth and disease. To complicate matters further there is a multiplicity of independent governments within these metropolitan areas and such jurisdictional proliferation is increasing. It has been estimated that in those metropolitan regions in the United States containing more than one million residents there is an average of 270 local governments and special purpose units such as transit authorities, sanitary districts, and water districts. The coordination of health activities of these local governments and promotion of uniform codes for the control of public health hazards are prime objectives of the United

States. Dirty, contaminated air and polluted streams do not recognize political boundaries and present such problems of control that even the more conservative recognize the important service which can be rendered by the Federal Government.

## Government Health Activities

The extremely diverse health activities of the Federal Government are scattered in more than 65 administrative units. It is not within the scope of this text to list all of the government health programs or to discuss them in detail, but from the following abridged list of some of the current programs there are major areas of interest and trends which are significant. The programs in this list provide technical assistance, research, planning, training, and financial assistance in furnishing services to maintain the physical and mental health of individuals.

Aid to permanently and totally disabled
Air pollution
Child welfare services
Chronic diseases and health problems of the aged
Community action program
Community health services for chronically ill and aged
Crippled children's services
Dental care for the chronically ill, aged, and mentally retarded
Development and expansion of community mental health programs
Environmental engineering and food protection
Experimental and demonstration projects for the mentally retarded
Grants for community health practice and research
Health insurance for the aged
Health Maintenance Organization
Health professions educational assistance
Health referral services for armed forces medical rejectees
Health services for American Indians and for migratory agricultural workers
Hospital improvement projects for the mentally disabled
Identification of mentally retarded American Indian children
Intensive community immunization program
Maternal and child health services
Medical library assistance
Mental health—research, training, and community centers
Mental retardation—research centers, and university affiliated clinical facilities

Narcotic drug problems
Nurse training
Research relating to maternal and child health and crippled children's services
Training of teachers for mentally retarded and other handicapped children
Veteran's domiciliary program, hospitalization, and restoration centers
Vocational rehabilitation (six programs)—facilities, workshops, services, research, demonstration, training grants, and training for disabled veterans.

These are merely some of the more direct programs which were in effect recently. No attempt has been made to exhaust the list or to record the numerous programs which merely touch upon some phase of public health. Certainly, more health programs have been added with each session of Congress since this list was compiled. The majority of the members of Congress, reflecting the will of their constituents, have determined that our National goal is the assurance of good health for all of our citizens, regardless of geographic location or financial status. To this end the Federal Government is rapidly expanding its activities and exerting its influence in the health field. Major contributions are being made to promote health knowledge, manpower, health protection, and health care and to improve mental health. Essentially all of the enacted health legislation has some effect on the majority of those in the allied medical professions.

A discussion of the Health Functions of HEW (Chapter II) presented a view of the structure and function of the nation's major health agency and provided a glimpse of its extensive operations. The amendments to the Social Security Act and the widespread effect of this legislation is another example of the mushrooming Federal participation in the field of health. Certainly, it must be recognized by all members of the allied medical professions that the Federal Government is a permanent and increasingly important partner in both the provision and use of health care, research, facilities, and manpower.

## Representative Effects of Government Participation

It is generally agreed that the overall effects of government activities in the health field have been highly beneficial, both for the recipients and for the ancillary medical providers. In striving toward the goal of total health care for all the people it will be assured that those who need medical attention will receive quality service, regardless of the individual's ability to pay. The elderly will be able to live out the remaining years of their lives with more dignity, assured that they will receive adequate care during chronic illness and convalescence. The mentally ill no longer face the bleak future that awaited them only a few short years ago. Thanks to government support, particularly the Hill-Burton program, both the quantity and quality of medical clinics and hospitals in the United States have vastly improved. Government assistance for construction of professional schools and the provision of scholarships and other incentives for students of medicine, pharmacy, nursing, dentistry, osteopathy, podiatry, and optometry have served to help alleviate the acute shortage in health manpower. Government funds to finance research have been a boon to the scientific community, particularly to colleges and universities, both public and private. Because of government grants these institutions are able to purchase expensive investigational equipment, to build new buildings to house this equipment, and to hire graduate students to work on research projects. The net results have been more scientists trained in investigational procedures and more completed research. Government funds also assure that the results of such financed research will be publicized and will be made available for adoption and utilization.

The many benefits accruing from government activities in the health field are accompanied by features which some health practitioners view with displeasure and others with alarm. Some of these features can be changed or removed by interested groups conferring with the appropriate agencies and working out differences. Others must evidently be accepted as an inevitable consequence of the dominant position and extensive participation of government in matters relating to the health of its citizens.

It must be emphasized that most of the Federal health programs did not emanate from the medical professions. The majority of these bills represent social legislation with varying degrees of political influence and controls. The drug price hearings and the thalidomide fallout are examples of sensationalism in this field. The war waging between trade names and generics,

The Drug Abuse Control activities, the regulations pertaining to new drug products, the liberal interpretation of social security and welfare provisions, and tighter restrictions from government regulatory agencies all have received their initial stimuli from sources outside the health professions.

Within a community, the transition from the customary health care pattern to that of a government health program is frequently accompanied by misunderstandings, frustrations, and hard feelings. The additional paperwork involved and the necessity to adhere to government regulations usually result in local changes, not all of which are pleasantly accepted as improvements. In addition, as government programs move into communities there have been charges of government competition with private enterprise. Fears have been expressed that physicians and private duty nurses serving low socio-economic neighborhoods must consider the options of either working for the government or of moving to a neighborhood higher on the economic scale. Pharmacy organizations are rightfully complaining that prescription drugs which are furnished through such programs as Family Planning and Neighborhood Health Centers frequently circumvent the local pharmacist and are supplied from other sources.

In the field of research there are charges that investigators have altered the design of their projects and have abandoned original goals in order to qualify for Federal grant money. It has been stated that some scientists have not achieved their greatest potentials because they were lured by financial support. Also, the major colleges and universities now receive such quantities of Federal funds in the forms of research grants and administrative overhead expenses that it is incumbent upon these institutions to conform to government regulations and to agree to free access and audit by government inspectors. In addition, all patents which are developed as a result of government-sponsored research remain the property of the Federal Government, not of the institution in which the research was conducted.

Within recent years there has been an accelerated evolution in thinking and in the philosophical positions assumed by traditionally conservative members of the allied medical professions. It is now being recognized that there is a spiraling government involvement in the health field. The commitments made by the Federal Government through Social Security Amendments and through literally dozens of other health programs have created acute shortages in health manpower and in health facilities. To answer these needs the government has developed additional programs to educate health professionals and to modernize hospitals, clinics, and teaching facilities.

As the potentials from these latter programs are realized, political observers forecast that even more commitments toward total health care for all the people will be made. The result appears to be that the Federal Government, along with state and local public health agencies, is emerging as the dominant factor in the field of health, exerting both influences and controls. Regardless of individual political leanings, all members of the allied medical professions should be aware of these trends and changes. Now, more than ever before, it is important to support professional organizations so that full, working partnerships can be established through government agencies. In this way the professions can help to assure the finest in health care for the people of this country.

## FINANCING HEALTH CARE

. We trust our health to the physician . . .Such confidence could not be safely reposed in people of a very mean and low condition. Their reward must be such, therefore, as may give them rank in society which so important a trust requires.

ADAM SMITH

That any nation, having observed that you could provide for the supply of bread by giving bakers a pecuniary interest in baking for you, should go on to give a surgeon a pecuniary interest in cutting off your leg, is enough to make one despair of political humanity.

GEORGE BERNARD SHAW

### Introduction

It is generally recognized that health care and services are better in the United States than in most of the other countries of the world. There is more medical research conducted in this country, the United States has more Nobel prize winners for medically related discoveries and developments, and longevity is among the highest in the world. This nation's people are healthier and their vitality is reflected in their productive efforts.

The growing concern and interest in matters of health is reflected in the fact that approximately $100 billion are spent annually in the average of over $274 million a day. Much of this money is spent for research, operating costs for insurance, and general public health programs, but the major portion of this sum represents direct service expenditures. Future medical costs probably will be even higher as additional techniques, more extensive vaccines, mechanical organs, and multiphasic computer analyses are further developed and more widely used. One such development is telediagnosis, which utilizes diagnostic instrumentation to reproduce closely the normal clinical setting, even though the physician and the patient are miles apart. Through the use of two-way audio-visual micro-wave circuits and electronic stethoscopes the physician can extend his services into medically disadvantaged areas.[34] Another development is the scalar electrocardiographic computer program which reads and interprets electrocardiograms with 97 per cent reliability.[35]

Despite the advances in the quality of health care the costs for such services have increased so much that many people have not sought medical assistance when it was needed. The lower the individual is on the economic scale, the more certain he is to experience serious illness. Because purchasing power determines the amount and quality of food consumed, how crowded the housing conditions may be, and the degree of exposure to or protection from the elements of nature, it is readily seen why there is such a positive correlation. If income is low there is an increased tendency toward self-treatment or complete neglect of care. Without the preventive care and early treatment, lower income groups experience more acute conditions which demand attention. Therefore, these groups not only have more frequent medical bills but they must also spend proportionately more of their incomes for medical care.

Although the overall pattern of illness in the general population is predictable the forthcoming experience of the individual cannot be foretold. For many years the lay public in

## Table 3.10

*Aggregate national health expenditures, by type of expenditure, selected calendar years, 1929-72 (in millions)*

| Type of Expenditure | 1929 | 1935 | 1940 | 1950 | 1955 | 1960 | 1965 | 1970 | 1971 | 1972 |
|---|---|---|---|---|---|---|---|---|---|---|
| Total | $3,649 | $2,936 | $3,987 | $12,662 | $17,745 | $26,895 | $40,468 | $71,619 | $79,658 | $89,516 |
| Health services and supplies | 3,436 | 2,875 | 3,868 | 11,702 | 16,884 | 25,185 | 37,087 | 66,405 | 73,864 | 83,173 |
| Hospital care | 663 | 763 | 1,011 | 3,851 | 5,900 | 9,092 | 13,605 | 27,528 | 30,850 | 34,215 |
| Physicians' services | 1,004 | 773 | 973 | 2,747 | 3,689 | 5,684 | 8,745 | 14,294 | 15,822 | 17,325 |
| Dentists' services | 482 | 302 | 419 | 961 | 1,508 | 1,977 | 2,808 | 4,419 | 4,860 | 5,200 |
| Other professional services | 252 | 153 | 174 | 396 | 562 | 862 | 1,038 | 1,466 | 1,557 | 1,635 |
| Drugs and drug sundries | 606 | 475 | 637 | 1,726 | 2,384 | 3,657 | 4,850 | 7,405 | 7,800 | 8,475 |
| Eyeglasses and appliances | 133 | 133 | 189 | 491 | 604 | 776 | 1,230 | 1,866 | 1,984 | 2,065 |
| Nursing-home care | – | – | 33 | 187 | 312 | 526 | 1,328 | 3,070 | 3,355 | 3,610 |
| Expenses for prepayment and administration | 110 | 95 | 167 | 316 | 624 | 861 | 1,293 | 2,098 | 2,647 | 3,680 |
| Government public health activities | 96 | 117 | 153 | 361 | 377 | 414 | 698 | 1,568 | 1,986 | 2,542 |
| Other health services | 91 | 64 | 112 | 666 | 924 | 1,336 | 1,492 | 2,691 | 3,003 | 4,426 |
| Research and medical-facilities construction | 213 | 61 | 119 | 960 | 861 | 1,710 | 3,381 | 5,214 | 5,704 | 6,343 |
| Research | – | – | 3 | 117 | 210 | 662 | 1,469 | 1,848 | 1,949 | 2,163 |
| Construction | 213 | 61 | 116 | 843 | 651 | 1,048 | 1,912 | 3,360 | 3,845 | 4,190 |

## Table 3.11

*Per capita national health expenditures, selected calendar years, 1929-72*

| Type of Expenditure | 1929 | 1935 | 1940 | 1950 | 1955 | 1960 | 1965 | 1970 | 1971 | 1972 |
|---|---|---|---|---|---|---|---|---|---|---|
| Total | $29.49 | $22.65 | $29.62 | $81.86 | $105.38 | $146.38 | $204.61 | $343.66 | $378.34 | $421.57 |
| Health services and supplies | 27.77 | 22.18 | 28.74 | 75.66 | 100.27 | 137.00 | 187.51 | 318.64 | 350.82 | 391.70 |
| Hospital care | 5.36 | 5.89 | 7.51 | 24.90 | 35.04 | 49.46 | 68.79 | 132.09 | 146.52 | 161.13 |
| Physicians' services | 8.11 | 5.96 | 7.23 | 17.76 | 21.91 | 30.92 | 44.21 | 68.59 | 75.15 | 81.59 |
| Dentists' services | 3.90 | 2.33 | 3.11 | 6.21 | 8.96 | 10.75 | 14.20 | 21.20 | 23.08 | 24.49 |
| Other professional services | 2.04 | 1.18 | 1.29 | 2.56 | 3.34 | 4.69 | 5.25 | 7.03 | 7.40 | 7.70 |
| Drugs and drug sundries | 4.90 | 3.67 | 4.73 | 11.16 | 14.16 | 19.89 | 24.52 | 35.53 | 37.05 | 39.91 |
| Eyeglasses and appliances | 1.07 | 1.03 | 1.40 | 3.17 | 3.59 | 4.22 | 6.22 | 8.95 | 9.42 | 9.72 |
| Nursing-home care | – | – | .25 | 1.21 | 1.85 | 2.86 | 6.71 | 14.73 | 15.93 | 17.00 |
| Expenses for prepayment and administration | .89 | .73 | 1.24 | 2.04 | 3.71 | 4.68 | 6.54 | 10.07 | 12.57 | 17.33 |
| Government public health activities | .78 | .90 | 1.14 | 2.33 | 2.24 | 2.25 | 3.53 | 7.52 | 9.43 | 11.97 |
| Other health services | .74 | .49 | .83 | 4.31 | 5.49 | 7.27 | 7.54 | 12.91 | 14.26 | 20.84 |
| Research and medical-facilities construction | 1.72 | .47 | .88 | 6.21 | 5.11 | 9.30 | 17.09 | 25.02 | 27.52 | 29.87 |

## TABLE 3.9

*Aggregate and per capita national health expenditures, by source of funds, and percent of gross national product, selected fiscal years, 1928-29 through 1972-73*

| Fiscal Year | Gross National Product (in Billions) | Health Expenditures | | | | | | | | |
|---|---|---|---|---|---|---|---|---|---|---|
| | | Total | | | Private | | | Public | | |
| | | Amount (in millions) | Per capita | Per cent of GNP | Amount (in millions) | Per capita | Per cent of total | Amount (in millions) | Per capita | Per cent of total |
| 1928–29 | $ 101.0 | $ 3,589 | $ 29.16 | 3.6 | $ 3,112 | $ 25.28 | 86.7 | $ 477 | $ 3.88 | 13.3 |
| 1934–35 | 68.7 | 2,846 | 22.04 | 4.1 | 2,303 | 17.84 | 80.9 | 543 | 4.21 | 19.1 |
| 1939–40 | 95.1 | 3,863 | 28.83 | 4.1 | 3,081 | 22.99 | 79.8 | 782 | 5.84 | 20.2 |
| 1949–50 | 263.4 | 12,028 | 78.35 | 4.6 | 8,962 | 58.38 | 74.5 | 3,065 | 19.97 | 25.5 |
| 1954–55 | 379.1 | 17,330 | 103.76 | 4.6 | 12,909 | 77.29 | 74.5 | 4,420 | 26.46 | 25.5 |
| 1959–60 | 495.6 | 25,856 | 141.63 | 5.2 | 19,460 | 106.60 | 75.3 | 6,395 | 35.03 | 24.7 |
| 1964–65 | 655.6 | 38,892 | 197.75 | 5.9 | 29,357 | 149.27 | 75.5 | 9,535 | 48.48 | 24.5 |
| 1965–66 | 718.5 | 42,109 | 211.56 | 5.9 | 31,279 | 157.15 | 74.3 | 10,830 | 54.41 | 25.7 |
| 1966–67 | 771.4 | 47,860 | 237.83 | 6.2 | 32,037 | 159.20 | 66.9 | 15,823 | 78.63 | 33.1 |
| 1967–68 | 827.0 | 53,563 | 263.38 | 6.5 | 33,523 | 164.84 | 62.6 | 20,040 | 98.54 | 37.4 |
| 1968–69 | 899.0 | 59,978 | 292.08 | 6.7 | 37,041 | 180.38 | 61.8 | 22,937 | 111.70 | 38.2 |
| 1969–70 | 954.8 | 68,082 | 328.17 | 7.1 | 42,851 | 206.55 | 62.9 | 25,232 | 121.63 | 37.1 |
| 1970–71 | 1,013.3 | 75,630 | 360.94 | 7.5 | 47,046 | 224.52 | 62.2 | 28,584 | 136.41 | 37.8 |
| 1971–72 | 1,100.6 | 84,710 | 400.36 | 7.7 | 51,319 | 242.55 | 60.6 | 33,391 | 157.82 | 39.4 |
| 1972–73 | 1,220.1 | 94,070 | 441.18 | 7.7 | 56,516 | 265.05 | 60.1 | 37,554 | 176.12 | 39.9 |

Source: Research and Statistics Note No. 24. DHEW Pub. No. (SSA) 74-11701, 1973.

general held the belief that good health was a matter of good luck. Who ever paid for good luck? The essence of good luck is that it costs nothing. However, the costs of medical care over the years, particularly hospital expenses, have risen much faster than the cost of any other item of personal expense. When the individual had the bad luck to get sick it was soon determined that acute medical expenses were greater than amounts budgeted for that purpose. Indeed, many households did not have any budgeted funds, and it was necessary to obtain loans from financial institutions. It became apparent that relying only on good luck was not worth the risk involved and that a prepaid share-the-risk program could offer a solution. Using the same type of predictions as do the life insurance companies, enough experience has been accumulated to make medical care insurable.

### Health Insurance

In keeping with social and industrial progress and in the quest for increasing security, various types of insurance have been developed. Workmen's compensation laws, which require employers to carry insurance on employees, are found in all states. These programs protect against hospital and medical costs and offer limited protection against wage loss if injury is sustained while the employee is on the job. Other types of insurance are offered in pension and retirement plans which contain illness and disability benefits. In addition, some labor unions and management provide extensive health services to members and their immediate families; frequently this is a bargaining point in labor-management contracts. Also, life insurance policies often contain disability clauses. Liability insurance on homeowners, automobile drivers, and businesses provide for specific hospital and medical expenses. Still the most prevalent, at the current time, is some type of voluntary health insurance, either on an individual or a group plan.

Approximately 91 per cent of the people in the United States have some form of health insurance.[36] Ninety-six per cent of the elderly are at least partially covered by Medicare. Among those under 65 years of age, 80 per cent have hospital insurance and 75 per cent have surgical insurance. As in other expenditures for

health there is a relation between annual income and the percentage of families possessing health insurance. For example, in families with annual incomes totalling $15,000 or more approximately 90 per cent have health insurance whereas in families with incomes of $3000 or less only about 39 per cent possess such protection.[37] Voluntary insurance coverage is also relatively poor among families of workers in agriculture, forestry, fishing, and construction, residents of rural farm areas, the unemployed and unemployable, and those over 65. In recent years, however, there has been a marked increase in health insurance among families with low incomes, rural farm residents, and the elderly.

For most of the uninsured, coverage is not available through group plans or places of employment. Some never had insurance and may not want it. Others do not need health insurance because the Federal Government assumes responsibility for providing health care. Representative of this sizable group are members of the armed forces, veterans (particularly those with service-connected disabilities), Indians, merchant seamen, Federal prisoners, and some government employees. In addition, victims of certain diseases or conditions that are of socio-economic importance may receive special care and privileges regardless of their ability to pay. These services are furnished either as a public health measure or as part of a voluntary health agency program. Special beneficiaries in this group may include victims of acute communicable diseases, tuberculosis, poliomyelitis, venereal disease, pregnancy, heart disease, and psychiatric disorders. Victims of cancer, multiple sclerosis, leprosy, and narcotic addiction may also receive special care regardless of ability to pay.

Approximately three-fourths of the families with hospital coverage are members of group plans, available through places of employment. These plans are usually cheaper than individual policies because of a broader risk base and because of reduced administrative expenses. However, even in a group plan the legal contract is between the individual and the carrier. The arrangements between the employer and employee for payment of premiums for group plans vary considerably.

An average of 45 per cent of all voluntary hospital insurance is furnished through the Blue

Cross Plan. The percentage is higher in urban areas and lower in rural areas. Blue Cross started with the Baylor Medical School Hospital in 1929. It provides for direct payment to the participating hospital for most charges incurred by patients who are policyholders. Blue Shield, a surgical plan, is closely aligned with Blue Cross and is similar in structure; Blue Shield calls for medical society rather than hospital approval. The charges under Blue Shield plan, both for surgery and postoperative care, are based on a sliding scale according to ability to pay. Those in a higher income bracket must pay an additional charge for such service.

Some of the private insurance companies pay money directly to the patient so that the individual may have more flexibility in taking care of the various expenses associated with the illness or injury. This has led to some abuse by people who have taken out policies with more than one company in anticipation of a prolonged period of hospitalization. With cash benefits received from two insurance companies or more the individual has actually made money, sometimes considerable amounts, as a consequence of his illness. Because the net result of this practice has been the necessity to increase health insurance premiums for all participants, the major carriers are cooperating in computerized data processing so that this duplication of policies can be eliminated. In the case of a person carrying multiple policies, Blue Cross has declared that they would pay only the residual expenses not covered by the other policies.

*Types of Health Insurance*

There are so many health insurance companies in existence, each one offering a variety of policies, that the combinations of coverage are almost limitless. These combinations are dependent, of course, upon the ability of the subscriber to pay premiums. Although many of the policies may have attractive fringe benefits, they are similar in many respects. Listed below are the primary benefits usually provided in the five most popular types of health insurance.

**Hospital Insurance.** This is the most popular type of health insurance in the United States both from subscription and use. Basic benefits provided in this coverage usually include the following:

Inpatient care in a participating hospital.

Appropriate care in a non-participating hospital when no participating hospital is reasonably available.

Emergency room care.

Diagnostic X-ray services.

Maternity benefits to a wife covered under a family contract which has been in effect at least nine months.

No waiting period required for treatment of traumatic wounds, coronaries, bacterial inflammations, acute diseases, and other emergencies.

The majority of hospital insurance policies provide very little or no coverage for such items as dental care and cosmetic surgery.

**Surgical Expense Insurance.** Policies providing coverage for expenses incurred for surgical procedures are almost as popular as hospital insurance. Under the terms of most of these policies, in addition to allowance made for operating room charges, a fee has been predetermined for each of the frequently encountered operations. If the policyholder has an income which falls below a specified level there is frequently no additional charge for surgery. With fees and cost spiraling upward, however, it is not unusual for the expense of a surgical procedure to exceed the benefits paid by the contract. If the policyholder has a relatively high income the charges for surgery will usually greatly exceed the basic fee, and the difference between the established fee and the surgeon's charges will be billed directly to the patient.

**Medical Expense.** A policy such as this covers expenses apart from hospital room and surgery. There is some overlapping with other policies but this type of coverage is usually more extensive, frequently including physician's charge. Once again, those in higher income brackets may come under an increased fee schedule for services rendered under the contract.

Characteristic benefits in a medical policy usually include the following:

Medical, surgical, or obstetrical care rendered for a hospitalized bed patient.

Postoperative care.

Anesthesia services.

Medications.

Diagnostic X-ray, and laboratory services.

Radium, X-ray, and isotope therapy.

Some services allowed by non-participating physicians or dentists.

No waiting period for coverage of emergencies such as acute attacks of crippling diseases, traumatic wounds, acute inflammations, and certain acute, reportable diseases.

There are perhaps more variations to the medical expense policies than there are to any other type. Generally, the added benefits such as physician house calls and non-institutional prescriptions are added with a significant increase in premiums.

**Major Medical Expense Insurance.** This form of insurance has been available only since 1949 and is the fastest growing of all types. Assuming that the patient can pay for normal medical expenses, usually through other types of health insurance, the major medical policy offers a protection against possible catastrophe. It has saved many families from economic ruin and long-term indebtedness.

There are three essential features of the major medical policy: (1) a maximum limit is placed upon the benefits payable, and this maximum usually ranges between $50,000 and $250,000; (2) a deductible amount ranging from $100 to $500 is included to allow for coverage payments provided by the usual base plans, to keep premiums relatively low and to reduce the possibility of duplicating benefits payable by other policies; (3) a coinsurance percentage is also added to keep the premium costs down. This latter feature stipulates that the insured must pay 20 or 25 per cent of ill health expenses above the deductible amount and the major medical policy pays the remaining 75 or 80 per cent.

Provisions of the major medical policies usually go far beyond the coverage supplied in the basic health insurance plans. The following benefits are characteristic:

Numerous long-term diseases such as chronic nephritis, muscular dystrophy, active tuberculosis, cancer, and fractures in the elderly.

Physicians' services for hospital visits and payments for hospitalization, both starting on the 121st day.

Nursing services for a hospitalized bed patient.

Outpatient medical and surgical services, under certain conditions.

Prescription drugs outside the hospital.

All X-ray therapy and laboratory examinations.

Hospitalization in a mental hospital.

The premium rates for major medical insurance are lower than one might imagine. Fortunately, catastrophic illnesses strike only a relatively small portion of the population so there is a broader base to share the risk. Also, the coinsurance, the deductible amounts, and the maximum payable are all features which keep the costs low enough so that this type of insurance is financially available to more people.

**Loss-of-Income Insurance.** A secret dread of many young, growing families is that the major breadwinner may become incapacitated for a prolonged period of time. Thus, he will be unable to support his family and to pay off outstanding indebtedness. As a partial protection against this wage loss there have been established policies which pay money during periods of illness-caused unemployment. The payments usually begin after the policyholder has been absent from work for at least one week; the amount and duration of payments are dependent upon the premiums paid for such protection. This is one of the oldest forms of voluntary health insurance and is the most expensive.

**Additional Types.** Another kind of health insurance which is gradually being incorporated into the standard types is "doctor's expense" benefit. These policies provide for physician's treatments which do not involve surgery or postoperative care. There are usually three types of contracts under this policy: physicians' hospital calls, physicians' house calls, and office calls.

Other types of insurance which are developing slowly are those of prepaid prescription insurance and dental care. Limited experience in each of these areas indicates that both a deductible amount and coinsurance are needed in order for these programs to prove successful. For prepaid prescriptions some carriers are testing the feasibility of either a deductible or coinsurance. With deductible, beneficiaries will usually get subsequent prescriptions free after paying the first $15 to $40 annually for prescription medications. Under the terms of coinsurance, beneficiaries pay a flat fee of $1 or $2 for every prescription. The usual dental policy, however, specifies that the beneficiary must pay the first $50 for dental work and the insurance policy will pay from 40 to 60 per cent of the remaining dental bill each year.

The average annual personal expenditure for

health in the United States is now approximately $140 for those under 19 years of age and $323 for persons between the ages of 19 and 64. The increase in these expenditures currently exceed 11 per cent each year.[38] Although Medicare, Medicaid, and Welfare are paying one-half of the Medical Services cost, the lowest income families still spend 14.5 per cent of their income for medical care. The highest income families spend 3.3 per cent. There have been significant increases in voluntary health insurance premiums in recent years, mainly to cover the increased cost of hospitalization. Yet, only about 10 per cent of the population use the inpatient facilities of hospitals each year. In 1972, the net cost of insurance, the difference between premium income and benefit expenditures, increased 47 per cent. These apparent excesses have stimulated certain Congressional committees to consider legislation to regulate health insurance as interstate commerce.[39]

The largest and most widely used segment of the American health care system is ambulatory medical care. The Commerce Department estimates an excess of one billion ambulatory visits a year, an average of 4.6 per person. Seventy-five per cent of these visits are to physicians' offices. The cost for the majority of these visits is paid by the patient or the patient's family and is not covered by insurance. More than 2 billion prescriptions are dispensed annually, an excess of 5 million per day.[40] Americans spend over $11 billion annually for drugs, drug sundries, eyeglasses, and health appliances, yet only about 5 per cent of these charges are covered by insurance. Because hospital and doctor's charges are necessary items of expense and must be paid, many people feel that they cannot afford to buy needed drugs, glasses, and dental work with the money that is left. As progress is being made in the health field progress is also being made in devising ways to finance these health needs. One of the newer and more exciting challenges is the wider use of an insurance that is designed to pay for services intent upon keeping a person well. Much of the concern over financing health care has been based upon the fact that disease rather than health is profitable; the physician, pharmacist, nurse, and other allied personnel are paid only when sickness occurs. By introducing more preventive services such as increased use of immunization and greater concern with nutrition and diets, it is anticipated that morbidity rates will decline and that the premiums paid for preventive insurance will be considerably less than that expended for sickness. It is becoming increasingly clear that we need to focus our attention on the causes of health, rather than on the causes of disease.

## HEALTH MAINTENANCE ORGANIZATIONS

It has long been recognized that certain inequities have existed in our health care delivery systems. Under the fee-for-service concept, payment is made to the provider for each individual service performed. This system has led to abuses involving multiple services and overutilization of facilities. Also, the individual must largely find his own way among various types and levels of service, sometimes partially diagnosing his own illness in order to choose the proper type of specialist. Commonly, no one takes the responsibility for determining the total appropriate level of care and for managing the patient to assure that such care, but no more, is supplied. In addition, of the total annual health-related expenditures in the United States approximately 92 per cent is spent for treatment after illness occurs. Of the remainder, about 5 per cent is spent for biomedical research and only 3 per cent of the total is spent on preventive health measures and health education. In an endeavor to help solve these and many other problems, several alternative methods of health care delivery have been proposed. The Health Maintenance Organization (HMO) concept received the widest support and most influential backing.

The official definition, as stated in the Health Maintenance Organization Act of 1973 (Public Law 93-222), describes an HMO as "...a private or non-profit entity which provides (1) basic health services to enrollees for a fixed amount on a prepayment basis, and (2) supplemental health services for additional payments." An HMO is an organized system of health care capable of bringing together the necessary components which a defined population might reasonably require. These include the services of all needed health professionals and of inpatient and outpatient facilities for all health services, including preventive care. This system accepts the responsibility to provide or otherwise assure the delivery of an agreed upon set of comprehensive health maintenance and treatment services for a voluntarily enrolled group of persons in a geographic area. The HMO is reimbursed through a prenegotiated annual sum. Monthly premiums are paid by each person or family unit enrolled in the plan. HMO's turn the traditional medical economic structure completely around. Instead of paying doctors and other health professionals more money for giving more treatments to more patients, the HMO pays for keeping their patients well. There is no incentive to provide unnecessary health care. HMO's can differ quite markedly and there are many different forms: non-profit, profit-making, union- or employer-sponsored, rural, urban poor, Medicaid, and group practice. Two basic types are the centralized plan and the decentralized or foundation model.[41] Newly successful HMO's are a mix of converted medical clinics, foundations, neighborhood health centers, prepaid group practices, and those started by associations or communities.

The concept of prepaid, group medical practice is not new in the United States. It was first recorded as a community hospital contract plan in Elk City, Oklahoma, during the late 1920's. The acknowledged prototype of HMO's is Kaiser-Permanente, which started in the early 1930's as a small prepaid group health plan providing care for workers building an aqueduct in the Southern California desert. The Kaiser-Permanente Medical Care Program now has a membership of 2.5 million persons, a current staffing complement of approximately 20,000 health workers including over 2000 doctors, a school of nursing, 21 hospitals ranging up and down the Pacific Coast and Hawaii, and region programs in Cleveland and Denver.[42] The modern HMO concept, however, proposing a national distribution of organizations as a method for maintaining health, assuring quality health care, and reducing spiraling medical care costs, is attributed to Dr. Paul Ellwood, Jr., a triple board-certified physician in Minneapolis. Experience with existing HMO's indicates that the concept has merit. While reported figures are not absolute proof, they do show that HMO members spend less on health care, are hospitalized less frequently, experience fewer deaths among the elderly, and have fewer babies born dead or prematurely.

The HMO Act of 1973 provided $375 million to assist in developing and expanding Health Maintenance Organizations. In order to qualify under this Act, an HMO must prove that it is financially sound, have an open enrollment period of 30 days annually, and must assure equitable representation on its policy-making board. In addition, the HMO must provide quality assurance programs, health education for members, and continuing education for the professional staff.

The basic health services which HMO's must provide include physician services; inpatient and outpatient hospital services; emergency health services; short-term outpatient mental health services, including crisis intervention; medical treatment and referral services for alcohol and drug abuse; diagnostic laboratory and therapeutic radiological services; home health services; and preventive health services including preventive dental care and eye examinations for children, and family planning. Also, the HMO's can provide supplemental health services including intermediate and long-term care, dental services, vision care, mental health services, physical therapy and other rehabilitative services, and prescription drugs. These supplemental services require an additional copayment by the patient. Other features of this Act override state laws which prohibit development of HMO's, require employers of 25 or more persons to offer an HMO option in their health plan, and provide for health services for beneficiaries under the Indian Health Service Act.

It is generally recognized that HMO's will continue to be a topic of concern for at least the next few years. With the hundreds of such organizations projected for the United States there is increased interest and activity displayed by allied health workers and vendor groups. Speculation is being raised concerning the continued economic security of some of the older health professionals who are reluctant to change their established patterns of health care delivery. Pharmacists are rightly concerned about the rising volume of prescriptions associated with HMO's and are wondering whether in-house pharmacies will be established or if the prescriptions can be filled by pharmacists in the community. In a considerable number of cities, Pharmacy Foundations are formed by local pharmacists. These foundations are non-profit corporations of pharmacists who retain their present practices but collectively contract to provide pharmaceutical services to HMO's. They develop standards of pharmacy practice for their geographic area, negotiate contracts on behalf of participating member pharmacies, provide all essential pharmaceutical services, and establish peer/ultilization review mechanisms for the programs they serve.

The future success of Health Maintenance Organizations depends largely upon their acceptance by the public. The HMO Act has provided for very comprehensive services, but administrators of group prepaid plans complain that some of the required services, particularly mental health care and dental care for children, will price them out of the market. Also, they state that the open enrollment requirement would force HMO's to take high-risk persons who have been turned down by private insurers and the HMO would have to spread the increased costs equally over all enrollees. The net effect of these requirements may place the HMO at an uncompetitive disadvantage and may raise the cost to such an amount that membership would not be attractive for many people. The *price* of health insurance is frequently more of a determinant than the *benefits* which are offered. At the time of this writing, it is too early to predict, but it is not unreasonable to expect alterations and compromises in order to make the program more acceptable.

## Social Medicine

More medical service is needed, particularly in early treatment and in convalescent care. Some of the medical care and services that are available are priced too high for widespread use by the average wage earner. In addition the large hospitals, modern clinics, and other similar facilities for quality health care are not equally distributed throughout the United States. There are relatively large geographic pockets which contain very few medical facilities and trained personnel, and even these may be of poor quality. Minority groups living within these regions have not had the care and services that they need. In certain areas of the country in the recent past, large segments of the population received little or no professional medical care.

Much progress toward more complete health care has been made in these regions but much remains to be done. Allied medical personnel are needed to establish clinics, but financial considerations are frequently influencing factors in determining whether or not clinics will be established. There has to be some assurance that patients will be able to pay their medical bills or that these expenses will be paid for them. Costs of equipment, facilities, and maintenance must be met. Also, the training and preparation of physicians, pharmacists, nurses, laboratory technicians, and other health professionals is such that adequate remuneration for their services must be expected. The attitude of medicine to society has changed and there are now some sociological positions that are generally accepted and others that still raise some controversy. Among those positions are the following: no one should be penalized because of illness; restoration to good health is both a community and a national obligation; medical care has now become a political as well as an economic and ethical issue; the poor and elderly need more medical care because of their position and age; in a civilized commonwealth the benefits of medical science should be available to all people; in a society as large, great, and complex as this the Federal Government should assume obligation for defense, education, and medical care.

For a number of years each session of Congress has seen the introduction of bills designed to provide government-sponsored health insurance. The Kerr-Mills Act of 1960 was an example of the nation's concern for its needy senior citizens. Under the terms of this Act, qualified states received Federal funds on a matching basis to provide health care for elderly people who were in financial need. To qualify, a state had to enact a health care law of its own and then appropriate funds to match those needed from the Federal Government. The Kerr-Mills Act, however, did not meet with complete success. Five years after passage of the Act, 10 states still did not have laws to implement it and some which had passed laws failed to appropriate funds to carry out an adequate program. Actually, full participation in the Kerr-Mills Act was found in only about one-half the states.

Social legislation in the health field continued. Large segments of the population, particularly those in the larger eastern metropolitan areas, urged their legislators to produce a bill which would provide health care for all people over 65, regardless of individual ability to pay. The result was the proposal for drastic ammendments to the existing Social Security Act of 1935. Because they represented by far the most active participation of Federal Government in direct health services, these proposed amendments were interpreted as representing a large, definite step toward total socialized medicine. As such, they were actively opposed, in varying degrees, by most of the organized allied medical associations in the United States.

Despite rather formidable opposition, support for the proposed amendments continued to grow until there was strong evidence that the bill would pass in both houses of Congress. Recognizing this, the American Medical Association withdrew most of its opposition and representatives from this group helped in the preparation of the final draft of the bill. As a result, features were amended which made the legislation more acceptable to physicians. The pharmaceutical profession, on the other hand, continued to oppose the bill until its passage. This may very well be an important reason why drugs and pharmaceutical services did not receive the emphasis which were needed and, indeed, expected in such a comprehensive plan. It is felt by many that, if the pharmaceutical organizations had offered more cooperation in preparing the bill and had actively supported its passage, adequate provisions for outpatient prescriptions in Title 18 and for prescription medications in Title 19 would have been included as essential features of the original bill. In view of the rapidly expanding tax-supported health care, perhaps a lesson may be learned from this experience.

*The Social Security Act of 1935*

During the years of the Great Depression the Federal Government was called upon to make more adequate provisions for needy people who were unable to maintain a minimal standard of health and well-being through their own efforts. Through the constitutional authority to "provide for the general welfare," the Social Security Act was passed by Congress and signed into law by President Roosevelt in 1935. This Act has been revised over the years to strengthen its original provisions, to include additional groups of individuals, and to broaden its services. Public assistance and child welfare

services were revised and greatly enlarged in the Public Welfare Amendments of 1962. Almost each year since 1962 other amendments have been added to reinforce the programs.

Various titles, or sections, of the Social Security Act contain provisions for supplying medical assistance to specialized groups. The sections which are particularly applicable are the following:

Medical Assistance for the Aged— Title I
Aid to Families With Dependent Children—Title IV
Maternal and Child Health, and Crippled Children's Services—Title V
Aid to the Blind—Title X
Aid to the Permanently and Totally Disabled—Title XIV
Aid to the Aged, Blind or Disabled—Title XVI (a single program)
Basic Hospital Insurance Plan for the Aged—Title XVIII-A
Supplementary Insurance for the Aged—Title XVIII-B
Medical Assistance—Title XIX

On July 30, 1965, President Johnson signed into law the 1965 Amendments to the Social Security Act. These amendments represented the most sweeping changes that had occurred to date in the Act, particularly in the area of comprehensive health care. Outstanding features of the Amendments were provisions for drastic changes in Title 5 and the addition of Titles 18 and 19.

**Title V.** The 1965 Amendments to Title 5 set up a program of special grants to improve the health care of school age and preschool children, especially in low income areas. This program covers the whole range of services, such as screening, diagnosis, preventive services, dental care, and remedial care and treatment. Under the provisions of these amendments, all children must have medical and social services reasonably available, regardless of where they live. Title 5 also allowed for Federal grants to be made to medical schools, teaching hospitals, crippled children's agencies, and state health agencies to pay for 75 per cent of such comprehensive health services. These amendments were designed to help speed up major changes in the organization and availability of community health services for children. They emphasized the need for preventive pediatrics while at the same time they provided for treatment and continuing supervision of health care.

**Title XVIII—Medicare.** This amendment to the social security act provided for the major portion of health care for the elderly, regardless of the individual's ability to pay. It is divided into two parts, the universal or basic insurance plan and the voluntary or supplementary insurance plan. The basic plan, part "A," included the following four types of services: inpatient hospital service, extended care services, home health services, and outpatient diagnostic services. Part "B" extended the coverage provided in part A and also included physician's services. The major benefits provided in Title 18 are the following:

*Basic Hospital Insurance.* Full hospital care coverage provided for up to 60 days for each period of illness; the patient must pay the first $92 of this charge. Thirty additional days of hospital care are provided but the patient must pay $23 per day for this extended period. A time limit of 190 days has been established for treatment in mental hospitals.

Posthospital care coverage is provided in convalescent sections of hospitals or in a nursing home for 20 days in each period of illness without charge. Extended care for 80 additional days is provided when the patient pays $11.50 per day.

Up to 100 home visits by nurses or technicians (doctors are not included) in each period of illness are provided at no cost to the patient. These visits are covered for a period of one year following release from a hospital.

The benefits payments under this basic plan cover room and board costs in semiprivate accommodations, ordinary nursing services, costs of medications and supplies, and such items of service which are usually provided patients by hospital or extended care facilities.

*Supplementary Medical Insurance (Title 18B).* This part of Medicare is semivoluntary; the beneficiaries of the basic plan have the opportunity to accept this portion or reject it. As a result of recent amendments, all persons who become eligible for the basic plan (Title 18A) are automatically enrolled for Supplementary Medical Insurance unless they specifically reject it. Approximately 97 per cent of the beneficiaries have subscribed to this plan. The monthly premium for this Medical insurance was initially set at $3, such sum to be deducted

from Social Security payments. The Federal Government contributed the same amount from general revenue. Initially, the premium rates were to be examined every two years to determine whether such rates were commensurate with the costs of the program. The monthly premiums have since been raised to $6.70 and there are indications that the rates will be scaled even higher unless an alternative program is introduced. Further increases in these rates, however, will be permitted only if there is an increase in Social Security payments.

Under provisions of Title 18B the beneficiary pays the first $85 of his total annual costs and 25 per cent of the costs of all services totaling more than $85. The medical insurance plan helps pay for such medical services as the following:

The services of physicians and surgeons in the hospital, doctor's office, home or elsewhere.

Up to 100 nursing visits each year in addition to those allowed under the hospital insurance plan (18A); prior hospitalization is not needed for this benefit.

Such services as X-rays and other diagnostic tests, radiological treatments, casts, splints, artificial limbs, ambulance services, and purchase or rental of medical equipment.

Outpatient hospital benefits and physical therapy services.

In view of a number of bills in Congress at the time of this writing, it is likely that prescription medications will be included as an added benefit.

In addition to the benefits established under Title 18, this amendment also sets standards and qualifications for medical facilities and for medical personnel providing health services. Regulations have been established and review committees and audits have been stipulated to assure the government that high quality medical care is being provided at a reasonable cost. Persons and organizations who attempt to give or secure discounts and who provide materials or service in conflict of interest will be suspect of acting in bad faith and will be closely audited.

Approximately 23 million people are eligible to receive benefits under Medicare and it was anticipated that large numbers of senior citizens would be admitted to hospitals and nursing homes shortly after the effective date. This marked increase in admissions did not occur immediately but has risen in recent years.

Given only one year to implement the plan the Federal Government and its agencies worked very diligently with insurance carriers, administrators of medical facilities, and with professional health personnel to place the plan in operation. There existed, however, confusions, misunderstandings, apathy, and natural reticences which slowed the processes of implementation. Forms were improperly filled out, patients were misdirected, some physicians would not take assignments and preferred to bill their patients directly, and payments for services were not promptly received. As these knotty problems were solved, there was increased utilization of Medicare. Early in the program it was estimated that Medicare would cost the nation approximately $3.5 billion annually. The current Medicare budget is $14.2 billion and is projected to rise to $24.5 billion by 1979.[43] Currently, there are approximately 7 million Medicare hospital admissions annually, or about 305 for each 1000 persons enrolled. Reimbursements average $590 per inpatient hospital claim and $122 per medical bill. The average length of hospital stay is 12 days and about one of every 15 persons hospitalized enters an extended care facility upon discharge from the hospital. The number of providers of services certified to participate in the Medicare program are approximately 6700 hospitals, 4000 skilled nursing facilities, over 2000 home health agencies, and 2900 independent laboratories. Ironically, the Medicare program was designed to finance medical care for the elderly. Yet, in 1972, Medicare accounted for only 42 per cent of personal health care expenditures for the over-65 population. The aged spent as much out-of-pocket for personal health services as they did before Medicare was enacted.

**Title XIX–Medical Assistance.** With earlier attention focused upon the implementation of Title 18, the importance of Title 19 had not been adequately recognized by many health workers. This latter amendment to the Social Security Act was even more comprehensive because it helped provide benefits for an estimated 35 million people, has cost the Federal Government at least $6.5 billion annually, and represents another major trend toward the development of a total health care program for all the people in the United States.

Title 19 is a Federal-state cooperative program, authorizing grants to states for medical assistance. The purpose of the grants is to assist the states in providing medical care for needy persons of all ages. To be eligible for these grants, states were required to establish health programs for large segments of the population. These programs were to be extended progressively to the point where medical care was to be available to substantially all persons who are medically indigent under the state's established definition of medical need. The cost of the program is shared between the state and Federal Government; the Federal share depends on the state average per capita income and ranges from 50 to 83 per cent of total costs.

The state has the primary responsibility for initiating and developing the Medical Assistance Program. Title 19 is enabling legislation; the decision to operate a program with Federal participation rested with the state. The relationship between the Federal Government and the state government was established voluntarily by a state. Once established, this relationship was a continuing one; as long as a state had an approved state plan and was complying with it, the state was eligible to receive Federal funds.

Strictly speaking, a state government did not have to subscribe to the provisions of Title 19, but there was considerable financial incentive to adopt the program. This has been termed "reverse blackmail" by some political observers.

Federal law established the groups of needy people that could be covered under the medical assistance program but within these groups each state set its own eligibility requirements. Aid was given to people whose incomes and resources were below the minimal level of need established by the state in which they live. For example, to receive benefits under Title 19 it had to be determined that the individual met the particular state's definition of either an indigent or of a "medical indigent." Generally speaking, an indigent is one who is absolutely unable to pay for medical care; this person must also be helped to pay for food and shelter. A medically indigent can pay for normal household living expenses and minor health disturbances but cannot pay for serious illnesses. With each state establishing its own criteria by which eligibility is determined, it would not be unusual for a family with a specified low income in one state to qualify as medically indigent whereas a similar family with the same annual income in another state could not meet the qualifications. Bills are now being introduced which will allow the Federal Government to determine the level of eligibility for all states.

Each state planned and operated its own programs, but to receive Federal support the state had to agree to meet basic Federal requirements. In addition, a broad Federal base was established whereby a state may extend medical care to categorically related groups if it elected to do so. With the use of this combination, the Title 19 program established a step-by-step progression leading to a full range and scope of services.

First, top priority had to be given to providing medical care for the people in the public assistance programs who receive money from the Federal Government. These people are grouped in the following categories: old age assistance, aid to the blind, aid to the permanently and totally disabled, and aid to families with dependent children. This was the minimal coverage that had to be provided by the states if they had a plan under Title 19.

Another phase was the so-called Ribicoff provision which authorized states, if they chose, to provide full and comprehensive medical care for all medically needy children under 21 years of age. Thus, the family income may cover all the basic daily needs of the children, but, if this family income is insufficient to meet the medical needs, the children could be made eligible for the Title 19 program. In addition, this coverage could be extended to mothers with dependent children whose fathers were dead, disabled, absent from the home, or unemployed.

The final phase of this progression specified that in order to meet Federal requirements and to get Federal funds, states had to provide a comprehensive program of medical care for all who could not afford the care they needed. This included those people between the ages of 21 and 64 whether they were recipients of public assistance or not.

A stipulation of Title 19 was that all states which adopted the program had to supply five basic services to their recipients.

*1. Inpatient Hospital Care.* This had to be administered in facilities which met Medicare standards so that a patient was not required to transfer from one hospital to another if his coverage was switched from Medicare to Medi-cal Assistance.

*2. Outpatient Hospital Care.* This included services for the diagnosis, prevention, and treatment of disease.

*3. Physician's Services Including Specialists and Consultants.* Calls at home, hospital, nursing home, office, or elsewhere when needed were allowed under this provision.

*4. Nursing Home Care for Persons over 21.* Skilled nursing services had to be provided and the facilities had to be comparable to those of Medicare.

*5. Additional Laboratory and X-ray Services.* These more extensive services were provided by certified laboratories when prescribed by a physician.

In addition to these five basic services a state could, at its option, provide any or all of 10 additional items which the Federal Government helped support.

1. Medical care, or any other type of remedial care recognized under state law and furnished by licensed practitioners within the scope of their practice.

2. Home health care services.

3. Private duty nursing services.

4. Clinic services.

5. Dental services.

6. Physical therapy and related services.

7. Prescribed drugs, dentures, prosthetic devices, and eyeglasses.

8. Other diagnostic, screening, preventive, and rehabilitative services including family planning.

9. Inpatient hospital services and skilled nursing home services for individuals aged 65 or over in an institution for tuberculosis or mental disease.

10. Any other medical care and any other type of remedial care, as specified by the Secretary of Health, Education, and Welfare, that was recognized by law.

The Title 19 Medical Assistance Program is not Medicare, although it can supplement Medicare by providing services in addition to those made available under the insurance provisions of Title 18. In addition, Title 19 also complements Medicare. Under the medical assistance program, the state had to pay the Medicare insurance premiums and the deductible amounts for the needy, aged persons who were insured.

Another important change from previous assistance programs is in the concept of the financial responsibility of relatives. No longer will states be able to hold adult children responsible for the medical expenses of their aged parents. However, states can still make husband and wife responsible for each other and for their children.

States could not impose a durational residence requirement as a condition of elibigility for the medical assistance program. Thus the states had to find eligible all those residents of the state who met the other requirements, without regard to the length of residency within the state. States also had to make arrangements to provide medical assistance to residents who were temporarily absent from the state.

Title 19 specified that hospital fees be based on reasonable costs as determined by commonly used accounting methods. It was intended that payment be made for the actual cost of the services. Although the law specified only the hospital costs, states were encouraged to follow the same principle in payments to physicians, pharmacists, other therapists, and suppliers of all kinds. Fee schedules were set by the state agency in consultation with its Medical Care Advisory Committee, because the Committee was able to speak authoritatively about the different specialty groups involved in the program. By this procedure it had been anticipated that fair and uncontroversial fees would be established in line with the economic position of the state.

The extent to which the Medical Assistance Program accomplished its purpose depended largely upon how well a state's public agencies, local Health Planning Councils, and medical and health communities coordinated their knowledge, skills, and resources. The role played by professional health and welfare people in the community was of utmost importance.

Unfortunately, Medicaid met with less than success. It was charged that organized medicine was against the concept of Medicaid and was determined that it would not work. The system was described as ". . . a hypochondriac's heaven and an unscrupulous health service provider's paradise."[44] Charges of waste and fraud were commonly made along with reports of unnecessary surgery, maltreatment, fraudulent billing, and excessive income or profits. Medicaid benefits have been substantially reduced in a number of states in response to a "taxpayer's revolt." The recipients of care provided under this program are reported to be

both bewildered and fearful as they are caught in the middle of a struggle between governmental administrators and health providers. Examples of these conditions were the case in which nursing-home operators collectively refused Medicaid patients while they were negotiating for higher rates, and another situation involving pharmacists who refused to fill telephone prescriptions in protest to regulations adopted by the Welfare Department.[45]

Medicaid was widely viewed as a welfare program which only incidentally provided health care. It remained a target of criticism because of the following deficiencies: the exclusion of low-income persons who were not categorically related to one of the public assistance programs; the wide variations in income eligibility levels and the generosity of each state's Medicaid program; and the seemingly uncontrollable annual increase in program expenditures. Steps are being taken to alleviate some of the more pressing problems. For example, in 1974 the Federal grants to states for aid to the aged, blind, and disabled were terminated and replaced by direct payments to the recipients through supplemental Social Security payments. This significantly altered the list of state public assistance beneficiaries and placed more responsibility on the Federal Government to determine the level of Medicaid eligibility. At the time of this writing, there are numerous bills in both houses of Congress that are designed either to drastically change Medicaid, remove it completely as a separate program, or absorb it into a larger, more comprehensive program, such as National Health Insurance.

## SOCIAL SECURITY AMENDMENTS OF 1972

As health care providers, beneficiaries, program analysts, and government auditors worked with programs under the Social Security Act, particularly Titles 2, 5, 18, and 19, it became apparent that certain changes were needed. In an effort to group all these changes into one package, a massive amendment bill was passed by Congress and signed into law late in 1972. In addition to the changes in Titles 2 and 5, the Social Security Amendments of 1972 (Public Law 92-603), contained 95 amendments to Medicare and Medicaid. Generally, the amendments were more restrictive in relation to administering the various programs and were more expansive concerning eligibility of beneficiaries and the wider range of health care coverage.

Although space does not permit a complete listing, these are some of the more prominent changes not discussed elsewhere in this chapter. Medicare is now available to a large percentage of those people under 65 years of age who are totally and permanently disabled. Also, people under 65 who need hemodialysis treatment or a kidney transplant because of a chronic kidney disease may be covered under Medicare. In addition, those people over 65 who previously were ineligible for Medicare because they had not worked long enough under Social Security can now purchase Medicare insurance. Other changes provide that advanced approval be obtained for posthospital care, the Medicaid Medical Advisory Council is abolished, family planning services are mandatory under Medicaid, the pressure is off the various states to continue expanding their Medicaid programs, and services of chiropractors, optometrists, and podiatrists are recognized and reimbursed under specified conditions.

As numerous and as comprehensive as these amendments of 1972 were, additional bills in both houses of Congress propose even further changes. Each progressive change attempts to focus on a more unified financing system and extend both coverage and eligible beneficiaries. Indeed, some observers of the current scene have stated that we are backing into National Health Insurance through Medicare.

## Professional Standards Review Organizations

Undoubtedly, the most controversial and perhaps the most significant provision of the 1972 amendments was Section 249F, the so-called Bennett amendment, that established Professional Standards Review Organizations (PSRO's). This provision is hailed by some in the health care field as the first major step toward public accountability in Federally financed programs. Other organized health care providers have gone on record as strongly opposing this program. Both factions agree, however, that this law promises to have a greater effect on health care delivery, to date, than any other legislation since Medicare.

A Professional Standards Review Organization is a group of at least 300 physicians working in a defined geographical area (a local medical society, for example) who has contracted with the Department of HEW to review the professional activities related to services provided under the Social Security Act. Among its duties, a PSRO determines whether institutional confinement is necessary and of appropriate duration, if the institutional care meets the recognized professional standards in the area, and if the care could be given as effectively in a less expensive facility or on an outpatient basis. Each health practitioner is monitored to determine that the care and treatment provided are in accordance with the criteria of the PSRO. The cost of services are not scrutinized but a PSRO has the authority to recommend an end of payments to a physician or hospital with a poor performance pattern. In extreme cases, practitioners could be recommended for removal from Medicare and Medicaid participation. It is anticipated that a PSRO will rotate virtually all its members through review panels. It can contract with hospital utilization review committees and with allied health consultants for specialized reviews. Pharmaceutical services and nurse practitioners services are examples of specialized reviews. PSRO's can review ambulatory care through provider and patient profiles, inspect health care facilities, and review provider records where pertinent. Under the law, physician-sponsored organizations are given first preference to organize a PSRO. If such organizations do not choose to assume these responsibilities in a given geographical area, the Secretary of HEW may designate another organization having professional medical competence as the PSRO for the area. At present, it is assumed that medical foundations will constitute the majority of PSRO's.[46]

## NATIONAL HEALTH INSURANCE

Certainly, to even the casual observer, there is a ferment in the reorganization of health services in the United States. In spite of earnest attempts by dedicated people to solve the problems associated with health care delivery, many of the efforts have been unsuccessful. Indeed, some of the attempted solutions actually developed additional problems. It would serve no useful purpose to list these shortcomings in this discussion but there is a fervent hope that a more positive national health policy will develop from some of these expensive lessons.

The first movement for governmental health insurance in the United States started in New York State in 1915. The State Health Insurance Bill had impressive backing from Labor, civic and women's groups, and the Governor but was opposed by manufacturers, merchants, and the State Medical Society. Although the bill passed the Senate it was blocked in the Assembly by the Speaker who denounced this and other welfare measures as "Bolshevistic."[4 7]

It would be redundant to say that times have changed, since it is almost certain that some form of National Health Insurance will be officially in existence sometime in the near future. The United States is now the only industrial nation which does not have either national health insurance or a national health service. With the public expecting more services from their rising tax dollar and the seeking of "cradle-to-grave" security, the legislators are responding by preparing government-sponsored health care financing to be available to essentially all citizens. This has been called "social medicine" by some and "political medicine" by others.

At the time of this writing there are ten bills in Congress that describe different forms of National Health Insurance and new bills are being introduced almost monthly. These bills are the following:

1. Comprehensive Health Insurance Program.
2. National Health Care Services Reorganization and Financing Act.
3. Health Security Act.
4. Health Care Insurance Act.
5. National Catastrophic Illness Protection Act.
6. National Health Insurance and Health Services Improvement Act.
7. National Health Care Act.
8. Catastrophic Illness Insurance Act.
9. National Comprehensive Health Benefits Act.
10. Catastrophic Health Insurance and Medical Assistance Reform Act.

According to professional observers of the legislative health scene, the eventual form of National Health Insurance probably will be a compromise between the Catastrophic Health Insurance and Medical Assistance Reform Act, which is primarily a comprehensive extension of the Social Security Act; the Administration-backed Comprehensive Health Insurance Program, that relies heavily on HMO's, plus private insurance companies, Blue Cross and Blue Shield as carriers; and the Kennedy–Griffiths' Health Security Act, the most liberal of all the proposals.

It must be remembered that each of these proposals, with the probable exception of the Health Security Act, is a method of financing health care and not a method of delivery. The natural question that is expected to rise after the passage of a National Health Insurance is, "Is this enough?" As stated by Dr. David Rogers at the 83rd Shattuck Lecture,

"Thus, I have the belief, shared by many, that any form of national financing of health services will create a series of expectations for Americans that are not likely to be fulfilled if we continue our current ways of delivering health care."[4 8]

As these expectations continue to rise, forces are created which promise to have a fundamental bearing on the future of health services in this country. Stemming from the concept that "health is a right and not a privilege," look for a new public attitude which states that the main issue is not the availability of medical care, as such, but the *national maintenance of individual health*. Thus, the United States may then be preparing to take yet another step toward National Health Service.

## REFERENCES

1. Haviland, J. W. Next steps in meeting the nation's health goals. *Bull. N. Y. Acad. Med., 41:* 1255-1267, 1965.
2. Health Resources Statistics, 1972-73. National Center for Health Statistics. DHEW Publication No. (HSM) 73-1509, 1973.
3. Magraw, R. M. *Ferment in Medicine: A Study of the Essence of Medical Practice.* Philadelphia: W. B. Saunders Co., 1966, pp. 152-153.
4. Medical News: Journal American Medical Association. *220:* June 12, 1971.
5. National Commission on Community Health Services. *Health Is a Community Affair.* Cambridge, Massachusetts: Harvard University Press, 1967.
6. *Meeting the Challenge of Family Practice.* The report of the *ad hoc* Committee on Education for Family Practice of the Council on Medical Education. Chicago: American Medical Association, 1966.
7. Education number. J.A.M.A., *226:* 986, 1973.
8. Somers, H. M., and Somers, A. R. *Doctors, Patients, and Health Insurance.* Washington, D. C.: The Brookings Institution, 1961.

9. *Group Practice–Guidelines to Joining or Forming a Medical Group.* American Association of Medical Clinics. Chicago: American Medical Association and Medical Group Management Association, Ed., 2, 1970.

10. Fein, R. *The Doctor Shortage–An Economic Diagnosis.* Washington, D.C.: The Brookings Institution, 1967.

11. National Conference on Group Practice. *Promoting the Group Practice of Medicine.* Public Health Service Publication 1750. Washington, D. C.: United States Public Health Service, 1968.

12. MacLeod, G. K., and Prussin, J. A. The continuing evolution of health maintenance organizations *N. Engl. J. Med., 288:* 439-443, 1973.

13. American Medical News: American Medical Association. December 24, 1973, p. 6.

14. Egdahl, R. H. Foundations for Medical Care. *N Engl. J. Med., 288:* 491-498, 1973.

15. American Association of Foundations for Medical Care. General Information, 540 E. Market St., Stockton, Cal. 95201.

16. American Medical News: American Medical Association. November 6, 1972; December 11, 1972.

17. *Doctor's Unions–Down and Out? Med. Econ.,* Sept. 17, 1973, pp. 45-58.

18. *Hospital Statistics, 1972.* Chicago: American Hospital Association,1973.

19. Sadler, A. M. Jr., *The Physician's Assistant–Today and Tomorrow.* Sadler, B. L. and Bliss, A. A. New Haven: Yale University Press, 1972.

20. Horowitz, S. M. Personal Communication. National Coordinator Physician's Assistant Program, Office of Special Programs, DHEW, Health Resources Administration, Bethesda, Md., November 12, 1973.

21. Kluge, D. N., Wegryn, R. L., and Lemley, B. R. The expanding emergency department. *J.A.M.A., 191:* 801-805, 1965.

22. Report for Fiscal Year 1972 of the Hill-Burton Health Care Facilities Service, DHEW Publication No. (HSM) 73-4034. Washington, D. C.: Health Service and Mental Health Administration, 1973.

23. Baehr, G. The hospital as a center of community medical care: facts and fiction. *Amer. J. Pub. Health, 54:* 1653-1660, 1964.

24. Manion, M. E. Rent an office from the hospital. *Med. Econ.,* 44: 73-76, 1967.

25. Elements of Progressive Patient Care, Public Health Service Publication 930-C-1. Washington, D. C.: United States Public Health Service, revised 1962.

26. Personal communication from Congressman Morris K. Udall, Representative from 2nd District of Arizona to the U. S. Congress. Information on the various government services was supplied to Congressman Udall by the Legislative Reference Service of the Library of Congress, November 15, 1973.

27. Personal communication from B. J. Dietz, CDR, MSC, USN, Director, Data Processing Division, Bureau of Medicine and Surgery, Department of the Navy, Jan. 3rd, 1974.

28. Cowen, D. L. Community health-a local government responsibility. *J. Amer. Pub. Health Assn., 61:* 2005-2009, 1971.

29. Hilleboe, H. E. Public Health in the United States in the 1970's. *J. Amer. Pub. Assn. 58:* 1588-1610, 1968.

30. Sbarbaro, J. A. *Local Health Departments and the Future: An Iliad or an Odyssey,* pp. 143-145. Cave. V. G. *Health Departments: An Ombudsman Role?,* pp. 149-151. Communicable Disease Control Conference, Houston, Texas, March 13-16, 1972. DHEW Publication No. (H.S.M.) 73-8172, U.S. Government Printing Office, 1973.

31. Pan American Health Organization, 1972 Annual Report of the Director, Document No. 124, 1973.

32. National Health insurance Reports, *3:* 26, Dec. 31, 1973.

33. Washington Newsletter, APHA, Jan. 1974.

34. Murphy, R. L. H., Jr., and Bird, K. T. Telediagnosis: A new community health resource. *Amer. J. Pub. Health, 64:* 2, 1974.

35. Crevasse, L. and Ariet, M. A new scaler electrocardiographic computer program. *J.A.M.A., 226:* 9, 1973.

36. National Health Insurance Reports, Feb. 11, 1974.

37. Hospital and Surgical Coverage among Persons under 65 Years of Age in the United States. Vital Statistics Report, 21: 9, Dec., 1972.

38. National Health Expenditures. Research and Statistics Note, DHEW Pub. No. (SSA) 74-11701, No. 3, 1974.

39. Washington Report on Medicine and Health, Jan. 28, 1974.

40. Weekly Pharmacy Reports, 23:8, 1974.

41. Carlucci, F. C. The future outlook for delivery of human services. Health Services Reports, *88:* 10, 1973.

42. Annual Report. Kaiser Foundation Health Plan, Inc., 1972.

43. Fiscal Year 1975 Health Program Memorandum of HEW. Congressional Record-Senate, 93rd Congress, 119:117, 1973.

44. Brownfield, A. Medicaid: The anatomy of a failure. *Private Practice,* Nov., 1973.

45. Callahan, J. J. Poor people and the medical care crisis. *N. Engl. J. Med., 286:* 23, 1972.

46. Mahoney, F. PSRO's: What they are, how they work. Mod. Med., Oct. 29, 1973.

47. Terris, M. Crisis and change in America's health system. *Amer. J. Pub. Health, 63:* 4, 1973.

48. Rogers, D. E. Shattuck lecture–The American health-care scene. *N. Engl. J. Med., 288:* 1377-1383, 1973.

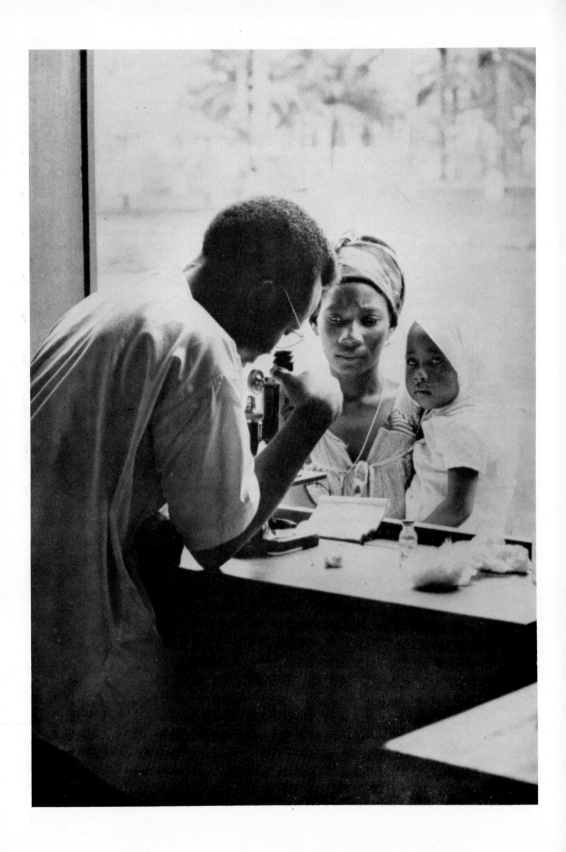

# 4

# The methodology of public health

To carefully observe the phenomena of life in all its phases, normal and perverted, to make perfect that most difficult of all arts, the art of observation, to call to aid the science of experimentation, to cultivate the reasoning faculty, so as to be able to know the true from the false—these are our methods.

WILLIAM OSLER

The reasonable man adapts himself to the world; the unreasonable one persists in trying to adapt the world to himself. Therefore all progress depends on the unreasonable man.

GEORGE BERNARD SHAW

---

Public health developed in response to the challenge of epidemic diseases. From time immemorial, man has sought ways to prevent the onslaught of the dread effects of plague, cholera, typhus, malaria, and a host of other devastating pestilences. Hippocrates was an acute observer of the natural history of disease. In "Air, Waters, and Places," he points out the danger of locating towns near marshes or swamps. Attempts to prevent the spread of epidemics by quarantine go back to ancient days. Isolation of contagious individuals also has a long history. It was not until the advent of Edward Jenner with cowpox vaccine near the end of the 18th century that a reliably effective method of preventing an important epidemic disease became available.

In the 19th century came the era of sanitary reform. Control of diseases spread through the intestinal discharges became possible. Cholera and typhoid fever began to wane in Europe and America as pure water supplies and sewerage systems became fairly common. Modern public health developed in the mid-19th century primarily to foster this sanitary revolution.

During the past 100 years, public health has grown and matured. While it still concerns itself with the control of infectious diseases, that responsibility now represents perhaps less than half of the total program. In reaching an assessment of the relative importance of the many health problems confronting a community, public health has developed and made use of two important methods. These highly regarded tools of public health workers are: (1) epidemiology, and (2) biostatistics.

## EPIDEMIOLOGY

Strictly speaking, epidemiology is the science treating of epidemics. Others have defined the term as the natural history of disease. Dr. John R. Paul of Yale University[1] defines epidemiology as the study of the circumstances under which diseases occur, where diseases tend to flourish, and where they do not. A more comprehensive definition has been provided by the late Dr. K. F. Maxcy, one of the distinguished American practitioners of the science. According to Maxcy[2] epidemiology is "that field of medical science which is concerned with the relationships of the various factors and conditions which determine the frequencies and distributions of an infectious process, a disease, or a physiological state in a community." In contrast to the physician, the unit of study for the epidemiologist is the group or population rather than the individual.

The purpose of epidemiology is to gain sufficient knowledge of the natural characteristics and distribution of a disease to enable the formulation of effective measures of prevention. It has been particularly valuable in leading to the discovery of causative agents of disease, in evaluating factors in susceptibility, in clarifying modes of transmission, and in demonstrating the importance of environmental influences on the development of disease.

Even in the days before Pasteur, Koch and other bacteriologists had clearly proved the "germ" theory of disease; pioneer epidemiologists using extraordinary powers of observation and analysis of data made important contributions to our knowledge of disease transmission. In 1842, Oliver Wendell Holmes of Boston[3] collected data on the incidence of puerperal, or childbed fever, from the practicing physicians of that city. His analysis of the information obtained showed that physicians and nurses attending one woman with the dread fever were likely to carry the infection to their next obstetrical case.

The contribution of a Danish physician, Peter Ludwig Panum, in the study of measles is outstanding. At 26 years of age and fresh from medical school, Panum was sent by his government to the Faroe Islands to report on a serious epidemic of measles then raging. These islands had been free of measles since 1781. When the 1846 epidemic struck, 6000 of the 7782 inhabitants came down with .the disease. By following the spread of measles from village to village and from island to island, Panum established the incubation period of measles at 13 to 14 days. He supplied good evidence of the long lasting immunity in measles, having interviewed 98 old people who had previous attacks in 1781 and all of whom escaped in 1846. Panum concludes that it was everywhere clear that the disease had spread from man to man as a result of some kind of contagious material. He also states that the contagium was transmitted in the early eruptive stage of measles.[4]

In London, John Snow[5] studied the outbreaks of cholera in 1848 and 1854 and clearly demonstrated that cholera occurred in an irregular distribution, which coincided with certain sources of water supply. He argued convincingly that the agent of cholera was taken in by drinking contaminated water.

William Budd from 1840 to 1860 investigated outbreaks of typhoid fever in England. He recognized the contagiousness of the disease and proclaimed that the infective agent was acquired by drinking water contaminated with intestinal discharges of a typhoid patient. He stated that the incubation period for typhoid fever is between 10 and 14 days and urged that all excreta and soiled linen from typhoid cases be thoroughly disinfected.[6]

As a result of the brilliant discoveries of the bacteriologists, parasitologists, and others during the years from 1860 on, emphasis came to be directed far too much to the specific infective agent of disease. In the pursuit of knowledge about the agent, the main objective—a thorough understanding of all aspects of a disease—was frequently lost. Many workers in the field of epidemiology contributed to rethinking of disease as it affects man. One of the best equipped minds in microbiology set himself the task of voicing the new philosophy of

infection. Theobald Smith in 1934 in his small volume, *Parasitism and Disease,*[7] translated epidemiology in the terms of biology. Infectious disease he explained as a manifestation of parasitism, an interplay between the host and infectious agent. Smith recognized disease as a resultant of the forces within a dynamic system consisting of the agent of disease, the host, and the environment. Whether infection with an agent results in disease depends on all three elements. Known agents of disease include those of physical, chemical, and biological nature. Some non-living agents may produce mass disease as readily as do microorganisms, for example, lead poisoning. On the other hand, mass disease may result from an absence or deficiency of an agent, as of nicotinic acid in pellagra or Vitamin C in scurvy.

An agent is usually classified as a pathogen if it is able to incite disease in a susceptible animal. Some strains of an agent are regarded as more virulent than others; that is, some strains of living agents possess greater disease-inciting powers. One measurement of virulence is the number of organisms required to kill selected groups of animals under standardized conditions within a certain time period.

Other important characteristics of pathogens are communicability and invasiveness. By communicability is meant the ability of the organism to spread from host to host. Invasiveness denotes the ability of the organism to spread throughout the tissues of the host.

Every living agent has its own biological and biochemical characteristics which give it the ability to multiply in the host tissue.

Successful parasitic agents do not ordinarily kill their usual hosts, since loss of a high percentage of host animals endangers the parasite's survival. It is important for the parasite to succeed in leaving the body of the host before death or recovery and to enter the tissues of a new host.

Contribution of the host factor in the causation of disease is partly through inherited characteristics and by age, sex, race, geographical isolation, and other considerations. Acquired host characteristics such as immunity resulting from previous infection or from artificial immunization are the most common factors. The physiological state of the host, for example, malnutrition or pregnancy, clearly affects response to the agent. Habits and customs, such as religious restrictions, affect the health of people. Some groups eat no pork or seafood; some drink no milk; some have high standards of personal hygiene; others are infested with lice.

The causative agent and the susceptible host are not carrying on their combat *in vacuo*. The environmental conditions affect the result. These environmental factors include living conditions, housing, nutrition, family size, occupation, and climatic and seasonal variations. Investigation of the environment is an essential feature in all epidemiological studies.

Recognition that there are multiple factors in play in determining the distribution and occurrence of each disease has greatly enlarged the scope of epidemiology. Indeed, the tendency now is to interpret disease phenomena in terms of ecology, an expression borrowed from the biologists. Ecology deals with the mutual relationships of organisms and their environment. The typhoid bacillus or the influenza virus have their life cycles, their requirements for reproduction, their nutritional necessities, and so on, as do bobcats, horses, or humans. To understand infectious disease, one must become familiar with the factors necessary for the continuity of the life cycle of pathogenic organisms.

The ecological situation determines the kinds of disease that could prevail should the specific disease agent be present or be introduced. The climate, soil, and flora in a region determine the fauna. In India there is a large monkey population. These monkeys are known to be susceptible to yellow fever virus. Mosquitoes known to be efficient transmitters of yellow fever are widely distributed throughout India. As far as is known, yellow fever has never been introduced into India, but it appears highly likely that the disease would flourish there, if given the opportunity. The government of India takes careful measures to prevent the entry of the yellow fever virus. As for yellow fever, man is not at all necessary to the maintenance of the disease in nature. In South America, yellow fever virus thrives in the monkey population, being carried from an infected monkey to a non-immune one by certain species of forest mosquitoes. It is suspected that other life cycles are also available in nature to the yellow fever virus.

## Methods of Epidemiology

Research physicians undertake their studies on individual patients or by the use of groups of experimental animals. The epidemiologist has the community for his laboratory. He is concerned with a population, large or small, at any rate, with groups of people. He brings modern clinical and laboratory methods into the field. Generally, a household or family is his unit for study. Disease in the field is seen in all degrees of severity, not only cases ill enough to require medical attention, but mild illnesses or inapparent infections that are not ordinarily seen by a physician. In field studies, disease is searched for, instead of being revealed when a patient seeks medical care.

Laboratory techniques are an essential element in epidemiology. Samples may be taken of the air, or the food, or the water used by the group under investigation. Indeed, the object of the inquiry is to understand disease as it occurs among humans, animals, birds, and the arthropod population in their natural environment.

This kind of field study has led to a team approach. Members of the team come from such professionals as physicians, nurses, laboratory experts, veterinarians, entomologists, zoologists, anthropologists, geneticists, and sanitary engineers. In dealing with people, the public health nurse has proved a highly valuable asset in all field studies.

In planning all field investigations and in the analysis of the data collected, the biostatistician is an irreplaceable team member. The epidemiologist, usually equipped with at least a rudimentary understanding of biostatistics, will, if he is wise, lean heavily on his expert associate in biometry in planning the project and at all stages of his field studies and for the analysis of all data. A number of highly useful treatises on the methods of the epidemiologist have appeared in recent years.[8-11]

The problems that epidemiolgoists are called upon to investigate vary greatly. Some study short-term, self-limited outbreaks of food poisoning. Others spend years on such slow moving diseases as rheumatic fever, tuberculosis, or leprosy. For some 30 years, scientists have studied the natural history of yellow fever as it occurs in the tropical forests. After this intensive and prolonged research on several continents, the puzzle of yellow fever remains only partially clarified.

Whatever may be the problem set for investigation in the field, the kinds of information required are basically the same. First comes the definition of the problem. If it be tuberculosis, which criteria constitute a case of tuberculosis?

What is meant by a tuberculosis death? If diphtheria or poliomyelitis, which criteria are required for diagnosis of a case?

*Time*

All epidemiological problems must be studied in respect to time. Some communicable diseases have a well-known, but poorly understood, seasonal variation. In the temperate zone, measles is most prevalent in spring and occurs less frequently in summer. Poliomyelitis, on the other hand, has its peak occurrence in late summer and early autumn. Of course, in the United States, mosquito-borne infections are confined to the warm months.

Other diseases show peaks of epidemicity at longer intervals. These diseases have years of high prevalence interspersed with years of low prevalence. This characteristic is common to scarlet fever and to influenza.

It is important to note any clustering of cases in respect to time. Outbreaks of food poisoning usually demonstrate a very short incubation period, so that a sharp rise in cases points to some recent common exposure, such as a school picnic or a wedding reception. In

situations in which the interval between the presumed cause and the effect is prolonged, interpretation is more difficult and less certain.

This clustering of cases can be graphically shown by charts showing numbers of cases by time intervals. In Figure 4.1, an outbreak of gastroenteritis at Morgantown, West Virginia, is depicted by hour of onset of cases. This outbreak occurred in September, 1967, following ingestion by hundreds of individuals of contaminated ice at a football game.

*Place*

Biological environment determines the geography of disease. Plague is endemic in the rodent population of most of the western United States. Cholera apparently is present continuously in northeastern India; yellow fever occurs in Brazil, some contiguous countries, and tropical Africa. Under certain favorable circumstances, these diseases have appeared in widespread epidemics in regions usually free of them. One does not expect to encounter epidemics of malaria in areas free of the anopheline mosquito.

Other diseases are extremely widespread and

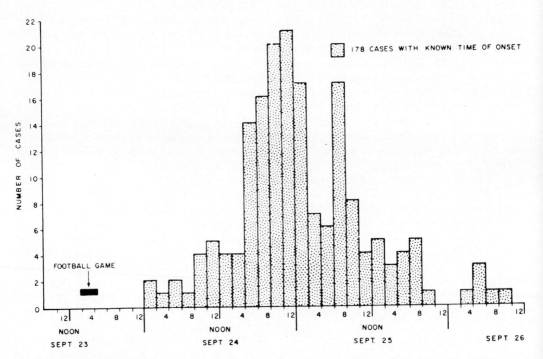

Fig. 4.1. Epidemic of gastroenteritis by hour of onset, Morgantown, West Virginia, September, 1967. Source: National Communicable Disease Center. *Mortality and Morbidity Report,* Vol. 16, no. 41. Public Health Service, October 14, 1967, pp. 346–347.

may occur in any part of the world, for example, influenza, syphilis, and rabies.

Chemical and physical environment may be significant. The degree of pollution of water or air in one place may play a role in disease. The lack of iodine in the soil results in thyroid disease in some areas.

The social environment as it affects housing, sanitation, level of education, and type of occupation is of profound importance in the distribution of communicable disease.

The distribution of cases by location in any outbreak under investigation is best shown on a spot map. Figure 4.2 provides an illustration of such a map.

### Characteristics of People

Age is a highly significant variable in the study of disease in a group. Association of age with disease frequency has been noted in all diseases. To compare disease incidence of one population with that of another, one has to take account of any age differences. Some diseases are known as "childhood diseases," for example, whooping cough and measles. The opportunity for infection early in life is so common that in all civilized countries infection and a resulting immunity occurs during the childhood years. When introduced to isolated peoples, these diseases attack adults as readily as children.

Adults are more subject to chronic diseases and degenerative processes, which may represent an accumulation of insults to the body over the years.

The age of individuals has a determining role on the range of activities. The infant is largely confined to his own household, the child joins the school population and ranges widely in the community; the adult has an occupation which strongly influences his health status; and the elderly are frequently confined to their homes in their last years.

### Sex

Differences in the distribution of disease by sex may be physiological or environmental. Pregnancy, menstruation, and varying biological

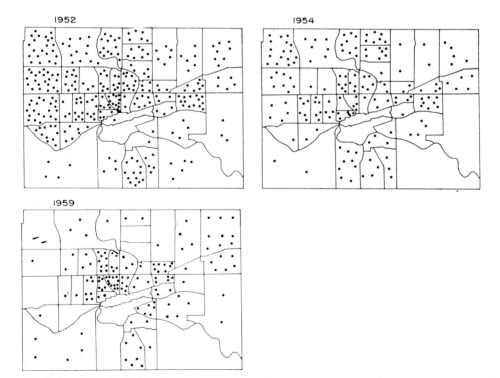

Fig. 4.2. Distribution of reported poliomyelitis cases, by census tract, Des Moines, Iowa, 1952, 1954, and 1959. Source: Chin, T. D. Y., Marine, W. M., Hall, E. C., Gravelle, C. R., and Speers, J. F. Poliomyelitis in Des Moines, Iowa, 1959. *Amer. J. Hyg., 74:* 67–94, 1961.

cycles exert definite influences on susceptibility to infections. Certainly women in all surveys of illness report more episodes of sickness than do men. On the other hand, life expectancy for men is less than for women. Also, death rates in females are falling more rapidly than in men.

Environmental factors play a role in influencing disease as related to sex. Women generally have different occupations than men. Their habit patterns vary from men's in a variety of ways, for example, recreations, food intake, alcohol consumption, and use of tobacco. Females are more likely to spend more time at home and in domestic occupations than do males. To some extent, this affects exposure to infectious agents.

### Ethnic Group

This term is used to denote groups of the population who have a greater degree of homogeneity than does the general population being considered. Race is also employed but has a less clear-cut significance. Ethnic groups may be selected on the basis of national origin, religion, local social units, or socially isolated groups.

Fruitful studies have been undertaken of the mortality from cancer among Japanese and Chinese groups living in the United States in comparison to the rates prevailing in their native lands. Similar studies have been done on tuberculosis as it occurs among Negroes in Philadelphia in comparison with Negroes of Jamaica.

Another illustration of the importance of ethnic groups in the study of disease is the low frequency of cancer of the uterine cervix among Jewish women in the United States as compared with the high rates prevailing among the women of Puerto Rican origin.

### Occupation

The kind of work an individual performs is an excellent measure of his socio-economic standard in the community. Knowledge of the precise daily occupation of people may identify hazards associated with exposure to toxic substances or to dangerous microorganisms. Such industrial poisons as phosphorus, lead, and benzene frequently have been causes of serious outbreaks of illness. Exposure to hides may lead to anthrax infections. Workers in poultry-processing plants are subject to expo-sure to psittacosis. Air pollutants in some industries are now recognized as health hazards.

### Marital Status

Married persons are more likely to be living in family groups than are the single, widowed, or divorced individuals of the community. In general, mortality rates for many diseases are more favorable for those living in the marital state than for others. The reasons for this are not altogether clear. Possibly those in a poor state of health are less likely to marry. At any rate, marriage brings changes in the way of life for most people.

### Analysis of Data

When the field studies have been completed, and the results of laboratory tests on material collected are available, the analysis of the data is undertaken. Of course, analysis of incomplete data may be carried out periodically in long-term studies. One undertakes to determine the distribution of the onsets of illness by time and by geographic location of cases. To express the pertinent data numerically, one calculates the attack rates to determine selectivity of the illness by age, sex, race, or other significant factors. By attack rate is meant[2]:

$$\frac{\text{No. of cases of a particular disease developing during a specified time period}}{\substack{\text{Average population present} \\ \text{during the same time period}}} \times 100$$

This attack rate or case rate provides knowledge of the incidence of the particular disease during a given time period. The term prevalence of a disease is used in epidemiology to give a cross-section of disease as it is occurring at a *specified point of time.*

All other pertinent data, such as from environmental studies on sanitation, water, and food and milk supplies, are considered as they possibly relate to frequency and distribution of the disease under investigation.

### Formulation of a Hypothesis

The information provided by the analysis of data must be weighed and all reasonable hypotheses to explain the epidemic must be considered. If at all possible, the epidemiologist should come up with a hypothesis to explain the causal factor of the disease and the mode by which the agent is transmitted to man. Also, definite information as to the time relationship between the cause and disease effect should be revealed.

It is obvious that other professional discipline—such as clinical medicine, with its careful detailed studies on individual patients, and that of the experimental microbiologist—provide advance knowledge to the epidemiologist for application in the field. Studies in the hospital of cases of the disease under investigation in the field frequently give the clue required for successful solution of the inquiry.

*Testing the Hypothesis*

It may be assumed that some kind of association exists between the suspected factor and the disease; otherwise, one would not have formulated the hypothesis. To test the hypothesis, additional information may be required, so that other field observations may be necessary.

In many investigations, the epidemiologist has had to conduct experimental procedures to prove the validity of the hypothesis. An illustration of such a situation is provided by Goldberger's studies on pellagra. His surveys of families in cotton mill villages and of institutional outbreaks of pellagra in southern United States convinced him that pellagra was due to dietary deficiency, and that it was not an infectious process, as previously believed. To prove the validity of this conclusion, Goldberger undertook experiments. He demonstrated that pellagra could be prevented by provision of balanced diets in institutions, and that by feeding deficient diets to volunteers in prisons pellagra could be produced among the men subjected to such inadequate food supplies. As described by Terris, it was many years later that the specific dietary substance essential to prevent pellagra was proved to be niacin, a member of the Vitamin B group.[12]

Another example of experimental epidemiology involved the testing of a hypothesis that intake of fluorides acts to prevent dental decay. Two large-scale studies enduring over a period of years have been carried out in the United States. In each instance, two towns have been selected; one had fluorides added to the water supply; the other had none, but served as a control population. Newburgh and Kingston in New York state and Grand Rapids and Muskegon, Michigan, were the sites of the investigations. In both studies, the population of the town receiving fluorides developed significantly less dental decay, especially among the children.

Other investigators have undertaken long-term studies of colonies of experimental animals to test epidemiological hypotheses. Such questions as the effect of nutritional deficiencies or the effect of crowding on infectious diseases have received careful attention by experimenters.

*Family Studies*

The family is the smallest unit of the community. Ordinarily, personal contact is more intimate and frequent in families than in any other group. Many useful studies of diseases spread by personal contact have been done by examination and continuous follow-up of selected families.

The first case that appears in the family is termed the "primary" case. By studying a sufficiently large group of families, it is possible to determine accurately the interval between the appearance of the primary case and the occurrence of secondary cases. This period is the incubation time of the disease and is a characteristic for each type of infection. From the occurrence of secondary cases, the attack rate by age and sex can be calculated. This rate indicates the degree of contagiousness of a communicable disease and also provides an opportunity for the assessment of preventive measures, such as $\gamma$-globulin or vaccination for the protection of exposed susceptibles.

A few diseases are notably associated with family groups. Tuberculosis has been studied most fruitfully as a familial disease. It is difficult to determine to what degree these familial aggregations of tuberculosis are due to inherited susceptibility or to greater opportunities for close and repeated exposure to infection. Other environmental factors such as crowding, nutrition, personal hygiene, and so on are of undoubted importance in rendering some families more liable to tuberculosis. However, evidence points to an enhanced susceptibility of some families on a genetic basis.

*Serological Surveys*

The testing for specific antibodies in serum samples is of great value in studying the distribution of communicable diseases. These tests can be rapidly done on a large scale and usually at a modest cost. When interpreted with care, these tests may give valuable information as to current infections in the population and also reveal the incidence of past infections. The techniques of these immunity tests vary widely. For some agents, complement fixation gives the best results; others are best revealed by neutralization, by hemagglutination inhibition, or by other tests. It is essential that the tests be carried out and be interpreted by technicians expert in their use.

If the immunity test is to be employed for the diagnosis of individual cases, it is necessary to obtain a serum in the early stages of the illness and a convalescent serum sample from two to six weeks later. The diagnosis is established by a significant rise in specific antibody titer in the interval between the acute phase serum specimen and the one taken in the convalescent period.

Surveys of immunity in population groups have been widely used. One of the first was undertaken by The Rockefeller Foundation in cooperation with a large number of national health agencies around the world to determine the distribution of immunity to yellow fever. During the period 1930 to 1941, thousands of sera were tested by the mouse protection method. It was established that yellow fever had been present in large areas of South America and Africa where it had previously been unsuspected. Likewise, it was clear from the survey that yellow fever had not been present in the Far East during the lifetime of those whose sera was tested.

Another disease in which immunity surveys have yielded highly useful information is poliomyelitis. Serological surveys of tropical cities revealed that virtually all children were infected by the virus of poliomyelitis. Serological surveys of tropical cities revealed that virtually all children were infected by the virus of poliomyelitis during the first years of life—an age at which few paralytic cases occur. The disease had been endemic and almost silent. This was the situation in cities like Bombay and Cairo and Manila, while epidemics of paralytic poliomyelitis were occurring in western Europe and North America with increasing frequency.

Two points must be considered in planning serological surveys. One is the specificity of the test to be used. All biological tests have their limitations. The limitations of usefulness of the tests to be employed in a given study must be thoroughly understood and kept in mind during planning of the survey and in the interpretation of results. The other important aspect of surveys is the selection of a representative sample to be tested. In this selection, the constant advice of a competent biostatistician is most valuable.

## Epidemiological Studies of Chronic Diseases

As the part played by acute diseases as a cause of death and sickness is diminishing, the importance of chronic infective and degenerative diseases has increased. This is in part due to the greater number of people living to middle and old age spans. Perhaps other causes of increase in chronic disease are environmental— greater stress, air pollution, toxic hazards, and over-rich diets.

In applying the epidemiological method to the study of chronic disease, the same questions are posed as in the study of acute problems. The principal inquiry is in respect to the distribution of the disease in the population and to those factors that influence this distribution. The epidemiologist investigating chronic disease studies the changes in frequency of the disease over a period, its occurrence by geographical areas, and the frequency of disease by sex, race, age, socio-economic class, occupation, individual living habits, and known exposure to harmful agents.

One chronic disease that has reached almost epidemic proportions in the United States is cancer of the lung. Many studies have indicated that most lung cancer patients are cigarette smokers. Of those who do smoke, a larger proportion of the lung cancer cases is found among the heavy smokers. This type of study is called retrospective, backward looking. One starts with cases of the disease and studies them for a history of the suspected cause.

Another approach to the study of this problem has been undertaken by Hammond and Horn.[13] In 1952, these investigators obtained histories of smoking habits of about 190,000 men aged 50 to 69 years; these men were traced for 44 months. Death certificates of all who died during the study period were obtained. During the period of the study,

11,870 men died. Primary cancer of the lung was recorded as the cause of 448 deaths. Of these men, 15 had never smoked and eight had smoked only occasionally, whereas 397 had smoked cigarettes regularly. Twenty-eight had smoked only pipes or cigars. Death rates from lung cancer increased markedly with the number of cigarettes regularly smoked in the last years of life. See Figure 4.3 for a graphic presentation of these data.

In Figure 4.4 are given additional data collected by Hammond and Horn in their study. In this figure, data on bronchogenic cancer in relation to urban or rural residence and in respect to a history of cigarette smoking are presented. Lung cancer death rates are higher among regular cigarette smokers than among non-regular smokers regardless of whether they lived in rural or urban areas. However, among those who resided in urban areas, the lung cancer death rates were higher for cigarette smokers than among corresponding rural smokers. The study shows definitely that the effect of smoking in the production of lung cancer is far greater than is the effect of urban residence alone.

Many other chronic disease problems are now being extensively investigated by epidemiological methods. Coronary heart attacks, cancer of the breast, and rheumatoid arthritis are among the most important now under study. Indications are that the team approach combining the methods of clinicians, laboratory researchers, statisticians, and epidemiologists along with many other professional groups will produce answers that have so long been sought to the knotty questions posed by these important diseases.[14,15]

## THE VALUE OF BIOSTATISTICS

The health officer and the epidemiologist deal with populations or with selected groups of a population. To obtain reliable information from the comparison of groups of people, it is necessary to have certain knowledge of the comparability of one group with another. One must know the distribution of the individuals making up the groups in respect to such important biological variables as age, sex, race, occupation, place of residence, and so on. No meaningful comparisons can be made of public health data from one community with those of another without adjustments to correct differences in these variables.

## Health Indices

The most common statistical terms used in public health are employed to express in a generally acceptable manner data relating to births, deaths, or the occurrence of disease. These data are expressed as rates and are stated for a definite period of time, usually one year, but any other convenient time period may be selected. Mortality rates are usually stated in terms of the number of deaths per 1000. Disease rates are commonly given as the number of cases per 100,000 of the population, although for diseases of extremely rare incidence the rate may be expressed as the number of cases per 1 million of the population. Custom and convenience determine the choice of method of expressing these data.

In the analysis of health data a great many different kinds of rates are used. Each serves to provide a different variety of information, but all are based on the same principles. A frequently used formula is the crude death rate. This rate is determined as follows:

$$\frac{\text{No. of deaths for one year}}{\text{Estimated midyear population}} \times 1000$$

The crude death rate means that for each 1000 of the population under consideration, an average of 9.0 or 12.0, or whatever the figure may be, individuals died during the period of observation, usually one year. The death rate is a composite of the rates affecting the various segments of the population. If there is a preponderance of elderly individuals in the population, the crude death rate may be expected to be higher than for a younger population. Death rates among non-whites are generally higher than among the white population. If there are large numbers of non-whites in the population being studied, one may expect to find the death rates affected toward the higher side. These factors make it clear that rates can be fruitfully compared only if the populations from which the data are drawn are comparable. For this reason, comparisons can best be made in terms of data from specific groups of the population.

Rates applying to selected segments of the population are known as specific rates. These rates may be made specific for any factor such as age, sex, race, occupation group or for any

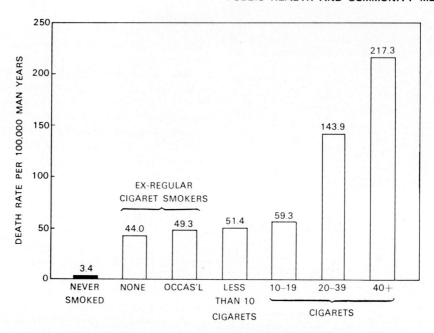

Fig. 4.3. Age-adjusted death rates of well-established cases of bronchogenic carcinoma (exclusive of adenocarcinoma) by number of cigarettes smoked daily. Source: Hammond, E. C., and Horn, D. Smoking and death rates. Report on 44 months of follow-up of 187,783 men. *J.A.M.A. 166:* 1294–1308, 1958.

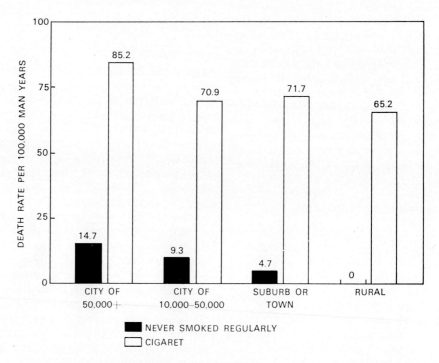

Fig. 4.4. Age standardized death rates due to well-established cases of bronchogenic carcinoma (exclusive of adenocarcinoma) by urban-rural classification. Rates for cigarette smokers are compared with those for men who never smoked regularly. Source: Hammond, E. C., and Horn, D. Smoking and death rates. Report on 44 months of follow-up of 187,783 men. *J.A.M.A., 166:* 1294–1308, 1958.

selected group being studied, as long as the number of deaths, the numerator, can be related to the population group being considered.

Such a specific rate of frequent interest is the maternal mortality rate. This rate expresses the risk of women dying in childbirth. The data for this rate are derived as follows: the total number of deaths due to causes related to childbirth occurring during the specified time period, usually one year, is the numerator. The denominator might be made of the segment of the population exposed to the risks of childbirth, *i.e.,* the total number of females who became pregnant during the year. This is a difficult or impossible number to obtain, so another figure is employed, that of the number of live births occurring in the population during the year. Stillbirths are not included as the stillbirth data are so unreliable. The maternal mortality rate for a particular population is defined as follows:

$$\frac{\text{Deaths due to maternal causes}}{\text{No. of live births}} \times 1000$$

Sickness rates are also widely employed. These rates are usually calculated on an annual basis using data derived from cases reported to health departments. Depending upon the frequency of the disease, the case rates for the disease may be expressed as cases per 100, per 1000, per 10,000, per 100,000, or per million of the population. The rate is computed as follows:

$$\frac{\text{No. of cases of the disease for one year}}{\text{Estimated midyear population}} \times 1000 \text{ or other unit}$$

Many other rates are used in expressing public health information relating to death and disease. These specific rates are highly valuable in permitting meaningful comparisons of data from one segment of the population with another. In addition to the rates already described, the following ones are frequently used in expressing health information:

*1. Crude Birth Rate*

$$\frac{\text{No. of registered births in one year}}{\text{Average population during the period}} \times 1000$$

*2. Age-specific Death Rate*

$$\frac{\text{No. of deaths in a certain age group } (e.g., 15-24)}{\text{Average population in same age group during the same period}} \times 1000$$

*3. Infant Mortality Rate*

$$\frac{\text{No. of deaths under 1 year of age in one year}}{\text{No. of live births during the year}} \times 1000$$

*4. Neonatal Mortality Rate*

$$\frac{\text{No. of deaths under 28 days of age in one year}}{\text{No. of live births during the year}} \times 1000$$

*5. Case Fatality Rate*

$$\frac{\text{No. of deaths from a specific cause}}{\text{No. of cases of the same cause}} \times 100$$

*6. Incidence Rate*

$$\frac{\text{No. of new cases occurring in one year (or other period)}}{\text{Midperiod population (usually midyear)}} \times 100,000$$

*7. Prevalence Rate*

$$\frac{\text{No. of existing cases at a particular time}}{\text{Population at the given time}} \times 100,000$$

See Tables 4.1 and 4.2 for examples of calculating attack rates and case fatality rates.

The terms "prevalence" and "incidence" are most useful expressions of the occurrence of various phenomena in a population. Their meaning, however, is often confused. Both terms take into account the estimated population at risk and are measures of the occurrence of a condition in the community. Incidence rates express the rate of occurrence of a phenomenon during a given period of time. Chronic diseases, such as tuberculosis or cancer, endure over a long period of time. Incidence rates are particularly useful in these diseases to express the number of cases newly discovered or diagnosed in a defined period of time related to the population exposed. Incidence then refers to the number of cases of a disease developing over a stated time period, usually one year, in a specified population group.[16]

TABLE 4.1

*Food histories of students consuming school lunch, Laredo, Texas, March 21, 1968*

| Food | Ate | | | | Did Not Eat | | | |
|------|-----|-----|-------|----------------|------|-----|-------|----------------|
| | Well | Ill | Total | Attack rate | Well | Ill | Total | Attack rate |
| | | | | % | | | | % |
| Chicken salad | 3442 | 1316 | 4758 | 27.7 | 734 | 48 | 782 | 6.1 |
| Lettuce and tomato | 3279 | 1103 | 4382 | 25.2 | 897 | 261 | 1158 | 22.5 |
| French fries | 3858 | 1252 | 5110 | 24.5 | 318 | 112 | 430 | 26.0 |
| Cupcakes | 3954 | 1264 | 5218 | 24.2 | 222 | 100 | 322 | 31.1 |
| Hot rolls | 3793 | 1261 | 5054 | 25.0 | 383 | 103 | 486 | 21.2 |
| Milk | 3547 | 1211 | 4758 | 25.5 | 629 | 153 | 782 | 19.6 |

Source: National Communicable Disease Center. *Morbidity and Mortality Weekly Report,* Vol. 17, no. 13, week ending March 30, 1968.

TABLE 4.2

*Relationship of case fatality ratio to type of C. diphtheria*

| Type of *C. diphtheria* | Cases | Deaths | Case Fatality Ratio |
|------|-------|--------|----------|
| Mitis | 72 | 9 | 12.5 |
| Gravis | 36 | 3 | 8.3 |
| Intermedius | 22 | 2 | 9.1 |
| Indeterminate | 8 | 1 | 12.5 |
| Total | 138 | 15 | 10.9 |

Source: National Communicable Disease Center. *Morbidity and Mortality Weekly Report,* Vol. 17, no. 12, week ending March 23, 1968.

The prevalence of a disease denotes the number of cases of that condition in a population at a given point of time. For example, on January 1, 1967, the prevalence of influenza in New York City might have been 110 per 100,000, whereas the incidence of influenza in 1967 for the same city might have been 980 per 100,000, or the incidence of diphtheria in Baltimore for December, 1937, might have been 30 per 100,000 whereas, the prevalence rate on December 31, 1937, may have been only 11 per 100,000.

In respect to a chronic disease, tuberculosis, Puffer[17] has pointed out the significance of incidence and prevalence rates. She gives 0.9 case per 1000 of white population per year as the incidence rate of new active cases of tuberculosis in Williamson County, Tennessee, in 1945 to 1946. On January 1, 1946, there were 94 known cases of active tuberculosis in

the white population of 20,000 in the same county or a prevalence rate of 4.7 per 1000. The prevalence rate then shows a cross-section of the population at a given time period in respect to a specific condition; the incidence rate gives a longitudinal picture over a selected period of time.

The final value of these health indices depends upon their accuracy. Errors due to faulty diagnosis, incomplete reporting, or mistakes in estimation of the population will greatly reduce the usefulness of the indices. Naturally, the better organized a nation or a community may be, the more reliable are the health statistics. In underdeveloped areas of the world, little credence can be put in the indices with the possible exception of the crude death rate. Even in the case of death rates, it is necessary to have reasonably accurate population figures.

Other sources of error may be attributed to special interest in one or another disease. This leads to a diagnosis of this disease more frequently and a tendency for physicians to attribute death to the disease currently in the spotlight; for example, coronary heart disease as a cause of death is now often reported. A few decades ago many of these deaths might have been assigned to "acute indigestion" or to arteriosclerotic heart disease.

Limitations on the value of health indices are imposed by the shifting makeup of the population base. The national census every 10th year is an invaluable source of information on the characteristics of the population, but the marked tendency of the people to migrate from one area to another soon leads to outdating of the census data. Various procedures are employed to estimate these population changes, but only an approximation of accuracy can be achieved.

Over a period of half a century, American cities have experienced remarkable changes in the composition of their populations in regard to age, and race particularly. In New York, the influx of Negroes and Puerto Ricans during recent decades has been accompanied by a transfer of a large segment of the urban population to the suburbs. These significant alterations in the composition of the population make it difficult to make long-time comparisons of mortality and morbidity experience even in the same city. (See Table 4.3 for differences in maternal and infant death rates in New York City by ethnic groups.)

The greatly increased life expectancy since 1900 has given more and more people the opportunity of dying old rather than young. This survival of a greater proportion of the population to the later decades of life affects the death rates. The crude death rates do not give a true indication of the relative health of the community. For this reason, age-specific rates are regarded as necessary to provide a more complete picture of current health conditions.

As an alternative to comparing a series of age-specific rates, an adjusted or standardized rate can be calculated for each population to be compared. To develop such an adjusted rate, one calculates the number of deaths that would occur in each population, if the age distributions were similar. A standard population is selected, usually that of the nation as a whole, and then the age-specific rates of the two populations are applied to each standard age grouping. The expected number of deaths for each age group is added together and divided by the total number in the standard population to give the adjusted rate for each of the groups to be compared.[18,19]

For the study of individual disease patterns, cause-specific rates are often used. Here again age-specific rates must be employed to make such data comparable with those from other communities. In the study of some diseases that show markedly different effects on people of various races, for example, tuberculosis, rates specific both for age and race are valuable. There may be sharp differences in the distribution of a disease between the sexes. Rates then specific for age, sex, and race may be of value.

Maternal and infant mortality rates are regarded as rough indices of the health status of a community. Infant deaths and deaths of women in childbirth frequently result from poor or inadequate medical services. Poor socio-economic conditions and cultural factors often are associated with such unfavorable rates.[20]

Health indices then are used as indicators of the state of public health and to make comparisons for different periods of time or for different population groups. These indices may serve to point out problems in the health field where preventive measures may be required. These health rates may also serve to indicate progress or lack of progress in disease control programs. Recently the Pan American Health Organization has completed a study of urban mortality in which data from 10 cities of Latin America are compared with two English-speaking urban areas. Table 4.4 provides an example of the kind of comparisons of mortality data undertaken in this study.[21]

## Evaluation of Health Programs

The health administrator must constantly ask himself whether the limited resources of money and personnel at his disposal are being used to best advantage. Programs that were highly important a short time ago are no longer of major significance in his community. New problems resulting from the current modes of life assume larger proportions. Community health is not static. To keep abreast of changing conditions, frequent assessments of the situation are required. Statistical data are needed to define current problems, to guide the establishment of appropriate programs, and to evaluate the results of these programs as they evolve.

In the past, data obtained from death reports were sufficient to orient health programs. With the great decline in infant deaths and deaths due to communicable disease in other age groups, mortality data are no longer reliable guides for program planning.

Reliable statistical data are needed regarding such matters as the amount and nature of illness, the availability of medical care, and hospital and nursing home facilities. Some areas of each community and certain groups of the population are lacking in suitable or convenient health and medical facilities. Planning for these needs can only be done intelligently on the basis of an adequate knowledge of the problems. Health statistics must now deal with

## TABLE 4.3

Infant and puerperal mortality by ethnic group, New York City, 1955 to 1965

| Ethnic Group | 1955 | 1956 | 1957 | 1958 | 1959 | 1960 | 1961 | 1962 | 1963 | 1964 | 1965 |
|---|---|---|---|---|---|---|---|---|---|---|---|
| Live births |  |  |  |  |  |  |  |  |  |  |  |
| Total | 165,150 | 165,553 | 166,977 | 167,775 | 168,138 | 166,300 | 168,383 | 165,244 | 167,848 | 165,695 | 158,815 |
| Puerto Rican | 18,365 | 19,545 | 20,553 | 21,863 | 22,894 | 24,022 | 24,746 | 24,975 | 25,563 | 25,081 | 24,498 |
| Non-white | 27,093 | 29,103 | 30,431 | 32,546 | 33,705 | 34,233 | 36,502 | 37,890 | 40,530 | 41,481 | 40,962 |
| Other | 119,692 | 116,905 | 115,993 | 113,366 | 111,539 | 108,045 | 107,135 | 102,379 | 101,755 | 99,133 | 93,355 |
| Infant deaths |  |  |  |  |  |  |  |  |  |  |  |
| Total | 4,268 | 4,052 | 4,176 | 4,435 | 4,458 | 4,328 | 4,307 | 4,510 | 4,334 | 4,438 | 4,076 |
| Puerto Rican | 641 | 562 | 632 | 673 | 734 | 682 | 749 | 705 | 722 | 742 | 653 |
| Non-white | 1,112 | 1,113 | 1,276 | 1,404 | 1,459 | 1,452 | 1,448 | 1,640 | 1,589 | 1,700 | 1,612 |
| Other | 2,515 | 2,377 | 2,268 | 2,358 | 2,265 | 2,194 | 2,110 | 2,165 | 2,023 | 1,996 | 1,811 |
| Infant mortality rates[1] |  |  |  |  |  |  |  |  |  |  |  |
| Total | 25.8 | 24.5 | 25.0 | 26.4 | 26.5 | 26.0 | 25.6 | 27.3 | 25.8 | 26.8 | 25.7 |
| Puerto Rican | 34.9 | 28.8 | 30.7 | 30.8 | 32.1 | 28.4 | 30.3 | 28.2 | 28.2 | 29.6 | 26.7 |
| Non-white | 41.0 | 38.2 | 41.9 | 42.1 | 43.3 | 42.4 | 39.7 | 43.3 | 39.2 | 41.0 | 39.4 |
| Other | 21.0 | 20.3 | 19.6 | 20.8 | 20.3 | 20.3 | 19.7 | 21.1 | 19.9 | 20.1 | 19.4 |
| Deaths under 28 days |  |  |  |  |  |  |  |  |  |  |  |
| Total | 3,235 | 3,072 | 3,211 | 3,286 | 3,347 | 3,186 | 3,263 | 3,310 | 3,192 | 3,319 | 3,044 |
| Puerto Rican | 469 | 413 | 463 | 486 | 522 | 492 | 578 | 512 | 529 | 551 | 487 |
| Non-white | 851 | 840 | 958 | 1,021 | 1,077 | 1,075 | 1,070 | 1,158 | 1,140 | 1,250 | 1,190 |
| Other | 1,915 | 1,819 | 1,790 | 1,779 | 1,748 | 1,619 | 1,615 | 1,640 | 1,523 | 1,518 | 1,367 |
| Neonatal mortality rates[1] |  |  |  |  |  |  |  |  |  |  |  |
| Total | 19.6 | 18.6 | 19.2 | 19.6 | 19.9 | 19.2 | 19.4 | 20.0 | 19.0 | 20.0 | 19.2 |
| Puerto Rican | 25.5 | 21.1 | 22.5 | 22.2 | 22.8 | 20.5 | 23.4 | 20.5 | 20.7 | 22.0 | 19.9 |
| Non-white | 31.4 | 28.9 | 31.5 | 31.4 | 32.0 | 31.4 | 29.3 | 30.6 | 28.1 | 30.1 | 29.1 |
| Other | 16.0 | 15.6 | 15.4 | 15.7 | 15.7 | 15.0 | 15.1 | 16.0 | 15.0 | 15.3 | 14.6 |
| Puerperal deaths |  |  |  |  |  |  |  |  |  |  |  |
| Total | 99 | 104 | 107 | 103 | 104 | 115 | 130 | 121 | 116 | 74 | 104 |
| Puerto Rican | 18 | 20 | 21 | 21 | 22 | 26 | 19 | 18 | 26 | 7 | 24 |
| Non-white | 39 | 45 | 42 | 45 | 47 | 47 | 61 | 68 | 48 | 52 | 51 |
| Other | 42 | 39 | 44 | 37 | 35 | 42 | 50 | 35 | 42 | 15 | 29 |

| Puerperal mortality rates[2] | | | | | | | | | | | |
|---|---|---|---|---|---|---|---|---|---|---|---|
| Total | 6.0 | 6.3 | 6.4 | 6.1 | 6.2 | 6.9 | 7.7 | 7.3 | 6.9 | 4.5 | 6.5 |
| Puerto Rican | 9.8 | 10.2 | 10.2 | 9.6 | 9.6 | 10.3 | 7.7 | 7.2 | 10.2 | 2.8 | 9.8 |
| Non-white | 14.4 | 15.5 | 13.8 | 13.8 | 13.9 | 13.7 | 16.7 | 17.9 | 11.8 | 12.5 | 12.5 |
| Other | 3.5 | 3.3 | 3.8 | 3.3 | 3.1 | 3.9 | 4.7 | 3.4 | 4.1 | 1.5 | 3.1 |

[1] Rates per 1000 live births.
[2] Rates per 10,000 live births.

Source: Bureau of Records and Statistics, New York City Department of Health, 1965.

illness rates and with provision of medical services, as well as with birth and death rates. To meet this requirement, every department of health of any size must have at least one staff member well trained in statistical methods.

To determine the need for new programs and to evaluate current activities, data must be obtained by special investigations. It is in the planning of these study programs that statisticians can be most helpful. The first stage of an investigation is the stating of the objective. After the objective has been defined, one can proceed to plan a program needed to reach that objective. For example, every health officer wishes to know the extent to which the population under his care has been immunized against the various infectious diseases that are likely to appear in the area. The objective is simple and clear. It would be impractical to survey every household in a large community to gather the desired information on the immunization status of each family. Statisticians have developed the science of accurate sampling to meet such situations. Thus, by selection of rather small numbers of households for interviews, properly distributed, a reasonably accurate picture of the whole community in respect to the matter under investigation can be obtained. With the collaboration of the Center for Disease Control, a survey to determine the immunization status of the population was recently undertaken in Tucson, Arizona. The design and procedure of the survey had been employed in a variety of epidemiological studies in cities around the country. The procedure required both census tract[22] and block statistics data. The first step was classification of the Tucson census tracts into broad socio-economic areas based on: (1) median school years completed by persons 25 years old and over; (2) percentage of housing units in sound condition; and (3) percentage of occupied housing units with less than 1.01 persons per room.

A sample of 600 housing units was determined to be an adequate one. This sample was to be chosen so that 150 units would be obtained in the upper and lower socio-economic areas and 300 housing units in the middle socio-economic area. On the average, 150 housing units were estimated to provide about 40 to 50 children in the 5-year age group.

Primary sampling units in the survey consisted of two city blocks as delineated in the census city block statistics.

## TABLE 4.4

*Deaths and annual crude and age-adjusted death rates per 1000 population at ages 15 to 74 years, by sex, in Latin American cities, in Bristol, England, and in San Francisco, California, 1962 to 1964*

| City | Total | | | Male | | | Female | | |
|---|---|---|---|---|---|---|---|---|---|
| | Deaths | Rate per 1000 population | | Deaths | Rate per 1000 population | | Deaths | Rate per 1000 population | |
| | | Crude | Age-adjusted | | Crude | Age-adjusted | | Crude | Age-adjusted |
| Bogotá | 3629 | 5.2 | 6.6 | 1628 | 5.2 | 6.8 | 2001 | 5.2 | 6.3 |
| Bristol | 4262 | 8.9 | 4.6 | 2547 | 11.1 | 6.3 | 1715 | 6.9 | 3.2 |
| Cali | 3298 | 4.9 | 5.6 | 1676 | 5.4 | 6.2 | 1622 | 4.5 | 5.1 |
| Caracas | 2999 | 4.1 | 5.0 | 1700 | 4.5 | 6.3 | 1299 | 3.6 | 4.0 |
| Guatemala City | 3422 | 5.4 | 5.8 | 1793 | 6.4 | 7.0 | 1629 | 4.6 | 4.9 |
| La Plata | 3556 | 7.1 | 5.1 | 2317 | 9.4 | 6.9 | 1239 | 4.9 | 3.4 |
| Lima | 4378 | 4.9 | 5.5 | 2417 | 5.4 | 6.5 | 1961 | 4.3 | 4.6 |
| Mexico City | 4191 | 5.9 | 6.0 | 2200 | 6.8 | 7.3 | 1991 | 5.1 | 5.0 |
| Ribeirão Preto | 1016 | 6.5 | 6.4 | 619 | 8.4 | 7.9 | 397 | 4.8 | 4.9 |
| San Francisco | 3865 | 10.5 | 5.5 | 2447 | 13.8 | 7.2 | 1418 | 7.5 | 4.0 |
| Santiago | 4321 | 7.7 | 7.3 | 2490 | 10.0 | 9.8 | 1831 | 5.8 | 5.4 |
| São Paulo | 4361 | 4.6 | 5.2 | 2532 | 5.4 | 6.2 | 1829 | 3.9 | 4.3 |

Source: Puffer, R.R., and Griffith, G.W *Patterns of Urban Mortality,* Scientific Publication 151 Pan American Health Organization, 1967.

The number of blocks in each socio-economic area was cumulated separately, and, on the basis of the average number of housing units per block, the estimated number of sample blocks necessary to yield the required number of sample households was calculated. Using as an interval the number of occupied blocks in each area divided by the number of sample blocks required, and beginning with a random number within that interval, the number of blocks for each census tract was determined by cumulation of the interval.

Within each census tract, the number of blocks required was divided by two to yield primary sampling units consisting of two "census blocks." Actual selection of the particular block pairs was accomplished by reference to a table of random numbers and selection of a number in the range from one to the total number of blocks in the census tract. With this number selected, the block was identified on the census block map. The number of blocks adjacent to the selected block was then counted and the order of counting was noted. By reference to a table of random numbers, a second block was selected. If the required number of blocks in a census tract was an odd number, one sampling unit consisting of only a single block was selected.

After the blocks were selected, the number of housing units in the block was obtained from the city block statistics and an estimate computed of the number of-interviews which the selected blocks yielded. If by chance fluctuation the estimated number of sample housing units differed considerably from the required number, adjustments were made by adding a block to a sampling unit consisting of a single block or reducing a block pair to one block[23] (see Table 4.5).

This method of sampling is particularly applicable for urban surveys. These surveys give valuable data regarding the prevalence of a disease or the current status of a problem in the community. This information is soon out of date. In many programs that include prevention and control of disease, the health officer is concerned with what happens over a period of time. Longitudinal studies with suitable statistical techniques for the analysis of results are required. Such studies are needed to assess the value of cancer prevention measures or the efficacy of BCG vaccine in protecting against tuberculosis.

## Experimental Procedures in Public Health

Of increasing importance in the application of biostatistical methods for public health is the so-called experimental trial. This method is used extensively in clinical medicine to determine the efficacy of new drugs. In public

## TABLE 4.5

*Data and calculations for selection of sample blocks
used in 1963 health index survey in
Tucson, Arizona*

| Item | Socio-economic Area | | | |
| --- | --- | --- | --- | --- |
| | Upper | Middle | Lower | All areas |
| 1. Population | 53,517 | 102,671 | 56,704 | 212,892 |
| 2. No. housing units | 17,376 | 34,407 | 17,266 | 69,049 |
| 3. No. sample housing units required | 151 | 299 | 150 | 600 |
| 4. Housing unit sampling ratio | 1/115 | 1/115 | 1/115 | 1/115 |
| 5. No. occupied blocks | 927 | 1,447 | 976 | 3,350 |
| 6. Average no. housing units per occupied block | 18.74 | 23.78 | 17.69 | 20.61 |
| 7. Approximate no. of blocks (census blocks) required | 32.23 | 50.29 | 33.92 | 116.44 |
| 8. Actual no. of census blocks in sample | 35 | 48 | 36 | 119 |
| 9. Block sampling ratio | 1/26.5 | 1/30.1 | 1/27.1 | 1/28.2 |
| 10. Percentage of Tucson housing units in sample | 0.86 | 0.87 | 0.87 | 0.87 |
| 11. No. of census tracts | 9 | 18 | 15 | 42[1] |

Source: *Health Index Survey, Tucson, Arizona,* National
Communicable Disease Center, Public Health Service,
1963.

[1] Excludes Tract 23, South Tucson; Tract 36, Davis-Monthan;
and Tract 42, San Xavier Reservation; includes portions of
Tracts 40, 41, 43, and 44 which lie within Tucson city
limits. Lines 1, 2 and 5 were obtained from 1960 Census
City Block data.

health, the material to be tested is most often a new vaccine or other immunizing product. For example, the protective value of immune human globulin against viral hepatitis has been subjected to evaluation tests. Also, the prophylactic value of a drug may be tested in certain situations.

Such studies must inevitably involve human experimentation; therefore, ethical questions arise and must be answered. It must be decided whether the procedure to be tested is too dangerous in relation to its possible value. Also, in respect to the control group, one must consider whether it is ethical to withhold a measure with a probable beneficial action. The evaluation program must be a reasonable one.

At the beginning it cannot be known whether the procedure to be tested has or has not a definite value. If this is already known, the evaluation test is unnecessary. In the rapidly changing technologies of the 20th century, controlled trials of new procedures are becoming ever more frequent. Not to experiment brings only the alternatives of using unproven measures or of declining the use of any new procedures.

In the past, new medical techniques were adopted without rigorous testing, because no precise methods of evaluation were then available. From now on, new procedures should not be accepted without proof of their value. In some instances, the new procedure cannot be compared with an alternative one, because none exists. Usually, the procedure to be tested is compared with the procedure previously employed for the purpose in the community. The object of the experiment is to determine whether the new procedure is more effective than the old.

Two large-scale evaluation experiments of vital interest to public health workers in recent years were: (1) the testing of the efficacy of poliomyelitis vaccine; and (2) tests on the value of fluoridated water supplies for the prevention of dental caries. In the poliomyelitis vaccine study, two types of control groups were provided: (1) in 127 areas of 33 states (mostly counties) vaccine was given to second grade students while first and third graders were kept under observation as controls; and (2) in 84 other areas of 11 states, students of first, second, and third grades were combined. One-half received vaccine; the other matching half, serving as controls, received a placebo, an injection of fluid similar in appearance to the vaccine but having no immunizing value[24] (see Table 4.6 for summary of results).

One large-scale program for testing the efficacy of fluorides in public water supplies for the reduction of dental caries was carried out over a 10-year period in Grand Rapids, Michi-gan. The people of Muskegon, Michigan, were studied in the same manner and served as a control population.[25] (See Table 4.7 for a summary of the results of the study and for the method used to present the comparative data from the study and the control populations.)

On planning evaluation experiments, the population to serve both for the testing and for comparison or control must be carefully selected. The group for the experiment may be: (1) the total population of geographical area or political unit; (2) selected age groups of the population of such an area; (3) the population of an institution or of a military unit or the employees of an industrial or commercial plant; (4) members of certain organizations or of insurance groups; and (5) groups exposed to high risks as household associates of sick individuals.[26]

The main purpose of evaluating procedures is to provide guidance for future programs to be applied more widely to other segments of the general population. Therefore, for many types of tests, it is important to select a population that is as widely representative as may be possible. Even of more consequence is the choosing of the experimental and control groups from the selected population. These two groups must be comparable in every respect as

TABLE 4.6

*Evaluation of the 1954 poliomyelitis vaccine trials: summary of the poliomyelitis cases by degree of severity and vaccination status (rate per 100,000)*

| Study Group | Study Population | All Reported Cases | | Poliomyelitis Cases | | | | | | Not Polio | |
| | | | | Total | | Paralytic | | Non-paralytic | | | |
| | | No. | Rate | No. | Rate | No. | Rate | No. | Rate | No. | Rate |
|---|---|---|---|---|---|---|---|---|---|---|---|
| All areas—total | 1,829.916 | 1013 | 55 | 863 | 47 | 685 | 37 | 178 | 10 | 150 | 8 |
| Placebo areas—total | 749.236 | 428 | 57 | 358 | 48 | 270 | 36 | 88 | 12 | 70 | 9 |
| Vaccinated | 200,745 | 82 | 41 | 57 | 28 | 33 | 16 | 24 | 12 | 25 | 12 |
| Placebo | 201,229 | 162 | 81 | 142 | 71 | 115 | 57 | 27 | 13 | 20 | 10 |
| Not inoculated[1] | 338,778 | 182 | 54 | 157 | 46 | 121 | 36 | 36 | 11 | 25 | 7 |
| Incomplete vaccinations | 8,484 | 2 | 24 | 2 | 24 | 1 | 12 | 1 | 12 | | |
| Observed areas—total | 1,080,680 | 585 | 54 | 505 | 47 | 415 | 38 | 90 | 8 | 80 | 7 |
| Vaccinated | 221,998 | 76 | 34 | 56 | 25 | 38 | 17 | 18 | 8 | 20 | 9 |
| Controls[2] | 725,173 | 439 | 61 | 391 | 54 | 330 | 46 | 61 | 8 | 48 | 6 |
| 2nd grade not inoculated | 123,605 | 66 | 53 | 54 | 44 | 43 | 35 | 11 | 9 | 12 | 10 |
| Incomplete vaccinations | 9,904 | 4 | 40 | 4 | 40 | 4 | 40 | | | | |

Source: Francis, T., Korns, R.F., Voight, R.B., Boisen, M., Hemphill, F.M., Napier, J.A., and Tolchinsky, E. An evaluation of the 1954 poliomyelitis vaccine trials. *Amer. J. Public Health, 45:* suppl. 1, 1955.

[1] Includes 8,577 children who received one or two injections of placebo.

[2] First and third grade total population.

## TABLE 4.7

*The effect of fluoridation of the water supply of Grand Rapids, Michigan, on dental caries, as expressed by the average number of DMF[1] permanent teeth per child by year of examination, compared to the results of examination of the teeth of children in Muskegon, Michigan, the control population*

| Age Last Birthday | Basic Examinations, 1944-1945 | 1945 | 1946 | 1947 | 1948 | 1949 | 1950 | 1951 | 1952 | 1953 | 1954 |
|---|---|---|---|---|---|---|---|---|---|---|---|
| **Grand Rapids** | | | | | | | | | | | |
| 6 | 0.78 | 0.56 | 0.23 | 0.37 | 0.26 | 0.38 | 0.26 | 0.26 | 0.23 | 0.12 | 0.19 |
| 7 | 1.89 | 1.72 | 1.11 | 1.09 | 1.04 | .76 | 1.03 | .84 | .90 | .71 | .69 |
| 8 | 2.95 | 3.27 | 2.54 | 2.62 | 2.30 | 2.16 | 1.77 | 1.58 | 1.50 | 1.41 | 1.27 |
| 9 | 3.90 | | 2.98 | 3.12 | 2.67 | 2.48 | 2.38 | 2.04 | 2.02 | 1.83 | 1.97 |
| 10 | 4.92 | | 3.70 | 3.56 | 3.51 | 3.56 | 3.17 | 2.93 | 2.71 | 2.41 | 2.34 |
| 11 | 6.41 | | 4.24 | 3.56 | 4.32 | 4.69 | 4.36 | 3.67 | 3.49 | 3.12 | 2.98 |
| 12 | 8.07 | 9.53 | 7.62 | 7.03 | 8.32 | 7.02 | 7.10 | 5.89 | 5.04 | 4.76 | 3.87 |
| 13 | 9.73 | 10.76 | 8.92 | 8.47 | 8.34 | 8.11 | 7.21 | 6.60 | 5.87 | 5.12 | 5.05 |
| 14 | 10.95 | 11.90 | 9.41 | 9.50 | 9.41 | 8.90 | 8.55 | 8.21 | 7.23 | 5.92 | 6.78 |
| 15 | 12.48 | 12.68 | 11.26 | 11.94 | 10.61 | 11.80 | 10.12 | 8.91 | 9.04 | 9.75 | 8.07 |
| 16 | 13.50 | 13.00 | 9.33 | 12.47 | 13.50 | 11.83 | 11.35 | 11.06 | 10.14 | 9.53 | 9.95 |
| **Muskegon[2]** | | | | | | | | | | | |
| 6 | 0.81 | | 0.48 | 0.66 | 0.79 | 0.63 | 0.75 | 0.80 | 0.52 | 0.35 | 0.45 |
| 7 | 1.99 | | 1.33 | 1.05 | 2.19 | 1.43 | 2.01 | 1.88 | 1.66 | 1.24 | 1.14 |
| 8 | 2.81 | | 2.83 | 2.15 | 3.50 | 2.58 | 2.96 | 2.63 | 2.49 | 2.66 | 2.18 |
| 9 | 3.81 | | 3.29 | 3.54 | 3.58 | 3.88 | 3.89 | 3.52 | 3.05 | 3.22 | 3.16 |
| 10 | 4.91 | | 4.27 | 3.60 | 4.87 | 4.44 | 4.53 | 4.32 | 3.90 | 3.64 | 3.72 |
| 11 | 6.32 | | 4.25 | 4.70 | 4.71 | 5.93 | 5.67 | 5.34 | 5.04 | 4.70 | 4.58 |
| 12 | 8.66 | | 8.43 | 6.79 | 7.82 | 7.21 | 6.88 | 7.71 | 7.00 | 6.53 | 6.12 |
| 13 | 9.98 | | 9.02 | 9.23 | 10.52 | 9.52 | 9.58 | 9.36 | 8.71 | 8.20 | 7.98 |
| 14 | 12.00 | | 11.09 | 12.00 | 12.27 | 11.08 | 12.11 | 11.36 | 10.06 | 10.35 | 10.74 |
| 15 | 12.86 | | 11.17 | 12.89 | 12.66 | 10.32 | 10.94 | 12.38 | 11.57 | 11.69 | 11.19 |
| 16 | 14.07 | | 19.00 | 12.77 | 14.31 | 12.51 | 13.91 | 13.16 | 12.36 | 11.48 | 12.55 |

Source: Arnold, F.A., Jr., Dean, H.T., Jay, P., and Knutson, J.W. Effect of Fluoridated Public water supplies on dental caries prevalence. *Public Health Rep., 71:* 652–658, 1956.
[1] Decayed, missing or filled permanent teeth. A decayed and filled tooth is counted only once.
[2] The basic examinations in Muskegon were not done until the late spring of 1945; therefore, no examinations were done in the fall of 1945.

far as may be possible. The identical procedure for the selection of the control group must be used in naming the study group. A frequent error in the sampling procedure is to allow individuals to volunteer for one group or the other. If volunteers are to be accepted, they should be willing to enter either the study or the control group. Another difficulty that may upset the strict comparability of the two groups is the failure of some individuals to cooperate with the program. This occurs especially in prolonged or tedious experiments. At any rate, the selection of samples is a highly complex affair for which the services of a competent statistician should be sought.

One frequent source of error in evaluation studies is the permitting of prior opinions of the investigators or of the group members to influence the course of the experiment or to bias the results. Experience has shown this fault can best be avoided by concealing the identity of both study and control groups. The technique of the double blind test has been developed to achieve this purpose. Neither does the investigator know to which group a member of the sample belongs, nor do the subjects of the experiment know whether they are members of the study or of the control group. The double blind test is useful when applicable, but in many evaluation procedures it cannot be used. However, in procedures not conducted on this basis, careful consideration must be given to the probability of bias in the interpretation of results.

When the data from the evaluation experiment are in hand, it becomes necessary to learn whether the observed differences between the study and the control group are greater than might be attributed to chance; that is, are the conclusions statistically significant? Statisticians have developed several tests to apply to the analysis of observed events for that purpose. Some commonly used tests are the $t$ test, the $F$ test, and $\chi^2$. By and large, it is advisable to employ the services of trained statistical personnel for these analyses. The methods to be employed are discussed fully in the many good biostatistical texts.[20]

## Presentation of Data

When data have been classified and tabulated, they are ready for presentation. It requires considerable thought to present such information in a concise and comprehensible form. The two most frequently used modes for the presentation of data are tables and graphs.

Tables are used to aid in rapid comprehension of the material and to make comparisons of data relatively easy. A good table is complete in itself and ought not to depend for clear understanding upon the text. The table should then be as simple as possible. Several small tables are preferable to one large complicated one. The title of the table should give a clear and concise description of the material presented therein. It should tell what data are given, the origin of the data, and when the data were collected. If abbreviations or symbols are used, they should be explained in the footnotes.

Graphs are employed to set forth the data in a simpler form capable of being rapidly grasped. Again, the graph should express the data in the simplest possible manner. The title of the graph and the labeling of the component parts should be clear and self-explanatory, so as to be understood without reference to the text. Graphs do not replace tables, and the tabular material should usually be made available for those who wish to examine the data in detail. There are many types of graphs. The choice of the particular one to be used is usually a matter of personal preference. Some of the more frequently used graphs are: [17,20,27]

### Bar Diagram

Bars may be represented vertically or horizontally. The length of the bar is determined by the size of the value to be reported. Bars may be divided to show more than one value. Bar graphs are particularly useful in comparing quantitative data of a discrete type, for example, the number of live births among Indian women as compared to white women. Sometimes two or three different bars, black, shaded, or cross-hatched may be used in the same graph to show different variables in the data.

### Line Graph

Points are plotted on a grid and are joined by lines. Time is represented on the horizontal axis and rates on the vertical axis. These commonly used graphs are suitable for plotting variables such as death rates over a period of time.

### Pie Diagram

A circle is divided into pie-shaped segments, whose areas and spaces occupied on the circumference represent proportional values. This type of graph is effective if the number of segments is small, and the area of each segment is large enough to permit easy comparison.

### Histogram

This is a type of bar graph without space between the bars. It is used like a line graph to express frequency distribution of quantitative data occurring in a continuous series. To construct a line graph from a histogram, the midpoint at the top of each bar may be connected.

### Statistical Maps

Maps of counties, cities, states, or other political units can be used to illustrate the geographical differences in the distribution of variables. For example, differences in death rates can be shown by varying the intensity of shading from white to black.

There are other and generally more complicated graphic methods in use, for instance, three-dimensional graphs. The correct type of graph suitable for the material to be presented should be chosen. The simpler the graph, the better.

## VITAL STATISTICS AND THE POPULATION

No accurate measurements of public health activities can be arrived at without a reasonable knowledge of the population being served, be it in the city, county, state, or nation, nor can meaningful comparisons be made with other areas unless the characteristics of the populations to be compared are known. For example, death rates of two countries cannot be compared satisfactorily if knowledge of the age distribution of the two populations is not available. In public health practice, it is important to know the characteristics of the population in respect to age, sex, race, marital status, occupation, and economic status. It is also helpful to have information on housing conditions, density of population, educational status, and so on. Most of this information is now provided in many countries by periodic census taking on the part of the responsible governments.

## Census

In olden times, census taking was employed by governments principally to get the population enrolled for assessment of taxes or for military service. Many eastern nations employed this method in olden times including the Babylonian, the Egyptian, the Persian, the Jewish, and the Chinese. Probably the Romans made the most effective and systematic use of the census. Having been in use in Rome itself for many years, the Emperor Augustus extended the census in 5 B.C. to all of the Roman Empire. A new census was carried out every 5th year.

Following the collapse of the Roman Empire, the census fell into disuse for a long interval. Some of the German states in the mid-18th century began periodic census-taking. The Scandinavian countries soon followed suit.

## Population of the United States

In the United States, the framers of the Constitution decreed that a national census be undertaken every 10 years beginning in 1790. The purpose of this enumeration of the people was to establish the number of members of the House of Representatives in Congress to which each state was entitled on the basis of population. For over a century after the first census, the census organization was a temporary one. In 1902, the Bureau of the Census was established as a permanent Federal agency.

The data collected by the census takers have proved so valuable to government, to business, and to educational, social, and health planners that there is always a demand to include more items in the questionnaires. Experiments are also being undertaken to keep up a flow of census information on a current basis. The Current Population Survey is a monthly nationwide survey of a scientifically selected sample of the population. The sample is located in 449 areas comprising 863 counties and independent cities with coverage in every state. About 58,500 houses or other quarters are designated for the sample.

Population estimates are made for intercensus years. Births and deaths, immigrants and emigrants, armed servicemen, and Federal employees serving abroad are all considered in arriving at the estimated number. Population projection of the approximate future population levels is made with given assumptions as to future birth and death rates and net immigration from abroad. Projected population figures by state make use of further assumptions about redistribution of people through interstate migration. The census provides information as to various characteristics of the population[28] as for example:

### Rural and Urban

According to the 1970 census definition, the urban population comprises all persons in (a) places of 2500 inhabitants or more incorporated as cities, villages, boroughs (except Alaska), and towns (except in New England, New York, and Wisconsin), but excluding persons living in the rural portions of extended cities; (b) unincorporated places of 2500 inhabitants or more; and (c) other territory, incorporated or unincorporated, included in urbanized areas. Some urbanized areas contain one or more incorporated places which are designated as "extended cities" because they have one or more large portions (normally at the city boundary) with relatively low population density. These portions are classified as rural (see Table 4.8).

### Color and Race

The population is divided into three major groups on the basis of race: White, Negro, and other. The 1960 and 1970 census obtained the information on race principally through self-enumeration; thus, the data represent essentially self-classification by people according to the race with which they identify themselves. Persons of Mexican or Puerto Rican birth or ancestry who did not identify themselves as of a race other than white were classified as white.

## TABLE 4.8

*Population, urban and rural, by race: 1950 to 1970*

[In thousands, except percent. An urbanized area comprises at least 1 city of 50,000 inhabitants (central city) plus contiguous, closely settled areas (urban fringe). Data for 1950 and 1960 according to urban definition used in the 1960 census; 1970 data according to the 1970 definition.]

| Year and Area | Total | White | Negro and other | Per Cent Distribution | | |
| --- | --- | --- | --- | --- | --- | --- |
| | | | | Total | White | Negro and other |
| 1950, total population | 151,326 | 135,150 | 16,176 | 100.0 | 100.0 | 100.0 |
| Urban | 96,847 | 86,864 | 9,983 | 64.0 | 64.3 | 61.7 |
| Inside urbanized areas | 69,249 | 61,925 | 7,324 | 45.8 | 45.8 | 45.3 |
| Central cities | 48,377 | 42,042 | 6,335 | 32.0 | 31.1 | 39.2 |
| Urban fringe | 20,872 | 19,883 | 989 | 13.8 | 14.7 | 6.1 |
| Outside urbanized areas | 27,598 | 24,939 | 2,659 | 18.2 | 18.5 | 16.4 |
| Rural | 54,479 | 48,286 | 6,193 | 36.0 | 35.7 | 38.3 |
| 1960, total population | 179,323 | 158,832 | 20,481 | 100.0 | 100.0 | 100.0 |
| Urban | 125,269 | 110,428 | 14,840 | 69.9 | 69.5 | 72.4 |
| Inside urbanized areas | 95,848 | 83,770 | 12,079 | 53.5 | 52.7 | 58.9 |
| Central cities | 57,975 | 47,627 | 10,348 | 32.3 | 30.0 | 50.5 |
| Urban fringe | 37,873 | 36,143 | 1,731 | 21.1 | 22.8 | 8.4 |
| Outside urbanized areas | 29,420 | 26,658 | 2,762 | 16.4 | 16.8 | 13.5 |
| Rural | 54,054 | 48,403 | 5.651 | 30.1 | 30.5 | 27.6 |
| 1970, total population | 203,212 | 177,749 | 25,463 | 100.0 | 100.0 | 100.0 |
| Urban | 149,325 | 128,773 | 20,552 | 73.5 | 72.4 | 80.7 |
| Inside urbanized areas | 118,447 | 100,952 | 17,495 | 58.3 | 56.8 | 68.7 |
| Central cities | 63,922 | 49,547 | 14,375 | 31.5 | 27.9 | 56.5 |
| Urban fringe | 54,525 | 51,405 | 3,120 | 26.8 | 28.9 | 12.3 |
| Outside urbanized areas | 30,878 | 27,822 | 3,057 | 15.2 | 15.7 | 12.0 |
| Rural | 53,887 | 48,976 | 4,911 | 26.5 | 27.6 | 19.3 |

Source: U. S. Bureau of the Census, Statistical Abstract of the United States: 1973, 94th Edition, Washington, D.C., 1973.

In 1970, the father's race was used for persons of mixed parentage who were in doubt as to their classification. In 1960, persons who reported mixed parentage of white and any other race were classified according to the other race; mixtures of races other than white were classified according to the father's race (see Table 4.8).

### Household

A "household" comprises all persons who occupy a "housing unit," that is, a house, an apartment or other group of rooms, or a room that constitutes "separate living quarters." A household includes the related family members and all the unrelated persons, if any, such as lodgers, foster children, wards, or employees who share the housing unit. A person living alone or a group of unrelated persons sharing the same housing unit as partners is also counted as a household.

### Family

The term "family" refers to a group of two or more persons related by blood, marriage, or adoption and residing together in a household. A primary family consists of the head of a household and all other persons in the household related to the head. A secondary family comprises two or more persons such as guests, lodgers, or resident employees and their relatives, living in a household and related to each other.

Most of the data yielded from the census

forms are useful to the public health worker in one way or another. This is especially true in urban areas where the cities are divided into small areas called census tracts. These tracts have definite and permanent boundaries and include a population of from 3000 to 6000. As a rule, these small populations are rather homogenous as to race, nativity, economic status, and general living conditions. Since 1940, census tract data have been made available on 60 of the larger cities or more. To public health officers, census tracts have proved most useful in spotting health problems on a geographical basis. Health data can be related to economical or other data available by census tract.[22]

In 1790, the United States had a population of almost 4 million. During 1967, it is estimated that the United States population passed the 200 million mark. Obviously, between 1790 and 1967 the population growth has not been uniform. The curve in Figure 4.5 shows how steeply the growth rate has increased since about 1850.

Not only has there been an accelerated growth of population during recent decades, but there are changes in the composition of the population of especial significance to public health. There were 16 per cent fewer children under five years of age in 1970 than in 1960, reflecting the lower birth rates pertaining in that period.

In 1900, only 4 per cent of our population was 65 years or older. The proportion has continued to grow steadily during the century, reaching 9.8 per cent by 1970, or 20 million persons. Depending upon future birthrates, the proportion of the population 65 years or over could reach 10.6 per cent by the year 2000.

The Bureau of the Census has compiled the following items of information describing some characteristics of the United States population as of 1970:

- 203,800,000 Americans
- 104,600,000 females
- 99,200,000 males
- 17,167,000 under five years of age
- 20,000,000 over 65 years of age
- 7,400,000 in college
- 60,400,000 in other schools
- 37,997,000 white collar workers
- 27,791,000 blue collar workers
- 178,800,000 white
- 25,000,000 not white

- 94,354,000 married
- 11,750,000 widows or widowers
- 124,498,000 old enough to vote
- 9,600,000 foreign-born
- 149,300,000 "city" dwellers
- 131,046,000 church members

By 1990, it is estimated that the figure for persons 65 years or over will reach 27,768,000. With this increase in the number of elderly people, the problems of chronic disease, hospitalization, and sheltered care will be greatly accentuated. (See Fig. 4.6 for the distribution of the population by age groups.)

There has also been a marked increase in the numbers of women entering the labor force. This increase is made up of young girls out of school, but, also, of many married women returning to work after their children reach school age.

Another important change in the population of the United States is the rapid increase of urban population at the expense of the rural. In Table 4.8 are summarized the urban and rural populations of the United States for the 1950 and 1970 census. It is apparent that there was a sharp rise in 'the urbanization of the white population, but an even greater increase of the non-white shift from rural to urban areas.

The total rural population in 1900 was 46 million, or 60 per cent of the population of the United States. By 1970, the rural population was only 26 per cent of the total. Paralleling the decline in rural percentage of the population has been a decline in the proportion of the population located in towns and cities of less than 50,000.

During the 20-year period between 1950 and 1970, there was a shift of population from one region of the United States to another. In the white population there was a movement from northeast and north central to the south, but more especially to the west. The non-white population left the south in large numbers, going to the other three regions of the country.

Nearly 40 million Americans, or one in five, change homes every year. Thirteen million migrate across a county line. Since World War II, large numbers of Blacks moved from rural to metropolitan areas. Seventy-four per cent of the Black population is now metropolitan, compared to 68 per cent of whites. In the 1960's, there was a net movement of whites out of the north to the west and south. Blacks moved to the north and west.

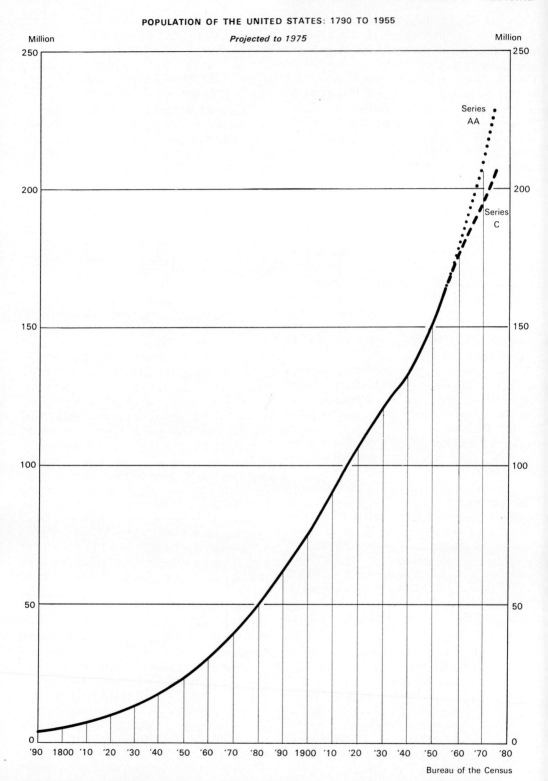

Fig. 4.5. Population of the United States: 1790 to 1955. Source: National Office of Vital Statistics. *Health and Demography*, Public Health Service Publication 502. Washington, D. C.: U. S. Public Health Service, 1956.

PERCENTAGE OF POPULATION IN SPECIFIED AGE GROUPS, 1880-1975

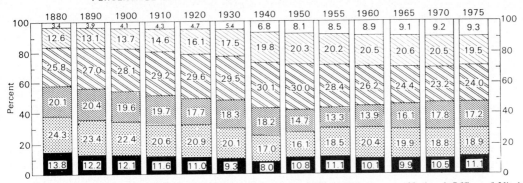

Fig. 4.6. Percentage of population in specified age groups, 1880–1975. Source: National Office of Vital Statistics. *Health and Demography*, Public Health Service Publication, 502. Washington, D. C.: U. S. Public Health Service, 1956. Key ■ under 5 years; ▨ 5 to 14 years; ◩ 15 to 24 years; ◪ 25 to 44 years; ▥ 45 to 64 years; □ 65 years and over.

## TABLE 4.9

*Sex ratio of the population, by age groups, 1910 to 1971, and by race, 1971*

[Data are for census dates; see table 24. Ratio represents number of males per 100 females. Total resident population]

| AGE | 1910 | 1920 | 1930 | 1940 | 1950 | 1960 | 1970 | 1971 Total | 1971 White[1] | 1971 Negro |
|---|---|---|---|---|---|---|---|---|---|---|
| All ages | [2]106.2 | [2]104.1 | [2]102.6 | 100.8 | 98.7 | 97.1 | 94.8 | 94.9 | 95.4 | 90.9 |
| Under 15 years | 102.2 | 102.1 | 102.6 | 103.0 | 103.7 | 103.4 | 103.9 | 103.9 | 104.5 | 100.5 |
| 15-24 years | 101.2 | 96.9 | 98.2 | 98.7 | 97.8 | 98.3 | 98.1 | 99.2 | 99.9 | 94.3 |
| 25-44 years | 110.5 | 105.3 | 101.0 | 98.7 | 96.5 | 95.7 | 95.5 | 95.7 | 97.3 | 83.4 |
| 45-64 years | 114.7 | 115.4 | 109.2 | 105.3 | 100.2 | 95.7 | 91.6 | 91.3 | 92.0 | 85.1 |
| 65 years and over | 101.2 | 101.5 | 100.6 | 95.7 | 89.7 | 82.8 | 72.2 | 71.6 | 71.2 | 75.5 |

[1] Includes "other races."
[2] Includes figures for "age not reported."
Source: U.S. Bureau of the Census, Statistical Abstract of the United States: 1973. (94th Edition) Washington, D.C. 1973.

In Table 4.9 is given the sex ratio of the United States population by age groups from 1910 to 1971. The proportion of males to females has been steadily declining until 1971. Females enjoy more favorable death rates. There has also been a decline in immigration which generally brings in a greater proportion of males. In urban areas, the ratio of males to females is much lower than in the rural. The increasing proportion of females in the population has some effect on the planning of health services for the community.

## World Population

The tremendous upsurge in the population of the world, which began around 1850,

presents the most difficult problem facing mankind. According to Harold F. Dorn,[29] the world's population is estimated to have reached 250 million at the beginning of the Christian era. This population had doubled at the time of the Pilgrim's landing in Massachusetts (1620 A.D.). Shortly before the beginning of the American Civil War, another 500 million people had been added. This doubling of the population required about 200 years. Since the mid-19th century, the population of the world has doubled at progressively shorter intervals. At current rates, only 6 to 7 years are required for another 0.5 billion to be added to the population of the world. In 1970, the figures for world population were 3.63 billion. Some estimates for the year 2000 (only 25 years ahead), place the number of humans in the world at 6.9 billion. The lowest estimate is about 4.8 billion people. In Figure 4.7 are projected curves illustrating the estimated world population up to the year 2000.

In the opinion of Dr. Dorn, the major cause for this great spurt in population growth is a decline in mortality. This has affected all nations. Present public health programs in underdeveloped countries will probably promote this decrease in the number of deaths, especially among the infants and children.

## Vital Statistics

To keep currently informed about population characteristics, it is essential to have good records of the births and deaths occurring in the area. These important human events have a determining effect on the population figures in any community.

### Registration of Births and Deaths

Data on births and deaths are obtained through a registration system set up by law in each state. Whenever a birth or death occurs, a certificate reporting the fact must be filed with a local registrar of vital statistics within a short interval after the event. In the case of a birth, the attending physician is responsible for filling the certificate of birth out and filing with the proper authority, usually in the local health department. Death certificates are filed by the funeral director after the physician has certified to the medical facts relating to the death (see Figs. 4.8 and 4.9).

Birth and death certificates are important legal documents. The certificate of birth is required to prove the individual's age for entrance to school, for licenses, for entering military services, for voter registration, for proof of citizenship, and for proof of family kinship. Death certificates are required for collection of life insurance, settlement of estates, pension claims, and use in analysis of public health data.

Usually, the certificates are forwarded directly by the local registrar to the state health department with a copy to the local health department. This system varies among the

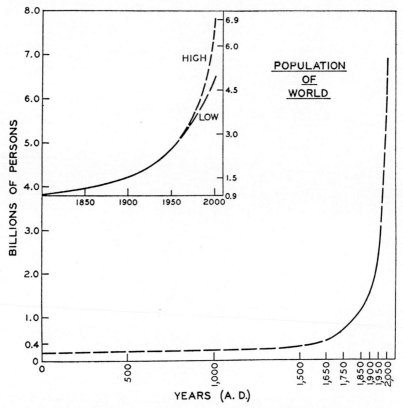

Fig. 4.7. Estimated population of the world, A.D. 1 to A.D. 2000. Source: Dorn, H. F. World population growth: an international dilemma. *Science, 135:* 283–290, 1962.

**ORIGINAL**
STATE COPY

**STATE OF ARIZONA**
DEPARTMENT OF HEALTH – DIVISION OF VITAL RECORDS
**CERTIFICATE OF DEATH**

STATE FILE NO.

**IDENTIFICATION OF DECEASED AND PLACE OF DEATH**

1. NAME OF DECEASED — A. FIRST — B. MIDDLE — C. LAST
2. SEX
3. RACE OR COLOR
4. DATE OF DEATH — MONTH — DAY — YEAR
5. PLACE OF DEATH — A. COUNTY — B. TOWN OR CITY — C. HOSPITAL OR INSTITUTION (IF RESIDENCE, GIVE STREET ADDRESS) — D. IN CITY LIMITS? ☐ YES ☐ NO
6. DATE OF BIRTH — MONTH — DAY — YEAR
7A. AGE (YEARS LAST BIRTHDAY) — B. IF UNDER 1 YEAR: MOS. DAYS — C. IF UNDER 1 DAY: HRS. MIN.
8. MARITAL STATUS ☐ MARRIED ☐ WIDOWED ☐ NEVER MAR. ☐ DIVORCED.
9. SURVIVING SPOUSE (IF WIFE, GIVE MAIDEN NAME)
10. PLACE OF BIRTH — STATE OR COUNTRY
11. CITIZEN OF WHAT COUNTRY? SPECIFY:
12. SOCIAL SECURITY NO.
13A. USUAL OCCUPATION
13B. TYPE OF BUSINESS

**RESIDENCE OF DECEASED AND NAME OF PARENTS**

14. USUAL RESIDENCE — A. STATE — B. COUNTY — C. TOWN OR CITY — D. ZIP CODE
14E. STREET ADDRESS OR R.F.D. (P.O. BOX NOT ACCEPTABLE) — 14F. IN CITY LIMITS? ☐ YES ☐ NO
HOW LONG LIVED IN ARIZONA? — 15A. IN THIS TOWN — 15B. IN STATE
16. PREVIOUS PLACE OF RESIDENCE — CITY AND STATE
17. FATHER'S NAME — A. FIRST — B. MIDDLE — C. LAST
18. MOTHER'S MAIDEN NAME — A. FIRST — B. MIDDLE — C. LAST

**INFORMANT**

19A. INFORMANT'S SIGNATURE ▶ — 19B. RELATIONSHIP TO DECEASED — 19C. ADDRESS — 19D. DATE SIGNED

**(ITEM 20) MEDICAL CAUSE OF DEATH**

CODE ____________

20. MEDICAL STATEMENT OF CAUSE OF DEATH
FILL OUT CAREFULLY
ENTER IMMEDIATE CAUSE ON LINE A. OTHER PRECIPITATING CAUSES SHOULD BE GIVEN ON LINES B AND C RESPECTIVELY. LIST UNDERLYING CAUSE LAST.

PART I. DEATH WAS CAUSED BY: (ENTER ONLY ONE CAUSE ON EACH LINE)
A. IMMEDIATE CAUSE
B. DUE TO OR AS A CONSEQUENCE OF:
C. DUE TO OR AS A CONSEQUENCE OF:

ESTIMATED TIME BETWEEN ONSET AND DEATH

21. IF DECEASED WAS ADULT FEMALE, WAS SHE PREGNANT AT DEATH OR ANY TIME IN PAST YEAR? YES, NO, UNKNOWN. SPECIFY:

OTHER CONDITIONS OF SIGNIFICANT MEDICAL IMPORTANCE CONTRIBUTING TO DEATH BUT NOT DIRECTLY RELATED TO IMMEDIATE CAUSE
PART II. OTHER SIGNIFICANT CONDITIONS
22A. AUTOPSY? ☐ YES ☐ NO
22B. IF YES, WERE FINDINGS CONSIDERED IN DETERMINING CAUSE OF DEATH? YES OR NO SPECIFY:

**MANNER AND CIRCUMSTANCES OF DEATH (FOR DEATHS FROM EXTERNAL FACTORS)**

23. MANNER OF DEATH ☐ ACCIDENT ☐ NATURAL CAUSES ☐ SUICIDE ☐ UNDETERMINED ☐ HOMICIDE
24A. DATE OF INJURY — MO. DAY YR. — 24B. HOUR M.
25. AT WORK WHEN INJURED? YES, NO, UNK.
26. HOW DID INJURY OCCUR? (CIRCUMSTANCES ONLY—NOT CAUSE)
27. PLACE OF INJURY (HOME, STORE, FACTORY, STREET, ETC.) SPECIFY:
28. WHERE LOCATED? STREET ADDRESS — CITY AND STATE

**CERTIFICATIONS: PHYSICIAN OR MEDICAL EXAMINER — CORONER (CROSS OUT WORDS NOT APPLICABLE)**

CERTIFICATION—PHYSICIAN OR MEDICAL EXAMINER
29A. I (ATTENDED) (EXAMINED) THE DECEASED (FROM) (ON): MO. DAY YEAR TO MO. DAY YEAR
29B. AND (SAW) (DID NOT SEE) HIM/HER ALIVE LAST TIME ON: MO. DAY YEAR HOUR M. — I (DID) (DID NOT) VIEW BODY AFTER DEATH.
DEATH OCCURRED AT: M. ON THE DATE AND AT THE PLACE LISTED ABOVE AND TO THE BEST OF MY KNOWLEDGE AND PROFESSIONAL JUDGMENT DUE TO THE CAUSES STATED.
SIGNATURE ▶ — TITLE
29C. (TYPE NAME HERE)
30. MAIL ADDRESS — 31. DATE SIGNED

CERTIFICATION—CORONER
FROM EXAMINATION OF THE BODY AND/OR MY INVESTIGATION, IN MY OPINION DEATH OCCURRED IN THE MANNER AND UNDER THE CIRCUMSTANCES STATED.
32A. DECEASED WAS PRONOUNCED DEAD ON: MO. DAY YEAR HOUR M. — I (DID) (DID NOT) VIEW BODY AFTER DEATH.
SIGNATURE ▶
33. PRECINCT OR DISTRICT
32B. (TYPE NAME HERE)
34. MAIL ADDRESS — 35. DATE SIGNED

**FOR STATE REGISTRAR'S USE**

36. SUPPLEMENTARY ENTRIES

**DISPOSITION AND REGISTRATION DATA**

37. DISPOSITION OF BODY—BURIAL, CREMATION OR REMOVAL SPECIFY:
38. DATE OF DISPOSITION
39. CEMETERY OR CREMATORY — NAME — STREET ADDRESS — CITY AND STATE
40. FUNERAL HOME — NAME — STREET ADDRESS — CITY AND STATE
41. FUNERAL DIRECTOR'S SIGNATURE ▶
42. CERT. NO.
43. DATE REGISTERED
44. REG. FILE NO.
45. REGISTRAR'S SIGNATURE ▶
46. REG. DISTRICT
47. DATE RCVD. IN STATE OFFICE

VS-2 REV. 9-67 30M 10-67

Fig. 4.8. Source: Division of Vital Records, Arizona State Department of Health, Phoenix, Arizona.

**ORIGINAL**
STATE COPY

STATE OF ARIZONA
DEPARTMENT OF HEALTH—DIVISION OF VITAL RECORDS
**CERTIFICATE OF LIVE BIRTH**

BIRTH NO.
102-

IDENTIFICATION OF CHILD AND PLACE OF BIRTH

1. NAME OF CHILD — A. FIRST — B. MIDDLE — C. LAST
2. SEX
3A. TYPE OF BIRTH SINGLE, TWIN, TRIPLET, ETC. — SPECIFY:
3B. IF MULTIPLE BIRTH BORN FIRST, SECOND, ETC. — SPECIFY:
4A. DATE OF BIRTH — MONTH DAY YEAR
4B. HOUR M.
5. PLACE OF BIRTH — A. COUNTY — B. TOWN OR CITY — C. HOSPITAL OR CLINIC (IF HOME BIRTH, GIVE STREET ADDRESS) — D. IN CITY LIMITS? ☐ YES ☐ NO

PARENTS

6. FATHER'S NAME — A. FIRST — B. MIDDLE — C. LAST
7. DATE OF BIRTH — MONTH DAY YEAR
8. PLACE OF BIRTH — STATE OR COUNTRY
9. MOTHER'S MAIDEN NAME — A. FIRST — B. MIDDLE — C. LAST
10. DATE OF BIRTH — MONTH DAY YEAR
11. PLACE OF BIRTH — STATE OR COUNTRY

RESIDENCE OF MOTHER

12. MOTHER'S USUAL RESIDENCE — A. STATE — B. COUNTY — C. TOWN OR CITY — D. ZIP CODE
12 E. STREET ADDRESS OR R.F.D. (P.O. BOX NOT ACCEPTABLE)
12 F. IN CITY LIMITS? ☐ YES ☐ NO
HOW LONG LIVED IN ARIZONA? — 13 A. IN THIS TOWN — 13 B. IN STATE
14. PREVIOUS STATE OF RESIDENCE

CERTIFICATIONS:

PARENT

15 THE INFORMATION LISTED IN ITEMS 1-14 IS TRUE AND CORRECT TO THE BEST OF MY KNOWLEDGE.
15A. ▶ PARENT OR INFORMANT'S SIGNATURE
16. RELATIONSHIP TO CHILD
17. DATE SIGNED

ATTENDANT

18. I ATTENDED THE BIRTH OF THIS CHILD WHO WAS BORN ALIVE AT THE PLACE, TIME, AND DATE ENTERED ABOVE.
▶ ATTENDANT'S SIGNATURE
18A. (TYPE NAME BELOW LINE)
19. TITLE ☐ M.D. ☐ D.O. ☐ OTHER (SPECIFY)
20. DATE SIGNED

FOR STATE REGISTRAR'S USE ONLY

21. SUPPLEMENTARY ENTRIES

REGISTRAR'S CERTIFICATION

22. DATE REGISTERED
23. REG. FILE NO.
24. ▶ REGISTRAR'S SIGNATURE
25. REG. DISTRICT
26. DATE RCVD. IN STATE OFFICE

IF MULTIPLE BIRTH, ENTER FILE NO'S. OF OTHER CERTIFICATES BELOW.

**MEDICAL AND HEALTH DATA SECTION – PLEASE COMPLETE ALL ITEMS BELOW**

27. RACE OR COLOR
28. EDUCATION–ENTER HIGHEST GRADE COMPLETED
29. SOCIAL SECURITY NO.
30. PREVIOUS DELIVERIES–HOW MANY OTHER CHILDREN

FATHER
27A. WHITE, NEGRO, INDIAN, ETC. — SPECIFY:
28A. ELEMENTARY (0,1,2...OR 8) — A. HIGH SCHOOL (1,2,3, OR 4) — A. COLLEGE (1,2,3,4 OR 5+)
29A. FATHER

MOTHER
27B. WHITE, NEGRO, INDIAN, ETC. — SPECIFY:
28B. ELEMENTARY (0,1,2,...OR 8) — B. HIGH SCHOOL 1,2,3, OR 4) — B. COLLEGE (1,2,3,4 OR 5+)
29B. MOTHER

30 A. ARE NOW LIVING?
30 B. WERE BORN ALIVE BUT ARE NOW DEAD?
30 C. WERE BORN DEAD AT ANYTIME AFTER CONCEPTION?
34. DATE LAST LIVE BIRTH
35. DATE LAST FETAL DEATH
36. DATE LAST NORMAL MENSES BEGAN

31. LENGTH OF PREGNANCY — WEEKS
32. SEROLOGY ON MOTHER? YES, NO, UNKNOWN — SPECIFY:
33. OPERATIVE PROCEDURES—DESCRIBE
37. DATE FIRST PRENATAL VISIT FOR THIS BIRTH
38. TOTAL NO. PRENATAL VISITS
41. IS MOTHER MARRIED OR WAS SHE MARRIED AT ANYTIME IN THE 10 MONTHS PRECEDING BIRTH OF THIS CHILD? YES OR NO — SPECIFY:
39. COMPLICATIONS OF LABOR—DESCRIBE
40. OTHER COMPLICATIONS — A. RELATED TO PREGNANCY — B. NOT RELATED TO PREGNANCY

CHILD
42. DROPS IN BABY'S EYES? YES, NO, UNKNOWN — SPECIFY:
43. LENGTH AT BIRTH — INS. OR CMS.
44. WEIGHT AT BIRTH — LBS. OZ. OR GMS.
45 A. DATE OF DEATH
45 B. PLACE OF DEATH
45 C. FILE NO.

STATE "NONE" WHERE NEGATIVE REPLY IS APPLICABLE TO ANY ITEM

46. CONGENITAL MALFORMATIONS OR ANOMALIES—DESCRIBE
47. BIRTH INJURIES—DESCRIBE
48. MOTHER'S MAILING ADDRESS (IF DIFFERENT FROM ITEM 12)

VS-1 REV. 9 67 65M 10-67

Fig. 4.9. Source: Division of Vital Records, Arizona State Department of Health, Phoenix, Arizona.

states. With the exception of the New England states, the original certificate is kept in the state division of vital statistics, but a photostatic copy is forwarded to the National Center for Health Statistics in Washington, where the data are compiled, analyzed, and published regularly in *Vital Statistics of the United States.*

To assure the dependability of these vital data, the Bureau of the Census established registration areas. The Federal registration area for deaths goes back to 1880, but at the beginning included only Massachusetts, New Jersey, the District of Columbia, and a few large cities. Data from other states were not regarded as acceptably dependable at that time. The birth registration area was established in 1915. By 1933, all states had become accepted for inclusion in both the birth and death registration areas.

There are certain defects in the system of registering births and deaths. Some of these events go unrecorded. The National Office of Vital Statistics carries out tests on the accuracy of reporting from time to time. Their conclusion is that among the white population approximately 98.6 per cent of the births are registered, whereas only 93.5 per cent of nonwhite births are reported[30] (see Fig. 4.10).

Problems are encountered with inadequate registration of stillbirths and of illegitimate babies. With the increasing use of hospitals for delivery of babies, the reporting of births has become more accurate.

Because of the legal requirement of a death certificate before burial, deaths are reported with a greater degree of accuracy. The value of the death certificate from the medical viewpoint depends upon the attending physician's knowledge of the case. If the patient had been thoroughly studied by all available diagnostic methods before death, or if the physician's statement of the cause of death has been substantiated by a postmortem examination, the stated cause of death has real value. All too often the physician has little knowledge of the case and must base his judgment as to the primary cause of death upon inadequate information.

Mortality data not only provide information on the number of deaths, but also data on mortality according to age, sex, geographical area, race, and a variety of other factors of economic or social significance. This source of information on the health status of a people is based on the entire population and does not depend on a sampling procedure. The mortality data are available for the whole nation or by

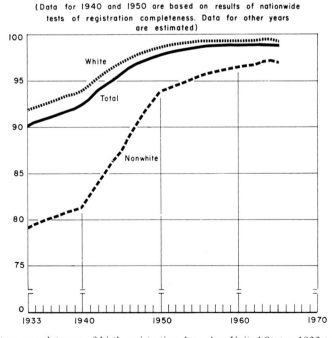

Fig. 4.10. Percentage completeness of birth registration, by color: United States, 1933 to 1964. Source: *Vital Statistics of the United States,* Vol. 1, 1965.

states, cities, counties, or even sections of cities. This detailed distribution of the data permits comparisons of one area with another.

In spite of its imperfections, the death registration system constitutes the most stable and basic element in the field of health intelligence. The system is essential.

To obtain standardization in disease terminology, most nations have adopted "The International Classification of Diseases" established by the World Health Organization.

### Death Rates

The average length of life of white males in the mid-19th century in the United States was about 33-40 years depending on the area of residence.[31]

According to a study by Moriyama,[32] the crude death rate in the 50-year period, 1900 to 1949, declined by over 40 per cent in the United States. The most rapid rate of decline was in the first years of the century, 1900 to 1917. Since 1954, there has been little change in the crude death rate which hovers around 9.5 per 1000 population. In Table 4.10 are given the number of deaths and death rates 1935 to 1968. In Figure 4.11 is shown a curve of death rates, 1930 to 1969. In 1972, the U. S. death rate was 9.4.

The mortality plateau experienced by the American population from 1954 to 1963 cannot be ascribed to death rates having reached the lowest possible level. At least 15 other nations have a longer life expectancy at birth than the United States. A report of the Department of Health, Education and Welfare suggests four factors as potentially responsible for our shorter period of life expectancy: (1) genetic and environmental factors; (2) the American style of life, including smoking, rich diets, lack of exercise, and the pressures of professional and business life; (3) unequal distribution of medical care; and (4) the deprivation suffered by the poor and underprivileged.

Differences in mortality may be taken as a significant indication of differences among the socio-economic levels of the population in life styles and in the potential to cope with the forces that affect life itself—the ability to survive.

Over the years mortality has declined due to a number of factors including increased productivity, higher standards of living, decreased internecine warfare, environmental sanitation, personal hygiene, public health measures, modern medicine climaxed by advent of pesticides and chemotherapy.

Further reductions in the United States death rates may be achieved more readily through improvements in socio-economic conditions for the underprivileged segments of the population than through advances in biomedical knowledge. The biomedical knowledge already available is not within the effective reach of the lower socio-economic elements of the population.[33]

If one examines the changes in the causes of death, a great shift can be seen in the disease spectrum. In Table 4.11, death rates for the 10 leading causes of death in 1900 and 1967 are compared.[34]

Tuberculosis, which ranked second as a cause of death in 1900, does not appear in the 10 most frequent fatal diseases of 1967. Diseases of the heart, which ranked fourth in 1900, rose to first place as a killer in 1967. In Fig. 4.12 are shown the leading causes of death of 1971.

In Table 4.11 there have been marked decreases in the deaths attributed to communicable disease. On the other hand, deaths from diseases of the heart and from malignant tumors have greatly increased.

As one might expect, deaths occur with greatest frequency in early infancy and in old age. Factors other than age affect death rates. Males for the most part have higher death rates than females. The white population in the United States has lower death rates than do non-white persons. Figure 4.13 depicts graphically the 1961 death rates in the United States by age, color, and sex.

In a study of deaths occurring in Houston, Texas, between 1940 and 1967, it was shown the males of Mexican descent had an excess of 400 deaths per 100,000 when compared with white Americans in 1950. Black males had 300 deaths per 100,000 per year more than did the white males. In 1960, the death rates among the Mexican-Americans had decreased to a level only slightly higher than the whites, but black males still experienced a death rate some 272 per 100,000 higher than prevailed among the whites.[35] (see Table 4.12).

### Maternal and Infant Mortality

Maternal mortality rates in the United States have declined steadily since 1915. The decline was slight until 1930, when the decrease

## TABLE 4.10

*Deaths, death rates, and age-adjusted death rates: 1935-68*

| Year | Number | Rate per 1,000 Population | | | | | Age-Adjusted rate per 1,000 Population | | | | |
|---|---|---|---|---|---|---|---|---|---|---|---|
| | | Total | White Male | White Female | All other Male | All other Female | Total | White Male | White Female | All other Male | All other Female |
| 1935 | 1,392,752 | 10.9 | 11.6 | 9.5 | 15.6 | 13.0 | 11.6 | 12.3 | 9.8 | 18.5 | 16.1 |
| 1940 | 1,417,269 | 10.8 | 11.6 | 9.2 | 15.1 | 12.6 | 10.8 | 11.6 | 8.8 | 17.6 | 15.0 |
| 1945 | 1,401,719 | 10.6 | 12.5 | 8.6 | 13.5 | 10.5 | 9.5 | 10.7 | 7.5 | 14.5 | 11.9 |
| 1950 | 1,452,454 | 9.6 | 10.9 | 8.0 | 12.5 | 9.9 | 8.4 | 9.6 | 6.5 | 13.6 | 11.0 |
| 1955 | 1,528,717 | 9.3 | 10.7 | 7.8 | 11.3 | 8.8 | 7.6 | 9.1 | 5.7 | 11.9 | 9.1 |
| 1956 | 1,564,476 | 9.4 | 10.8 | 7.8 | 11.4 | 8.8 | 7.6 | 9.1 | 5.7 | 11.9 | 9.1 |
| 1957 | 1,633,128 | 9.6 | 11.0 | 8.0 | 11.9 | 9.1 | 7.8 | 9.2 | 5.7 | 12.4 | 9.4 |
| 1958 | 1,647,886 | 9.5 | 10.9 | 8.0 | 11.6 | 9.0 | 7.6 | 9.1 | 5.6 | 12.2 | 9.2 |
| 1959 | 1,656,814 | 9.4 | 10.8 | 7.9 | 11.3 | 8.6 | 7.5 | 9.0 | 5.5 | 11.9 | 8.8 |
| 1960 | 1,711,982 | 9.5 | 11.0 | 8.0 | 11.5 | 8.7 | 7.6 | 9.2 | 5.6 | 12.1 | 8.9 |
| 1961 | 1,701,522 | 9.3 | 10.7 | 7.8 | 10.9 | 8.4 | 7.4 | 8.9 | 5.4 | 11.6 | 8.6 |
| 1962[2] | 1,756,720 | 9.5 | 10.8 | 8.0 | 11.2 | 8.5 | 7.5 | 9.0 | 5.4 | 12.0 | 8.7 |
| 1963[2] | 1,813,549 | 9.6 | 11.0 | 8.1 | 11.5 | 8.7 | 7.6 | 9.2 | 5.5 | 12.5 | 8.9 |
| 1964 | 1,798,051 | 9.4 | 10.8 | 8.0 | 11.1 | 8.3 | 7.4 | 9.0 | 5.3 | 12.2 | 8.6 |
| 1965 | 1,828,136 | 9.4 | 10.8 | 8.0 | 11.1 | 8.2 | 7.4 | 9.1 | 5.3 | 12.4 | 8.5 |
| 1966 | 1,863,149 | 9.5 | 10.9 | 8.1 | 11.3 | 8.3 | 7.5 | 9.2 | 5.3 | 12.7 | 8.6 |
| 1967 | 1,851,323 | 9.4 | 10.8 | 8.0 | 10.9 | 7.9 | 7.3 | 9.0 | 5.2 | 12.4 | 8.2 |
| 1968 | 1,930,082 | 9.7 | 11.1 | 8.2 | 11.6 | 8.3 | 7.5 | 9.2 | 5.3 | 13.3 | 8.6 |

[1] Adjusted to age distribution of U. S. population as enumerated in 1940.
[2] Figures by color exclude data for residents of New Jersey.
Source: Facts of Life and Death, Public Health Service Publication, No. 600, Revised 1970.

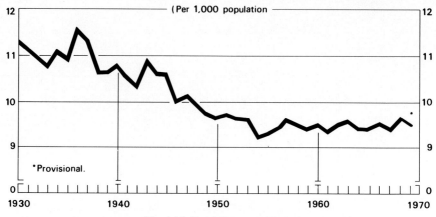

Fig. 4.11. Death Rates: 1930–69

Source: Facts of Life and Death, Public Health Service Publication, No. 600, Revised 1970.

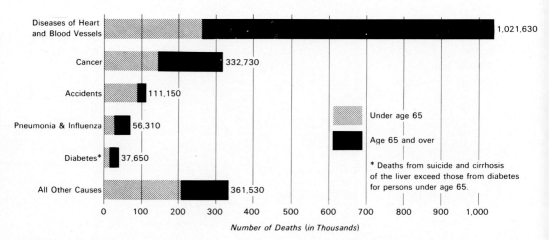

Fig. 4.12. Leading causes of death. United States: 1971 estimates. Source: *Heart Facts–1974*. The American Heart Association, New York, 1974.

became more rapid. From 1963 through 1971, deaths from causes related to pregnancy and delivery declined from 35.8 to 20.5 (preliminary figure) per 100,000 live births. The figures for 1968 (last year available) were 13.8 for white women and 25.6 per 100,000 live births among non-white women.

In Figure 4.14 are presented the curves of maternal mortality rates from 1941 to 1967 both in the white and non-white populations. It will be seen that the rates among non-whites, although declining, are substantially higher than are the rates for whites.

Many non-whites have no medical attendant during childbirth. This will account, at least partially, for the higher maternal mortality rates among the non-white population.

The infant mortality rate declined rapidly for many years. In the period 1933 to 1949, the rate for all races decreased about 4.3 per cent per year.[36],[37] Between 1950 and 1963, the average annual decline in the infant mortality rate was 1.0 per cent. See Figure 4.15 for the graph showing this trend from 1915 to 1963, and Fig. 4.16 for 1969 to 1973.

Infant deaths in the lowest socio-economic group are higher than those among the more prosperous segments of the population. Three indices of socio-economic status have been found significant: education of the father; education of the mother; and family income in the year prior to the infant death[38] (see Table 4.13 for infant mortality rates by education of parents, color, and family income).

The infant mortality rate in 1972 was the lowest ever recorded in the United States—18.2 per 1000 live births. The figure for July 1973 stood at 16.7[39] (see Figure 4.16). The weight at birth appears to be a most important factor in determining when a newborn infant will survive. In one study of 142,017 infants in those weighing 2500 gm. or less at birth, the mortality rate was 140.5 per 1000. The rate was 8.4 per 1000 for all infants who weighed more than 2500 gm.[40]

A number of other countries have achieved lower infant mortality rates than has the United States. The reasons for these more favorable experiences are not altogether clear. The National Center for Health Statistics has initiated studies on a contract basis to determine these reasons.

Of the infants who die, the period of greatest danger is the first weeks after birth. Usually these deaths are recorded separately and classified as neonatal deaths. From the number of infants dying during the first four weeks of life in relation to each 1000 live births, the neonatality rates are calculated. The chief causes of death in this early period are prematurity, birth injuries, congenital abnormalities, and respiratory infections. Since 1967, the neonatality rates have declined steadily reaching 12.9 per 1000 live births for whites in 1971 and 20.8 for non-whites (see Fig. 4.17).

*Expectation of Life at Birth*

The increase in expectation of life at birth during the past century has important social consequences for the nations so affected. It increases the period of family life and lengthens the years of the work span. The number of elderly and aged persons in the population has grown, introducing many socio-economic and health problems.

Life expectancy is a statistical measure used to indicate health conditions in a population. According to Lerner and Anderson,[41] life expectancy "shows for a given period of time the average lifetime to be expected by a population, if at each successive age it exper-

TABLE 4.11

*Deaths and death rates for the 10 leading causes of death in 1967 and death rates for these same causes in 1900*

| Rank 1967 | Cause of Death and Category Numbers of the Seventh Revision of the International Lists, 1955 | Number of deaths, 1967 | Rate per 100,000 Population | |
|---|---|---|---|---|
| | | | 1967 | 1900 |
| | All causes. . . . . . . . . . . . . . . . . . . . . . | 1,851,323 | 935.7 | 1,719.1 |
| 1 | Diseases of heart . . . . . . . . . . . 400-402,410-443 | 721,268 | 364.5 | 137.4 |
| 2 | Malignant neoplasms, including neoplasms of lymphatic and hematopoetic tissues . . . . 140-205 | 310,983 | 157.2 | 64.0 |
| 3 | Vascular lesions affecting central nervous system . . . . . . . . . . . . . . . . . . . . . 330-334 | 202,184 | 102.2 | 106.9 |
| 4 | Accidents. . . . . . . . . . . . . . . . . . . . E800-E962 | 113,169 | 57.2 | 72.3 |
| 5 | Influenza and pneumonia, except pneumonia of newborn . . . . . . . . . . . . . . . . . . 480-493 | 56,892 | 28.8 | 202.2 |
| 6 | Certain diseases of early infancy[1] . . . . . . . . 760-776 | 48,314 | 24.4 | 62.6 |
| 7 | General arteriosclerosis . . . . . . . . . . . . . . . . .450 | 37,564 | 19.0 | |
| 8 | Diabetes mellitus . . . . . . . . . . . . . . . . . . . .260 | 35,049 | 17.7 | (2) |
| 9 | Other diseases of circulatory system . . . . . . 451-468 | 29,944 | 15.1 | 12.0 |
| 10 | Other bronchopulmonic diseases . . . . . . . 525-527 | 29,360 | 14.8 | 12.5 |

[1] Birth injuries, asphyxia, infections of newborn, ill-defined diseases, immaturity, etc.
[2] Not comparable because of change in classification.

Source: *Facts of Life and Death.* Public Health Service Publication No. 600, Revised 1970.

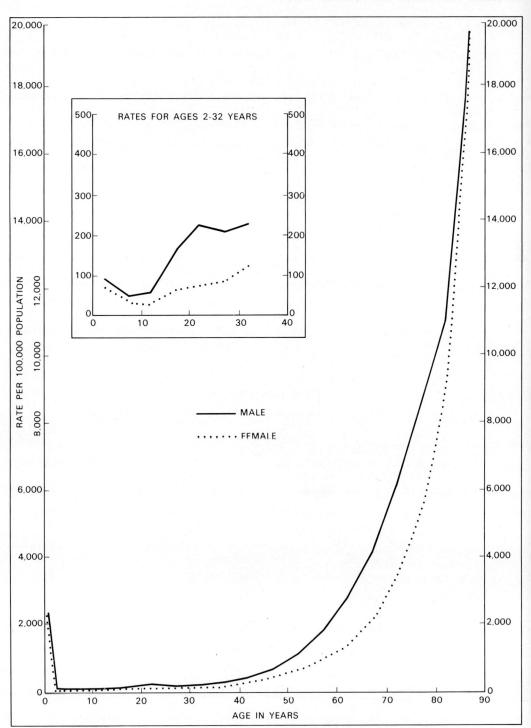

Fig. 4.13. Death rates by age and sex: United States, 1969.

Source: Mortality Trends: Age, Color, and Sex. United States—1950-69. National Center for Health Statistics, Public Health Service, Health Resources Administration, DHEW Publication No. (HRA) 74-1852. November, 1973.

TABLE 4.12

*Mortality from all causes, by sex and ethnicity, Houston, Tex.,*
*1950 and 1960*

| Sex and Ethnic Group | 1950[1] | | 1960[1] | |
|---|---|---|---|---|
| | Age-adjusted rate per 100,000[2] | Ratio of male to female | Age-adjusted rate per 100,000[2] | Ratio of male to female |
| Anglos: | | | | |
| Male | 990 | 1.58 | 951 | 1.75 |
| Females | 625 | | 543 | |
| Blacks: | | | | |
| Males | 1,291 | 1.20 | 1,223 | 1.33 |
| Females | 1,077 | | 921 | |
| Chicanos: | | | | |
| Males | 1,395 | 1.08 | 979 | 1.21 |
| Females | 1,296 | | 806 | |

[1] 3-year average deaths for 1949-51 and 1959-61.
[2] Age-adjusted rates computed by the direct method, using the total
U.S. population in 1950 as the standard.
Source: Roberts, R. E., and C. Askew, *A Consideration of Mortality in*
*Three Subcultures,* Health Services Reports 87: 262–279.
March, 1972.

iences the mortality rates that were prevalent during the given period of time."

In Table 4.14 are given the life expectancy figures by color and sex for the period between 1900 and 1970. In Table 4.15 are given the years of life expectancy at specified ages and by color and sex in the United States in 1970.

*Birth Rates*

There are many factors in a population that affect the birth rate. The age distribution of the population, the economic status of the people, and the prevailing views of people as to the value of rearing children are some of the controlling influences. Currently, one might add the availability of efficient contraceptive methods is an important factor in birth control.

The birth rate was about 32 births per 1000 population, and declined fairly steadily to about 18 per 1000 in the depths of the depression. Following World War II, a substantial rise in the birth rate occurred, the figure reaching 25.0 in 1955. Then a decline in the birth rate set in; the figures were 23.7 in 1960, 19.4 in 1965, and 15.6 (preliminary figure) in 1972. See Figure 4.18 for a graph depicting the annual birth rate and general fertility rate for the years from 1930 through 1972.

The U. S. Bureau of the Census has supplied the following figures for the birth rates and numbers of births in the United States since 1910:

| Year | Birth Rate | No. of Babies |
|---|---|---|
| 1910 | 30.1 | 2,777,000 |
| 1920 | 27.7 | 2,950,000 |
| 1921 | 28.1 | 3,055,000 |
| 1933 | 18.4 | 2,307,000 |
| 1940 | 19.4 | 2,570,000 |
| 1947 | 26.5 | 3,834,000 |
| 1957 | 25.2 | 4,332,000 |
| 1967 | 17.8 | 3,521,000 |
| 1969 | 17.7 (est.) | 3,571,000 (est.) |
| 1970 | 18.2 (est.) | 3,718,000 (est.) |
| 1972 | 15.6 (est.) | 3,256,000 (est.) |

## MEASUREMENT OF HEALTH STATUS OF THE POPULATION

Mortality data, while extremely useful in determining the health status of a population, provide only a partial view of the prevalent disease picture. Indeed, as the life span has been lengthened, the necessity for more exact information on ill health, both acute and chronic, becomes more pressing. The planning of health services and medical facilities requires knowledge of the extent and nature of sickness in the community. In addition to health agencies, other groups are keenly interested in sickness

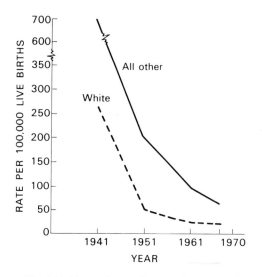

Fig. 4.14. Maternal mortality rates by color: United States, 1941–67.
Source: *The Health of Children–1970.* Selected Data from the National Center for Health Statistics Public Health Service Publication No. 2121.

data, among them are the medical research scientist, life and health insurance companies, manufacturers of drugs, the economist, and the sociologist.

The following list of sources of information on the health spectrum of the population is provided by the World Health Organization Expert Committee on Health Statistics, 1952.[42]

1. Sickness surveys by home visitation of: all persons in selected area, or representative sample of selected area or representative sample of whole population.

2. Mass diagnostic and screening surveys.

3. Census enumeration of sick persons.

4. Census enumeration of certain defects.

5. Records of notifiable communicable diseases.

6. Registration of certain diseases, with or without follow-up survey.

7. Certification of certain conditions for special benefits.

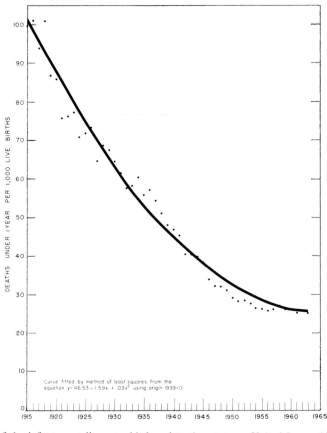

Fig. 4.15. Trend of the infant mortality rate: birth registration states or United States, 1915 to 1963. Source: Public Health Service Publication 1000, series 20, no. 3, National Center for Health Statistics, 1966.

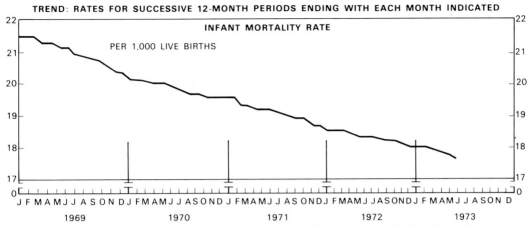

Fig. 4.16. Source: National Center for Health Statistics as published in American Medical News, November 5, 1973, page 21, American Medical Association.

TABLE 4.13

*Infant mortality rates by education of parents, color, and family income:*
*United States, 1964-66*

| Subject | Total | Years of School Completed | | | | |
|---|---|---|---|---|---|---|
| | | None or elemen-tary | High school | | College | |
| | | | 1-3 years | 4 years | 1-3 years | 4 years or more |
| *Infant mortality rate* | | | | | | |
| by education of mother | 22.8 | 34.8 | 27.4 | 19.2 | 15.7 | 19.7 |
| by education of father | 22.8 | 32.7 | 27.1 | 18.8 | 20.4 | 17.1 |
| *Index of infant mortality* | | | | | | |
| by education of mother | 1.00 | 1.53 | 1.20 | .84 | .69 | .86 |
| by education of father | 1.00 | 1.43 | 1.19 | .82 | .89 | .75 |

| Subject | Total | Family Income | | | | |
|---|---|---|---|---|---|---|
| | | Under $3,000 | $3,000-4,999 | $5,000-6,999 | $7,000-9,999 | $10,000 or more |
| Infant mortality rate, total | 22.8 | 31.8 | 24.9 | 17.9 | 19.6 | 19.6 |
| White | 20.5 | | | | | |
| Nonwhite | 37.1 | | | | | |
| Index of infant mortality, total | 1.00 | 1.39 | 1.09 | .79 | .86 | .86 |

Source: National Center for Health Statistics, *The Health of Children - 1970* (Washington: Government Printing Office, 1970).

8. Records of road accidents.

9. Records of industrial and occupational accidents and diseases.

10. General hospital inpatient records.

11. General hospital or clinic outpatient records.

12. General home visiting and nursing services.

13. Records of special clinics, hospitals, and agencies.

14. Continuous records of doctors' practices.

15. Social security schemes, compulsory and

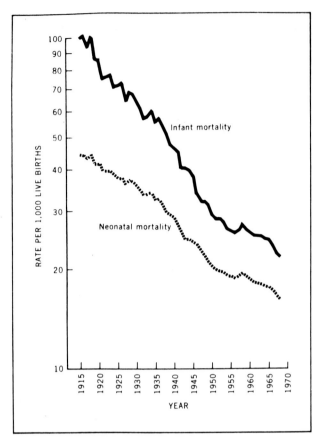

Fig. 4.17. Source: A Study of Infant Mortality from Linked Records: Comparison of Neonatal Mortality from Two Cohort Studies. United States National Center for Health Statistics, DHEW Publication No. (HSM) 72-1056. 1972.

TABLE 4.14
*Selected life table values, by color and sex: Death-registration areas, 1970,*
*1969, 1960, 1950, 1900-1902*

| Life Table Value and Year | Total | White | | All Other | |
|---|---|---|---|---|---|
| | | Male | Female | Male | Female |
| Life expectancy at birth: | | | | | |
| 1970 | 70.9 | 68.0 | 75.6 | 61.3 | 69.4 |
| 1969 | 70.4 | 67.8 | 75.1 | 60.5 | 68.4 |
| 1960 | 69.7 | 67.4 | 74.1 | 61.1 | 66.3 |
| 1950 | 68.2 | 66.5 | 72.2 | 59.1 | 62.9 |
| 1900 | 47.3 | 46.6 | 48.7 | 32.5 | 33.5 |
| At age 20: | | | | | |
| 1970 | 53.1 | 50.3 | 57.4 | 44.7 | 52.2 |
| 1900-1902 | | 42.2 | 43.8 | 35.1 | 36.9 |
| Percent reaching age 65: | | | | | |
| 1970 | 71.9 | 66.2 | 81.5 | 49.9 | 66.3 |
| 1900-1902 | | 39.2 | 43.8 | 19.0 | 22.0 |

Source: Vital Statistics of the United States, 1970, Volume II, Section 5,
        Life Tables, National Center for Health Statistics.

TABLE 4.15
*Selected life table values, by age, color, and sex: United States, 1970*

| Life Table Value and Age | Total | White | | All Other | |
|---|---|---|---|---|---|
| | | Male | Female | Male | Female |
| Expectation of life: | | | | | |
| At birth | 70.9 | 68.0 | 75.6 | 61.3 | 69.4 |
| At age 1 | 71.3 | 68.4 | 75.8 | 62.5 | 70.4 |
| At age 21 | 52.2 | 49.4 | 56.4 | 43.9 | 51.2 |
| At age 65 | 15.2 | 13.1 | 17.1 | 13.3 | 16.4 |
| Percent surviving from birth: | | | | | |
| To age 1 | 98.0 | 98.0 | 98.4 | 96.5 | 97.2 |
| To age 21 | 96.6 | 96.3 | 97.5 | 94.0 | 95.8 |
| To age 65 | 71.9 | 66.2 | 81.5 | 49.9 | 66.3 |
| Median age at death | 74.9 | 71.5 | 79.4 | 64.9 | 72.9 |

Source: Vital Statistics of the United States, 1970, Volume II, Section 5,
Life Tables, National Center for Health Statistics.

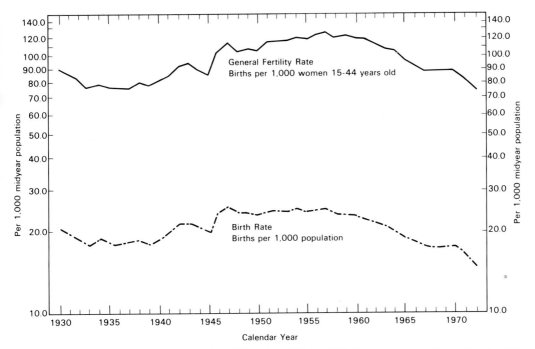

Fig. 4.18. Annual birth rate and general fertility rate: 1930 to 1972. Source: Current Population Reports, Bureau of the Census, Series P-60, No. 89, July 1973.

voluntary.

16. Voluntary health plans and funds.

17. Pensions and veterans' records.

18. Life insurance and sickness insurance records.

19. Records of health welfare centers (maternity, infant, and preschool child).

20. Medical records in educational institutions.

21. Records of physical examinations and sickness absenteeism in various occupational groups.

22. Sickness and recruitment records of the Armed Forces.

All of these sources serve important needs and provide information of varying degrees of usefulness. For example, a survey of hospital records will yield information on the disease conditions that are leading to hospital admissions.

## Reporting of Notifiable Diseases

Physicians on a local basis, as far back as the colonial period, were required to report to the authorities cases of epidemic diseases that came to their attention. It was hoped that when the great pests appeared steps might be taken early to prevent their spread. Compulsory notification of communicable diseases on a state-wide basis was not introduced until 1883 when Michigan made it mandatory for physicians and householders to report certain diseases to the boards of health. Within 30 years, the other existing states adopted similar laws.

As the state laws now stand, there is considerable uniformity in the requirements for disease notification, but there are some wide variations in the laws from state to state. The number of notifiable diseases ranges from 40 to nearly 70. All states require notification by physicians, hospitals, or householders. Usually, the reports are made to the local health department, or, if none exists, to the state department of health. Reports received by the state are tabulated and serve to orient the activities of the health department in disease prevention. Each state sends a weekly report of a selected list of diseases to the U. S. Public Health Service. The Center for Disease Control of the Public Health Service publishes a weekly list of 25 notifiable diseases in its *Mortality and Morbidity Report.* Annual summaries are also published. Information on the occurrence of quarantinable diseases is transmitted promptly to the World Health Organization by the Public Health Service as a part of the world-wide epidemiological reconnaissance service.

This system of notifying diseases has its defects. Some physicians fail to make their reports. In some cases, the diagnosis may not be correct. Many patients are not seen by a physician. With all of its defects, the system has proved useful in all countries, especially in the control of the more severe epidemic diseases such as smallpox, typhoid fever, and cholera.

## Health Surveys

As valuable as may be the registration of deaths and the notification of communicable diseases as sources of information on the health status of the population, these methods have failed to supply many kinds of data that are useful in understanding the health profile. A number of attempts to obtain such information by the survey method have been made, the most notable of which was conducted by the Public Health Service in 1935 and 1936.[43]

Following World War II, there was a growing interest in the lack of current data on chronic disease, disability, and the provision of medical care. These growing pressures for better sources of health information led Congress in 1956 to pass the National Health Survey Act. This Act provides for the establishment of a permanent, continuous health survey program to be directed by the National Center for Health Statistics. All of the surveys are on samples of the population. The samples are selected to obtain a cross-section of the nation. "The purpose of the survey is to provide data on the incidence of illness and accidental injuries; the prevalence of diseases and impairments; the extent of disability; the volume and kinds of medical, dental, and hospital care received; and other health related topics."[44] This information is related to age, sex, family status, and urban-rural residence.

Three types of survey are employed: (1) the health interview survey; (2) the health examination survey; and (3) the health records survey.

### The Health Interview Survey

The data in these surveys are obtained by household interviews of a selected sample of the population. Some 44,000 households containing about 134,000 persons throughout the United States are interviewed annually. The survey is continuous; about 800 households are covered each week. Trained interviewers follow a prescribed form which requires an average of 45 to 60 min. for completion at each interview.

The information obtained on reports of unattended illnesses is of an approximate nature. However, the individual involved is the best source of accurate data on the social and economic aspects of health and on the effects of illness on his own life and that of his family.

The data obtained from these interviews are compiled continuously and published periodically as sufficient data on particular items become available by the National Center for Health Statistics.

*The Health Examination Survey*

In this type of survey, data are collected by physical examination and clinical tests of a population sample. Of necessity, this survey covers fewer people and moves more slowly. In the first cycle of this survey terminating in 1962, examination of 6672 adults between 18 and 79 years of age was completed. This task was accomplished by two mobile units that sampled 42 locations throughout the United States.

Cycle II of the survey, conducted from July 1963 to December 1965 involved examination of selected samples of children aged 6 to 11 years. Ninety-six per cent of the 7417 children in the sample were examined. Factors relating to growth and development were determined and a variety of somatic and physiological measurements made.

A comparable examination of data collection for Cycle III, youths aged 12 to 17, was completed in 1970. To give a longitudinal aspect to the survey, the same sample areas and housing units of Cycle II were used again. In both cycles, 2271 youths were examined.

The caravan containing the clinical facilities for these examinations is staffed by two physicians, two nurses, one dentist, a psychologist, two X-ray and laboratory technicians, and a field staff trained in choosing the sample to be examined, bringing them to the examination center, and obtaining the necessary data for completion of the survey forms. The mobile unit provides space for interviews, examining rooms, a soundproof room for hearing tests, and X-ray and other facilities.

All examinations are limited to one visit. Special attention is given to discovering evidence of chronic diseases and impairments, of determining blood pressure levels and blood cholesterol content, and to tests for hearing defects or impairment of visual acuity. Measurements of height, weight, and physical development are taken. The smallness of the samples prevents the establishment of the frequency of rare conditions.

With the increasing concern over malnutrition, it was decided to merge the Health Examination Survey with a Nutrition Examination Survey—the new program designated HANES. Before the amalgamation, HES had already begun Cycle IV. This cycle centered around the problems of current and unmet needs of the United States adult population with heavier sampling of older persons and minority groups.

Planning for HANES surveys contemplates that each cycle will cover approximately a two-year period based on a sample of about 30,000 persons aged one through 74 years. All persons are to receive a designated nutrition examination with a portion of the sample to receive a more detailed examination based on HES methods. Three mobile examination centers are to be used.[45]

*The Health Records Survey*

The basic function of this survey is to create and maintain a master list of all hospitals, nursing homes, clinics, physicians' and dentists' offices, industrial and union dispensaries, homes for the aged, and a variety of other residential and correctional institutions. From this list, survey samples may be selected to provide continuous information on such matters as the use of hospitals, on services provided in hospitals, on the kinds of cases being hospitalized, and on methods of financing hospital care.

Another function of the Health Records Survey is to collect data on the institutionalized population which constitutes about 1 per cent of the total population. Many of the most severely disabled persons are found in resident institutions of one kind or another. This survey of resident institutions covers all types in the United States, both medical and non-medical. This includes long-stay hospitals, penal institutions, orphanages, nursing homes, and homes for the aged.

*Research on Methods*

The National Health Survey Act provides for studies on the methods and survey techniques in the health statistics field with a view of their continued improvement. The primary purposes of these studies are to evaluate the degree to which the various aspects of the survey program are meeting their objectives, to develop new and improved methods of collecting the required data, and to conduct pilot projects to prepare new methods for full use in the survey.

The National Health Survey has been in operation over 10 years. Already the great value of the data produced has become apparent. That there are limitations to the surveys as now employed is freely acknowledged; for example, the sample sizes are such as to permit estimates for major geographic areas only. In spite of this and other limitations, the survey is likely to remain as a permanent feature of the health resources of the United States and has already proven to be a valuable asset to all interested in health data.

## REFERENCES

1. Paul, J. R. *Clinical Epidemiology,* rev. ed. Chicago: University of Chicago Press, 1966.
2. Maxcy, K. F. Principles of epidemiology. In *Bacterial and Mycotic Infections of Man,* edited by R. Dubos, Ed. 3. Philadelphia: J. B. Lippincott Company, 1958.
3. Holmes, O. W. On the contagiousness of puerperal fever. *N. Engl. Quart. J. Med. Surg., 1:* 503–530, 1842–1843.
4. Panum, P. L. *Observations Made During the Epidemic of Measles on the Faroe Islands in the Year 1846,* translated from Danish and reprinted by Delta Omega Society. New York: American Public Health Association, 1940.
5. Snow, J. On Cholera. New York: The Commonwealth Fund, 1936.
6. Budd, W. *Typhoid Fever, Its Nature, Mode of Spreading and Prevention.* New York: The Commonwealth Fund, 1931.
7. Smith, T. *Parasitism and Disease.* Princeton, New Jersey: Princeton University Press, 1934.
8. Morris, J. N. *Uses of Epidemiology,* Ed. 2. Baltimore: The Williams and Wilkins Company, 1964.
9. Taylor, I., and Knowelden, J. *Principles of Epidemiology,* Ed. 2. Boston: Little, Brown & Company, 1964.
10. MacMahon, B., Pugh, T. F., and Ipsen, J. *Epidemiological Methods.* Boston: Little, Brown & Company, 1960.
11. *Trends in Epidemiology. Application to Health Service Research and Training.* Edited by G. T. Stewart. Springfield, Ill.: Charles C Thomas, 1972.
12. Terris, M. The scope and methods of epidemiology. *J. Amer. Pub. Health Assn., 52:* 1371–1376, 1962.
13. Hammond, E. C., and Horn, D. Smoking and death rates. Report on 44 months of follow-up of 187,783 men. *J.A.M.A., 166:* 1294–1308, 1958.
14. Lilienfeld, A. M. Epidemiological concepts applied to studies of chronic diseases. In Genetics and the Epidemiology of Chronic Diseases, Public Health Service Publication 1163, edited by J. V. Neel, M. W. Shaw, and W. J. Schull. Washington, D. C.: United States Public Health Service, 1965.
15. *The Community as an Epidemiologic Laboratory.* Edited by I. I. Kessler and M. L. Levin. Baltimore: The Johns Hopkins Press, 1970.
16. Siegel, M. Indices of community health. In *Preventive Medicine,* edited by D. W. Clark and B. MacMahon. Boston: Little, Brown & Company, 1967.
17. Puffer, R. R. *Practical Statistics in Health and Medical Work.* New York: McGraw-Hill Book Company, 1950.
18. Ipsen, J. and Feigl, P. *Bancroft's Introduction to Biostatistics.* Ed. 2. New York: Harper & Row, 1970.
19. Kilpatrick, S. J., Jr. *Statistical Principles in Health Care Information.* Baltimore: University Park Press, 1973.
20. Densen, P. M. Statistical reasoning. In *Rosenau Preventive Medicine and Hygiene,* edited by K. F. Maxcy, Ed. 7. New York: Appleton-Century-Crofts, Inc., 1951.
21. Puffer, R. R., and Griffith, G. W. *Patterns of Urban Mortality, Scientific Publication 151.* Washington, D. C.: Pan American Health Organization, 1967.
22. Dunn, H. L. Health and social statistics for the city. *Amer. J. Pub. Health, 37:* 740–743, 1947.
23. Brady, F. J., Farner, L. M., Nighswonger, W. H., Rasmussen, W., and Serfling, R. E. *Health Index Survey.* Tucson, Arizona: National Communicable Disease Center, U. S. Health Service, 1963.
24. Francis, T., Korns, R. F., Voight, R. B., Boisen, M., Hemphill, F. M., Napier, J. A., and Tolchinsky, E. An evaluation of the 1954 poliomyelitis vaccine trials. *Amer. J. Pub. Health, 45:* suppl. 1, 1955.
25. Arnold, F. A., Jr., Dean, H. T., Jay, P., Knutson, J. W. Effect of fluoridated public water supplies on dental caries prevalence. *Public Health Reports, 71:* 652–658, 1956.
26. Hutchison, G. B. Evaluation of preventive measures. In *Preventive Medicine,* edited by D. W. Clark and B. MacMahon. Boston: Little, Brown & Company, 1967.
27. Kinch, S., and Amos, F. B. Vital statistics. In *Preventive Medicine,* edited by H. E. Hilleboe and G. W. Larrimore, Philadelphia: W. B. Saunders Company, 1965.
28. U. S. Bureau of the Census, Statistical Abstract of the United States: 1973, 94th edition. Washington, D. C., 1973.
29. Dorn, H. F. World population growth: an international dilemma. *Science, 135:* 283–290, 1962.
30. Schachter, J. *Birth Registration Completeness in United States and Geographic Areas, 1950.* Vital Statistics Special Report, Vol. 45, No. 9. Washington, D. C.: National Office of Vital Statistics, 1956.
31. Taeuber, I. B. Growth of the population of the United States in the twentieth century. Commission on Population Growth and the American Future, Vol. 1. *Demographic and Social Aspects of Population Growth,* Edited by C. F. Westoff and R. Parke, Jr. Washington, D. C.: U. S. Government Printing Office, 1972.
32. Moriyama, I. M., Preliminary observations on recent mortality trends. *Public Health Rep., 76:* 1056–1058. 1961
33. Kitagama, E. M., Hauser, P. M. *Differential Mortality in the United States: a Study in Socioeconomic Epidemiology.* Cambridge, Mass.: Harvard University Press, 1973.
34. *Mortality Trends: Age, Color and Sex.* United

States, 1950–69. National Center for Health
Statistics, DHEW Publication No. (HRA)
74–1852, November, 1973.

35. Roberts, R. E., Askew, C., Jr. A Consideration
of Mortality in Three Subcultures. Health
Services Reports, 87: 262–270, 1972.

36. National Center for Health Statistics. Infant,
Fetal, and Maternal Mortality, United States,
1963. Public Health Service Publication 1000,
series 20, no. 3, 1966.

37. National Center for Health Statistics. *Infant
Mortality Trends, United States and Each
State, 1930–1964.* Public Health Service Pub-
lication 1000, series 20, no. 1, 1965.

38. *Infant Mortality Rates: Socioeconomic Factors.*
United States National Center for Health
Statistics, DHEW Publication No. (HSM)
72–1045, March, 1972.

39. U. S. Infant Mortality Rate at a Record Low, but
Experts Note Its Not Best Index of Nation's
Health. American Medical Association. Amer-
ican Medical News, p. 21, Nov. 5, 1973.

40. MacMahon, B., Kovar, M. G., and Feldman, J. J.

*Infant Mortality Rates: Socio-economic Fac-
tor.* National Center for Health Statistics.
DHEW Publication No. (HSM) 72–1045,
March, 1972.

41. Lerner, M., and Anderson, O. W. *Health Progress
in the United States, 1900–1960.* Chicago:
The University of Chicago Press, 1963.

42. World Health Organization, Expert Committee on
Health Statistics. WHO Technical Report,
series 53, Geneva, 1952.

43. Perrott, G. St. J., Tibbetts, C., Britten, R. The
national health survey (1935–36). *Public
Health Reports, 54:* 1663–1687, 1939.

44. National Center for Health Statistics. Plan and
initial program of the health examination
survey. Public Health Service Publication, No.
1000, Series 1, No. 4, July, 1965.

45. National Center for Health Statistics. Plan and
operation of the health and nutrition examination survey United States, 1971–1973.
DHEW Publication No. (HSM) 73–1310. Vital
and Health Statistics, Series 1–no. 10b, Feb.,
1973.

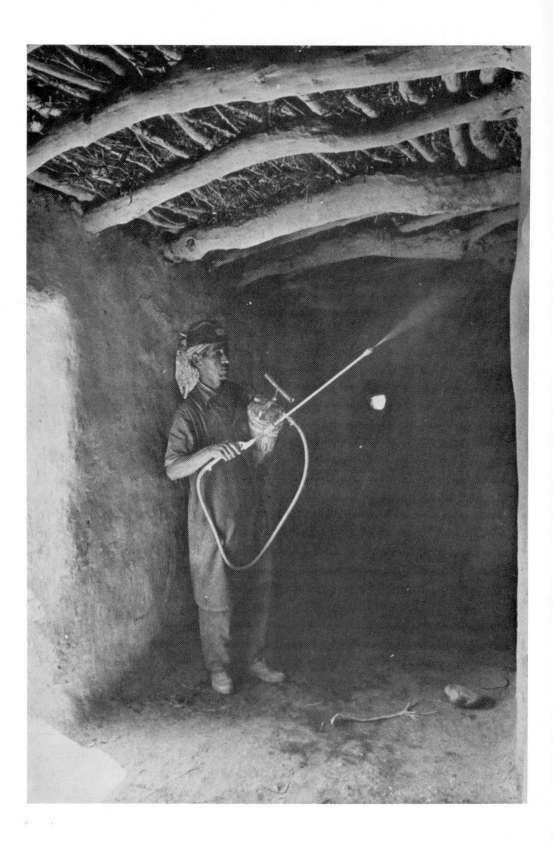

# 5
# *Factors contributing to ill health*

If man could see
The perils and diseases that he elbows
  Each day he walks a mile; which catch at him,
  Which fall behind and graze him as he passes;
    Then would he know that Life's a single
    pilgrim,
    Fighting unarmed amongst a thousand
    soldiers.
          THOMAS L. BEDDOES (1798-1851)
*Death's Jest Book*

Life is an adventure in a world where nothing is static; where unpredictable and ill-understood events constitute dangers that must be overcome, often blindly and at great cost; where man himself, like the sorcerer's apprentice, has set in motion forces that are potentially destructive and may someday escape his control. Every manifestation of existence is a response to stimuli and challenges, each of which constitutes a threat if not adequately dealt with. The very process of living is a continual interplay between the individual and his environment, often taking the form of a struggle resulting in injury or disease.
          RENE DUBOS, *The Mirage of Health* *

Disease and health are polar words: that is, like hot and cold, they have meaning only in relation to each other. Disease is ordinarily defined as "a departure from a state of health"; contrarily, health is "the absence of disease." To give hot and cold more precise meaning, we devise a scale of changes with reference to particular events, such as the freezing and boiling of water. The many efforts to establish a comparable sort of a scale for measuring "degrees" of health have all failed. One suggestion is that zero, the absolute lower limit of health, is death, that as long as there is some life, there is some degree of health. With such a scale, the upper limit, the maximum level, of health would be the perfect functioning of the organism in all respects, but no satisfactory

criterion for this maximum has ever been founded.
          MARSTON BATES, *Man in Nature*†

Any precise definition of health is difficult. Webster's *New International Dictionary* defines health as the "state of being hale, sound or whole, in body, mind or soul; well-being, especially the state of being free from physical disease or pain." To others, "the real measure of health is not the Utopian absence of all disease, but the ability to function effectively within a given environment."[1] In 1950, Dr. John Romano gave his concept of the relationship of health and disease as follows[2]: "Health and disease are not static entities but are phases of life, dependent at any time on the balance maintained by devices, genically and experientially determined, intent on fulfilling needs and adapting to and mastering stresses as they may arise from within the organism or from without. Health, in a positive sense, consists in the capacity of the organism to maintain a balance in which it may be reasonably free of undue pain, discomfort, disability or limitation of action, including social capacity."

In essence, disease represents "failures or disturbance in the growth, development, functions, and adjustments of the organism as a whole or of any of its systems."[3]

As early as 1859 to 1860, the great French physiologist Claude Bernard stated in his lectures that living beings are concerned with two environments—an outer environment that surrounds the organism as a whole and an internal environment in which the living elements of the body are exposed. Plasma of the blood and lymph constitute the major factors in the *"milieu interne."* "It is the fixity of the *'milieu intereur'* which is the condition of free and independent life", postulated Bernard. "All the vital mechanisms, however varied they may be, have only one object, that of preserving constant the conditions of life in the internal environment."[4] Bernard listed water, oxygen,

---

uniform temperature, and nutrient supplies (including salts, fats, and sugar) as the necessary constants.

The fundamental biological concept was forgotten for years, until the Harvard University physiologist, Walter B. Cannon, summarized the results of his laboratory experience in 1932 in a book titled *The Wisdom of the Body*.[5] Cannon supported Bernard's concept, filling out the details of the body's mechanisms for stabilizing its internal environment with the results of recent research. He demonstrated that the necessary processes in the body's economy are largely controlled by the autonomic nervous system and by hormones which mediate the activities of the various organs and organ systems. Cannon gave the combined Greek words of "homeostasis," a term whose exact meaning is "staying the same," to this state produced in the healthy body by the constant physiological adjustments. When all of the homeostatic mechanisms are properly functioning, the body meets changes in the external environment efficiently.

Homeostasis is not well developed in the newborn baby. In the womb, the developing infant is protected by the mother's regulatory systems. After birth, the baby comes into contact with environmental changes that demand constant adjustment. Little by little its own regulatory mechanisms become developed. At the other extreme of life, aged individuals tend to lose some of their ability to cope with the marked changes in temperature, both cold and heat. Other mechanisms of their internal stability are also more easily disarranged.

In considering the nature of diseases, physicians like to regard them as separate entities, classifiable on this basis of either causative factors or similarity of their manifestations. Actually, diseases represent patterned responses or adaptations to harmful forces in the environment. A great variety of diseases share similar manifestations, but frequently in different combinations. Some of the phenomena appearing as indications of disease include vomiting, malaise, headache or other pains, muscular weakness, depression or excitement, loss of consciousness, alteration in the amount and composition of the blood, the plasma and excretory products, shifts in electrolyte concentration in various body fluids, immunological changes involving capillary permeability, excessive cell reproduction, and changes in the

tissues such as hyperemia, edema, and necrosis.[6]

In the latter part of the 19th century came proof that certain microorganisms are agents of disease. This led to effective methods of treatment and of control of a number of man's most feared enemies, including plague, cholera, typhoid fever, diphtheria, yellow fever, and typhus. The very success of the campaigns against these and other communicable diseases led physicians to think in terms of one disease-one cause. If the causative factor could be discovered, the method of control was sure to follow. As the public health movement progressed and one after another infectious disease was greatly reduced in importance, more people began to live longer lives. Instead of dying from typhoid fever or pneumonia, they survived to acquire the chronic illnesses of advanced life—cardiovascular disease, diabetes, or cancer. It soon became apparent that such complex forms of ill health were not at all likely to result from one specific causal agent but are the result of a combination of many noxious factors. Indeed, in recent years it is becoming generally recognized that even the microbial diseases rarely are the result of a single agent. Thousands of individuals harbor such germs as those of tuberculosis, *Staphylococcus* infections, influenza, and others but do not develop the disease. Such other factors as malnutrition, severe exposures to inclement weather, or stresses due to strains in the social environment may provide the additional stimuli that cause the infection to proceed to disease. Every illness, of whatever kind, is the consequence of a variety of causes.

In a challenging little book edited by Iago Galdston and published by the New York Academy of Medicine called *Beyond the Germ Theory*, the roles of deprivation and stress in health and disease are emphasized.[7] Man must have a supply of the important chemicals required to maintain the constancy of his internal environment. If these "balancing factors" are missing, disease, due to their lack or inadequacy, results. Vitamins provide a well-known example of materials essential to body health. Deprivation of such biological essentials causes ill health. As for stress, man can maintain his inner balance in the face of external variations if these changes are not excessive in degree or do not come on too suddenly. Men do break down when subjected to physical or emotional stress in excess of their tolerance. It is the purpose of this chapter to discuss the above-mentioned and other important factors that contribute to human ill health.

## INHERITED DISEASE

### Genetic

The principles which have provided the basis for the studies on heredity and disease were propounded by Gregor Mendel in 1866 after prolonged investigations of the inherited characteristics of peas. These classic experiments were promptly forgotten and remained to be brought to light by three botanists in 1900. Each of the three who were working independently in different countries reported that Mendel had preceded his own discoveries by 34 years.

In 1905, a British botanist, William Bateson, coined the word "genetics" and urged Cambridge University to create an institute for the study of heredity. This proposal was rejected, but he did succeed in interesting his friend, a physician, Archibald Garrod, in beginning biochemical investigations on hereditary conditions. Garrod described the first example of a hereditary chemical defect in man. This condition was a rare one, known as alkaptonuria, a metabolic disorder characterized by the excretion of urine that turns black upon standing. Garrod summarized his studies in a series of lectures in 1908 under the title "Inborn Errors of Metabolism." As frequently happens, Garrod was ahead of his time.

In the 66-year period following Garrod's early studies, great progress has been made in the understanding of the mechanisms underlying the inheritance of human characteristics. Much of the basic research has been carried out on *Drosophila* (fruit flies), on fungi, on bacteria, and on bacterial viruses (bacteriophage), although in recent years fruitful studies on human chromosomes are common.

The current concept of the hereditary mechanism is that each individual originates from the union of two parental cells, the ovum and the spermatozoon. The bearers of the hereditary elements are called chromosomes. These are present in the cell nucleus. Both the ovum and the spermatozoon contain 23 chromosomes which upon union form the usual complement of 23 pairs or a total of 46 chromosomes. It is believed that the chromosomes are the bearers

of the hereditary elements present in the cell nucleus. The chromosomes are visible under the microscope as discrete particles during the mitotic process of cell division.

Each pair of chromosomes has its own characteristics and differs from others in size and form. These variations provide a basis for classifying chromosomes into seven separate groups. One of the most important features for classification of chromosomes is the position of the connecting bond, called the centromere. If the centromere is located in the middle, the chromosomes are called metacentric; if below the center, submedian; and if at or near the ends, acrocentric. In Figure 5.1 is shown the distribution into groups of a normal male set of chromosomes. Twenty-two of the pairs are called autosomal chromosomes. The other two are the sex chromosomes—in the female (see Fig. 5.2), the two chromosomes are designated XX; in the male, there is an X and a Y chromosome. In Figures 5.1 and 5.2, the chromosomes are presented in a systematized array arranged in pairs in descending order of size and according to the position of the centromere. This scheme of chromosome presentation is designated as the karyotype of an individual. To prepare a karyotype, the chromosomes are arranged in order of decreasing size as shown in Figures 5.1 and 5.2. By international agreement, the human autosomes are arranged in seven groups, designated A to G. Chromosomes, although they appear to be short and thick, are quite long thin filaments. These are coiled tightly in a spiral formation which gives the appearance seen in the process of cell division. Normally, as cell division takes place in the growth of the embryo and throughout life, the chromosomes split in two to provide a full complement of the chromosomal pattern to the daughter cells.

Therefore, the normal body (somatic) cell contains 46 chromosomes, of which 44 are autosomes and two are sex chromosomes. In the female, the sex chromosomes are represented by two X chromosomes. In addition to 44 autosomes, the male has an X chromosome and a shorter Y chromosome. The genes, or mendelian units of inheritance, are located on the chromosomes. Each has a definite place or locus. They number between 20,000 and 40,000 and are of molecular size. Genes have two properties: first, capacity for exact reproduction of themselves and, second, the ability

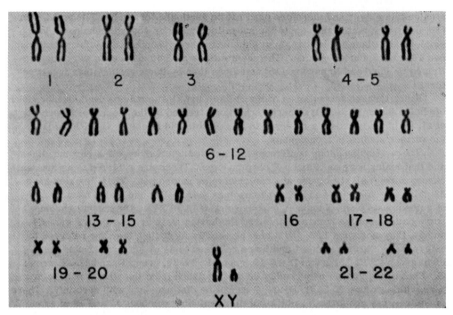

Fig. 5.1. Karyotype of a normal human male. Source: M. Neil Macintyre, Department of Anatomy, Western Reserve University. Appeared in *Preventive Medicine,* edited by D. W. Clark and B. MacMahon. Boston: Little, Brown, and Company, 1967.

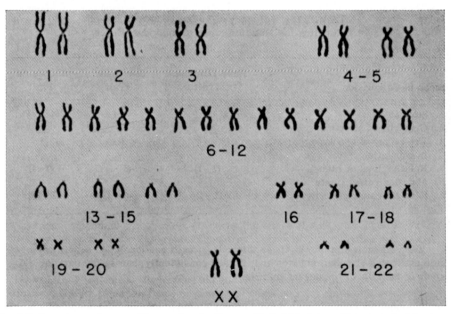

Fig. 5.2. Karyotype of a normal human female. Source: M. Neil Macintyre, Department of Anatomy, Western Reserve University. Appeared in *Preventive Medicine,* edited by D. W. Clark and B. MacMahon. Boston: Little, Brown, and Company, 1967.

to stimulate formation of enzymes and other proteins. Both chromosomes and genes are made up of deoxyribonucleic acid (DNA) combined with protein. Genes are subject to frequent mutations which change or destroy their usual function. X rays and atomic radiations are frequent sources of gene mutations.[8] Genes may be located on either the autosomal or the sex chromosomes. Also, the genetic trait may be either dominant or recessive. An inherited characteristic may result from the action of a single gene or result from a combination of genetic factors.

Most diseases can be considered as "constituting a spectrum of the relative importance of genetic and non-genetic factors in their causation."[8] At one end of the spectrum are diseases predominantly genetic but which are still influenced slightly by environmental factors. At the other extreme are found such disorders as hypertension, otosclerosis, and peptic ulcer where environmental factors predominate, but at least some genetic factors are also involved. In chronic illnesses, especially degenerative diseases, there is evidence that hereditary constitutional characteristics are often important factors in determining individual susceptibility to such conditions. Probably, even the rate of aging depends on the inherited constitution.

## Abnormalities of the Chromosomes

Since 1956, techniques for the study of human chromosomal patterns have been available. Dividing cells may be observed in cultures of human tissues, in scrapings of epithelial cells from the mucous membranes, from bone marrow tissue, or from leukocytes in the blood. Spreading of cells may be achieved by squashing between glass slides. Appropriate stains are used to bring out the details of form and structure of the chromosomal material.

A considerable number of congenital malformations have been shown to have their basis in abnormalities of structure or in the number of the chromosomes. Mongoloid idiocy (Down's disease) is known to be accompanied by a chromosome count of 47 rather than the normal number of 46. The extra chromosome is usually located together with the number 21 pair, resulting in three number 21 chromosomes, or one extra. This condition is known as "trisomy." Women who become pregnant in the latter part of the child-bearing period give birth more frequently to mongoloid children than do younger mothers. Mongolism is thought to occur once in every 500 births.[9] It accounts for about 15 per cent of mental deficiencies that require institutionalization in the United States.

An abnormality of the sex chromosome may be associated with children having both masculine and feminine characteristics. One such condition that has been extensively studied is Klinefelter's syndrome. Patients with this defect are male in appearance with external male genitalia. The testes are quite small and biopsies reveal abnormal tissue structure. Sterility is common. Breasts of female type may develop. Mental retardation is frequent. These patients usually show a chromosome count in their body cells of 47 with an extra X sex chromosome.[10]

Other chromosomal abnormalities have been described as resulting in aberrant development of sexual organs and of sexual secondary characteristics. Probably, abnormal chromosomes are responsible too for a considerable portion of spontaneous abortions and stillborn infants.

## Abnormalities of the Genes

From the point of view of hereditary factors in their causation, human diseases tend to fall into two categories. On one hand are several relatively rare conditions in which the hereditary factor weighs more heavily than environmental influences. In such conditions, the genetic factor is frequently a relatively simple one. In the case of many common conditions which have a complex or multifactorial causation, there may be a wide range of genetic and environmental factors contributing to their development. The hereditary basis for such complex conditions may involve many genes. For a long time it has been known that some congenital abnormalities are inherited along the mendelian pattern. Many such abnormalities are attributable to a change in a single gene. It is estimated that this type of defect accounts for nearly 10 per cent of human malformations.

Both chromosomes of a pair may carry the same gene. In this case, the individual is called homozygous for the particular gene. One chromosome of a pair may carry an abnormal gene while the other may have a normal gene for a certain character. This situation is termed heterozygous. In the case where a gene produces its effect whether present on one or both the chromosome pair, it is designated as dominant. If the effect is produced only if the same gene is present on both chromosomes, it is referred to as recessive. An intermediate situation is sometimes encountered when neither gene is dominant. One abnormal gene in such an individual produces an abnormal effect, while the presence of two in the same individual results in a greater degree of the defect.

In the inheritance of dominant characteristics, every affected individual has an affected parent (except in the case of a gene mutation). Normal children of affected parents have normal children. If one parent is affected and the other is normal, affected and normal children are born in equal proportions.

The form of dwarfism called achondroplasia is a well-known example of the dominant inheritance pattern. The metabolic anomaly, porphyria, in which the body fails to break down porphyrin properly, an essential component of hemoglobin, is another of the diseases transmitted by dominant genes.

Inherited biochemical disorders of metabolism occur with an estimated frequency of one in 100 live births. More than 40 different inborn errors of metabolism have been described. Some are associated with profound mental defects and/or a fatal outcome; others are mild. The mutant gene responsible for these birth defects is located on an autosomal chromosome. Several different types of metabolic defects are known:

1. Disorders of lipid (fatty) metabolism.
2. Disorders of mucopolysaccharide metabolism.
3. Amino acid and related disorders.
4. Miscellaneous biochemical disorders.

In abnormalities based on recessive inheritance, the affected individual must have received the gene for the particular trait from both parents. Harmful recessive genes are relatively common. Probably every person carries at least one and maybe several potentially injurious recessive genes. Only such individuals as chance to mate with another person with the same recessive gene pass the hereditary trait on to offspring.

Possibly, the most common recessive disease in the United States is fibrocystic disease of the pancreas. This serious affection occurs in about one in 2000 births.

In recessive inheritance, most affected persons have parents who are normal in appearance. There is a familial history of similar affectations. In general, the number of normals in family relationships is 3:1. Affected persons who marry unaffected spouses usually have normal children. Consanguinous marriages are more common in the rarer types of abnormali-

ties. Some genetic defects are limited to one sex. In the human, this type of inherited abnormality denotes a gene that is regularly dominant in one sex and regularly recessive in the other. More frequently, partial sex linkage is found. This means that the gene is expressed more frequently in one sex than in the other or to a greater degree in one than in the other. Complete sex linkage is rare, but sex limitation to a partial degree is quite common. The males show a higher incidence of sex-linked defects. This is the case with harelip, congenital pyloric stenosis, and hemophilia.[11]

Another genetically controlled physiological system of great medical importance is the blood groups. The group to which an individual belongs is determined by heredity. The antigens that a person possesses on the surface of the red blood cells determine the group to which an individual belongs. These antigens react with their appropriate antibodies. There are three genes controlling the ABO blood group system. An individual with two O genes belongs to Group O; a person with two A genes or an A and an O belongs to Group A; one with two B genes or a B and an O is in Group B; and a person with one A and one B gene is in Group AB. It thus appears that both A and B genes are dominant to O.

This ABO system was discovered at the beginning of the century. It was relatively easy to demonstrate as the corresponding antibodies are found to occur naturally in the blood. Blood cells of Group A injected into the vein of a Group B or Group O person are rapidly destroyed, frequently producing a severe reaction; the same reaction occurs if cells of a Group B are injected into individuals of Groups O or A, or if cells of a Group AB are introduced into the bloodstream of any other group.

Other blood group systems of lesser importance were subsequently discovered. The so-called Rhesus system was not demonstrated until 1940. This group system has proved to be of great importance in the production of a severe, often fatal, anemia in newborn infants. This occurs when an Rh negative woman has children by an Rh-positive man. This situation results in many stillbirths and in the birth of severely ill infants. Fortunately, many of these affected newborns can be saved by prompt exchange transfusions. Diseases due to a single gene abnormality are generally very rare. Perhaps the most common is sickle cell anemia.

The mutant gene responsible for sickle cell disease leads to formation of an abnormal form of hemoglobin. Persons suffering from this anemia frequently die at an early age. The sickle cell gene is widely distributed throughout the Negro races both in Africa and in the Americas. The incidence is about nine per cent among Negroes in the United States. Of the simply inherited conditions in the United States, fibrocystic disease of the pancreas occurs most frequently.

In a great many diseases, infectious and otherwise, inheritance plays some part. Usually, many factors are involved of which inheritance is only one. For example, congenital dislocation of the hip tends toward familial occurrence. Several non-genetic factors have been noted, however. The occurrence of this condition is about twice as frequent among first-born infants as among infants born subsequently in a family. Occurrence is also much higher among infants born in the winter as in those born during summer months. These observations indicate a multifactorial causation of this instability of the hip joint.

Many causes of ill health display some familial incidence. The occurrence among family members may not be high but is more than expected by chance, suggesting a causal relationship. It is difficult to determine whether this apparent relationship is based on a common inheritance or on shared environmental conditions. Probably the explanation for the great majority of diseases is that both factors have an influence.

### Congenital Anomalies

In addition to the chromosomal and genic factors outlined in the preceding section, there are many agents that may affect the developing embryo and fetus *in utero* during the period of gestation. These may be infectious, chemical, or physical in nature. The injury to the tissues of the embryo or fetus may be so severe as to cause death or it may produce only mild effects. The stage of pregnancy at which the injury occurs is of great importance in determining the tissues affected. The limb buds of the embryo are developing during the fourth week of pregnancy; at six weeks, the palate is beginning to fuse; at the fifth to the sixth week, the primary fibers of the optic lens are developing; at the eighth week, the septal wall

in the heart is forming; and at the eighth to the ninth week, the organ of Corti, the hearing apparatus, is becoming differentiated. The type of malformation that may result from an intrauterine injury depends rather precisely upon the day or week of embryonic development that the damage is received.[12]

If the noxious agent acts in the first stage of embryonic development, it either causes death or only mild injuries which are readily repaired. In the next stage of intensive differentiation of organs, many agents are highly effective and produce malformations readily. Each organ is most susceptible to injury during the early stages of its development. As the weeks of embryonic or fetal life go by, organ susceptibility rapidly diminishes. Each agent acts in a specific way on a particular aspect of cell metabolism.

Between 10 and 20 per cent of all infant deaths in highly developed countries are ascribed to congenital malformations. Chromosomal abnormalities occur in about 1 in 200 live births, accounting each year for over 20,000 births in the United States. In a study being conducted by Metropolitan Atlanta Congenital Defects Program, among a total of 27,158 births, there were 704 cases with malformations; 526 of these were major and 178 had only minor malformations. Approximately 2.59 per cent of the infants born in this study had some malformation.[13]

Unfortunately, little progress has been made in the prevention of congenital malformations. Methods are now becoming available to make accurately a prenatal diagnosis of some gross congenital defects (see Table 5.1).

Putting a needle into the uterus during pregnancy (amniocentesis) to withdraw a sample of amniotic fluid is widely used in the management of Rh disease. The procedure is usually carried out during the period between the 14th and 16th weeks of pregnancy or later, if Rh studies alone are contemplated.

Biochemical tests on the fluid may reveal prenatal disorders of metabolism. Culture of cells found in the amniotic fluid may show abnormal fetal chromosome patterns.

Examinations for congenital malformations may be performed by ultra-sound, X rays, direct observation of the fetus with a fiberoptic endoscope, or by other techniques.

Knowledge that the fetus is severely affected by a genetic or other disorder gives the

Table 5.1

*Prevalance of common birth defects each year in the U.S.*

| Condition | Number under Age 20 |
|---|---|
| Mental retardation of prenatal origin | 1,170,000[1] |
| Congenital blindness and lesser visual impairment | 300,000[2] |
| Congenital deafness and lesser hearing impairment | 300,000 |
| Genitourinary malformations | 300,000 |
| Muscular dystrophy | 200,000 |
| Congenital heart and other circulatory diseases | 200,000 |
| Clubfoot | 120,000 |
| Cleft lip and/or cleft palate | 100,000 |
| Diabetes | 80,000 |
| Spina bifida and/or hydrocephalus | 60,000 |
| Congenital dislocation of hip | 40,000 |
| Malformations of the digestive system | 20,000 |
| Speech disturbances of prenatal origin | 12,000 |
| Cystic fibrosis | 10,000 |

[1] Includes an estimated 250,000 with mongolism.

[2] Includes congenital cataract, strabismus, and certain refractive errors.

Source:  Congenital Malformations and Environmental Influence: The Occupational Environment of Laboratory Workers, J.W. Yager. *Journal of Occupational Medicine* *15:* 724–728, September 1973.

physician a sound basis for counselling the parents on the best course of action—should the pregnancy be interrupted or allowed to proceed.

*Infectious Agents*

Syphilis, caused by a spirochete, *Treponema pallidum* (see Fig. 5.3), if present in the maternal system, will frequently attack the fetus *in utero*. Miscarriages and stillbirths may result. Some infants, born with congenital syphilis, may show signs of it at birth or develop such signs later. If the mother receives adequate treatment early in pregnancy, the child will be born free of syphilis. During the past 25 years, the rates for congenital syphilis have progressively declined. Still there were 1758 such cases reported in 1972 in the United States.[14]

Infections with toxoplasma, a protozoan, *in utero* lead to death of the fetus or to widespread severe disease evident at birth. Infections in later life are generally mild. The infection passes through the placenta about the fourth month but not later in pregnancy. Only when the mother acquires the infection during pregnancy can it be passed on to the fetus.[15]

In 1941, an Australian physician, Dr. Norman M. Gregg, reported that congenital cataracts and heart disease were associated with maternal infections with rubella during the early months of pregnancy.[16] Numerous investigators in various parts of the world have confirmed Gregg's observations. The embryo or fetus itself becomes infected with rubella virus. Spontaneous abortions and stillbirths are two to four times as frequent in women whose pregnancies are complicated by rubella as in those who were free of that infection. The malformations resulting from rubella during the first three months of pregnancy include anomalies of the eye, the ear, the teeth, the heart, and the nervous system. The ear and heart are most frequently involved.[17] It is estimated that, if rubella attacks the mother during the first four weeks of pregnancy, 47 per cent of the infants are affected. This figure declines progressively, so that with maternal rubella between the 13th and 16th weeks of pregnancy only 6 per cent of the children are adversely affected. The type of abnormality is determined by the week of pregnancy in which the rubella occurs.[12]

During the 1964 epidemic of rubella in the United States an estimated number of 30,000 infants were born with congenital defects to mothers who had the infection early in pregnancy. Probably a larger number of pregnancies ended by either spontaneous or therapeutic abortions.

Since the rubella story has become known, careful observations have been made in order to learn whether other infectious illnesses during pregnancy might have similar effects. Prenatal infection with the cytomegalo virus does lead

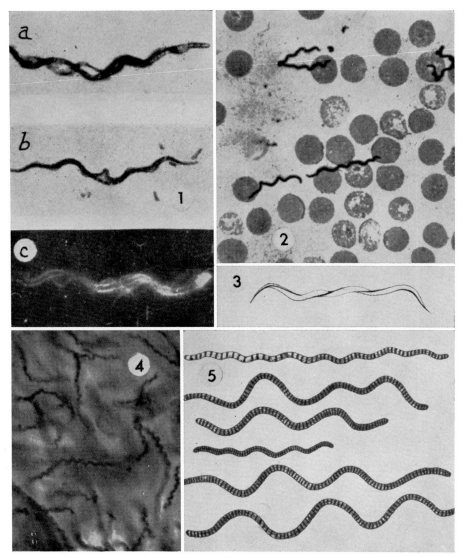

Fig. 5.3. *Treponema pallidum.* Photomicrograph. X 2500. Source: *Genera of Bacteria,* V. B. D. Skerman. Baltimore: The Williams & Wilkins Company, 1967.

to such malformations as hydrocephalus, microcephaly, and other changes in the central nervous system. Several reports have been published stating that Asian influenza virus (see Fig. 5.4) has caused congenital anomalies following maternal infection in pregnancy. These observations are not generally accepted. It has been reported from Australia that mongoloid children appear in greater frequency at appropriate periods following epidemics of infectious hepatitis.[18] Infections of the mother during pregnancy with Coxsackie and ECHO viruses have also been reported to have caused congenital abnormalities. Probably other infec-

tious agents will be incriminated of having teratogenic effects in the years ahead.[19]

Among the physical agents capable of producing congenital defects, ionic radiation is probably the most important. A study of the outcome of pregnancy in women exposed to the effects of the atomic bomb in Nagasaki, Japan, revealed that, among 30 pregnant women who were within 2000 m. of the bomb hypocenter and who suffered major radiation injuries, there were seven fetal deaths and six neonatal or infant deaths. Among the surviving children, four gave evidence of mental retardation.[20]

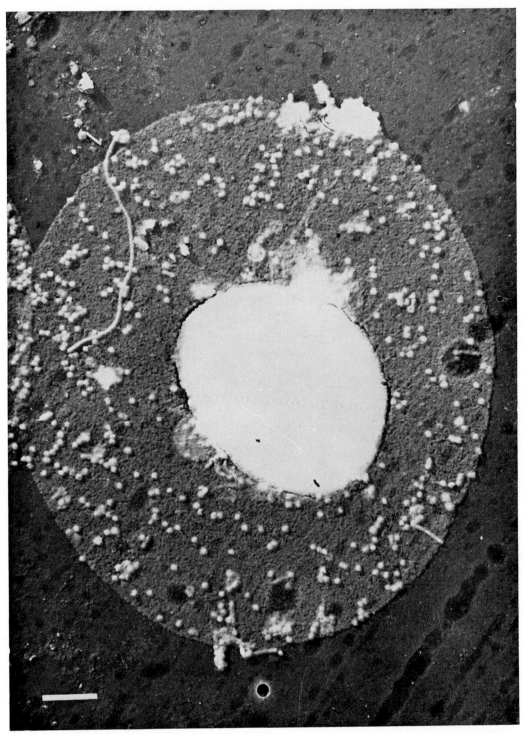

Fig. 5.4. Influenza virus type A2 attached to lysed fowl red cells. × 15,000. Source: *Textbook of Virology*, A. J. Rhodes and C. E. van Rooyen. Baltimore: The Williams & Wilkins Company, 1962.

Of the 68 pregnant women who were within the 2000 m. zone around the hypocenter, but who did not receive severe radiation injuries, three lost their babies by abortion or stillbirth.

Among 113 pregnant women who were located at 4000 to 5000 m. from the hypocenter at the time of the explosion, there were two abortions and one stillbirth.

The intense radiation experienced by those individuals exposed near the hypocenter of the bomb may also have caused gene mutations that will be revealed in future years.

Overexposure of pregnant women to X rays or radium is likely to cause injuries to the developing embryo.[21]

Medical-dental X-rays are the largest source of man-made radiation affecting the human population. A survey in 1964 indicates that 66 million persons were given medical radiographic examinations, 46 million received dental X-ray examinations, 7.8 million were given fluroscopic examinations, and 600,000 persons received radiation therapy. It is estimated that by 1977 these numbers will have doubled.

Experts estimate that congenital anomalies are most likely to follow X-ray examinations during the first six weeks of a pregnancy, but there is danger of harmful effects due to irradiation of the fetus at any time.

Injury of the uterine contents by trauma may produce death or anomalies of the embryo. Blows on the abdomen, automobile accidents, or falls are not uncommon and may result in congenital malformations.

The importance of drugs and chemicals as teratogenic agents was pointed up in a startling manner by the thalidomide episode. This drug, with no other toxic effects and having been tested in some animal pregnancies without untoward results, proved capable of producing severe congenital defects if given early in human pregnancies over a very short time period. The defect most commonly produced by thalidomide was an absence of all or part of the arms and legs.

Cortisone and other steroids are believed to be dangerous for the developing embryo. Aminopterin, sometimes used to produce abor-

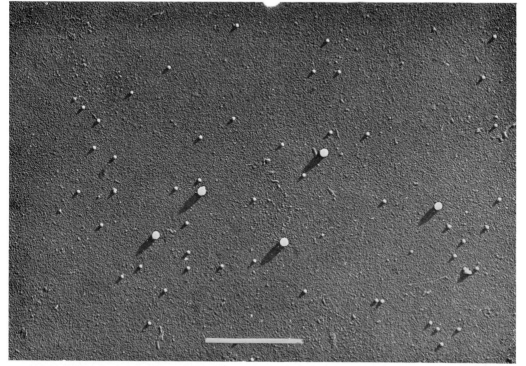

Fig. 5.5. Suspension of elementary bodies of polio virus type 1, with larger latex particles (88 m$\mu$ in diameter) for comparison. Shadowed × 34,000. Source: Courtesy of Mr. L. Pinteric, Connaught Medical Research Laboratory, University of Toronto, in *Textbook of Virology*, A. J. Rhodes and C. E. van Rooyen. Baltimore: The Williams & Wilkins Company, 1962.

Table 5.2
*Effects of medication on the intrauterine and newborn patient*

| Maternal Medication | Fetal or Neonatal Effect | Maternal Medication | Fetal or Neonatal Effect |
|---|---|---|---|
| Oral progestins<br>Androgens<br>Estrogens | Masculinization and advanced bone age | Hexamethonium bromide | Neonatal ileus |
| | | Intravenously administered fluids (excessive amounts) | Fluid and electrolyte abnormalities |
| Potassium iodide<br>Propylthiouracil<br>Methimazole | Goiter | Heroin and morphine | Neonatal death, convulsions and tremors |
| Iophenoxic acid (Teridax) | Elevation of serum protein-bound iodine | Phenobarbital (excessive amounts) | Neonatal bleeding |
| | | Smoking | Premature births |
| Aminopterin<br>Amethopterin<br>Chlorambucil | Anomales and abortions | Orally administered hypoglycemic agents:<br>Sulfonylurea derivatives | Anomalies[1] |
| Bishydroxycoumarin (Dicumarol) | Fetal death | Phenformin (D.B.I.) | Lactic acidosis[1] |
| Ethyl bicoumacetate | Hemorrhage | Phenothiazines | Hyperbilirubinemia[1] |
| Salicylates (large amounts) | Neonatal bleeding | Meprobamate | Retarded development[1] |
| Tetracyclines | Deposition in bone<br>Inhibition of bone growth in premature infants<br>Discoloration of teeth | Chloroquine | Retinal damage or death[1] |
| | | Quinine | Thrombocytopenia |
| | | Thalidomide | Phocomelia and fetal death; hearing loss |
| Sulfonamides | Kernicterus | Vaccination | Fetal vaccinia |
| Chloramphenicol | Death ("gray" syndrome) | Influenza vaccination | Increased anti-A and anti-B blood-group titers in mother[1] |
| Novobiocin | Hyperbilirubinemia | | |
| Erythromycin | Liver damage[1] | | |
| Nitrofurantoin (Furadantin) | Hemolysis | Antihistamines | Anomalies[1]<br>Prevention of pregnancy[1] |
| Vitamin K analogues (excessive amounts) | Hyperbilirubinemia | Insulin shock | Fetal loss |
| Ammonium chloride | Acidosis | | |
| Reserpine | Nasal congestion and drowsiness | | |

[1] Indicates results based on animal studies only.

Source: Lucey, J. F. Drugs and the intrauterine patient. In *Birth Defects*, original article series, Vol. 1, no. 1. Symposium on the Placenta. The National Foundation, March of Dimes, New York, 1965.

tions, is known to cause abnormalities in the embryo in cases in which the abortion did not occur. Congenital defects have resulted also in women being treated for leukemia with drugs and is suspected following use of other drugs (see Table 5.2).

As for the frequency of congenital abnormalities, accurate figures are difficult to obtain. It is estimated that about 1 million spontaneous abortions occur in the United States each year. Most of these result from abnormal development of the embryo. Probably 2 to 3 per cent of all live-born infants show evidence of one congenital malformation or more. By the end of the first year of life, this figure is doubled by the manifestation of defects not discovered at birth.[22-24]

## INFLUENCE OF ENVIRONMENT ON HEALTH

All human disease is largely determined by both the inherited characteristics of the individual and the environmental experience to which that individual is subjected. It is sometimes difficult to evaluate separately the extent to which these all important factors affect the onset of any specific type of illness.

Rene Dubos[25] says "To a surprising extent, modern man has retained unaltered the bodily constitution, physiological responses, and emotional drives which he inherited from his Paleolithic ancestors. Yet he lives in a mechanized, air-conditioned, and regimented world radically different from the one in which he evolved." Man modifies his environment continuously and frequently changes his way of life, bringing about a resulting change in the prevalence and severity of various diseases. These diseases are always closely related to his responses to environmental stimuli. In modern affluent societies, heart diseases now constitute the leading cause of death, with cancer in second place, vascular disease of the brain third, and accidents fourth. These are the diseases of modern civilized life.

It is estimated that, by 1980, 80 per cent of the population will be urban (see Fig. 5.6). This increasing urbanization of the population of the United States is creating a new disease pattern. Crowding, almost anonymous existence, and problems of air, water, and food pollution are increased. Stresses and anxieties due to unsettled social conditions lead to psychogenic disorders. Increased leisure, overeating, sedentary mechanized life, addiction to alcohol, tobacco, and drugs, and emotional strains all combine to bring on the chronic, degenerative diseases of middle and old age.

It is difficult to measure the effects on human health of such alterations in our way of life as are produced by central heating and air conditioning, by technological improvements in food preservation and distribution, by jet plane travel, and by almost constant exposure to food additives, pesticides, and powerful drugs. Without question, these factors do affect health adversely. In a recent report, Lave and Seskin present data indicating a close association between mortality rates and air pollution. They argue that mortality rates could be lowered by abating pollution.[27]

Man introduces new technologies at such a rapid rate and on such a wide scale that there is no opportunity to evaluate the consequences. It appears easier to develop new technologies than to determine the long-range biological effects of such innovations. Our current pattern of diseases is an expression of the effects of new environmental forces to which the human has not had time to become adapted.

Contamination of water and of food is a well-known source of disease, especially of intestinal infections. Typhoid fever (see Fig. 5.7), cholera, and infectious hepatitis may be waterborne, while food may also serve as the source of these diseases as well as of Salmonella infections, staphylococal poisoning, and amebic dysentry. The water supplies of the country are being increasingly polluted by industrial wastes, detergents, pesticides, and other noxious material. Purification of water for household use becomes ever more difficult.

In most large cities, the refuse disposal problem has reached such proportions that available landfill area is almost exhausted. Today's waste includes everything from dead

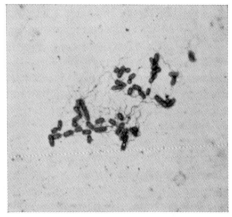

Fig. 5.7. *Salmonella typhosa* with flagella. X 1200. Source: *Oral Microbiology and Infectious Disease*, G. W. Burnett and H. W. Sherp. Baltimore: The Williams & Wilkins Company, 1968.

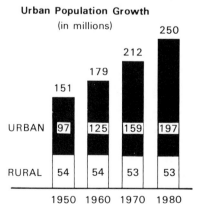

**Urban Population Growth**
(in millions)

Fig. 5.6. Source: *A Strategy for a Livable Environment*. Washington, D. C.: Government Printing Office, 1967.

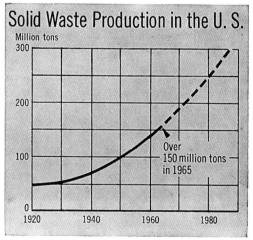

Fig. 5.8. Source: A strategy for a livable environment. Washington, D.C.: Government Printing Office, 1967.

animals, construction refuse, old appliances, industrial discharges, and non-returnable containers to hazardous refuse from hospitals or nuclear power plants. In New York City, solid wastes consist of 75 per cent paper or paper derivatives, 10 per cent garbage, and 8 to 10 per cent metal, plastic, glass, or other non-combustible material; the remainder is demolition debris and miscellaneous materials.[28] The national per capita consumption of packaging materials was 404 pounds in 1958, 525 pounds in 1966 and will be 661 pounds by 1976[29, 30] (see Fig. 5.8).

Many sources contribute to pollution of the air, but the internal combustion engine appears to be the most universal and persistent offender. The large metropolitan areas have the worst atmospheric pollution. While proof is difficult, evidence is mounting to show that such pollution is associated with higher incidence of chronic lung conditions such as emphysema and bronchitis (see Fig. 5.9 and Table 5.3). Lung cancer also is more prevalent in urban than in rural areas. Bronchial asthma is aggravated by air pollution. Radiation is now recognized as an extremely hazardous threat to health.[31] X rays, radium, nuclear explosions, use of nuclear materials for industry, and cosmic rays are among the known sources of radiation. Lung cancer is a hazard of uranium miners; bone cancer developed in luminous watch dial painters; physicians and dentists overexposed to X rays have developed skin

cancer; leukemia occurs more commonly than expected in those repeatedly exposed to X ray and among the survivors of the atomic bombs in Japan. It is believed that radiation damages the genes and may produce harmful mutations affecting the newborn in various undesirable ways.

Occupational health hazards are numerous and complex. Industrial dusts, chemicals, heat, cold, noise, and vibration are potential sources of injury. Most large industrial plants give careful attention to protecting their workers from health hazards, but small plants are generally not so concerned. Recent evidence indicates that the numbers of job-related injuries and deaths have been grossly understated. Injuries probably exceed 20 million rather than the reported 2 million a year, and deaths may be nearly twice the reported 14,000.

New technical advances are frequently introducing new health problems so that health workers must be constantly on guard for unforeseen bad effects on the health of those exposed. The rapid discovery of new chemicals and their application greatly outpaces the rate at which their toxicology can be investigated by all concerned with this responsibility.

With the enactment of the Federal Coal Mine Health and Safety Act of 1969 and the Occupational Safety and Health Act of 1970 the legal basis for improvements in safety for workers is now available. A study by one of

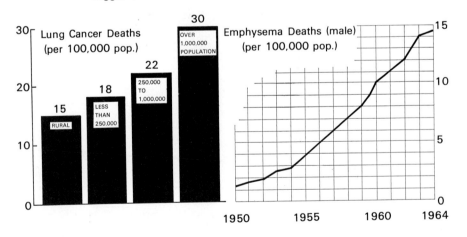

Air pollutants—135 million tons per year

Fig. 5.9. Emphysema deaths (male, per 100,000 population) Source: *Strategy for a Livable Environment.* Washington, D. C.: Government Printing Office, 1967.

Table 5.3

*Prevalence of selected chronic respiratory conditions reported in health interviews, number per 1000 persons, per cent of conditions by measures of impact, and disability days in past year: United States, 1970*

| | Chronic Condition and ICDA Code | | Prevalence | |
|---|---|---|---|---|
| | | | Number in thousands | Number per 1000 persons |
| 1 | Chronic bronchitis | 490,491 | 6,526 | 32.7 |
| 2 | Emphysema | 492 | 1,313 | 6.6 |
| 3 | Asthma, with or without hay fever | 493 | 6,031 | 30.2 |
| 4 | Hypertrophy of tonsils and adenoids | 500 | 4,359 | 21.8 |
| 5 | Chronic sinusitis | 503 | 20,582 | 103.0 |
| 6 | Deflected nasal septum | 504 | 798 | 4.0 |
| 7 | Nasal polyp | 505 | 546 | 2.7 |
| 8 | Chronic laryngitis | 506 | 1,149 | 5.7 |
| 9 | Hay fever, without asthma (includes upper respiratory allergy) | 507 | 10,826 | 54.2 |
| 10 | Pleurisy | 511 | 686 | 3.4 |
| 11 | Pneumoconiosis | 515,516 | 126 | 0.6 |
| 12 | Other chronic interstitial pneumonia | 517 | 403 | 2.0 |
| 13 | Bronchiectasis | 518 | 116 | 0.6 |
| 14 | Tuberculosis, active | 010-018 | 157 | 0.8 |
| 15 | Tuberculosis, arrested or inactive | . . . | 137 | 0.7 |

Source:   Prevalence of Selected Chronic Respiratory Conditions – United States 1970. National Center for Health Statistics, DHEW Publication No. (HRA) 74-1511. September 1973. Vital and Health Statistics–Series 10-No. 84.

Ralph Nader's study groups charges that the government is dragging its feet in the implementation of meaningful measures to control the harmful work environments of many large industrial plants.[32,33]

Before the Industrial Revolution few people were exposed to excessive noise. The advent of power-driven machinery has changed all that. Today noise has become omnipresent. Little has been done by industrial firms to reduce noise levels in their plants, although it is well known that constant exposure to noise causes marked impairment of hearing. Probably prolonged exposure to excessive noise may affect human health in other ways. Certainly it causes loss of attention and work efficiency. Thus, it may contribute to industrial accidents.[34]

Reactions to drugs and drug poisoning are common occurrences leading to ill health and some fatalities. Between 1960 and 1971, 260 new drugs were officially approved for clinical use by the Food and Drug Administration. This flow of new pharmaceutical products continues. Unpredicted responses to drugs are

usually rare occurrences; they do not develop in more than one of several thousand patients treated with the drugs. Reactions to drugs may result from: (1) intolerance, (2) idiosyncrasy, (3) allergy, (4) drug interaction,[35] or (5) over dosage.

In spite of efforts to control depressant and stimulant drugs—barbiturates and amphetamines in particular—huge amounts of these psychotoxic substances are consumed by the public each year. Abuse of such drugs as marijuana, lysergic acid diethylamine tartrate (LSD), and the narcotics continues widely to the detriment of the public's health.

The National Clearing House for Poison Control Centers reports that, in 1972, 160,824 cases of ingestion of poisonous substances were recorded from 548 centers in 47 states. According to figures of the Metropolitan Life Insurance Company as many as 1 million Americans swallow toxic substances each year.[36] Of these 1692 died in 1968, this number being about one sixth higher than in 1965. This increase was due primarily to a sharp rise in drug fatalities among adolescents and young adults. The tranquilizers, the analgesic and soporific drugs, rose accounting for 44 per cent of all accidental deaths due to drug poisoning among males and 28 per cent among females[37] (see Table 5.4). Children under 5 years of age continue to experience danger from ingesting poisonous substances greater than at any other period of life.

In addition to defects in physical environment, citizens of a modern industrial society are plagued with a whole series of grave social problems. The rapid growth of cities has led to a deterioration of living conditions in urban areas. Those able to do so have moved to suburban areas in large numbers. This desertion of the city by substantial taxpayers has created difficult financial situations for municipal authorities. Our society is marked by instability. People move their homes far more frequently. Families are broken up by divorce at an increasing rate. Racial tensions have become more acute, especially in cities. Confidence in government at all levels appears to have declined. Unemployment and shorter working hours are posing difficulties in providing healthful recreational activities. Juvenile delinquency and adult convictions for crime pose distressing situations for all communities. The pace of living has been accelerated by the ubiquitous telephone and the constant use of the automobile. Radio, television, and movies can scarcely be said to promote emotional equilibrium.

All of these social influences and many more

TABLE 5.4

*Deaths from accidental poisoning by drugs*
*United States, 1965 and 1968*

| Drug Category, by Sex | 1965 All Ages | 1968 All Ages | Under 5 | 5-14 | 15-24 | 25-34 | 35-44 | 45-64 | 65 and over |
|---|---|---|---|---|---|---|---|---|---|
| **Barbiturates** | | | | | | | | | |
| Male | 212 | 151 | 7 | 2 | 45 | 23 | 29 | 33 | 12 |
| Female | 332 | 170 | 4 | 2 | 16 | 21 | 32 | 78 | 17 |
| Total Persons | 544 | 321 | 11 | 4 | 61 | 44 | 61 | 111 | 29 |
| **Aspirin and related salicylates** | | | | | | | | | |
| Male | 89 | 63 | 37 | 4 | 2 | | 3 | 8 | 9 |
| Female | 86 | 57 | 24 | | 2 | 7 | 8 | 10 | 6 |
| Total Persons | 175 | 120 | 61 | 4 | 4 | 7 | 11 | 18 | 15 |
| **Opiates and synthetics** | | | | | | | | | |
| Male | 59 | 198 | 2 | | 74 | 75 | 35 | 10 | 2 |
| Female | 10 | 31 | 1 | | 11 | 10 | 6 | 2 | 1 |
| Total Persons | 69 | 229 | 3 | | 85 | 85 | 41 | 12 | 3 |
| **Tranquilizers, analgesics, soporific and related drugs** | | | | | | | | | |
| Male | 202 | 467 | 21 | 3 | 176 | 143 | 66 | 46 | 12 |
| Female | 148 | 179 | 8 | 2 | 22 | 31 | 42 | 53 | 21 |
| Total Persons | 350 | 646 | 29 | 5 | 198 | 174 | 108 | 99 | 33 |
| **Other and unspecified** | | | | | | | | | |
| Male | 114 | 184 | 22 | 5 | 50 | 29 | 22 | 26 | 30 |
| Female | 138 | 192 | 24 | 2 | 18 | 19 | 38 | 56 | 35 |
| Total Persons | 252 | 376 | 46 | 7 | 68 | 48 | 60 | 82 | 65 |
| **Total** | | | | | | | | | |
| Male | 676 | 1,063 | 89 | 14 | 347 | 270 | 155 | 123 | 65 |
| Female | 714 | 629 | 61 | 6 | 69 | 88 | 126 | 199 | 80 |
| Total Persons | 1,390 | 1,692 | 150 | 20 | 416 | 358 | 281 | 322 | 145 |

Source : Statistical Bulletin. Metropolitan Life Insurance Company 53: page 5, February 1972.

that are part and parcel of modern living affect human health in ways that are impossible to measure. The increases of stresses and tensions without doubt promote many types of disease such as duodenal ulcer, high blood pressure, and diabetes. Other conditions such as allergies, asthma, and skin eruptions are made worse by stressful living. Psychiatric problems characterize modern society. Large numbers of people consult psychiatrists, and even larger numbers consume tranquilizing drugs. Suicide rates are going up slightly in recent years. Suicide has been among the 12 leading causes of death in the United States since 1954. In 1964, the suicide rate of the United States was 10.8 per 100,000. This figure rose to 11.1 in 1965 and has remained at that figure through 1971. There can be little doubt that adverse social conditions tend to bring individuals to the point of taking their own lives.

## THE INFECTIOUS PROCESS

Man constantly lives in an environment of soil, air, and water and is, therefore, exposed to a large variety of bacteria, viruses, and other microorganisms. Fortunately, most of these organisms cannot successfully establish a foothold in competition with the normal flora of the body.

Since bacteria flourish on dead organic matter, one can expect many species of the organisms to find habitation in or on the bodies of living animals. On the skin, surface cells are continuously dying to provide a food supply. The moist portions of the skin between fingers and toes and in skin folds are favorable as bacterial habitats. The mouth, nose, and throat are bathed with saliva and mucus containing the dead cells constantly being shed from the epithelial linings. These accessible openings provide maximum opportunity for entrance of microorganisms from the air or in food and water. In the lower intestinal tract, there are residues of partially digested food to provide highly favorable conditions for the maintenance of a rich fauna of microorganisms. Probably about half of the bulk of feces consist of bacteria. The relative freedom of the normal conjunctivae from infection is probably due to the washing effect of tears. These secretions contain lysozyme, an antibacterial substance.

Among this great natural fauna living in or on the body, only a very few organisms have developed the capacity to invade normal tissues

and become disease producers or pathogens. It is of interest to note that those bacteria that have become pathogens usually attack the areas of the body which normally harbor those harmless bacteria that most resemble the pathogenic species. All individuals have a certain degree of resistance to those microorganisms classified as pathogenic; therefore, only a portion of those who become infected actually develop signs of illness. Also, each disease-producing organism has its own peculiar characteristics which make it capable of invading and multiplying in the tissues of the host. Usually successful parasites must find a means to leave the host before death to find entry to a new host.

When microorganisms enter the tissue of the body, one of three results may follow. The organisms may multiply unimpeded by the body's defenses and cause a fatal infection; they may become established in the tissues and remain localized indefinitely; or the defenses of the individual may prove effective in overwhelming the invading organisms so that they are destroyed and eliminated. Usually the infection results in recovery. The result of the contest between invader and host will depend on the nature of the organism and the degree of resistance of the host. For each infection that results in obvious symptoms in the host there are hundreds of incipient infections that are overcome by the body without production of symptoms or in which only trivial discomfort is experienced.

### Defenses of the Body Against Infection

The intact skin and mucous membranes provide considerable protection against entry of organisms to susceptible tissues. The glandular secretions of the skin have some protective action against bacteria and fungi. The tears, saliva, and urine wash away many bacteria and have some antibacterial activity through such natural compounds as lysozyme. Nasal secretions, bronchial secretions, and saliva have a cleansing action and may contain other antibacterial agents.

The little hairs of the epithelial lining of the bronchial tree, called cilia, have a wave-like motion, carrying foreign particles to the throat for elimination in the sputum. Organisms that are swallowed are subjected to the acid of the gastric juice, which destroys many.

Once pathogenic organisms have gained entrance to the tissues, the defense mechanisms of the body tend to limit their spread from the local site of infection. A walling-off process by deposition of fibrin and collagen is begun.

Organisms, as they multiply in the tissues, produce toxic substances which injure the adjacent cells. These cells as they die provide food for the invader, but also through chemical stimuli call forth the body's defense mechanisms. The lymph becomes clotted in the local lymph channels, thus impeding spread of the organisms. Histamine is released from the damaged cells. This substance acts on the walls of capillaries, so that they dilate and allow a greater blood flow. The capillary walls become more porous, allowing white blood cells to pass through to the infected area. These phagocytes engulf bacteria and usually destroy them, or at least prevent further multiplication. The local activity of thousands of these phagocytes and of the ensuing inflammatory response produces an environment in the tissues unfavorable to multiplication of the invading organisms.

Some types of organisms, such as the staphylococcus, produce a powerful toxin which destroys the phagocytes. As the dead tissue cells and killed phagocytes accumulate, the resultant material is known as pus.

In ordinary circumstances, these defense mechanisms prove effective and the invaders are overcome. Repair processes quickly get underway and the damaged area slowly returns to its normal state.

If the local defenses are not adequate, the invading organisms spread beyond the local site. This spread is usually accomplished through the lymph vessels to the regional lymph glands. These glands may become swollen and tender as a result of an accumulation of white blood cells assembled to combat the infection. The invaders may be overcome at this point and the tissues involved will then return gradually to their normal state. In the event that the infection is not contained by the regional lymph glands, the invading organisms continue to spread along the lymph channels until they reach the bloodstream and are disseminated throughout the body, thus producing a generalized infection.[38]

Each pathogenic organism has certain biochemical requirements for its growth. These individual characteristics determine the kinds of tissue and the location of the tissues that it is most likely to invade. For example, the gonococcus attacks no other animal than man.

This organism requires moist, warm conditions that are provided best by the genital membranes of the human. The gonococcus will also invade the conjunctival membranes around the eyes and rarely produces severe acute inflammation of the lining of the heart or of the joints. The meningococcus, an organism similar in some respects to the gonococcus, produces its characteristic damage to the membranes surrounding the brain and spinal cord.

The portal of entry and mode of transmission bring some organisms into almost immediate contact with their "target" organs. The pneumococcus, a natural inhabitant of the upper respiratory tract, can reach the lung tissues almost directly to produce its characteristic symptoms. The typhoid bacillus swallowed with contaminated food or water arrives directly at its favorite locus, the lower, small intestine. From the tissues in the intestinal wall, the typhoid bacilli spread to regional lymph glands and finally to the bloodstream for widespread distribution.

Streptococci (see Fig. 5.10) may penetrate the skin through traumatic breaks and cause either localized inflammation or, in preantibiotic days, severe septicemia or blood poisoning. The frequent route of entry for streptococci is by way of the mouth and throat with tonsillitis being a common result of infection.

The tuberculosis bacillus (see Fig. 5.11) may be ingested with milk from a tuberculous cow. The initial infection in such cases occurs in the intestinal tract and generally the abdominal lymph glands become quickly involved. More commonly these days, tuberculous infection is acquired by breathing in contaminated dust or aerosols, so that the organism reaches the lining of the bronchioles or air sacs, thus setting up the infectious process in the lung.

In the case of virus diseases, a virus particle must make contact with a susceptible cell. Natural infections are acquired by deposition of virus on a suitable surface cell of the conjunctiva, the throat, the respiratory epithelium, or the intestinal mucosa. A large group of viruses are transmitted by the bite of an appropriate arthropod, such as a mosquito or tick.

The incubation period of a disease is a reflection of the complexity of the infective process or pathogenesis of that particular illness. Influenza usually has an incubation period of one to three days. This virus enters the body by inhalation of infected aerosols and is deposited immediately upon susceptible cells

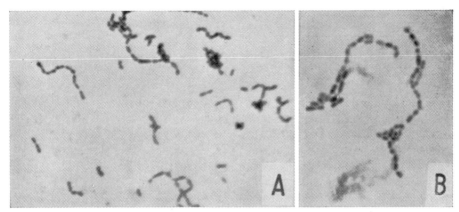

Fig. 5.10. *A*, Oral aerobic streptococci. *B*, oral anaerobic streptococci. Source: *Oral Microbiology and Infectious Disease*, G. W. Burnett and H. W. Sherp. Baltimore: The Williams & Wilkins Company, 1968.

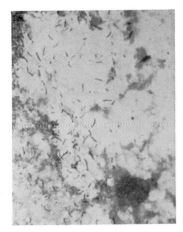

Fig. 5.11. *Mycobacterium tuberculosis* in sputum. Source: *Oral Microbiology and Infectious Disease*, G. W. Burnett and H. W. Sherp. Baltimore: The Williams & Wilkins Company, 1968.

lining the respiratory tract. Virus enters such cells rapidly and begins multiplication without delay. As infected cells discharge new virus particles on the surface of the bronchial tree, other cells become infected until a considerable portion of the lung may be involved. As toxic materials from the damaged and necrotic cells are absorbed, symptoms occur.

Other virus diseases, such as smallpox, measles, mumps, and chickenpox, have incubation periods of from about 10 to 21 days. It is thought that in these diseases initial growth of virus occurs in a localized area, perhaps the throat. After some days, virus becomes disseminated through the bloodstream reaching the target organs characteristically involved in the particular type of infection.[39]

## Immunity

Immunity to disease is usually described as (1) natural or hereditary immunity, and (2) acquired immunity (see Table 5.5). Fatal diseases among people in the child-bearing age groups tend to eliminate those having a high degree of susceptibility. This tends to ensure the survival of that portion of the population having more than average innate resistance. Gradually, the average inherited resistance of that population repeatedly exposed to the same infection is built up. Through some such process of evolutionary adaptation between hosts and their parasites, a state of biological equilibrium may be approached.

Innate immunity refers to the mechanisms that render the body resistant to infection which has not been acquired after the birth of the individual. These innate mechanisms are concerned with species and race and are probably dependent on reactions genetically controlled. The properdin system of the blood appears to be such an important natural defense factor.

Acquired immunity is directed against specific pathogenic organisms. This type of immunity may be based on either active production of antibodies in response to a stimulus or provided by supplying antibodies produced by another. The second type of immune protection is known as passive immunity. The mechanisms of antibody formation are still not clearly understood. The fetus *in utero* does not have the capability of responding to the introduction of foreign protein, that is, antigen, by the production of antibodies. If antigen is introduced to the body of the fetus, a tolerance

TABLE 5.5

*Natural or innate immunity*

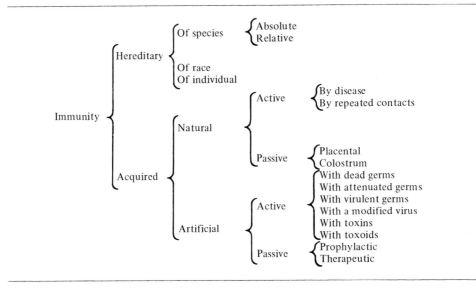

Source: *Zinsser Microbiology,* edited by D.T. Smith, and N. F. Conant, Ed. 12. New York: Appleton-Century-
Crofts, Inc., 1960.

generally develops to the new protein in the same manner as the body has tolerance of its own cells and tissues. Shortly after birth, the newborn infant develops the capacity to respond to contact with foreign proteins with its tissues by production of specific antibodies capable of assisting the body in the rejection of the foreign matter. In the case of bacteria, the specific antibodies apparently act on the invaders in such a manner as to make them more readily taken up or phagocytized by the appropriate white blood cells. In viral infections, it is probable that the antibodies react with the receptor areas of susceptible cells to prevent the entry of virus particles into the cells in which they might multiply.

From recent studies, it appears that the cells of the body principally involved in the immune response are those of the lymphocyte cell group.[40] These cells are found for the most part, in lymph glands, the spleen, the bone marrow, and local accumulations of cells in inflamed areas. All the lymphocytes that circulate in the body have arisen from precursor cells in the bone marrow. About half of these lymphocytes, the T cells, have passed through the thymus gland on their way to the tissues; the other half, the B cells, have not. Only B-type lymphocytes and their progeny secrete

antibody molecules. T cells are also highly important as they can attack cancer cells, transplanted tissues, or other cells of foreign origin.

The immune system consists of about a trillion lymphocytes and about 100 million trillion molecules called antibodies that are produced and secreted by the lymphocytes. Foreign substances that stimulate antibody formation are known as antigens.[40,41]

Antibodies are $\gamma$-globulin in nature and thus are to be found in that protein fraction of the blood. The antibody molecule is made up of multiple polypeptide chains. Until recently, four major classes of circulating human immunoglobulins had been defined. Probably at least one other type exists. The most studied one has been gamma globulin G (IgG) which makes up about 70 per cent of normal human immunoglobulins in the serum. The gamma globulin A (IgA) is found in the serum as well as in saliva and other external secretions. IgM molecules tend to appear in the early stages after the introduction of an antigen and may be designed for rapid protection. Two other immunoglobulins are present in low concentrations in the serum IgD and IgE. The latter, IgE, appears to be largely responsible for allergic reactions.

Knowledge of resistance to infection has been

enriched by the study of those occasional individuals who through a genetic defect are incapable of producing γ-globulins. These unfortunate individuals are highly susceptible to repeated bacterial infections and develop no specific defense in consequence. Some protection is afforded by regular injections of concentrated pooled γ-globulins. These persons do handle virus infections such as measles and chickenpox quite successfully. This observation suggests that some mechanism other than antibody is responsible for recovery from these viral infections and for any subsequent resistance to new infections with the same organisms.[4 2]

While the immune response is invaluable in protecting an individual against dangerous infections, it does pose a difficult problem in other life-saving measures such as blood transfusion, skin grafts, and, more recently, organ transplants. It is impossible to find an identical twin as donor in most cases requiring a kidney or heart transplant. At present, the surgeons must depend upon measures designed to suppress the immune reactions until the transplant is accepted by its new host.

In addition to the production of specific antibodies, the body frequently responds to infection by the development of a delayed-type hypersensitivity. The tissue cells develop and retain for long periods this specific sensitivity to the antigens of microbial agents. The tuberculin test gives noteworthy evidence of this type of immune response to the proteins of the tubercle bacillus. The immune response to smallpox vaccine in vaccinated individuals is another such evidence of cellular sensitivity. It is believed that this immune mechanism plays a significant role in the defense of the body.

Chick embryos, which neither produce antibodies nor manifest delayed hypersensitivity, do recover from some viral infections. Interferon, a protein produced by cells in response to foreign nucleic acids, especially those of viruses, has been proposed as the substance affording protection to these chick embryos. Possibly, interferon is an important factor in recovery of animals from many virus infections.

Interferon, which was discovered in 1957, is produced by many different viruses and many viruses are sensitive to the interferon which has been stimulated by other viral agents. There is evidence that interferon does not inactivate the infective virus particle, nor does it prevent absorption of the particle to susceptible cells. It does inhibit the synthesis of new virus particles in the cell. In the course of many virus infections, the production of interferon does proceed steadily, and it seems a reasonable conclusion that there may be a causal relationship between these two processes so that recovery from these infections may occur on that basis.

Naturally acquired immunity may result from a frank attack of a particular disease or be produced by a mild infection with the disease. In many cases, this infection may be so mild that it is not recognized or indeed not noted. These mild episodes are designated as subclinical or inapparent infections. The immunity resulting from such mild attacks may be as effective and as enduring as results from severe disease.

Passive immunity of the natural type is seen in every newborn infant and is effected by transmission *in utero* of antibodies from the mother's blood to the blood of the fetus by passage through the placenta. Antibodies may also be transmitted through the mother's milk in the early stages of lactation. No such immunity can be transmitted unless the mother has experienced previous immunization.

This congenital passive immunity safeguards the infant during the first months of life and frequently enables the infant to develop its own active immunity through infections occurring while it still has a partial protection from the maternal antibody umbrella.

Artificially produced immunity is assuming more and more importance in prevention of communicable disease. Vaccines produced with attenuated living organisms or with dead organisms have received ready acceptance for mass use. Toxoids produced by modifying chemically the powerful toxins of tetanus (see Fig. 5.12), diphtheria, and other toxin-producing microorganisms have also proved their value. New immunizing agents are appearing for general use almost every year. Indeed the very multiplicity of products presents problems to parents and pediatricians faced with giving infants and young children a large number of immunizing injections. Attempts to purify the antigen components of vaccine and to combine all possible vaccines into a single product have already been partially successful and will probably be even more acceptable in the years to come.

Another important feature of the immune system is complement. This term refers to a

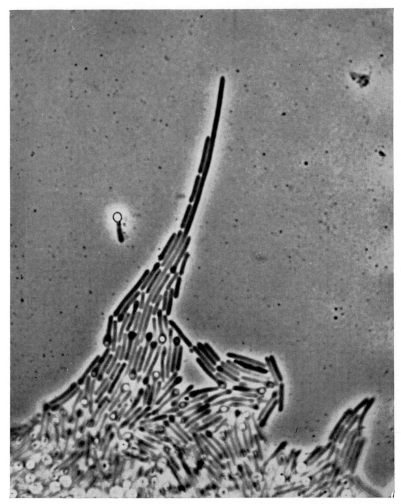

Fig. 5.12. *Clostridium tetani.* Slide culture. Original. × 1800. Source: *Genera of Bacteria,* V. B. D. Skerman. Baltimore: The Williams & Wilkins Company, 1967.

complex group of enzymes in normal blood serum that, working together with antibodies, plays an important role in immune reactions that occur in blood serum or in other body fluids. Antibody serves to recognize the foreign invader; to activate complement; and to fix complement on the surface of the invading cell.

Artificial passive immunity has also been widely used in the prevention and treatment of infectious diseases. Serum from horses, rabbits, or other animals carefully immunized with appropriate antigens was first used for this purpose. Many lives were saved with such an antitoxin to diphtheria. Immune horse serum was widely employed to treat pneumococcus infections and to prevent tetanus. Immune human sera were frequently used to prevent

attacks of measles among children who had been exposed to the infection. Since blood transfusion centers have developed a considerable supply of γ-globulin as a by-product of their operations, this material is being used to provide passive immunity whenever possible.

Passive immunity has been a valuable asset to those concerned with control and treatment of infectious diseases. The main limitation of this method is the short duration of the protection. Depending upon the concentration of antibodies and the dosage of γ-globulin administered, the protective effect varies from about one to six weeks after the inoculation. In the case of infectious hepatitis, immune globulin is thought to provide some protection up to six months.

Ordinarily an individual is tolerant of his own tissue antigens, but an increasing number of diseases have been shown to fall into the category of autoimmune disease. These include some types of hemolytic anemia, lupus erythematosus, membranous glomerulonephritis, Hashimoto's thyroiditis, rheumatoid arthritis, myasthenia gravis, and scleroderma. In these disease states an autoantibody or a sensitized lymphocyte reacts with the host's tissue.[43]

Mutation is a constant phenomenon among lymphocytes. These "abnormal" lymphocytes and their progeny will carry new antigens. When these antigens do not call forth an antibody response from normal lymphocytes, such mutants multiply and attack normal host cells. The mechanisms involved are not well understood, but there appears to be no doubt that such self-destructive processes do occur with some frequency especially in older age groups.

## Latent Infections

Most of the infectious illnesses result from contact with a virulent agent from outside the body, for example, measles, smallpox, yellow fever, syphilis, and malaria. Other infections arise from infectious agents already harbored in the body as persisters from a prior contact. Many of these persisting agents are highly virulent and fully capable of producing endogenous disease. When the general resistance of the host diminishes, these organisms again begin to flourish and produce signs and symptoms of disease. Tuberculosis is a prime example of an important disease that may remain quiescent or latent in the body for many years and which may readily become reactivated as a result of a period of physiological stress.[44]

Another well-known example of latent infection is that of herpes simplex. This virus most frequently remains in a latent state in the cells around the margins of the lips and breaks out actively as fever blisters in response to such stimuli as fever, sunburn, or other physical stresses.

Following attacks of epidemic typhus fever, the individual appears to make a complete recovery from the infection. It is known that a few such individuals suffer a relapse or recrudescence of the typhus infection many years later. This reappearance of typhus was described in New York City among immigrants from eastern or central Europe who gave a history of experiencing the original disease as long as 20 years previously. The name of Brill's disease has been given to this form of typhus.

As many as 30 to 50 per cent of the general population harbor virulent staphylococci in their nasal-pharyngeal spaces. These pathogenic agents may produce abscesses, pneumonia, or other serious infections when the body's defenses become lowered through surgery or other physical stresses.

Pathogens may persist in the body in different states. In some instances, the presence of the agent in the tissues may be demonstrated by the usual laboratory procedures. Typhoid bacilli, for example, are readily recovered from carriers of that disease. In other types of latent infection, the organism is most difficult or impossible to demonstrate with currently available techniques. The term "masked" infections has been applied to such situations.

This phenomenon of organisms remaining in the tissues has become more significant as a result of widespread employment of antibiotics. These drugs are frequently highly successful in restoring the patient to health but usually do not succeed in eliminating the pathogen completely from the tissues. Even after infections with tuberculosis have been brought under control by isoniazid, the causative organisms persist in the tissues. The same is true of gonococcal infections treated with penicillin. In many cases, the persisting agents are still susceptible to the drug. Probably, they remain walled off inside cells of the previously infected tissues.[45] Since the introduction of antibiotics, the importance of infections arising from microbes persisting in the body has greatly increased. The colon bacillus, the common fungus *Candida albicans,* a common inhabitant of the mouth, the influenza bacillus, and other organisms relatively low in virulence are now responsible for many fatalities, especially in hospital practice.

Many kinds of physiological stress may activate latent infections and diminish the ability of the body to combat them. Diabetes is a well-known form of physiological derangement that is favorable to infections. Hunger, fatigue, and emotional stress are other stressful conditions that are known to lower the defense mechanisms of the body. A variety of hormonal stimuli, such as large doses of cortisone, has been used to activate latent infections in experimental animals.

## LIVING DISEASE AGENTS

The living agents of disease that affect man are primarily concerned with preservation of their own biological cycle. They seek favorable conditions for multiplication in human tissues or on the body's surface and an efficient means of leaving the infected host, so that a successful transfer to a new host may be effected. For the parasite to affect the host fatally is not usually the most successful result, as the infecting agent may perish with the host. Long continued association of parasite with a host population results in the evolution of a biological balance, satisfactory to the parasite and generally tolerable to the host. The truth of this observation is demonstrated by the importation into isolated populations of an infection of mild character in civilized regions. The isolated population reacts violently to the new agent, so that many fatalities may result from an infection considered to be a mild childhood disease in its usual habitat. This principle was illustrated by introduction of measles to the American Indians and by the infection of the South Pacific Islanders with many new agents.[46]

The host range of different disease agents varies widely. Some are primarily parasites of animals with man as only an occasional host. Other parasites affect only humans in their natural distribution. With some parasites, animals and humans may serve as hosts with almost equal facility. The life cycle of a few parasites is so complicated that more than one host species is necessary to fulfill all of the requirements for the complete maturation of the agent.

The living agents of human disease vary tremendously in their size and in their complexity. The principal characteristics of these parasites are discussed below, beginning with the smallest—the viruses.

### Viruses

Although the diseases caused by viruses have been well known clinically for many years, the existence of the viral agents and knowledge of their characteristics have only been realized within the past few decades. Yellow fever was shown by the U. S. Army Commission in 1901 to be caused by an agent that passed through filters capable of holding back all known bacteria. Following this demonstration of a human viral agent, progress in research continued to be slow until about 1930, when new techniques for isolation and study of viruses in the laboratory began to be available. Since that time and especially since World War II, when human tissue cultures and other continuous cell culture lines were perfected, the rate of progress in accumulation of new knowledge of viruses has been greatly accelerated.[47] Viruses are characterized by smallness in size, ranging from about 300 m$\mu$ for some of the largest forms to about 17 m$\mu$ for some of the smallest. By comparison, the staphylococcus ranges in size from about 800 to 1200 m$\mu$.

A second general characteristic of viruses is that multiplication only occurs in the presence of living susceptible cells. This inability to multiply in lifeless media requires that, for culture in the laboratory, animal viruses must be grown in tissue culture or in a susceptible laboratory animal, such as the mouse or the chick embryo.

Viruses are inactivated by high temperatures similar to those used to kill bacteria. They withstand low temperatures and are preserved in deep freeze units at $-70°$ C.

The smallest and simplest viruses have an outer coat of protein and an inner core of nucleic acid which may be of the deoxyribonucleic acid (DNA) or the ribonucleic acid (RNA) type. No virus has been found to possess both types of nucleic acids. The protein of the outer coat is antigenic and accounts for most of the immunological reactions induced by viruses. The role of the virus protein which surrounds the nucleic acid component appears to be protective, although it may also aid in the penetration of the virus particle into the susceptible cell. The nucleic acid fraction of the virus particle carries the genetic material and accounts for the transmission of the heritable characters in virus multiplication. Viruses show no evidence of independent metabolism and appear to have no life of their own outside susceptible cells. Viruses become absorbed to cells by receptors on the cell wall. The protein coating remains outside the cell while the nucleic acid portion penetrates into the interior of the cell. New virus particles are produced in the cell; in some viruses this process occurs in the cytoplasm, and in others this replication takes place inside the nucleus. When the process is complete, the new virus particles emerge from the cell.

Cells infected by viruses may show different responses. They may degenerate and die or be transformed to a malignant state. Other cells survive but continue to harbor virus particles from one cell generation to another. These effects on cells account for the basic pathological reactions to virus infections. These primary pathological changes are: (1) hyperplasia alone, i.e., increased proliferation of cells; (2) hyperplasia followed by necrosis; and (3) necrosis alone. If inflammation occurs, it is generally a secondary response to the materials released from damaged cells.

Virus infections alone account for probably about 60 per cent of all episodes of human illness. Eight major groups of virus with more than 300 different immunological types are now recognized. The classification of viruses is based on the chemical composition, the size, and the structural characteristics of the virus particle. Because essential information is lacking, a number of important animal viruses remain unclassified. Among these are the viruses of infectious hepatitis and rubella.

*Laboratory Tests in Virus Infections*

Isolation of virus from the patient may frequently be accomplished by inoculation of susceptible animals or tissue cultures with material taken from the patient. Usually, there is more likelihood of virus isolation early in the course of infection or from tissues obtained at autopsy in the case of fatal infections. Virus so isolated may be identified in the laboratory by neutralization with specific immune serum.

Virus infections may also be identified by demonstration of a significant rise in antibody titer during the course of an illness. Two serum specimens must be collected. The first specimen is obtained during the early stage or acute phase of the illness; the second specimen is obtained in the convalescent stage, usually two to four weeks after the day of onset of symptoms. These sera are tested for antibodies against the viruses suspected of being the cause of the particular outbreak. Depending upon the viruses selected, the sera may be tested by neutralization, complement fixation, or the hemagglutination inhibition test. Generally speaking, a four-fold rise in antibody between the acute and convalescent sera is regarded as highly significant.

In some viral infections, diagnosis may be confirmed by examination of tissue at autopsy. Yellow fever, for example, causes a typical liver damage that can be readily identified by experienced pathologists.

*Immunity to Viral Infections*

As a result of infection and the subsequent multiplication of virus in the susceptible host, the antibody-producing mechanism is stimulated to produce immune globulins. In addition to these specific immune bodies, the host may develop a delayed-type hypersensitivity.

The protective action of antibodies appears to be by interfering with the adsorption and penetration of virus into tissue cells. Once the virus has entered a susceptible cell, antibody can no longer prevent its activity or interfere with its multiplication.

With a number of viral and rickettsial diseases, one attack generally results in a lifetime immunity to that disease. Those diseases characterized by viremia almost always result in a long-term immunity. Examples of this are smallpox, measles, yellow fever, and epidemic typhus.

It seems clear that antibodies have an important role in overcoming viral infections in the host and in the prevention of subsequent reinfections. It has been demonstrated, however, that those children who are agammaglobulinemic and incapable of producing antibodies do recover readily from viral infections. This indicates that the body has other means of resistance than antibodies to these infections.

One aid to recovery from viral infections may be interferon. This substance is a protein produced by cells as a response to infection by viruses.

Many different viruses have the ability to produce interferon. A remarkable property of interferon is a lack of virus specificity. Interferon produced by one type of virus may prevent multiplication of another type of agent. This inhibitory action of interferon may play an important role in the process of recovery in viral infections.

## Psittacosis-Lymphogranuloma-Venereum Organisms

This group of disease agents was formerly classed as viruses because of their dependence on living host cells for multiplication and cultivation only in tissue cultures in the laboratory. Now the group is distinguished from "true viruses" as they contain both DNA and RNA. Also they are enclosed in a cell wall closely resembling that of bacteria. The diseases they cause are susceptible to treatment by sulfonamides and many antibiotics. In size this group is comparable to rickettsiae. Three diseases caused by member of this group of organisms are of considerable importance to man: (1) a venereal infection (lymphogranuloma venereum); (2) trachoma, affecting the eyes; and (3) psittacosis, usually contracted from birds of the parrot family.[39]

## RICKETTSIAE

The rickettsiae were first described by Howard T. Ricketts in 1909. They appear to be intermediate between viruses and bacteria. Like viruses, rickettsiae multiply only in certain cells of susceptible animals. Rickettsiae resemble in many ways the agents of the psittacosis-lymphogranuloma venereum group. Multiplication of both groups is by binary fission. Both possess enzymes and contain both RNA and DNA.

Rickettsiae may be readily seen by the light microscope. They are generally shaped like small cocci.

One important characteristic of rickettsiae is their frequent occurrence in fleas, lice, mites, or ticks under natural conditions.

The rickettsial diseases are usually considered to form four main groups on the basis of clinical symptoms, their epidemiologies, and their immunological reactions. These are:

1. Typhus group
   A. Epidemic (louse-borne) typhus
   B. Recrudescent typhus (or Brill-Zinsser disease)
   C. Murine (flea-borne) typhus
2. Spotted fever group
   A. Rocky Mountain spotted fever
   B. Rickettsial pox
   C. Tick-borne rickettsioses of the eastern hemisphere
3. Scrub typhus (Tsutsugamushi disease)
4. Q fever (see also Table 5.6)

Another rickettsia, apparently not fitting into the above four groups, is the cause of louse-borne trench fever so prevalent during both world wars. Rickettsiae grow in laboratory-reared lice and ticks, in tissue cultures, and in the yolk sac of developing chick embryos. They are susceptible to heat, drying, and chemical agents, but can be readily preserved for long periods at low temperatures. It has been noted that the rickettsia of Q fever may persist for months in dust of barns contaminated with the feces of infected ticks.

All rickettsiae are susceptible to broad spectrum antibiotics. The diagnosis of rickettsial infections may be confirmed by serological tests. Most rickettsiae contain an antigen shared by certian strains of the *Bacillus proteus*. Therefore, sera from patients convalescent from rickettsial infections will usually agglutinate *Proteus* organisms of strains OX19, OX2, or OXK In some of the rickettsial infections the agent may be isolated from the blood or other material from the patient early in the illness by inoculation of suitable susceptible animals.[39]

### Bacteria

Bacteria are small, unicellular, plant-like organisms containing no chlorophyll and usually multiplying by binary fission. Individual bacterial cells in culture are physiologically independent. As noted by Leeuwenhoek in the 17th century, these organisms occur in three main forms: (1) spherical (cocci), (2) rod-like (bacilli), and (3) the spiral (spirilla). Bacteria, as they multiply, may separate into single cells or remain attached together in pairs (diplococci or diplobacilli) or form multiple aggregates. These aggregates may be in chains (for example, streptococci) or in squares of four cells (tetrads) or in irregular clusters (staphylococci). Most bacteria of medical importance have a dimension around 0.15 to 2.0 $\mu$ in diameter. There is considerable variation in size from the small *Haemophilus influenzae* (about 0.5 $\mu$ in length by 0.2 $\mu$ in width), to *Bacillus anthracis* (which may be 5 to 10 $\mu$ in length and 1 to 3 $\mu$ in width). Spirilla are, of course, much longer.

When suspended in one drop of fluid, many bacteria are recognized to be actively motile. Motility is due to movement of filament-like appendages (flagella). The number and location of these flagella aid in classification of bacteria.

Some bacilli produce spores within their cell walls called endospores. Such spores are formed in response to unfavorable environmental conditions. Spore formation renders the bacterium resistant to heat, desiccation, and chemicals that would injure the organism in its vegetative form. This ability to survive in the endospore stage is an important epidemiological characteristic in several infections that afflict

| Disease | | Natural Cycle | | | | Serological Diagnosis | |
|---|---|---|---|---|---|---|---|
| Group and type | Agent | Geographic distribution | Arthropod | Mammal | Transmission to man | Weil-Felix reaction | Complement fixation |
| Typhus Epidemic | R. prowazeki | Worldwide | Body louse | Man | Infected louse feces into broken skin | Positive OX-19 | Positive group and type-specific |
| Brill's disease | R. prowazeki | N. America; Europe | Recurrence years after original attack of epidemic typhus | | | Usually negative | Positive group and type-specific |
| Endemic | R. mooseri | Worldwide | Flea | Rodents | Infected flea feces into broken skin | Positive OX-19 | |
| Scrub | R. tsutsugamushi | Asia; Australia; Pacific Islands | Trombiculid mites | Wild rodents | Mite bite | Positive OX-K | Positive in about 50% of patients |
| Spotted fever Rocky Mountain spotted fever | R. rickettsi | Western Hemisphere | Ticks | Wild rodents; dogs | Tick bite | Positive OX-19, OX-2 | Positive group and type-specific |
| Boutonneuse fever | R. conori | Africa; Europe; Middle East; India | Ticks | Wild rodents; dogs | Tick bite | Positive OX-19, OX-2 | |
| Queensland tick typhus | R. australis | Australia | Ticks | Marsupials; wild rodents | Tick bite | Positive OX-19, OX-2 | Positive group and type-specific |
| North Asian tick-borne rickettsiosis | R. sibiricus | Siberia; Mongolia | Ticks | Wild rodents | Tick bite | Positive OX-19, OX-2 | |
| Rickettsialpox | R. akari | North America; Europe | Blood-sucking mite | House mouse and other rodents | Mite bite | Negative | |
| Q fever | R. burneti | Worldwide | Ticks | Small mammals; cattle; sheep and goats | Inhalation of dried, infected material | Negative | Positive |
| Trench fever | R. quintana | Europe; Africa; North America | Body louse | Man | Infected louse feces into broken skin | Negative | None available |

Source: Smadel, J. E. Rickettsial infections. In *Diagnostic Procedures for Viral and Rickettsial Diseases*, edited by E.H. Lennette and N. J. Schmidt, Ed. 3. New York: American Public Health Association, 1964.

man, tetanus being a notable example. Culture of bacteria in or on artificial media requires that the proper nutrients be available and that factors such as moisture, temperature, and available oxygen be appropriate for the particular organism. For the isolation and cultivation of most of the bacteria of medical interest, it is sufficient to use meat infusion base which has been enriched with special nutritive substances such as blood, ascitic fluid, amino acids, or carbohydrates. Special media are required for intestinal pathogens and other disease-producing agents.

Bacteria may be inoculated on the surface of a solid medium so that isolated colonies are formed. The pigmentation of these colonies, their size, the character of the surface and margins, and their shape and contour are useful in the identification of organisms.

Most bacteria are seen clearly under the microscope only when stained. The reaction to stains is helpful in identifying bacteria. Two of the best known differential stains are Gram's stain and Ziehl-Neelsen acid fast stain.

Classification of bacteria is still in an unsatisfactory state. In addition to morphology, staining reactions, and colony formations, other properties such as biochemical activity, antigenic structure, and pathogenicity are employed for purposes of differentiation.

Man living in an environment containing soil, water, and air is constantly in contact with a great variety of bacteria. Fortunately, most of these bacteria do not find favorable growth conditions on or in the human body. Cultures from the skin, the nose, mouth, and throat do show the presence of many different bacteria. Ordinarily, these organisms do not cause disease unless introduced into the tissues by cuts or other breaks in the skin or mucous membranes.

Pathogenic bacteria attack human tissues in various ways to overcome the defenses of the body and to produce harmful effects. Some bacteria have a substance on the cell surface or in their surrounding capsules that attack the white cells of the blood so as to prevent phagocytosis. All disease-producing bacteria elaborate enzymes that are excreted during growth. These enzymes are numerous and produce specific changes in the tissues of the host. Examples of such enzymes are: (1) streptokinase, which brings about digestion of fibrinogen and breaks up fibrin clots; (2) collagenase, capable of disintegrating muscle in

infected animals in gas gangrene infections; and (3) hyaluronidase, which facilitates spread of organisms in the tissues by destroying intercellular connective substances.

Many bacteria produce toxic substances. These may be exotoxins or endotoxins. The exotoxins are extremely potent and are responsible for the lethal effects of diphtheria, tetanus, and some food poisonings. These toxins are excreted into the tissues as the organisms multiply.

Endotoxins are liberated only after the death and disintegration of the bacteria. These toxins produce local inflammation at the site of their release, as well as general reactions of the body such as fever and malaise. Bacteria and their antigenic products frequently serve to sensitize the tissues of the body in such a manner that renders them allergic to subsequent contact with the same organism. Acute rheumatic fever is currently explained on the basis of resulting from repeated infections with certain strains of hemolytic *Streptococcus*. Some manifestations of tuberculosis are interpreted also on an allergic basis.

On the whole, it may be said that immunity to bacterial infections is not so complete or so enduring as it appears to be in many virus diseases. A number of vaccines have been developed that produce a reasonably effective defense against some bacterial diseases. The antityphoid fever vaccine can be cited as one. In two serious diseases in which the chief effect results from a powerful exotoxin, the population can be effectively immunized by toxoids. These are diphtheria and tetanus.

Great assistance to epidemiologists has been rendered by recent progress in identifying specific types of organisms by appropriate methods. Streptococci have been divided into groups on the basis of serologically active polysaccharides they contain. Nearly all human infections result from Group A strains. In Group A, no less than 40 types are recognized. These types are designated by number. The enteric group are divided into types by means of special agglutination tests for the Vi (virulence) antigen. The salmonellae that are commonly associated with food poisoning can be typed by serological tests. Staphylococci are frequently typed by the use of specific bacteriophages. These techniques enable the epidemiologist to know the precise type of organism responsible for the individual's infection and to trace positively the probable source of the infection.[39] Fortunately, many of the bacterial diseases have proved responsive to drugs that have become available in increasing numbers since 1935.

In recent years much study has been devoted to a class of microorganisms now called mycoplasmas. These are very tiny organisms ranging in size between viruses and bacteria. Mycoplasmas can be cultivated on lifeless media. They also contain both DNA and RNA.

Mycoplasmas are suspected to play a role in 21 human diseases. Yet, only one, the agent of atypical primary pneumonia, has been demonstrated to cause a major human disease. A great deal of research on this group of organisms is now underway.[48]

## SPIROCHETES

Several diseases of importance to humanity are caused by spirochetes. Among these are syphilis, yaws, relapsing fever, and hemorrhagic jaundice. Under the general term spirochetes are grouped a diverse assortment of spiral and actively motile microorganisms, most of which multiply by transverse fission. Classification is based mainly on morphology. There are both pathogenic and non-pathogenic species in each group. Spirochetes vary in length from 5 to 30 $\mu$ and in width from 0.1 to 0.5 $\mu$. One group of spirochetes, designated the treponema (meaning the turning thread), is the causative agents of syphilis, yaws, pinta, and a group of non-venereal syphilis-like infections.

Another group of spirochetes is known as the *Borrelia.* Relapsing fever is caused by *Borrelia recurrentis.* These fevers are prevalent in many parts of the world and are mostly transmitted by the body louse or by certain ticks. Another species of *Borrelia* is responsible for infections of the mouth, throat, genitalia, and cause ulcers on the skin.

The third group of spirochetes are the *Leptospira.* Spirochetal jaundice, or Weil's disease, is the most important disease caused by this spirochete. It is probable that wild rodents are the natural reservoir of all *Leptospira.* Man usually becomes infected by contact with soil or water contaminated by the excreta of infected rodents.

Spirochetes, with the exception of *Leptospira,* are difficult to cultivate on artificial media. Most laboratory isolations are done by inoculation of experimental animals.

Most spirochetal infections are treated successfully by antibiotics, penicillin being the drug of choice. Again leptospiral infections are an exception as treatment of them is not too successful.[39]

## Yeast and Molds

Only a few organisms in this large and complex group are known to cause human disease. The *Actinomyces* show some relationships to bacteria and to the higher fungi or molds. Actinomycosis in man is characterized by chronic abscesses with multiple draining sinuses most frequently located around the neck or face, but occasionally in the abdomen. Another member of this group, the *Nocardia,* most often causes abscesses in the lungs, but may affect other tissues. The *Streptomyces,* a third member of the group, occasionally cause deep tissue abscesses. These actinomycetes are free living in nature and are transmitted to man by air-borne contamination or by introduction into the tissues through breaks in the skin. Organisms of these groups grow readily at 37°C or at room temperature on a variety of simple media. They grow as branching filamentous forms that may break up into bacillary or coccus-like elements. Sulfonamides and broad spectrum antibiotics usually produce good therapeutic results.

*Cryptococcus neoformans* (see Fig. 5.13), a yeast-like fungus, frequently affects the lungs

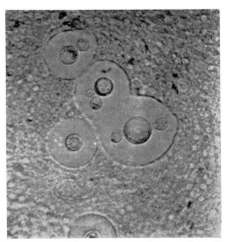

Fig. 5.13. *Cryptococcus neoformans* in culture, showing the characteristic large capsule. Source: *Oral Microbiology and Infectious Disease,* G. W. Burnett and H. W. Sherp. Baltimore: The Williams & Wilkins Company, 1968.

184

PUBLIC HEALTH AND COMMUNITY MEDICINE

simulating tuberculosis. It commonly affects the central nervous system causing a chronic meningitis and sometimes nodules or abscesses in the brain. This organism, formerly known as torula, is easily grown on ordinary laboratory media. It produces neither mycelia nor spores. *Cryptococcus* is worldwide in distribution. It has been cultivated from the soil and is found in association with pigeon-roosting areas. Amphotericin B is apparently effective in the treatment of patients.

Another yeast-like fungus that causes human illness is *Candida albicans (Monilia)*. This species inhabits the mouth, intestinal tract, or genital membranes of about 35 to 40 per cent of the population. It can be readily cultured on ordinary laboratory media. *Candida* may cause infections of the oral mucous membranes (thrush). It may also affect the skin. Serious illness is caused by internal infections, especially of the lungs. These infections are becoming more common in patients undergoing prolonged treatment with antibiotics which upset the normal balance of the body's microbiological flora.

Occurrence of *Monilia* infection is worldwide. Man is the reservoir. *Monilia* produces budding forms, asexual spores in culture, but not true filamentous growth.

Blastomycosis is a comparatively rare disease in man. It is usually a tuberculosis-like disease of the lungs, but may also cause chronic skin ulcerations. The agent is *Blastomyces dermatitidus* which grows easily on laboratory cultures. When cultures are kept at room temperature, the organism appears as a mold with filamentous forms; at 37° C , it appears in a spherical, yeast-like form. The reservoir of the organism is in the soil. It is probably transmitted by spore-laden dust. For treatment, amphotericin B is the current drug of choice.

Another form of blastomycosis occurs in South America. This disease is due to *Blastomyces braziliensis* and chiefly affects the mucous membranes of the mouth and the facial tissues. Fortunately, the sulfonamides are quite effective in the treatment of this disease.

A fungus disease only recently described is being recognized with increasing frequency in this country as a cause of ill health. This disease, known as histoplasmosis, is caused by a soil fungus *Histoplasma capsulatum* (see Fig. 5.14). Infections due to this fungus are widely distributed around the world, but in the United

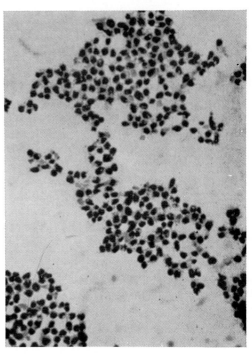

Fig. 5.14. The yeast form of *Histoplasma capsulatum*. Source: *Oral Microbiology and Infectious Disease*, G. W. Burnett and H. W. Sherp. Baltimore: The Williams & Wilkins Company, 1968.

States they are found to be concentrated in the eastern and central sections. Infection in these areas as shown by positive skin reactions increases from childhood to about 30 years of age; sometimes as much as 80 per cent of a local population has been infected. Severe disease usually affecting the lungs occurs in only a small percentage of those infected.

The reservoir of *Histoplasma* is in the soil around old chicken houses, bird or bat roosts, in caves, and other areas having a high organic content in the soil.

*H. capsulatum* may be cultured on all ordinary laboratory media. In the soil, the organism grows as a mold; in the human, it assumes a yeast-like form. The mouse is a useful laboratory animal for isolation of *Histoplasma*.

Man is infected by breathing in the highly infectious spores in contaminated dust. Many outbreaks of the disease have appeared among groups exploring caves, cleaning out chicken houses, or among children playing in areas where birds roost. Treatment of this disease is not too effective. Amphotericin B has been recommended by some physicians.

During the past 30 years, increasing attention has been focused on another fungus infection in the United States. Coccidioidomycosis or valley fever was first described in Argentina in 1892.[49] Although sporadic cases were discovered in the United States, it was not until the 1930's that it became clear that this infection was a common one among the inhabitants of the hot, interior valleys of California and in the desert areas extending from southern Nevada to south Texas. The agent causing this disease is known as *Coccidioides immitis* (see Fig. 5.15). It grows in the soil, especially around rodent burrows, and in regions with suitable temperature and moisture requirements. In the soil and in cultures, it grows as a filamentous mold, but in animal tissues it assumes a spherical, yeast-like form.

Transmission is by breathing in dust contaminated by spores of the fungus. Infection may be entirely asymptomatic, but in some individuals, there may be an influenza-like illness. About one-fifth of those who develop symptoms get painful, red nodules on the lower extremities; generalized skin rashes also appear in many individuals.

A progressive, highly fatal disease, affecting

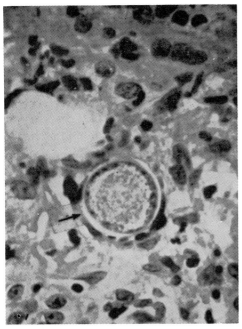

Fig. 5.15. *Coccidioides immitis.* Source: *Oral Microbiology and Infectious Disease,* G. W. Burnett and H. W. Sherp. Baltimore: The Williams & Wilkins Company, 1968.

the lungs and other organs, occurs in a small per cent of those infected. This generalized type of disease is more prevalent among colored peoples, including Negroes, Filipinos, and other Orientals.

Amphotericin B has been found to be somewhat effective in the severe cases, but must be given near the level of toxicity to produce results.

A localized fungus disease of the skin, characterized by ulcerations and nodules, is seen in many parts of the world. It often appears as an occupational disease of farmers and gardeners. Many animals, both wild and domestic, are susceptible. The agent is *Sporotrichum schenkii.* The reservoir is in the soil or on wood. Infection is transmitted through breaks in the skin. The organism is a budding, round, yeast-like fungus in animal tissues, but on culture it becomes a filamentous form.

A common problem, especially in hot countries, is ringworm. This is a general term covering various types of fungal infections of the skin, nails, and hair. The causative agents belong to several genera of fungi but are collectively known as dermatophytes. They do not cause systemic disease and rarely invade the subcutaneous tissues.

Some pathogenic species of dermatophytes affect man only. Others are found infecting man and animals. The diseases caused by these agents are divided by the sites of infection:

*Tinea capitis—Ringworm of the Scalp.* The agents are various species of the genera *microsporum* and *trichophyton.*

*Tinea corporis—Ringworm of the Body.* The agents the *Epidermophyton floccosum* and various species of *Microsporum* and *Trichophyton.*

*Tinea pedis—Ringworm of the Foot.* The agents are *Epidermophyton floccosum* and various species of *Trichophyton.*

*Tinea unguium Ringworm of the Nails.* The agents are *Epidermophyton floccosum* and various species of *Trichophyton.* Probably extends from infections on the feet.

Griseofulvin, an antibiotic discovered in 1958, has proved effective in treatment of the dermatophytoses.

Dermatophytes are readily cultivated on ordinary media, but the use of Sabouraud's glucose agar with antibiotics to suppress bacterial growth greatly aids in isolation of strains from infected tissues.[39]

## Protozoa

Parasitic protozoa are one-celled organisms of animal nature. They are composed of a nucleus, or multiple nuclei, and cytoplasm. The cytoplasm is divided into endoplasm, an inner portion concerned mainly with nutrition, and an outer portion, the ectoplasm, whose function is a protective one. Food from the environment is taken in by the ectoplasm. Motility is the function of small appendages of the ectoplasm. These may be flagella, cilia, pseudopodia, or undulating membranes. Protozoa range in size from 1 to 2 $\mu$ to more than 100 $\mu$. These parasites, when in the body of the host, are found chiefly either in the intestinal tract or in the blood. Blood parasites rarely, if ever, are found free in nature. Intestinal parasites, by contrast, are frequently able to exist outside the body in the form of resistant cysts.

Four classes of protozoans of medical importance are recognized. This division is based mainly on the means of locomotion. The classes are:

1 Rhizopoda—motility through pseudopodia.

2. Mastigophora—motility by flagella.

3. Sporozoa—possess no specialized means of motion.

4. Ciliata—move by cilia.

The protozoa usually develop through a series of stages, called the life cycle of the parasite. Intestinal protozoa pass through the trophozoite stage and the cystic stage. In the vegetative or trophozoite phase, the organism is active, feeding, growing, and reproducing, and in this stage causes the tissue damage that produces symptoms in the host. In the cystic stage motility ceases, the parasite becomes reduced in size, and a cyst wall is secreted as a protective coat. The organism passing out the intestine in the cystic stage can survive any reasonably favorable conditions outside the body until it is taken in with water or food by a new host. Desiccation, sunlight, and heat are inimical to the cysts and may destroy their viability.[50]

Protozoans responsible for blood infections generally have a more complex life cycle. Blood parasites depend upon bloodsucking arthropods for their dissemination.

Protozoa reproduce in various ways. Asexual multiplication is a division of the cell without fertilization by simply splitting to form two or more new organisms. Sexual reproduction is a division of the cell following fertilization. Frequently, sexual multiplication is associated with an alternation of generations, an asexual cycle taking place in man with a sexual cycle of reproduction occurring in the arthropod vector.

Of the protozoal diseases of the intestine, amebiasis is by far the most common and is responsible for a great deal of human disease. Ameba cause both acute and chronic diarrheal disease. It also commonly produces severe abscesses in the liver. Ameba move by pseudopodia and are classified among the Rhizopoda.

Of the protozoal parasites of the blood, malaria is the most widely spread and over the centuries was perhaps the most important disease affliction of man. Happily, through the various means of control, malaria has been reduced to a relatively small problem for man. It still persists in many tropical regions and will no doubt continue to collect its toll of human suffering for many years to come. There are four species of malaria parasites that affect man. They are classed among the Sporozoa.

Of the Mastigophora or flagellates, the trypanosomes are of great medical importance. *Trypanosoma gambiense* and *Trypanosoma rhodesiensi* are the agents of African sleeping sickness which has devastated large areas of Central Africa. The tsetse fly, which transmits these infections, lives along the streams. It may become infected by feeding on wild game, such as antelopes, or may transmit from man to man.

Another serious disease caused by a flagellate is visceral leishmaniasis (kalaazar). It is characterized by fever, enlargement of liver, spleen, and lymph glands, and progressive emaciation and weakness. Untreated, it is a highly fatal disease. The agent is *Leishmania donovani*. The disease occurs in the rural areas of most tropical and subtropical regions. It is transmitted by the bites of infected sand flies.

The only ciliate that parasitizes man is *Balantidium coli*. It is the largest of the protozoa found in man. This parasite prefers the cecal area of the large intestine and may produce shallow ulcerations causing diarrhea. Usually, the agent can be readily detected and effective treatments are available.

## Helminths (Worms)

There are some numerous multicelled animals, sometimes called Metazoa, that parasitize man. These organisms are much larger than the parasitic agents already discussed. They vary in length from 1 mm. to over 6 m. The helminths have a complex and distinctive structure; some even require two or three successive hosts to complete their life cycles. These organisms are found in all parts of the world as parasites of almost all vertebrates. A few species are sharply limited in their geographical distribution; others occur very widely indeed. Most of the helminths are obligatory parasites, but some have ability to live for at least part of their lives as free agents, usually in water or soil. A few species, if no host is available, are able to adapt completely to a free living state (see Table 5.7).

The helminths of medical importance belong to two classes: (1) roundworms—the nematodes, and (2) flatworms—the trematoda and cestoda.

The Nematoda have an elongated, unsegmented, cylindrical body. They are covered by a cuticle and have a complete digestive tract with a mouth and anal pore. Male and female individuals differ characteristically in shape and appearance, the males being almost invariably smaller than the females. The life cycles of

## TABLE 5.7

*Prevalence of Helminth infections in man*[1]

| Parasite | Source of Infection | United States and Canada | World-wide |
|---|---|---|---|
| Nemathelminthes (roundworms) | | | |
| *Trichinella spiralis* | Pork | 21,100,000 | 27,800,000 |
| *Enterobius vermicularis* | Human feces | 18,000,000 | 208,800,000 |
| Hookworm | Human feces | 1,800,000 | 456,800,000 |
| *Ascaris lumbricoides* | Human feces | 3,000,000 | 644,400,000 |
| *Trichuris trichiura* | Human feces | 400,000 | 355,100,000 |
| *Strongyloides stercoralis* | Human feces | 400,000 | 34,900,000 |
| *Trichostrongylus* spp. | Human feces | [2] | 5,500,000 |
| *Dracunculus medinensis* | Cyclops | | 48,300,000 |
| *Onchocerca volvulus* | Black fly | | 19,800,000 |
| *Mansonella ozzardi* | Culicoides | | 7,000,000 |
| *Acanthocheilonema perstans* | Culicoides | | 27,000,000 |
| *Loa loa* | Mango fly | | 13,000,000 |
| *Wuchereria bancrofti* and *malayi* | Mosquitoes | | 189,000,000 |
| Platyhelminthes (flatworms) | | | |
| Cestoda (tapeworms) | | | |
| *Taenia saginata* | Beef | 100,000 | 38,900,000 |
| *Taenia solium* | Pork | [2] | 2,500,000 |
| *Echinococcus granulosus* | Dog feces | [2] | [2] |
| *Hymenolepis nana* | Human feces | 100,000 | 20,200,000 |
| *Diphyllobothrium latum* | Fish | [2] | 10,400,000 |
| Trematoda (flukes) | | | |
| *Clonorchis sinensis* | Fish | | 19,000,000 |
| *Opisthorchis felineus* | Fish | | 1,100,000 |
| *Fasciolopsis buski* | Water nuts | | 10,000,000 |
| *Paragonimus westermani* | Crabs-crayfish | | 3,200,000 |
| *Schistosoma japonicum* | Water through skin | | 46,000,000 |
| *Schistosoma haematobium* | Water through skin | | 39,200,000 |
| *Schistosoma mansoni* | Water through skin | | 29,200,000 |
| Total infections | | 44,900,000 | 2,257,100,000 |
| Population | | 143,500,000 | 2,166,800,000 |
| Percentage infections of population | | 31 | 104.2 |

[1] The world's population has increased nearly 50 per cent since the data in the above table were collected. The prevalence of most of the parasites has increased correspondingly.

[2] Represents less than 100,000 infections (from Stoll, N.R.: *J. Parasit, 33:* 1, 1947).

Source: Brown, H. W. Diseases caused by metazoa. In *Cecil-Loeb Textbook of Medicine,* edited by P. B. Beeson and W. McDermott, Ed.12. Philadelphia: W.B. Saunders Company, 1967.

nematodes vary greatly from one species to another, but in general, they tend to conform to the following pattern:

1. The typical adult nematode is found in the intestinal lumen.

2. Eggs are discharged in the stools of the host.

3. Eggs develop to a larval stage either as free living organisms or may reinfect man while still in the egg stage.

4. Larvae may enter a new host by mouth or by penetration of the skin.

5. Larvae enter the blood of the host, pass through the lung tissue to reach the esophagus, and reach the intestine where they grow to adult worms.

There are several diseases of importance to man caused by nematodes. Ascariasis, a chronic infection of the intestine most common in tropical regions, is due to large round-worms—15 to 35 cm. in length. These worms live unattached in the small intestine. Large numbers of eggs are produced. Fertilized eggs require two to three weeks to develop to an infective stage after elimination in the feces. Infective eggs, under favorable conditions, may remain viable in the soil for many months. These eggs reach the mouth of man through contamination of food. The eggs hatch out in the small intestine. The larvae penetrate the inner lining of the gut, getting into the blood stream. In the lungs, they molt and form other larval stages, finally reach the esophagus, and are swallowed, setting up the intestinal infection. Light infections usually cause few symptoms, but a heavy worm load in the intestine deprives the host of his food and may cause obstruction of the gut or bile ducts. The larvae, if numerous, may cause irritation and inflammation of the lung tissue.

Another widespread and serious disease of man caused by nematodes is hookworm. These nematodes are quite small ranging from 8 to 13 mm. in length. Hookworms have specially adapted mouth parts for fastening themselves to the walls of the small intestine in order to suck blood from the capillaries. Fertilized eggs are produced in large numbers. When deposited on the soil in suitable conditions of moisture, shade, and temperature, the eggs hatch within 24 to 48 hr. These larvae develop by molting through to the third stage. At this stage, the larvae have a sharp tail capable of penetrating

human skin. In the host, the larvae get to the lungs through the blood stream and finally to the small intestine where they complete their life cycle.

Hookworm occurs widely in tropical and subtropical regions. Symptoms of hookworm disease result from loss of blood resulting in a profound anemia in heavily infected individuals. Improvement in sanitary practices has greatly reduced the number and severity of infections during recent decades.

The larvae of dog and cat hookworms, *Ancyclostoma caninum* and *Ancylostoma brasiliense,* may cause a creeping eruption of the skin, most commonly found in young children. The larvae penetrate the skin of individuals playing in the sand. As the larvae migrate through the skin, reddish colored streaks appear that cause intense itching. If infection is heavy, severe illness may be caused.

A nematode disease of great interest and of some public health importance is trichinosis. The worm causing this disease, *Trichinella spiralis* (see Fig. 5.16), is principally a parasite of hogs. Garbage containing uncooked or undercooked pork scraps is the most common source of transmitting the infection to hogs. Man becomes infected by eating inadequately cooked, infected pork. This disease is more prevalent in Europe and the United States than in the remainder of the world.

The parasite has no free living stage in its life cycle. Man ingests the larvae encysted in the muscle tissue of swine. Gastric juice frees the larvae which penetrate the wall of the small intestine where development occurs to the adult stage. The females are fertilized in the intestinal mucosa and begin to release new larvae within five days after infection occurs.

These small larvae enter the blood stream and are disseminated throughout the body entering striated muscle fibers where they become encysted and remain viable for years.

Symptoms may occur as a result of irritation and tissue destruction caused by the adult worms in the intestinal wall or later by the waves of larvae causing inflammation of muscle fibers. Muscle pains and toxic effects causing fever and weakness may cause severe or even fatal illness.

Trichinosis may be prevented by freezing pork products. The time of storage and temperature depends upon the thickness of the

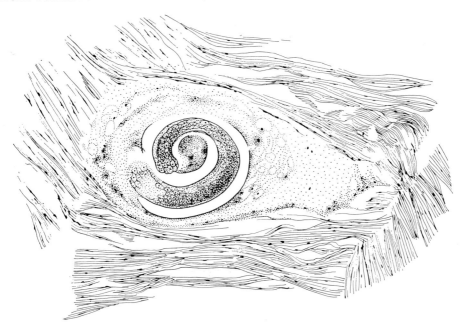

Fig. 5.16. *Trichinella spiralis;* encapsulated larva in muscle section. Source: *Textbook of Medical Parasitology,* H. H. Najarian. Baltimore: The Williams & Wilkins Company, 1967.

cuts. Regulations vary from 20 days at 5° to six days at –20° F. Another preventive measure is to ensure thorough cooking of all pork before its consumption. In 1972, only 96 cases of trichinosis occurred in the United States. There was one death reported. This contrasts with the 1947 figures when 6200 cases of trichinosis were reported with 126 deaths.[51]

Filariasis is a nematode disease of importance in many tropical regions around the world. There are at least six species of filaria which parasitize the lymphatic or subcutaneous tissues of man. Female worms give rise to larval microfilariae (see Fig. 5.17), which reach the blood stream. There is usually a definite periodicity for the larvae to appear in the blood. Man is the reservoir of infection. Mosquitoes transmit the parasite from man to man.

Prolonged and repeated infections result in obstruction to lymph drainage with a resulting chronic swelling of the extremities or genitalia known as elephantiasis.

A rather rare and localized form of filariasis produces a disease, onchocerciasis, which occurs mostly in central Africa but is found in a few foci of the American tropics, probably brought over in the slave trade. This organism frequently affects the eyes causing blindness. It thrives in the subcutaneous tissues of man and is transmitted by the black fly, *Simulium.*

The trematodes have complicated life cycles involving alternation of generations and of hosts. The schistosomes, or blood flukes, are of very considerable public health importance. The adult worms are usually found in pairs attached to the walls of the large veins in the abdominal cavity. They vary from 0.16 to 1.1 mm. in width and from 10 to 20 mm. in length. After copulation, they give off eggs in considerable numbers over a long period. These eggs pass through from the veins to either the urinary bladder or the lower intestine, thus leaving the body in the urine or feces. Upon reaching fresh water, the eggs hatch, freeing the larvae or miracidia. The intermediate hosts for the schistosome are certain snails. The miracidium enters the snail's soft tissues and over a period of several weeks passes through three stages. The final stage, cercaria, has a forked tail. It escapes from the snail and swims about in the water. Man becomes exposed to infection when he enters the water. The cercariae, upon contact with the skin, discard their tails and digest their way through the skin to enter the blood stream reaching maturity after 16 days.

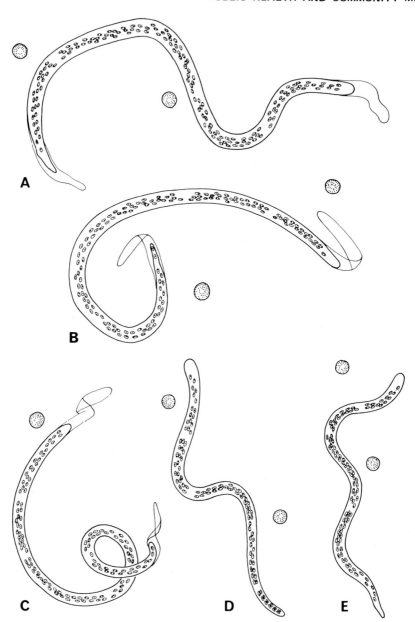

Fig. 5.17. Microfilariae from blood smears: *A, Wuchereria bancrofti; B, Brugia malayi; C, Loa loa; D, Acanthocheilonema perstans; E, Mansonella ozzardi.* Source: *Textbook of Medical Parasitology,* H. H. Najarian. Baltimore: The Williams & Wilkins Company, 1967.

Finally, the parasites become anchored in the portal veins to repeat the sexual cycle.

There are three main species of schistosomes that cause human disease. Each has its own geographical distribution in the tropics and subtropics.[52]

Schistosomiasis affects the urinary system, the intestinal tract, and the liver principally. It is a chronic and debilitating disease of great importance in the regions where it is endemic.

The three major species of schistosomes which infect man, *S. haematobium, S. mansoni* and *S. japonicum* are widely distributed. The first is found in Africa and Southwest Asia mainly; the second in the same areas and in South America and the Caribbean; the third is found only in the Far East. WHO estimates there are 200 million people in the world suffering from schistosomiasis.

The cestodes, or tapeworms (see Fig. 5.18), in the adult stage are segmented flatworms, made up of a head, a neck, and a series of segments. The head is adapted for attachment to the intestinal wall. The neck is a budding zone which produces the segments forming the rest of the worm. The parasite may reach a length of over 6 m. Tapeworms have simple nervous and excretory systems. No digestive system is required. Each segment is hermaphroditic, possessing both male and female reproductive organs.

The eggs are discharged in the feces. In the case of the beef tapeworm, these are taken up by cattle grazing in contaminated pastures. In cattle, the only intermediate host, larvae escape from the eggs to eventually reach the blood stream from the intestine. Most of them reach muscle tissue where over a period of 60 to 75 days they develop into cysticircal form. Man, eating raw or undercooked beef, becomes infected. The head of the larva attaches to the lower small intestine and the worm develops to maturity. It may live for several years.

The pork tapeworm has a similar life cycle, except that the hog is the intermediate host. The main difference between the pork and beef tapeworm infection is that in man, if the eggs of the pork parasite are ingested, they develop larval forms in the intestine (cystercerci) which get into the blood and are scattered throughout the body. These larval forms become encysted and often are located in parts of the body that cause great damage, *e.g.*, the eye, the brain, or the heart.

Two other types of tapeworm infection frequently involve man. The fish tapeworm infection is acquired through eating fish. It is not usually a severe disease but may produce a troublesome anemia. When eggs from feces get into fresh water, they hatch and the first stage larvae are taken up by the first intermediate host, small crustaceans. Fish eat these infected crustaceans and become the second intermediate hosts. Man acquires the parasite by eating raw fish.

A fourth type of tapeworm that occasionally affects man is that of the dog. The eggs are expelled in the feces and infect other dogs or wild animals. Humans usually are infected by getting the hands contaminated with dog feces. Taken in by mouth, the eggs hatch in the intestine and larvae migrate to various organs to produce cysts. The liver and lungs are most frequently involved. If in vital areas, the cysts may cause death. Echinococcosis, or hydatid disease, is the term used for the human infections. This disease is rare in the United States.

## Arthropods (Jointed Legs)[53]

Arthropods have segmented bodies, are covered by an external skeleton, and are distinguished by the presence of jointed appendages

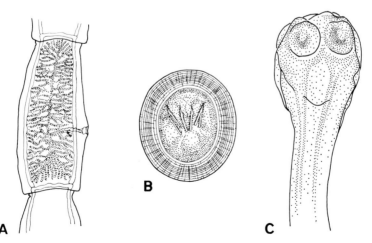

**A**      **B**      **C**

Fig. 5.18. *Taenia saginata: A,* gravid proglottid; *B,* egg; *C,* scolex, or head. Source:*Textbook of Medical Parasitology,* H. H. Najarian. Baltimore: The Williams & Wilkins Company, 1967.

in the form of legs, mouth parts, and antennae. Although the number of species of arthropods is vast, relatively few affect human health. Some of these transmit communicable diseases to man and are in that way highly important links in the life cycles of many infectious agents. Malaria, yellow fever, typhus, and plague are familiar examples of arthropod-borne diseases. Many arthropods add to human discomfort (see Table 5.8).

There are two main types of transmission of disease by arthropods. One type is mechanical transmission. Typhoid fever by the common housefly is an example of this. The housefly feeds upon and lays its eggs in human feces, thus contaminating its feet and mouth parts with material laden with intestinal bacteria. This contaminated material may be transferred shortly thereafter to food being prepared for human consumption.

Another illustration of mechanical transmission of infection is the role of mosquitoes in

TABLE 5.8

*Some arthropods affecting human comfort*

| Common Name | Scientific Name of Arthropod | Effect on Man |
|---|---|---|
| Mites | | |
|   Chigger | *Trombicula alfreddugesi* | Intense itching; dermatitis |
|   Rat mite | *Ornithonysseus bacoti* | Intense itching; dermatitis |
|   Grain itch mite | *Pyemotes ventricosus* | Dermatitis and fever |
|   Scabies mite | *Scarcoptes scabiei* | Burrows in skin, causing dermatitis |
| Ticks | | |
|   Hard ticks | *Amblyomma* spp. | Painful bite |
| | *Dermacentor variabilis* | Tick paralysis; usually fatal if ticks not |
| | *D. andersoni* and *Ixodes* spp. |   removed |
|   Soft ticks | *Ornithodoros* spp. | Some species very venomous |
| Black widow spider | *Latrodectus mactans* | Local swelling; intense pain and occasional death |
| Scorpions | Order: Scorpionida | Painful sting; sometimes death |
| Centipedes | Class: Chilopoda | Painful bite |
| Mayflies | Order: Ephemerida | Asthmatic symptoms from inhaling fragments |
| Caddis flies | Order: Trichoptera | Asthmatic symptoms from inhaling hairs and scales |
| Lice | *Pediculus Humanus* and *Phthirus pubis* | Intense irritation, reddish papules |
| Bugs | | |
|   Bed bugs | *Cimex lectularius* | Blood suckers; irritating to some |
|   Kissing bugs | Family: Reduviidae | Painful bite; local inflammation |
| Beetles | | |
|   Blister beetles | Family: Meloidae | Severe blisters on skin from crushed beetles |
|   Rove beetles | Family: Staphylinidae | Delayed blistering effect |
| Caterpillars | Order: Lepidoptera | Rash on contact with hairs or spines |
| Bees, wasps, and ants | Order: Hymenoptera | Painful sting; local swelling |
| Fleas | Order: Siphonaptera | Marked dermatitis frequent |
| Flies | | |
|   Punkies or Biting midges | *Culicoides* spp. | Nodular swelling, inflamed |
|   Black flies | *Simulium* spp. | Bleeding punctures; pain, swelling |
|   Sand flies | *Phlebotomus* spp. | Stinging bite; itching; whitish wheal |
|   Mosquitoes | Family: Culicidae | Swelling; itching |
|   Horse flies and deer flies | *Tabanus* spp. and *Chrysops* spp. | Painful bite |
|   Stable flies | *Stomoxys calcitrans* | Painful bite |

Source:   Pratt, H.D. *Introduction to Arthropods of Public Health Importance.* National Communicable Disease Center. Public Health Service Publication 772, Atlanta, 1960, reprinted 1967.

spreading myxomatosis. This disease, a mild chronic skin disease of South American rabbits, is a highly fatal systemic disease in the rabbits of Europe. It is caused by a viral agent. To aid in the control of the pest in Australia, this infection was introduced to the wild rabbit population in 1950. The mosquito acts as a "flying pin" in the spread of the disease, carrying the virus on its mouth parts.

The more usual mode of transmission of disease by arthropods involves biological mechanisms. At least two forms of biological transmission are recognized. The parasite may undergo developmental changes in the arthropod but does not multiply. This type of relationship is exemplified by microfilariae in mosquitoes. Another form of biological relationship between parasite and arthropod is that of the malaria organism in the mosquito. Here the parasite undergoes both a developmental cycle and multiplication in the mosquito. Other infectious agents such as the yellow fever virus in appropriate mosquitoes multiply but do not show changes in their development.

Each arthropod has its characteristic life cycle. In general, the individual begins with the egg stage, passing through a series of changes of form before attaining adulthood. The biological requirements of each species as it moves through its life cycle present man with opportunities to introduce control measures. For example, the requirement of mosquito larvae and pupae for an environment of water permits antilarval methods of control.

The life expectancy of arthropods in nature is also significant in disease control. The average life span of mosquitoes in nature is perhaps a few weeks, while that of ticks may be several years. Mobility is another important consideration. Mosquitoes can fly for only short distances but may be blown for miles by strong winds. They may also be carried great distances by trains, ships, or airplanes.

Ticks and mites possess certain characteristics that provide distinctive features to the diseases that they transmit. These arthropods pass through four stages of development: (1) egg, (2) larva, (3) nymph, and (4) adult. The tick is long-lived and may remain viable for years without feeding. The female is highly prolific and is known to produce, depending on the species, from several hundred to 18,000 eggs during one period of oviposition.

Both ticks and mites have the ability to pass some infectious agents to the next generation, thus greatly prolonging their capability for transmission of the agent to a new host.

Many species of ticks and mites tend to remain fixed in favorable habitats year after year. Thus, diseases in which these species are chief factors are geographically limited. Endemic foci, e.g., in Rocky Mountain spotted fever, have persisted for several human generations.

In addition to their importance as transmittors of disease, many arthropods are capable of producing human illness on their own. Many people suffer from skin irritations resulting from mosquito, flea, or louse bites. Almost everyone has felt the itching resulting from the larvae of certain mites, chiggers, or redbugs burrowing into the skin after an outing in the woods.

Powerful venoms are introduced to the body through the bites of some spiders, scorpions, bees, or wasps. These have been known to cause death in small children or in individuals allergic to the toxic material.

A most serious form of acute paralysis results from the bite of some ticks. This so-called "tick paralysis" has been reported in Canada, Australia, and the United States. Children are most often affected and girls more than boys. One female tick, usually hidden in the hair, can produce an ascending paralysis which may be fatal unless the tick is quickly discovered and removed. Symptoms clear up rapidly once the tick is taken off. Several genera of ticks are capable of producing a paralysis, but, in North America, the genus *Dermacentor,* or "wood ticks" is usually the responsible agent.

## NUTRITIONAL DEFICIENCIES

In this search for valid bases of our value judgments, I think that nutritionists would do well to recall the great lesson now receding in the history of their science. That lesson, of forty years ago, was that nutrition was not then, and may never be, a closed deductively formulated science. Forty years ago, chemists wrestled with the problem of a diet supporting life and growth, and found the solution to their problem, not in quantitative manipulation of the items they knew, but in an appeal to the natural world for new, qualitatively important items, the vitamins. Lest we commit the same blunder and the ultimate nutritional heresy, let us be aware that "nutrition" embraces the whole world of natural foods, and let us remember that there may lie in wait for us new nutritional entities that, if we but properly seek them out, may well be the real bridge into the world of infectious disease.

In these words, Howard Schneider warned his colleagues in 1955.[54]

Current belief is that a diet, in order to be adequate to maintain health, must contain appropriate amounts of protein, fat, carbohydrate, water, and the numerous essential minerals and vitamins. The requirements for these substances vary. Many of them have interrelated physiological functions, so that the amount required of one nutrient depends upon the proportion of the diet supplied by other substances; for example, the iron requirement is related to the amount of Vitamin C in the diet.[55]

In order to maintain an equilibrium in body weight, it is necessary that the diet provide sufficient caloric content to meet the body's basic metabolic needs and to allow for the physical activities of the individual.

The study of nutritional deficiencies indicates that they result from a variety of factors complexly interrelated. They are generally not due to a deficiency of a single essential nutrient. Some essential elements of diet are not stored in any large amounts in the body, so the available supplies are rapidly depleted unless provided in the daily diet. This is the case with the water-soluble vitamins of the B complex and of Vitamin C. On the other hand, Vitamins A and K, which are fat-soluble, are usually stored by the body in larger amounts. Prolonged dietary deficiency of these food substances is required before signs of depletion appear. The kind and severity of the signs and symptoms of nutritional deficiency depend upon the nature and degree of the multiple dietary inadequacies, the extent to which each essential nutrient is deficient, and the duration of the deficits.

In highly developed nations, there is relatively little nutritional deficiency. The poor and ignorant in some disadvantaged segments of society are still exposed to deficiencies, but public health programs to enrich basic foods with minerals and vitamins have reduced this threat to health. Certain individuals are more vulnerable to deficiencies because of increased physiological requirements. Women during pregnancy and the lactation period require special dietary consideration. Infants at the time of weaning from the mother's milk generally need dietary supplements. Those recuperating from extensive surgical procedures or suffering from chronic diseases require special dietary attention. The aged and, of course, food faddists may encounter nutritional disorders on account of restricted choice of foods. Alcoholics frequently develop liver disease or other signs of nutritional depletion resulting from replacement of normal food intake by alcoholic beverages.

Populations of certain localities obtain insufficient minerals from the foods grown in the area. This is well illustrated by the endemic goiter belts where iodine in the soil is in low concentration or in regions with high incidence of dental caries which can be largely corrected by fluoridation of water supplies.

The situation among the major proportion of the human race is vastly different, especially in those regions of the tropics and subtropics in which the population pressures have so greatly increased during the past century. Caloric shortages as well as unbalanced diets are all too common. In some regions, malnutrition has resulted when cash crops, such as cotton or sugar cane, have been substituted for the previous food crops. It has been estimated that between 10 and 15 per cent of the world population suffers from undernutrition. At least one-third of the human race probably show signs of some dietary deficiency. This high prevalence of nutritional disease is aggravated by widespread parasitic infections. Intestinal worms, malaria, tuberculosis, yaws, and diarrheal diseases intensify the effects of undernourishment.[56]

Throughout the underdeveloped regions, major reliance is placed upon rice, wheat, corn, cassava, or millet as the principal source of calories. Adults are able to supplement their diets with fruit, yams, or other vegetable foods. In these countries, malnutrition is likely to be particularly severe in women during pregnancy and the nursing period. Infants after being weaned and young children are especially vulnerable. The chief nutritional problem among children is due to protein deficiency or to an imbalance of amino acids resulting from a low protein intake. The name now generally used for this condition is the African word kwashiorkor. This severe form of malnutrition is exceedingly common in Africa, Asia, and Latin America. The growth rate of the children is impaired, the hair and skin become pale, feet and legs are swollen, and the patient is apathetic. These patients appear prone to all kinds of infections and, unless the diet is improved, they frequently die. Relief of symptoms is rapid when milk or proper mixtures of amino acids are given to the victims. This form of malnutrition is probably the most serious cause of ill health in the underdeveloped areas of the world.[57]

As previously mentioned, most cases of nutritional disease are of multiple causation. Rarely is there found a depletion of only one specific nutrient. This is particularly true of the B complex vitamins. Pellagra (a name derived from the Italian words meaning rough skin) results from a lack of niacin (one of the Vitamin B complex). This vitamin can be produced in the body by conversion of the amino acid tryptophan to niacin. Diets high in corn and containing little or no milk, meat, or other good protein sources are pellagragenic. Wheat eaters usually obtain sufficient tryptophan to prevent this disease.

Pellagra is common in parts of Italy, Spain, Rumania, and recently in the southern United States. As is true of other B vitamin deficiencies, pellagra often accompanies poverty, chronic alcoholism, dietary fads, fever, and other physiological stresses. In advanced cases, pellagra is characterized by dermatitis made worse by sunlight, diarrhea, and dementia. Early symptoms are sore red tongue, loss of appetite, weakness, burning sensations in various parts of the body, numbness, forgetfulness, and dizziness.

Beriberi is a disease resulting from Vitamin B1 (thiamin) deficiency. It may be either acute or chronic. Characteristic signs are painful neuritis of the extremities and in severe cases heart failure. In the past, beriberi was a frequent scourge in the Far East where polished rice is a main dietary constituent. It has also been a health problem in Labrador, Iceland, and Newfoundland during winter months when the diet is made up largely of white flour. Beriberi is most common in men subjected to hard physical labor. In women, pregnancy may be a precipitating factor. The heart and nervous system are most frequently affected. Death may ensue if the thiamin deficiency is not relieved.

In the United States, mild forms of beriberi sometimes occur among poverty stricken people or among alcoholics and food faddists.

Another well-known deficiency disease is scurvy, a hemorrhagic condition arising from lack of Vitamin C or ascorbic acid. This disease was a scourge of sailors in the days of the slow voyages in sailing ships. Inmates of jails and orphanages whose diet was devoid of fresh fruits and vegetables were also frequent scurvy victims. The disease is now seen mainly in infants on cow's milk without supplements or among those on restricted ulcer diets or among aged individuals.

In infants, scurvy prevents normal gain in weight, causes irritability, pain upon movement because of hemorrhages around the long bones, and swollen tender bleeding gums. Patients quickly recover when given fresh fruit juice or synthetic Vitamin C.

Rickets is also a deficiency disease largely confined to children but may occur in adults as osteomalacia. This disease is due primarily to lack of Vitamin D. It is characterized by a negative balance of calcium and phosphorus, resulting in deficient calcification of the bones. Rickets was formerly highly prevalent in Europe and North America but is now mostly found in northern India, China, and Japan.

Rickets may occur at any time during the growing period, but most cases develop before two years of age. The first signs may be skeletal deformities, especially of the pelvis, head, thorax, and long bones. The bones become soft and flexible. Symptoms are weakness, bone pains, and in severe cases, convulsions due to calcium deficiency. If the disease progresses, it leads to great deformity. In the adult, X ray of bones shows rarification in osteomalacia.

Rickets is most likely to occur in urban areas where infants and young children receive little exposure to sunlight. Vitamin D is produced in the body by action of ultraviolet light on the sterols of the skin. Rickets has been about eliminated in advanced countries by the introduction of Vitamin D supplements in the formulas of infants and young children.

Iron is a necessary component of the diet. Ordinarily, the average human diet contains sufficient iron for health unless there occurs an unusual demand for this mineral due to blood losses.

All cells of the body require iron, but the chief use of iron in body metabolism is for the production of hemoglobin. Iron from outworn red blood cells is used over and over again. Any excess of body requirements is stored in the liver, spleen, or bone marrow. Iron deficiency anemia is apt to occur in adolescence, during pregnancy and lactation, or in conditions characterized by continuous blood losses, for example, hookworm, bleeding hemorrhoids, or excessive menstruation.

Another important cause of anemia may result from deficiency in the three vitamins especially involved in formation of new red blood cells—Vitamin B12, folic acid, and Vitamin C. Pernicious anemia, formerly a highly fatal disease, is due to a deficiency of Vitamin B12.

A goodly number of other vitamins is known and has been studied in laboratory animals. It is thought that they are of importance in the maintenance of health in humans, but definite deficiency states are not well established. These are pyridoxine, pantothenic acid, biotin, Vitamin E, choline, and *para*-aminobenzoic acid.

In addition to nutritional deficiencies that result from inadequate diets or primary deficiency disease, such states may be secondary to physiological disturbances or abnormalities in the individual which interfere with intake of food, its absorption, or in the utilization of nutrients in the body's metabolism. Disease of the gastrointestinal tract frequently causes poor appetite. Conditions that produce nausea and vomiting also reduce food intake. Even loss of teeth may interfere with a proper nutritional state.

Lack of acid in the stomach, interference with normal bile flow, and diseases of liver or pancreas may reduce the efficiency of the absorptive process. Overdosing with mineral oil may interfere with absorption of the fat soluble vitamins.

Larger amounts of essential nutrients are required in certain conditions. In periods of delirium, fever, or heart failure, in leukemia patients, or in individuals with hyperactive thyroid glands, nutritional requirements are increased.

In diabetes and in cirrhosis of the liver, utilization of nutrients is disturbed. In the care of patients with such conditions, physicians must attempt to correct the responsible factors as well as to ensure supplementary dietary factors.

In addition to disease caused by a deficiency of one specific nutrient or more, malnutrition may lower resistance to infections, thus promoting the development of any one of a number of communicable diseases. It has proved difficult to establish a convincing relationship between any specific infection and a particular dietary factor, probably because poor nutrition lowers resistance through several different mechanisms. One such mechanism is that protective antibodies are less readily produced and more rapidly lost in malnourished individuals. Also the state of nutrition apparently has an effect on the phagocytic white blood cells. The quality of the inflammatory reaction to tissue infection is affected by malnutrition. Quite likely, the nutritional state affects susceptibility to infection through other channels.[58]

There is good evidence to show that certain kinds of malnutrition and nutritionally related diseases can cause mental retardation and severe mental illness. Probably protein deficiency and low caloric intake are the most common factors in producing this mental retardation in children.

Dietary deprivation affects the developing human, if it takes place during the critical stages of its rapid growth. The brain is extremely vulnerably during this early period of life. Electroencephalograms of malnourished children show striking abnormalities which do not revert to normal if the food deprivation is long continued.[59,60]

One great change in the eating habits of Americans is the increasing use of eating places outside the home. About $35 billion, or 23 per cent of the food dollar is spent for meals away from home with predictions that the amount spent will rise to $75 billion by 1980. Food service is the third largest industry in the nation.[61]

Two events of importance for the improvement of nutrition in the United States' have occurred recently. In response to a mandate from Congress, the Department of Health, Education, and Welfare, set up the National Nutrition Survey to carry out a careful study of the prevalence of malnutrition in selected areas of the country. Ten states were chosen and samples of the population in each were selected for examination. Emphasis was placed on low-income groups. Altogether 24,000 families composed of 86,000 members were included in the study. Dietary histories were taken, biochemical tests were done, and medical examinations were carried out on some 40,000 persons of the selected samples.[62]

Most signs of malnutrition were discovered among adolescents from 10 to 16 years of age. Low hemoglobin levels were widespread. Many pregnant women had low serum protein levels. Evidence of Vitamin A deficiency was common in some groups. Signs of goiter (thyroid disease), possibly due to iodine deficiency, were frequently encountered in the survey.

The second important event was the White House Conference on Food, Nutrition, and Health, held in Washington in December 1969. This meeting brought together some 800 participants for three days of constructive discussions. Definite recommendations for action by government and community groups were strongly pressed to wipe out the remaining pockets of malnutrition in the nation.[63,64]

## METABOLIC DISTURBANCES

Every individual is biologically unique. This implies a distinctive pattern of metabolic processes which affects every chemical reaction of the body. This individuality is based on inherited characteristics determined by the distribution of the 20,000 to 40,000 pairs of genes in the chromosomes. Biochemical individuality may be demonstrated "in the composition of tissues and body fluids, enzyme levels in cells and blood, quantitative needs for specific nutrients, pharmacological responses to specific drugs, and numerous other ways."[65] Environmental factors are also of great importance in determining the effects of the genetic inheritance in metabolic conditions as in all other biological systems.

Knowledge of inherited metabolic defects goes back to Garrod's work in England in the early years of this century. His monograph *Inborn Errors of Metabolism*, appearing in 1908 and again in 1923, established definitely that certain defects in the biochemical activities of the body were inheritable. Subsequent workers arrived at the principle that each enzyme is related to one gene. This concept led to the formulation by Tatum[66] of the following principles:

1. All biochemical processes in all organisms are under genic control.

2. These biochemical processes are resolvable into series of individual stepwise reactions.

3. Each biochemical reaction is under the ultimate control of a different single gene.

4. Mutation of a single gene results only in an alteration in the ability of the cell to carry out a single primary chemical reaction.

The one gene-one enzyme concept has recently been expanded to apply to proteins in general. Complex proteins are composed of polypeptides. Genetic changes may result in an alteration of structure of specific proteins or may affect the quantity of proteins. In the final analysis, all inherited disorders are affected through changes in kind or amount of one or more specific proteins. The best known example of a modified protein due to genetic mutation is sickle cell hemoglobin. The alteration of protein is in only one among the several hundreds of amino acids composing the globin component of the hemoglobin. Other variant hemoglobins have been found to have similar single substitutions of altered amino acids. Known inherited disorders of metabolism affect a wide variety of metabolic systems, including: (1) carbohydrates; (2) amino acids; (3) lipids; (4) purines; (5) porphyrins; (6) erythrocyte proteins; (7) plasma proteins; and (8) bloodclotting mechanisms.

Many metabolic disorders are without consequence and produce no symptoms. An example is inherited differences in ability to taste thiourea derivatives. Other such defects become known only as a result of some accidental environmental factor, for example, the effect of certain drugs on patients with porphyria. Some disorders produce mild to moderate symptoms, but many others have severe consequences and even prove a threat to life. Phenylketonuria may cause irreversible damage to the nervous system. Possibly, many fetal deaths are due to, as yet, unknown inherited disorders of metabolism.

Some of these disorders are sex-linked. Hemophilia occurs almost always in males but is transmitted by female carriers.

Diabetes is by all odds the most important of the metabolic disorders. It appears quite definite that susceptibility to diabetes is dependent on genetic factors. The overall incidence of diabetes is difficult to determine, but the evidence presented by surveys in the general population of the United States indicates that at least 3.5 per cent of the population show signs of the disease. According to the American Diabetes Association, at least 45 million persons in the United States are believed to be diabetes carriers in a genetic sense. Today, diabetes is largely a disease of middle and old age. The disease is on the increase as the number of persons in the older age groups has grown so markedly. Each year 325,000 Americans learn that they have diabetes. There is evidence that the prevalence of the disease in this country may be considerably higher. In 1967, there were 35,049 deaths in the United States attributed to diabetes; and in 1971, the number was 37,650 (provisional figure).[67] Diabetes now ranks among the 10 leading causes of death in this country. In the United States diabetes is described as the third leading cause of blindness. It is now considered that predisposition to diabetes is inherited on a simple mendelian recessive basis. This is indicated by the fact that there is a greater incidence of diabetes among the siblings than among the children of diabetic persons.

The major condition found in diabetes is considered to be a deficiency of insulin. This deficiency of insulin appears to depend upon a decreased number of pancreatic insulin-producing $\beta$ cells or to an abnormality of such cells of the pancreas. To an unknown degree, dysfunctions of the pituitary and adrenal glands may be of causal importance in some cases of diabetes. A low output of insulin might result from cells normal in appearance but abnormal in their insulin-producing ability or the insulin produced might be incomplete in some respect. Most of the features of diabetes can be explained as dependent upon decreased glucose utilization by certain body tissues.

Diabetes mellitus ordinarily appears in two recognized clinical forms—the juvenile (or youth-onset) type or the more common maturity-onset type. The disease in early life is related to an absolute insulin deficiency and is more severe, as a rule, than is the malady in older age groups, which is more often the result of a delayed release of insulin following the intake of carbohydrates.

Another common and disabling disease of metabolic origin is gout. This condition is a genetically determined disorder of the purine metabolism. A high level of uric acid in the blood is the characteristic biochemical feature of gouty individuals.

Gout may be asymptomatic, but in many persons it manifests itself clinically by periodic attacks of an acute arthritis or by kidney stones or both. Over a period of years, the disease may become chronic and produce destructive changes in the affected joints.

Males are far more frequently attacked by gout than are females. Most gouty patients produce uric acid at an excessive rate. They also show a lower rate of uric excretion. These two factors account for the high blood uric acid levels found in gout. A number of genes appears to be involved in the determination of uric acid metabolism.

The acute gouty arthritis is thought to depend upon the formation of urate crystals. This occurs in body fluids having a high concentration of uric acid. The real prevalence of gout is not known. From the National Health Survey Interview data, it is indicated that from 100,000 to 120,000 persons report annually in the United States that they have gout.[68]

A third metabolic disease of importance is phenylketonuria. In 1934, a series of 10 patients who were mentally deficient were found to excrete phenylpyruvic acid in their urine. The essential metabolic defect is an inability to oxidize phenylalanine to tyrosine, thus allowing phenylalanine to accumulate in the tissues. This defect depends upon the absence or inactivity of the appropriate enzyme. Infants born with this metabolic defect show an increased level of blood phenylalanine. After the sixth month, signs of mental retardation due to the noxious action of this chemical on the brain can be observed. The majority of the infants so affected become idiots.

Other effects of this condition are eczematous skin eruptions and a failure to develop normal pigmentation of skin and hair.

The disease is inherited as a genetic recessive trait. The incidence of phenylketonuria is about one in 25,000 of the population stemming from northern European ancestors. Most of the affected children are found in institutions and account for about 1 per cent of mentally retarded children.

All of the major abnormalities of a biochemical nature are relieved by a diet low in phenylalanine. The skin eruption promptly clears up but returns, if larger amounts of phenylalanine are restored to the diet. Treatment does not restore lost intelligence to older children but can prevent intellectual impairment in early life and even reverse impairment of short duration (see Chapter 6).

## ALLERGIC DISORDERS

Allergy as employed in this chapter represents an altered response by the body on re-exposure to certain foreign substances. The allergic reaction is due to the combination of the foreign substance with the protective antibodies formed by the body following the first exposure. Depending upon many factors, such antibodies show considerable variation in structure and in their activity. If the sensitizing substance is an infectious or toxic agent, the antibodies generally combine with it to prevent its harmful action.

In addition to reacting to harmful substances, the body may produce antibodies to other materials, for example, grass, pollen, or horse dander. This type of reaction results in the common symptoms of hay fever or eczema. Thus, an immune mechanism evolved by man as a protection against many common infectious diseases, under other circumstances, results in inconvenient and even dangerous reactions.

Allergic conditions are usually of two kinds: (1) those in which test material injected into or applied to the skin produces immediate response, that is, within 20 to 30 min.; and (2) those in which the skin reaction is delayed for 24 to 48 hr. The blood of individuals who manifest the immediate type of skin reaction contain antibodies which can be transferred from man to man by an injection of the allergic individual's serum. The antibodies of persons demonstrating delayed skin response cannot be so transferred. A patient with hay fever, sensitive to ragweed pollen, is an example of the immediate type of reaction; an individual reactive to tuberculin possesses a delayed type of sensitivity (see Table 5.9). At least four

TABLE 5.9

*Allergic diseases classified by type of skin reaction*

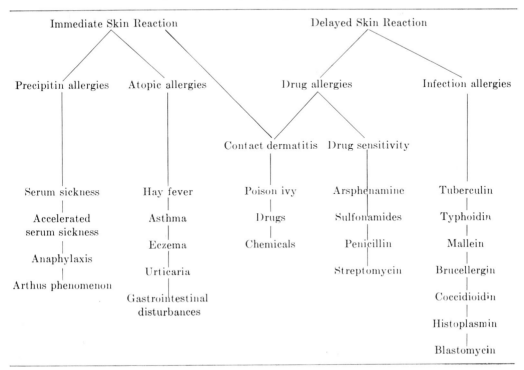

Source:   Smith, D. T., Conant, N. F., and J. R. Overman, Editors. *Zinsser Microbiology*, Ed. 13. New York: Appleton-Century-Crofts, Inc., 1964, p. 200.

clinical types of allergic reactions are recognized. Although the terms are unsatisfactory, these types of allergic reaction have been designated as: (1) precipitin allergies; (2) atopic allergies; (3) drug allergies; and (4) allergies of infection. Some allergic conditions are not readily classifiable and perhaps overlap these somewhat artificial groupings.[39]

Of the precipitin allergies, perhaps the best known is serum sickness. This condition was quite common in the presulfonamide era when immune sera were employed frequently in the treatment of several infectious diseases. Antibodies known as precipitins appear in the serum a few days following an injection of horse serum given to patients. As the antibody rose in the serum, the patient often rather suddenly developed fever, a red, blotchy skin rash, and painful sensitive joints. The explanation usually given for this reaction is that the foreign material, horse serum, had lodged widely throughout the body in the various tissues. As the blood level of antibody rose, reaction of antibody and foreign protein in the tissues produced the varied symptoms of serum sickness. The unpleasant reaction subsided within a few days as a rule.

Another form of precipitin allergy is fortunately rare, as its results may be fatal. An individual having received one injection or more of horse serum develops a high level of precipitin antibodies in the blood. A subsequent injection of this foreign protein may produce an immediate profound shock with difficulty in breathing and swelling of tongue and tissues of the throat. Death may ensue during this overwhelming reaction. This condition is known as anaphylaxis.

Severe anaphylaxis may result from stings of wasps or bees in previously sensitized individuals. Usually, persons reacting in this manner are known to suffer from previous allergic conditions such as hay fever or asthma.

The atopic allergies are to a considerable extent conditioned by genetic factors. Diseases of this type frequently are distributed in families. Hay fever, asthma, urticaria (hives), eczema, and some kinds of gastrointestinal disorders belong in the atopic allergies. Similar allergies are very common with the near relatives of patients with this type of disability. Inheritance, however, is not the only determining factor. Some individuals develop their allergic response only late in life. Others may experience only one episode of an allergic reaction. Hay fever and asthma are highly prevalent in the American population. Perhaps between 5 and 10 per cent of the general population have experienced one or more attacks of hay fever, hives, eczema, or asthma. The total effect of these illnesses is great. The National Health Survey reports that over 1,159,000 persons have some limitation of activity due to asthma and hay fever while 148,000 individuals are unable to carry on with their work.[69]

Antibody in the blood of hay fever patients is usually not discovered by laboratory methods, but it can be demonstrated by inoculation into another individual. This type of antibody adheres to tissue cells with which it comes in contact. When the appropriate foreign substance enters the body of an individual so sensitized, the union of substance and antibody on the cell surface releases a compound known as histamine. This liberation of histamine in the tissues produces the reaction characteristic of hay fever. Histamine-blocking drugs, or antihistamines, often give almost complete relief from these symptoms.

There are innumerable substances which can sensitize these unfortunate people. Among these are grass and tree pollens, dander, feathers, hair, eggs, milk, dust, bacteria, or fungi. Skin tests with a large series of these substances may reveal those to which a given individual is most reactive. Desensitization by injections of gradually increasing amounts of the offending substance may reduce the frequency and severity of the attacks.

Allergic reactions to drugs are becoming an increasingly important threat to health. These reactions may take the form of various types of skin rashes, hives, serum sickness, joint pains, or asthmatic attacks. With other drugs, there may be a localized or fixed eruption as in contact dermatitis.

Sensitivity to drugs is not the same as drug intolerance. Intolerance of individuals to specific drugs means an exaggerated reaction to the usual pharmacological action of the drug.

Drugs that most commonly cause allergic responses are: opiates; salicylates; barbiturates; iodides; bromides; arsenicals; sulfonamides; and antibiotics.

Penicillin interacts with certain amino acids of the serum protein to form a potent agent for stimulation of antibodies. Sensitivity to this drug is becoming more common in the general population. Between 100 and 200 severe anaphylactic-type reactions, of which many prove fatal, are reported to result from penicillin each year.

Contact dermatitis may be due to drugs, chemicals, or plant juices. Poison ivy is a well-known example. The toxic substances of poison ivy form compounds with host proteins which serve to sensitize some persons so that subsequent contact with the plant produces marked reactions of the skin.

Allergies resulting from infectious processes are well exemplified by those occurring in tuberculosis. Circulating antibody of the usual type in response to the invasion of the tubercle bacillus occurs at best in small amounts. The characteristic antibody of tuberculous infection cannot be transferred from animal to animal by tranfer of serum or by injection of serum from a tuberculous animal into the skin of a normal animal. These antibodies are fixed to tissue cells and white blood cells. Sensitivity to tuberculin may be transferred to a normal animal by injecting large amounts of white blood cells from a tuberculous subject. In persons infected with tuberculosis, skin reactions are obtained after a 24- to 48-hr. delay by inoculation of tuberculin.

A similar type of allergic response is recognized in several other diseases where there is localization of inflammation to hold the antigenic substances *in situ.* Typhoid fever, brucellosis, pneumococcal pneumonia, and streptococcal infections are examples. Some investigators have considered these allergic responses as protective and advantageous for the recovery of the patient from his infection. Opinion is gradually turning to the view that much of the damage done in the body by these infectious agents is a direct result of the harmful allergic reactions to the proteins of the agents in the tissues.

In general, individuals rarely form antibodies against the cells of their own bodies. Antibody-forming tissues are in contact with their own internal environment from early fetal life and presumably learn to distinguish between self and non-self. Certain individuals do produce antibodies to selected cells of their own organs. More and more this so-called autoimmune process is being recognized as a factor, if not the principal cause, of some human diseases. This process will be understood if one recalls

that skin grafts can readily be made from one part of an individual's body to another with great success. The body, however, sternly rejects skin grafts from another individual. The body has the ability to recognize its own tissues but regards the tissues of others as something foreign and to be rejected. It has been suggested that a genetic fault allows autoantibody-forming cells to break free from the mechanisms that usually keep them under control.[70] Autoimmune disorders may be produced readily in laboratory animals by inoculating extracts of homologous tissues such as brain, thyroid, or adrenal. One form of chronic inflammation of the thyroid gland in the human is considered to be an autoimmune disease. It is suspected that autoimmune disease plays an important factor in a number of other important diseases such as pernicious anemia, ulcerative colitis, glomerulonephritis, multiple sclerosis, and rheumatoid arthritis. Intensive research is underway in many centers on the mechanisms underlying such disease processes.Probably both genetic and environmental factors are involved.[43]

## AGING AND DEGENERATIVE PROCESSES

The staggering increase in the number of persons of 65 years and over in the United States has brought the health problems that result from an aging population into sharp focus. The population aged 65 and over in this country increased from about 3 million in 1900 to over 20.9 million in 1972, or from 4.1 to 10.0 per cent of the total population. The increase in survivorship has been greater among females than males. As of 1972, there is a female excess of about 2.6 million at ages 65 and over.

This rise in the older groups of the population explains to some degree the increased prevalence of chronic illness and various impairments such as blindness. There has also been a considerable rise in the use of personal health services as well as an increase in consumer spending for these services. According to data from the National Health Survey, not only are more physician visits required per year, but the number of days of confinement to bed due to disability is about 2½ times greater in those of 65 years or over than in younger adults.

The characteristic changes of the aging process are poorly understood. Certainly they vary markedly from one individual to another. One person appears old at 55 years of age; another is vigorous and well preserved at 70 years of age. Biological aging depends upon heredity, environmental experiences, and the individual's ability to adapt to the stresses of life. Perhaps the infectious diseases that have been encountered along the way may also have had deleterious effects upon the functioning of vital organs (see Table 5.10).[71]

As is well known, life expectancy at birth in the United States has been greatly increased since 1900. This tremendous increase in life expectancy is mainly due to the great reduction of mortality in the younger age groups. The life expectancy for an individual at age 65 years has risen at most from 12 years in 1900 to 14 to 15 years in 1965. A considerable part of this increased life expectancy in the older ages merely reflects a prolongation of survival time by expensive and complicated medical care rather than more years of healthful living—a kind of "medicated survival."[25] In fact, people of the current generation have little more chance to enjoy a long and healthy life than did their ancestors.

In 1969-70, the leading causes of disability in the age group of 65 years and over were: (1) heart conditions, (2) arthritis and rheumatism, (3) impairments of back or spine, (4) asthmahayfever, (5) impairments of lower extremities and hips, (6) visual impairments, (7) hypertension without heart involvement, and (8) mental and nervous conditions.

It is estimated that 815,130 people were residents in nursing homes in 1969. Almost 90 per cent of these were 65 years of age or over.[72]

## TABLE 5.10

*Work days lost due to acute conditions*
*In the United States, 1971*

| Acute Conditions | Number of Work Days Lost (000,000 omitted) | | | Work Days Lost per Employed Person | | |
|---|---|---|---|---|---|---|
| | All ages 17 and over | Age 17-44 | Age 45 and over | All ages 17 and over | Age 17-44 | Age 45 and over |
| **Both sexes** | | | | | | |
| All acute conditions | 262 | 168 | 94 | 3.4 | 3.6 | 3.1 |
| Infective and parasitic diseases | 23 | 16 | 8 | 0.3 | 0.3 | 0.3 |
| Respiratory conditions | 105 | 67 | 38 | 1.4 | 1.4 | 1.3 |
| Digestive system conditions | 17 | 12 | 5 | 0.2 | 0.3 | 0.2 |
| Injuries | 76 | 49 | 28 | 1.0 | 1.0 | 0.9 |
| All other acute conditions | 40 | 25 | 15 | 0.5 | 0.5 | 0.5 |
| **Male** | | | | | | |
| All acute conditions | 152 | 97 | 55 | 3.2 | 3.3 | 2.9 |
| Infective and parasitic diseases | 13 | 8 | 5 | 0.3 | 0.3 | 0.2 |
| Respiratory conditions | 57 | 36 | 21 | 1.2 | 1.2 | 1.1 |
| Digestive system conditions | 10 | 7 | 3 | 0.2 | 0.2 | 0.1 |
| Injuries | 53 | 35 | 19 | 1.1 | 1.2 | 1.0 |
| All other acute conditions | 19 | 11 | 8 | 0.4 | 0.4 | 0.4 |
| **Female** | | | | | | |
| All acute conditions | 111 | 71 | 39 | 3.8 | 4.0 | 3.5 |
| Infective and parasitic diseases | 10 | 7 | 3 | 0.4 | 0.4 | 0.3 |
| Respiratory conditions | 48 | 30 | 18 | 1.6 | 1.7 | 1.6 |
| Digestive system conditions | 8 | 5 | 3 | 0.3 | 0.3 | 0.2 |
| Injuries | 23 | 14 | 9 | 0.8 | 0.8 | 0.8 |
| All other acute conditions | 21 | 14 | 7 | 0.7 | 0.8 | 0.6 |

Note: The data refer to the civilian, noninstitutional population. In some cases the sum of the items does not equal the total shown, because of rounding.

Source:   Source Book of Health Insurance Data 1973-74. Health Insurance Institute, 277 Park Avenue, New York, New York 10017.

Cardiac and vascular disease in old age are largely dependent upon arterial degeneration characterized by atherosclerosis. This disease process may begin early in life and is frequently far advanced by middle age but, among the elderly, it is very common indeed (see Fig. 5.19). From evidence now available, it appears that atherosclerosis is a disease of civilization and that it may be dependent upon the characteristics of the diet, especially upon the intake of saturated fats. Other factors, such as physical exercise and mental stress, may also be of importance in influencing the blood levels of cholesterol. This condition of high blood cholesterol is thought to be intimately related to atherosclerosis.

In those 65 years of age and over, about two of every three deaths are due to cardiovascular disease. Of these, approximately 95 per cent are

due to atherosclerosis and high blood pressure.[73]

The respiratory system in old age becomes less efficient as a result of changes in the muscles and bones. Deaths from respiratory infections are frequent, especially among individuals confined to bed by other disabilities. The influenza-pneumonia infections are especially dangerous to the old.

Tuberculosis has the highest attack rate in persons 65 years and over than in any other age group. Among elderly males, tuberculosis case rates are more than three times higher than in females. Probably, these currently high attack rates are a reflection of tuberculous infections acquired in the earlier decades of life when tuberculosis was far more widespread than at the present time. Emphysema, asthma, and bronchitis are other forms of troublesome respiratory conditions common in the older age groups.

Three diseases of bone are common in old age. Most prevalent is osteoarthritis. Almost 90 per cent of people over 60 years suffer from some form of arthritis (see Table 5.11). Osteoporosis and osteitis deformans are less common but equally disabling. Because the bones are more brittle, fractures are likely to result from falls that would only cause bruises at an earlier age.

Accidents are a major cause both of deaths and of disability among the aged. About 10 per cent of the population is 65 years or over, but 24 per cent of all who die of accidents are in that group. From 65 to 74 years, deaths from accidents occur at the rate of 87 per 100,000 per year while in the group 75 years and over the rate rises to 232 per 100,000.[74]

Mental disease due to tissue changes in the brain or of the blood vessels supplying the brain is common. A survey by the American Psychiatric Association in 1960 revealed that in public mental hospitals in the United States 30 per cent of the patients were 65 years or over. Twenty-seven per cent of the first admissions were from that group. Of course, financial insecurity, loneliness, and boredom contribute to emotional instability of the aged and probably lead to depression in some individuals.[75]

Common diseases of the genitourinary tract in the elderly are associated with infection and interference with the flow of urine. Stones in the kidney and tumors of the bladder are relatively common. Benign hypertrophy of the

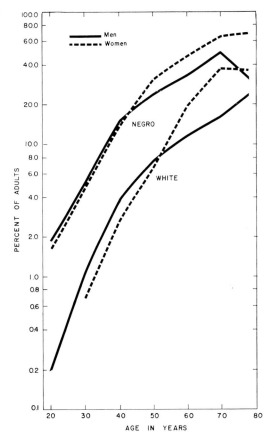

Fig. 5.19. Percentage of adults with hypertensive heart disease, by age, race, and sex. Source: National Center for Health Statistics. *Hypertension and Hypertensive Heart Disease in Adults,* Public Health Service Publication 1000, series 11, no. 13, 1966.

## TABLE 5.11

*Arthritis, by age, race, and sex, United States, July 1961 to June 1963*

|  | Age | Total | Race | | Sex | |
|---|---|---|---|---|---|---|
|  |  |  | White | Non-white | Male | Female |
| Number (in thousands) | All ages | 12,668 | 11,315 | 1,353 | 4,400 | 8,268 |
|  | Under 45 | 1,957 | 1,717 | 240 | 635 | 1,322 |
|  | 45-64 | 5,702 | 5,044 | 657 | 2,020 | 3,681 |
|  | 65+ | 5,009 | 4,554 | 455 | 1,744 | 3,265 |
| Rate per 1000 population | All ages | 69.6 | 70.4 | 63.6 | 49.9 | 88.2 |
|  | Under 45 | 15.2 | 15.3 | 14.5 | 10.1 | 20.2 |
|  | 45-64 | 154.7 | 151.1 | 189.3 | 113.6 | 193.0 |
|  | 65+ | 304.4 | 299.3 | 368.4 | 237.9 | 358.0 |

Source: *Arthritis Source Book.* Public Health Service Publication 1431, 1966. Original source: Arthritis reported in interviews, July 1961 to June 1963. Estimated annual average. Unpublished data. Division of Health Interview Statistics, National Center for Health Statistics, U.S. Public Health Service. (Civilian non-institutional population.)

prostate gland frequently occurs in the male. This interferes with complete emptying of the bladder.

In women, prolapse of the uterus and malignant growths of the uterus are not infrequent.

The skin problems of the older person are dependent upon the aging and degenerative processes. These include dryness, abnormal pigmentation, itching, malignant growths, and chronic ulcers, especially on the lower legs.[76]

Impairment of vision and of hearing are severe trials of the elderly. Cataracts, glaucoma, and degeneration of the macula are the three most common eye defects causing impaired sight. More than two-thirds of those with cataracts are in the 65 years and over age group. Impaired hearing is found in about 13 per cent of those 65 to 74 years of age and in twice that number in those 75 years and over.[77]

Problems with the teeth are extremely common in old age. They are largely based on previous neglect of good dental care. Examination of selected population samples by the United States National Health Survey staff reveals that, while only one in every 100 persons 18 to 24 years has no natural teeth, by age 65 to 74 years, nearly one in two had lost all teeth (see Fig. 5.20). Periodontal disease, which accounts for many lost teeth, also increases in prevalence and severity with age. At ages 75 to 79 years, about nine of every 10

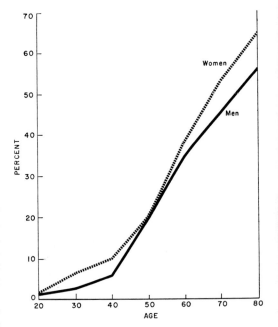

Fig. 5.20. Percentage of men and women who are edentulous, by age. Source: National Center for Health Statistics. *Selected Dental Findings in Adults, by Age, Race, and Sex.* U.S. Public Health Service Publication 1000, series 11, no. 7, 1965.

such persons had serious periodontal disease. Dental caries and periodontal disease are the two main causes of tooth loss. Nutritional deficiency may play some role in individual cases. The great majority of the aged require dentures.[78]

In general, less food is required to maintain body weight in older people. This is due to some lowering of the metabolic rates and to a decline in physical activity. In those living alone, the appetite is likely to falter. Absorption of food from the intestinal tract may be less efficient so that even if the diet contains sufficient nutrients they may not become available for use in the body.

Nutritional deficiencies are then more common among old people. Anemias and vitamin deficiencies must always be kept in mind by physicians charged with the care of aged.

## ACCIDENTAL INJURIES

The Medical Director of the World Health Organization, Dr. M. G. Candau, has estimated that accidents rank third among the causes of death in the world.[79] In the United States alone, 117,000 accidental deaths occurred in 1972. Approximately one-half of these fatalities are caused by motor vehicular accidents, about 27,000 of the fatal accidents occurred in the home, and some 14,100 occurred in occupational situations. In the United States, accidents are the leading cause of death among the population aged from 1 to 44 years.[74]

The severity of injury resulting from non-fatal accidents can now be assessed in the United States through the National Health Survey. These data indicate that in the year 1972 approximately 67.8 million persons were injured by accidents. Of these, about one-half required medical attention. The disabilities suffered by many of the injured are permanent or require extended medical care at great cost to the public.[80]

Accidents do not affect the population equally. Males account for about three-fifths of those who suffer accidents. Injuries sustained by children of school age and by young adult males were responsible for most of the sex difference. Rates for both sexes are high in infancy but decrease sharply by the fifth year. Accidental death rates for females remain low until about the 65th year. At that period, the female rates rise sharply and even exceed those in males at the 85th year.[81] Accident rates vary greatly from one occupation to another. In coal mining, the highest rates prevail.

Geographically also there is a variation in accident rates among states. In 1966, death rates from accidents ranged from 42.5 per 100,000 in the Middle Atlantic States to 74.8 per 100,000 in the Rocky Mountain region. Twelve states, mostly in the East and Northeast, had rates in 1966 below 52.0 per 100,000, while 12 states mostly in western mountain areas had death rates from accidents of 72.0 per 100,000 or greater.

From the point of view of human health, the fatalities of such a large number of persons, many of whom are in their early years of life, present a terrifying burden of recurring slaughter. The growing ranks of the permanently impaired is equally distressing. Visual and hearing impairments, paralysis, complete or partial loss of extremities, and other crippling disorders must now be measured in the millions in the population.

Since 1903, when the toll from the automobile began to assume significance, through 1965, there have been more than 6.5 million deaths from accidents in the United States. Of these, 1,690,000 were from accidents involving automobiles. Thus, loss of life due to automobiles far exceeds the number of Americans killed in all of the military operations of the United States.[82]

## CANCER AND OTHER NEOPLASMS

By reason of its common occurrence, its high fatality rate, the expense of treatment, and frequent long-term disability, cancer ranks high as a cause of illness. There will be about 655,000 newly discovered cases of cancer in the United States in 1974 and about 355,000 deaths from cancer (see Table 5.12). For 30 years, cancer has ranked second as a cause of death in this country.

There was a steady rise in the age adjusted national cancer death rate until 1950. Since that year the curve has flattened out. In 1930 the number of cancer deaths per 100,000 population (age adjusted) was 112; in 1940 it was 120; by 1950 it had risen to 125; and in 1969 the number was 130. Except for cancers of the lung, ovary, and pancreas, age-adjusted cancer death rates in general are leveling and in some cases falling off.

For almost 40 years—since 1936—the age-adjusted cancer death rate among American women has slowly declined, a drop of about 8 per cent. During the same period the male death rate has increased about 40 per cent. The decline among women is due to a reduction in

TABLE 5.12

*Trends in age-adjusted cancer death rates per 100,000 population*
*1952-54 to 1967-69*

| Sex | Site | 1952-54 | 1967-69 | Percent Changes | Comments |
|---|---|---|---|---|---|
| Male | All sites | 136.0 | 155.1 | + 14 | Steady increase mainly due to lung cancer, |
| Female | All sites | 118.5 | 109.6 | − 8 | Slight decrease. |
| Male | Breast | 0.2 | 0.2 | − | Constant rate. |
| Female | Breast | 21.8 | 22.9 | + 5 | Slight fluctuations: Overall no change. |
| Male | Colon rectum | 19.3 | 18.8 | − 3 | Slight decrease in both sexes. |
| Female | Colon rectum | 18.0 | 15.8 | − 12 | |
| Male | Lung | 22.7 | 44.5 | + 96 | Steady increase in both sexes due to cigarette |
| Female | Lung | 4.0 | 8.1 | + 103 | smoking. |
| Male | Oral | 4.6 | 4.9 | + 7 | Slight fluctuations: Overall no change in |
| Female | Oral | 1.4 | 1.4 | − | both sexes. |
| Male | Skin | 2.4 | 2.5 | + 4 | Slight fluctuations: Overall no change in |
| Female | Skin | 1.5 | 1.5 | − | both sexes. |
| Female | Uterus | 17.2 | 10.6 | − 38 | Steady decrease attributed in part to widening acceptance of regular checkup with "Pap Test". |
| Male | Esophagus | 3.8 | 4.1 | + 8 | Slight fluctuations: Overall no change in |
| Female | Esophagus | 1.1 | 1.1 | − | both sexes. |
| Male | Stomach | 16.9 | 9.1 | − 46 | Steady decrease in both sexes: Reasons unknown |
| Female | Stomach | 8.7 | 4.5 | − 48 | |
| Male | Pancreas | 6.9 | 8.8 | + 28 | Steady increase in both sexes: Reasons unknown. |
| Female | Pancreas | 4.3 | 5.2 | + 21 | |
| Male | Prostate | 14.0 | 13.5 | − 4 | Early increase, later decrease, again increasing. |
| Female | Ovary | 7.2 | 7.6 | + 6 | Steady increase. |
| Male | Kidney | 2.9 | 3.5 | + 21 | Steady slight increase. |
| Female | Kidney | 1.7 | 1.7 | − | Slight fluctuations: Overall no change. |
| Male | Leukemia | 6.8 | 7.3 | + 7 | Early increase, later leveling off. |
| Female | Leukemia | 4.7 | 4.6 | − 2 | Slight early increase, later leveling off. |

Source:   1974 Cancer Facts & Figures, American Cancer Society.

mortality from cancer of the cervix or the uterus. The rise among men is largely due to a 1400 per cent increase for lung cancer.[83]

There are a number of different types of cancer, but all cancer is characterized by an unrestrained, irregular growth of cells that, in most cases, builds up into tumors that compress, invade and destroy normal tissues. Cancer cells spread through the blood stream or the lymphatic system to form new growths in other parts of the body. This process is called metastasis.

The great majority of cancer originates on the surface of some tissue such as the skin, inner surface of the uterus, lining of the mouth, stomach, intestines, bladder, bronchi, or in a duct in the breast, prostate gland, or elsewhere. After a time, some of the cancer cells grow into the tissues below the surface. The cancer continues to grow locally after this invasion, spreading through the adjacent tissues.

Eventually, cells from this local growth get into lymph or blood channels and are carried to other organs of the body. Once the disease becomes widely disseminated, successful treatment becomes unlikely. Some cancers grow and spread slowly while others maintain a rapid growth rate.

Deaths by age groupings show that cancer is the cause of death in more than half of all mortality among persons over 65 years. Among women from 30 to 54 years cancer is the leading cause of death, and more school children die of cancer than from any other disease. In 1974, it is estimated that over 3500 children under the age of 15 years will die of cancer. About half of these childhood deaths will be due to leukemia.

Cancer of the breast is the leading cause of cancer disease and death among women in the 1970's. There has not been any great reduction in the mortality from breast cancer in the past 35 years. However, when found early the survival rate is high.[84]

Nearly all forms of cancer are more common among people residing in urban than in rural areas. This is especially the case for cancer of the respiratory tract and esophagus among urban men.

Although it is not too satisfactory to compare cancer rates of one country with another, the information available indicates sharp differences in cancer death rates. There are clear-cut differences in the anatomical sites affected by cancer from one country to another. Stomach cancer is five times more common in Japan than among the American white population. On the other hand, cancers of the breast, ovary, and intestine are more than five times as frequent in the United States while cancer of the prostate is 10 times more common. In Iceland, cancer of the stomach accounts for half of all cancers among men. Cancer of the lung is the most common cause of cancer deaths among men in the United States, England, and Wales. Breast cancer is over eight times more common among Israeli women than among the women of Japan. Surveys have shown that many of these patterns change on migration, the migrating peoples developing a cancer pattern more closely identified with that of the host country. The great geographical and social variations in cancer rates point to the importance of environmental and perhaps gen-

TABLE 5.13

*Agents which cause cancer*

Chemical
  Exogenous
    Aromatic polycyclic hydrocarbons and related heterocyclic compounds (with substitution of nitrogen, oxygen, or sulfur for carbon)
    4-Nitroquinoline oxide
    Aromatic amines
    Azo compounds
    Urethane (ethyl carbamate) and closely related compounds
    Alkylating agents
    Nitrosamines
    Polymers
  Endogenous
    Hormones–esp. estrogens
    Cholesterol
Physical
  Ionizing radiation
  Ultraviolet radiation
  Burns
  Other wounds(?)
Genetic
  Gross and visibly recognizable chromosomal abnormalities
  Genetic defects not visible cytologically
Viral
  Leukemia and lymphosarcoma viruses in mouse, fowl, and cattle
  Papillomatosis viruses in man, dog, horse, rabbit, cat, rat, and cattle
  Mammary tumor virus in mouse (Bittner)
  Kidney tumor virus in frog (Lucke)
  Fibroma virus in rabbit (Shope)

Source: Roe, F.J.C., Cancer as a disease of the whole organism. In *The Biology of Cancer,* edited by E.J. Ambrose and F.J.C. Roe. London: D. Van Nostrand Co., 1966.

etic factors in the causation of the disease.

Knowledge about the nature of the specific environmental factors that are concerned in the causation of cancer is still very scanty. The effect of radiations, certain viruses, and coal tar products in carcinogenesis is well known. The eating of smoked meat and fish in Iceland has been suggested as the explanation of their high incidence of stomach cancer. Cigarette smoking is associated with the rising incidence of lung cancer in many countries. It has recently been discovered that certain substances may act in conjunction with other compounds as potentiating agents in the causation of cancer. In mice, citrus oils enhance the action of benzpyrene in producing cancer of the stomach.[85]

The inheritance of increased susceptibility to cancer in man has been postulated but is not yet established. It has been possible to develop gene-determined susceptibility to cancer in some inbred strains of mice. It appears that the genetic basis of susceptibility to cancer is complex, involving many different genes. Even with increased disposition to cancer, the overriding importance of environmental factors appears definite.[86,87]

In Table 5.13 are listed agents known to cause cancer. This is an incomplete listing of carcinogenic agents. In the modern world, new physical and chemical agents are being released for use in the home or in industry at an ever-increasing rate.

## REFERENCES

1. Dubos, R. and Pines, M. *Health and Disease.* New York: Time, Inc., 1965.
2. Romano, J. Basic orientation and education of the medical student. *J.A.M.A., 143:* 409–412, 1950.
3. Engel, G. L. A unified concept of health and disease. In *Life and Disease,* edited by D. J. Ingle. New York: Basic Books, Inc., 1963.
4. Bernard, C. *Les Phenomenes de la Vie.* Paris: J. B. Bailliere and Fils, 1878-1879.
5. Cannon, W. B. *The Wisdom of the Body,* rev. ed. New York: W. W. Norton and Co., Inc., 1939.
6. Wolf, S. Disease as a way of life: neural integration in systemic pathology. In *Life and Disease,* edited by D. J. Ingle. New York: Basic Books, Inc., 1963.
7. *Beyond the Germ Theory,* edited by I. Galdston. A New York Academy of Medicine Book. New York: Health Education Council, 1954.
8. Knudson, A. G., Jr. *Genetics and Disease.* New York: The Blakiston Division, McGraw-Hill Book Co., 1965.
9. McKusick, V. A. *Heritable Disorders of Connective Tissue,* Ed. 4. St. Louis: C. V. Mosby Co., 1972.
10. McKusick, V. A. Genetic aspects of epidemiology and preventive medicine. In *Preventive Medicine and Public Health,* edited by P. E. Sartwell, Ed. 9. New York: Appleton-Century-Crofts, 1965.
11. *Advances in Human Genetics and Their Impact on Society.* Proceedings of a Symposium of the American Association for the Advancement of Science held in Chicago, Ill. Ed. by D. Bergsma. Birth Defects: Original Article Series, Vol. VIII, No. 4, July, 1972.
12. Langman, J. Congenital malformations and their causes. In *Medical Embryology,* edited by J. Langman. Baltimore: Williams and Wilkins Co., 1963.
13. *Congenital Malformations Surveillance.* Public Health Service, Center for Disease Control. July-August, 1973. Issued November, 1973, Atlanta.
14. National Communicable Disease Center. Morbidity and Mortality Weekly Report, Annual Supplement, Summary 1972. Atlanta: U. S. Public Health Service, 1973.
15. *Control of Communicable Diseases in Man.* Edited by A. S. Benenson. Ed. 11. American Public Health Association, 1970.
16. Gregg, N. M. Congenital cataract following German measles in mothers. *Trans. Ophthal. Soc. Aust., 3:* 35-46, 1941.
17. *Rubella.* First Annual Symposium of the Eastern Pennsylvania Branch of the American Society for Microbiology. Edited by H. Friedman and J. E. Prier. Springfield, Ill.: Charles C Thomas, 1973.
18. Stolles, A., and Collman, R. D. Relationship between infectious hepatitis and Downs syndrome. *Lancet, 2:* 1221-1223, 1965.
19. *Viral Etiology of Congenital Malformations.* Symposium of the National Heart Institute and the National Institute of Child Health and Human Development, Bethesda, Md., May 19-20, 1967. U. S. Government Printing Office, 1968.
20. Yamazaki, J. N., Wright, S. W., and Wright, P. M. Outcome of pregnancy in women exposed to the atomic bomb. *Amer. J. Dis. Child., 87:* 448-463, 1954.
21. Gaulden, M. E. Genetic effects of radiation. In *Medical Radiation Biology,* by G. V. Dalrymple, M. E. Gaulden, G. M. Kollmorgen, and H. H. Vogel, Philadelphia: W. B. Saunders Co., 1973.
22. Yager, J. W. Congenital malformations and environmental influence: the occupational environment of laboratory workers. *J. Occupational Med., 15:* 724-728, 1973.
23. Potter, E. L. Editorial. In *Notes on Teratology,* Vol. 2, no. 3. Stamford, Connecticut: Wampole Laboratories, 1966.
24. McKeown, T., and Record, R. G. Malformations in a population observed for five years after birth. In *Ciba Foundation Symposium on Congenital Malformations,* edited by G. E. W. Wolstenholme and C. M. O'Connor. Boston: Little, Brown, and Co., 1960.

25. Dubos, R. *Man Adapting.* New Haven: Yale University Press, 1965.
26. Hilleboe, H. E. Public Health in the United States in the 1970's. *Amer. J. Pub. Health, 58:* 1588-1610, September, 1968.
27. Lave, L. B., and Seskin, E. P. Air Pollution, climate, and home heating—their effects on U. S. mortality rates. *J. Amer. Pub. Health Assn., 62:* 909-916, July, 1972.
28. *Solid Waste/Disease Relationships: A Literature Survey.* Public Health Service Publication, No. 999-UIH-6, 1967. Bureau of Disease Prevention and Environmental Control. National Center for Urban and Industrial Health: Cincinnati, Oh.
29. Darnay, A., and Franklin, W. E. *The Role of Packaging in Solid Waste Management, 1966-1976.* Public Health Service Publication No. 1855. DHEW, Environmental Control Administration, 1969.
30. *Solid Waste Disposal and Control.* Report of a WHO Expert Committee WHO Technical Report Series #484. WHO, Geneva, 1971.
31. *Health Hazards of the Human Environment.* World Health Organization, Geneva, 1972.
32. Page, J. A., O'Brien, M. W. *Bitter Wages. Ralph Nader's Study Group Report on Disease and Injury on the Job.* New York: Grossman Publishers, 1973.
33. Kerr, L. E. Occupational health—A discipline in search of a mission. *J. Amer. Pub. Health Assn., 63:* 381-385, 1973.
34. Bell, A. *Noise—An Occupational Hazard and Public Nuisance,* Public Health Papers, No. 30. World Health Organization, Geneva, 1966.

35. Modell, W. Chairman's Opening Remarks. A Ciba Foundation Volume: *Drug Responses in Man,* edited by G. E. W. Wolstenholme and R. Porter. Boston: Little, Brown, and Co., 1967.
36. *National Clearing House for Poison Control Centers.* Bulletin, May-June, 1973. Food and Drug Administration.
37. Statistical Bulletin—Metropolitan Life Insurance Co., 49: 8-9, February 1968; 53:2-6, February 1972; 53:5, February 1972.
38. Burnet, F. M. and White, D. O. *Natural History of Infectious Diseases.* Cambridge, Eng.: Cambridge University Press, 1972.
39. Burrows, W. *Textbook of Microbiology,* Ed. 20. Philadelphia: W. B. Saunders Co., 1973.
40. Jerne, N. K. The immune system. *Sci. American, 229:* 52-60, 1973.
41. *Cell-mediated Immunity and Resistance to Infection.* Report of a WHO Scientific Group, Technical Report Series, No. 519, WHO, Geneva, 1973.
42. *Viral and Rickettsial Infections of Man,* edited by F. L. Horsfall and I. Tamm. Ed. 4. Philadelphia: J. B. Lippincott Co., 1965.
43. Burnet, F. M. *Auto-Immunity and Auto-Immune Disease.* Philadelphia: F. A. Davis Co., 1972.
44. McDermott, W. Microbiological persistance. *Yale J. Biol. Med., 30:* 257-291, 1958.
45. Smadel, J. E. Intracellular infection. *Bull. N. Y. Acad. Med., 39:* 158-172, 1963.

46. Smith, T. *Parasitism and Disease.* Princeton, N. J.: Princeton University Press, 1934.
47. Fenner, F. J. *Medical Virology.* New York: Academic Press, 1970.
48. *Pathogenic Mycoplasmas.* A Ciba Foundation Symposium. New York: Elsevier-Excerpta Medica-North Holland, 1972.
49. Ajello, L. The Medical Mycological Iceberg—A Study of Incidence and Prevalence. *HSMHA Health Reports, 86:* 437-448, 1971.
50. Faust, E. C., Russell, P. F., and Jung, R. C. *Clinical Parasitology.* Lea & Febiger, Ed. 8, Philadelphia: 1970.
51. *Trichinosis Surveillance.* Center for Disease Control, Public Health Service, Annual Summary, 1972. Atlanta, Georgia, August, 1973.
52. *Schistosomiasis Control.* Report of a WHO Expert Committee, Technical Report Series, No. 515. WHO, Geneva, 1973.
53. Pratt, H. D., Littig, K. S., and Marshall, C. W. Training guide. Insect Control Series, parts I to XII. Atlanta: National Communicable Disease Center, Public Health Service, 1960-1967.
54. Schneider, H. A. Recapitulation and prospects, *Ann. N. Y. Acad. Sci., 63:* 314-317, 1955.
55. Mayer, J. Nutritional aspects of preventive medicine. In *Preventive Medicine,* edited by D. W. Clark and B. MacMahon. Boston: Little, Brown, and Co., 1967.
56. Wohl, M. G., and Goodhart, R. S. *Modern Nutrition in Health and Disease,* Ed. 3. Philadelphia: Lea and Febiger, 1964.
57. Beaton, G. H., and McHenry, E. W. *Nutrition—A Comprehensive Treatise.* New York: Academic Press, 1966.
58. *Malnutrition and Disease.* Geneva: World Health Organization, 1963.
59. Latham, M. C., and Cobos, F. The effects of malnutrition on intellectual development and learning. *Amer. J. Pub. Health, 61:* 1307-1324, 1971.
60. Manocha, S. L. *Malnutrition and Retarded Human Development.* Springfield, Ill.: Charles C Thomas, 1972.
61. Henderson, L. M. Nutritional problems growing out of new patterns of food consumption. *Amer. J. Pub. Health, 62:* 1194-1198, 1972.
62. *Ten-State Nutrition Survey, 1968-70.* Center for Disease Control, Atlanta, 1972. DHEW Publication No. (HSM) 72-8130-8133.
63. *White House Conference on Food, Nutrition and Health—Final Report.* U. S. Government Printing Office, Washington, D. C. 1970.
64. *Proceedings of a Workshop on Problems of Assessment and Alleviation of Malnutrition in the United States.* Held at Vanderbilt University, January 13-14, 1970. Nashville, Tenn., 1970.
65. Stanbury, J. B., Wyngaarden, J. B., and Frederickson, D. S. *The Metabolic Basis of Inherited Disease,* Ed. 3. New York: Blakiston Division, McGraw-Hill Book Co., Inc., 1972.
66. Tatum, E. L. A case history in biological research. *Science, 129:* 1711-1715, 1959.
67. *Diabetes Mellitus Mortality in the United States, 1950-1967.* National Center for Health Statis-

tics. Public Health Service Publication. No. 1000-Series 20-No. 10, 1971.

68. *Arthritis Source Book.* Public Health Service Publication 1431, Washington, D. C.: Government Printing Office, 1966.

69. *Limitation of Activity Due to Chronic Conditions, United States, 1969 and 1970.* National Center for Health Statistics. Public Health Service Publication, Series 10, No. 80, 1973.

70. *Immunobiology.* Edited by R. A. Good and D. W. Fisher. Stanford, Conn.: Sinauer Associates, Inc., 1971.

71. Burch, P. R. J. *An Inquiry Concerning Growth, Disease and Aging.* Edinburgh: Oliver and Boyd, 1968.

72. *Chronic Conditions and Impairments of Nursing Home Residents, United States, 1969.* National Center for Health Statistics. DHEW Publication No. (HRA) 74-1707, December, 1973.

73. *Facts on the Major Crippling Disorders in the United States,* New York: National Health Education Committee, 1964.

74. *Accident Facts.* Chicago: National Safety Council, 1973.

75. *Report on Patients over 65 Years in Public Mental Hospitals.* Washington, D. C.: American Psychiatric Association, 1960.

76. Agate, J. N. *Medicine in Old Age, Proceedings of a Conference Held at the Royal College of Physicians, London, June 18-19, 1965.* Philadelphia: J. B. Lippincott, 1966.

77. Bakst, H. J. Prevention in geriatric practice. In *Preventive Medicine,* edited by D. W. Clark, and B. MacMahon. Boston: Little, Brown, and Co., 1967.

78. *Selected Dental Findings in Adults by Age, Race, and Sex – U. S. 1960-62.* Public Health Service, Health Statistics Series II, no. 7, Washington, D. C.: Government Printing Office, 1965.

79. Backett, E. M. *Domestic Accidents.* Public Health Papers No. 26. Geneva: World Health Organization, 1965.

80. *Current Estimates from the Health Interview Survey – United States, 1972.* Public Health Service Publication 1000, series 10, no. 85. Washington, D. C : Government Printing Office, 1973.

81. *Accidental Death and Injury Statistics.* Public Health Service Publication IIII. Washington, D. C : Government Printing Office, 1964.

82. *Accidental Death and Disability: The Neglected Disease of Modern Society.* Washington, D. C : National Academy of Sciences, National Research Council, 1966.

83. *Cancer Facts and Figures.* New York: American Cancer Society, 1974.

84. *End Results in Cancer.* Report No. 4. National Cancer Institute DHEW Publication No. (NIH) 73-272. Bethesda, Md. 1972.

85. Bailar, J. C., III, King, H. and Mason, M. J. *Cancer Rates and Risks.* Public Health Service Publication 1148. Washington, D. C.: Government Printing Office, 1964.

86. National Advisory Cancer Council. Progress Against Cancer, 1967, Public Health Service Publication 1720. Washington, D. C.: Government Printing Office, 1970.

87. *The Biology of Cancer,* edited by E. J. Ambrose, and F. J. C. Roe. London: D. Van Nostrand Co., Ltd., 1966.

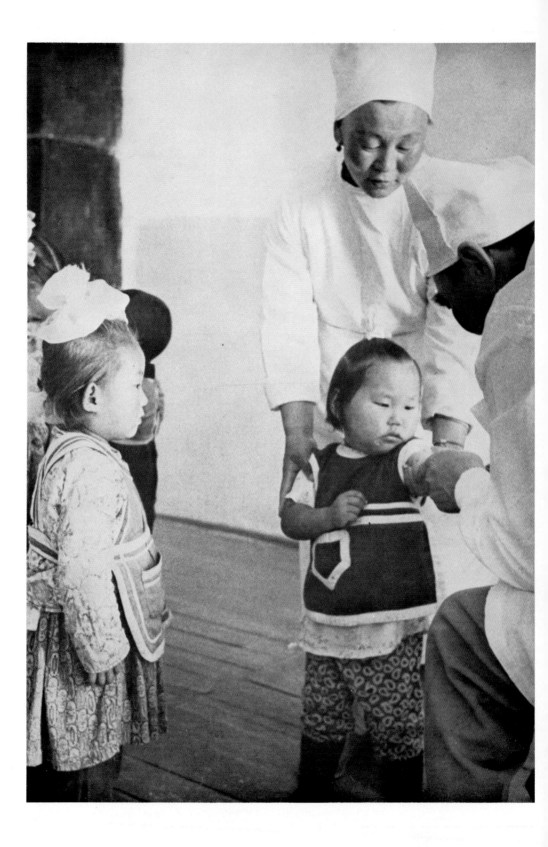

# 6

# *Some characteristic diseases of man*

Medical theories have changed greatly in the course of time, but not according to a continuous and orderly process of evolution. Rather the changes have occurred as discontinuous steps, the direction of which was determined by the prevailing view of man's nature and of his relation to the cosmos. Emphasis has been placed at times on the whole man and on his relationship to demons or to God. In contrast, the focus under other circumstances has been on fragments of man's nature, either on his mind or on the components of the body machine. Throughout the history of medicine, the "ontological" doctrine, which regards diseases as specific entities, has alternated with the "physiological" view, according to which disease is simply an abnormal state experienced by a given individual organism at a given time. In one form or another, the ontological attitude has been the most consistently dominant among both laymen and physicians. It assumes that disease is a thing in itself, essentially unrelated to the patient's personality, his bodily constitution, or his mode of life. This concept reasserts itself repeatedly in everyday language when it is said that the patient has *a* disease or that the physician treats *a* disease.

R. DUBOS, *Man Adapting**

In approaching the writing of this chapter, the authors were concerned about what material to include and what to omit. Obviously, one could not discuss, even briefly, the whole range of human disease. The popular current text on clinical medicine of Cecil and Loeb requires almost 2000 pages to survey in a succinct fashion the medical problems of man.[1] As mentioned in the "Preface," the valuable outline of communicable diseases published by the American Public Health Association is frequently revised and is readily available to students at a very reasonable price. Our objective, then, is to discuss a few characteristic disease problems of man selected because of their current interest. It is hoped that the material presented in the description of these representative problems of man will illustrate most of the general principles required for an understanding of the broad aspects of human disease.

Every student of disease from ancient times has tried to formulate an acceptable theory to account for the observed phenomena. Such theories have varied greatly from time to time in accordance with the prevailing view of the nature of man and his relation to the world at large. Since the time of Hippocrates, fifth century B.C., man has never completely lost the concept that disease can be explained in terms of natural laws, on the basis of careful observation and analysis. This view of the disease process encourages the development of therapeutic measures on a rational basis. Another important teaching of the Hippocratic School was that the health of man is strongly influenced by his environment, including the state of the atmosphere, the available water supply, and the location of his habitation. Low swampy areas were known to be unhealthy. A third basic concept taught by the ancient Greeks was that health depends upon a harmonious balance between the various elements of man's nature, his environment, and his way of living. They fully recognized that mind and body are inseparably united. The healthy functioning of the body depends upon a good mental equilibrium. The idea is preserved today under the term "psychosomatic," or mind-body, diseases.

Many physicians of previous centuries have contributed to the concept that each disease has a specific etiology or causation. Rhazes, in the ninth century, distinguished measles from smallpox as separate disease entities. Plague and

*©Yale University Press, New Haven, 1965.

leprosy were well known and carefully described in medieval Europe. In recent times,
perhaps the strongest impetus to this view came
from a great French clinician, Pierre-Fidele
Bretonneau (1778–1862) of Tours.[2] His
studies of diphtheria and scarlet fever were
particularly fruitful. At the same time, other
French physicians made equally clear-cut descriptions of all phases of phthisis, or consumption, giving a unified view of tuberculosis for
the first time. An American physician, William
Gerhard (1809–1872), provided data from
postmortem studies by which typhus fever and
typhoid fever could be differentiated.

By the time of Pasteur and Koch, these
significant contributions and many others had
prepared men's minds for the age of bacteriology with the concept that every disease has a
specific causative agent and that every harmful
organism produces its own characteristic effect
in the body.

Following soon after the advent of bacteriology, the demonstration that a number of
clear-cut clinical conditions resulted from a
deficiency of certain specific nutrients, for
example, beriberi, scurvy, rickets, and pellagra,
gave additional impetus to the doctrine of
specific etiology of disease. This doctrine has
proved a powerful force as a unifying theme in
the development of medicine for the past
century.

There has been a growing realization that
many diseases probably do not have specific
etiologies and that in general ill health may be
the consequence of a number of determining
factors acting more or less simultaneously. It is
recognized that individuals react differently to
the same specific agent and that the characteristics of a disease may be determined more by
the response of the individual as a whole than
by the qualities of the causative organism. One
person responds to the agent by developing an
inapparent or latent infection while another
dies, victim of a fulminating attack of the
disease.

The human body has only a limited range of
pathological responses that it can make. Therefore, agents of varying characteristics may
produce quite similar responses. Many diseases
of different etiologies give almost identical
symptomatology and can only be differentiated
by precise laboratory studies; hence the term
"influenza-like" disease describing the numerous infections with different organisms which
produce symptoms closely resembling those of
influenza. The body's responses also are affected by various stress conditions. The state of
nutrition, fatigue, anxiety, and other physiological and psychological factors may profoundly influence the outcome of the encounter of
an individual with a disease-producing agent.

The doctrine of specific causation of disease
has served and will continue to serve a most
useful function in our understanding of conditions of ill health. It appears as though the time
has come to enlarge that concept to include
factors of man's internal environment which
control the body's responses to injurious
influences. Each person responds to the environmental forces around him in a highly
individual pattern. The mechanisms of these
individual differences are poorly understood
and are necessarily complex. Investigation of
the significance of the many internal mechanisms by which the body and mind respond
adaptively to the stimuli and stresses of life will
provide a better understanding of human
disease. The very simplicity of the cause and
effect relationships of specific agents to disease
was an attraction which must now be relin-
quished in favor of multifactorial causation.

Evidence is accumulating to show that
chronic and degenerative diseases are not a
necessary concomitant of survival to old age,
but rather that their increasing incidence in
western countries may result from modern
technological and social innovations that adversely affect western man. Studies to define
these noxious influences of industrialized urban
living are certain to be difficult, but are
nevertheless essential for the discovery of
methods of reducing the health hazards to
which civilized man is now exposed.

These diseases of modern society are, to a
large extent, due to the effects of new
environmental impacts on man to which he has
not become adapted. It appears certain that as
one set of circumstances is met and overcome a
new and perhaps more ominous set of environmental forces will come into play. Man can
avoid these threats only by existing in a fixed,
stable state, which he has never been willing or
able to arrange.

To some extent man could alter the environment which threatens him in so sinister a
manner. These alterations would depend upon
personal effort and involve some loss of his
individual freedom of action. To accomplish

this, man will have to change his way of life, to curtail his smoking and drinking, to change his diet, to develop his body through exercise, to avoid the pollution of the air that he breathes and the water that he must use, and perhaps to modify many other facets of which modern urban living is composed. From past human experience, the likelihood of man changing his ways for the sake of health appears unrealistic whenever these changes demand a long continued individual effort.

## DISEASES OF INFECTIOUS ORIGIN

### Tuberculosis

*Historical*

Tuberculosis is one of the ancient scourges of man. Archaeologists have discovered evidence of tuberculosis in the bones and have found tuberculous adhesions in the chests of Egyptian mummies. The Greeks gave good clinical descriptions of the disease as early as the fifth century B. C. Tuberculosis was well known to the Romans. Continuing as a major disease, tuberculosis probably rose to its greatest prevalence in Western Europe during the Industrial Revolution and the concurrent rapid growth of urban populations.

In the 17th century, Sylvius de la Boe (1614–1672), in Holland, was the first to report careful studies on the morbid anatomy of tuberculous patients. He clearly described the characteristic tubercles, tuberculous cavities in the lung, and tuberculous lymph nodes.

At the beginning of the 19th century, there was still no generally accepted concept of tuberculosis. Physicians were all too familiar with scrofula characterized by swollen lymph glands of the neck and frequently with ulceration of the skin and involvement of bones. They also knew all the manifestations of consumption or phthisis, a wasting disease of the lungs. Many other frequent complications of tuberculosis, loss of the voice resulting from tuberculosis inflammation of the larynx, or the always fatal tuberculosis of the meninges, were commonly observed. Each of these symptom complexes was regarded as a separate disease and not related by a common denominator.

Perhaps the greatest student of tuberculosis of all time was Rene Theophile Hyacinthe Laënnec (1781–1826), of Paris, who labored intensively during his life to understand the relationship of the clinical picture of the disease with the results of meticulous observations at the autopsy table. After Laënnec, tuberculosis became a clearly unified concept, one integrated disease with different manifestations.

Although the infectious nature of tuberculosis had been suspected by many, the majority of physicians considered it hereditary. In 1865, Jean-Antoine Villemin (1827-1892), a French army surgeon, demonstrated that rabbits could be infected with material taken from tuberculous lesions of humans or cows. Infection could also be transferred from tuberculous rabbits to healthy rabbits. Thus, Villemin proved that tuberculosis was indeed a communicable disease. He had apparently been led to perform these experiments by observing that healthy young army recruits from the country often came down with tuberculosis within one year after coming to army posts for training.

Within a few years, in 1882, Robert Koch isolated the tubercle bacillus in cultures and produced proof that it is the causative agent of tuberculosis. Shortly afterward, in 1890, Koch announced the discovery of tuberculin, which is an extract of the tubercle bacillus. Koch thought that tuberculin would be useful in the treatment of tuberculosis. This hope proved unfounded, but Koch's tuberculin has been a valuable tool for discovery of new cases of the disease and for use in studying the epidemiology of tuberculosis.

Another important event in the tuberculosis story was the discovery of X rays by Wilhelm Röntgen (1845-1923) in 1895. The use of this technique has greatly aided in the diagnosis of cases and in the assessment of therapeutic measures.

Advances in the treatment of tuberculosis came with the institution of sanitorium care. Herman Brehmer (1826-1899) organized the first successful sanitorium for the treatment of tuberculous patients at Gorbersdorf, Silesia, Germany, in 1859. In 1876, Peter Dettweiler (1837-1904), also of Germany, became director of a sanitorium at Falkenstein. Here he introduced the rest cure in reclining chairs on open porches. By 1886, England had 19 hospitals for consumptives.

At Saranac Lake in New York State, Dr. Edwin L. Trudeau (1847-1915) founded the first sanitorium in America in 1884. This small institution grew to be an influential center for the treatment and teaching of tuberculosis as well as for research on the disease.

The use of collapse treatment for tuberculosis by pneumothorax was introduced in Italy by Carlo Forlanini (1847-1918) in 1894.[3]

Thus, at the close of the 19th century, all the necessary knowledge and skills were available to health workers to make a successful attack on tuberculosis possible. New advances during recent years have led to intensified efforts to conquer "the white plague." These recent events are described below.

### Description of the Disease

Tuberculosis is a chronic, relapsing disease that is an important source of ill health and of fatalities in most parts of the world. Primary infection usually produces no symptoms or only mild ones. The inflammatory reactions around primary foci heal spontaneously, leaving little residual changes except small calcified nodules in the lungs or in the lymph glands around the trachea and large bronchi.

Occasionally, primary tuberculosis leads to pleurisy or to disseminated disease with miliary, meningeal, or other extrapulmonary involvement. Primary infection, however, may progress directly to pulmonary tuberculosis. Sensitivity to tuberculin, determined by skin tests, appears within a few weeks after first infection occurs. Serious manifestations of primary tuberculosis develop most frequently in infants.

Pulmonary tuberculosis generally runs a chronic, variable, and often asymptomatic course, with exacerbations and remissions. Activity of the disease process is determined by demonstration of tubercle bacilli in the sputum, by extension or retrogression of infiltration in the lungs, as measured by serial chest X-ray examinations, or by symptoms. Three stages of disease are recognized: minimal, moderately advanced, and far advanced, according to the extent of lung tissue that is affected. Cough, fatigue, fever, loss of weight, chest pain, and blood-tinged sputum are the common symptoms, but are frequently absent until the disease is well advanced.

Extrapulmonary tuberculosis is much less common than is the pulmonary form. Any organ or tissue of the body may be affected. Meningitis, miliary tuberculosis, involvement of bones and joints, lymph nodes, skin, kidneys, intestines, or larynx are often encountered. Each of the types of disease has its own particular set of symptoms and may present quite unique clinical pictures.

### Pathogenesis and Pathology

When tubercle bacilli are introduced into the tissues, the first reaction is one of acute inflammation characterized by large numbers of polymorphonuclear leukocytes. These cells are unable to destroy the bacilli, but are themselves destroyed. Quickly, other phagocytic cells with a single large nucleus infiltrate the area. These come both from the blood and the tissues. These monocytes ingest the bacilli and are able to destroy them.

In the process of ingesting the bacilli, the monocytes undergo changes and begin to appear like epithelial cells. These "epithelioid" cells are characteristic of the primary tuberculous lesion.

Some of the large monocytes in the center of the tubercle unite to form multinuclear giant cells (see Fig. 6.1). Around the zone of giant cells and the surrounding epithelioid cells is a dense infiltration of small round cells, probably lymphocytes, and fibrin-forming cells.

By the second week, the center of the tubercle becomes necrotic, resulting in the production of cheesy-like material. This process is known as caseation. The current explanation of this phenomenon is that the cells in the center of the tubercle are destroyed by the development of allergy to products of the bacilli as they are broken down.[4]

This type of reaction to tubercle bacilli is designated as proliferative, since the response to the infection is cellular in character. Another type of tuberculous reaction is the exudative form. This type is characterized by an outpouring of fluid, rich in fibrin and containing many lymphocytes. Tuberculosis of the serous membranes such as the pleurae produces an exudative reaction with pleural effusion.

The localized area of tuberculous infection may heal, the caseous center being gradually calcified and walled off by scar tissue. On the other hand, the infection may spread along the lymphatic channels to the nearby lymph glands, usually transported by infected monocytes. These lymph nodes become greatly enlarged and eventually caseous. In turn, these tuberculous glands may heal and calcify or the infection may overcome local defenses and spread by means of the blood stream, causing generalized miliary tuberculosis with meningitis.

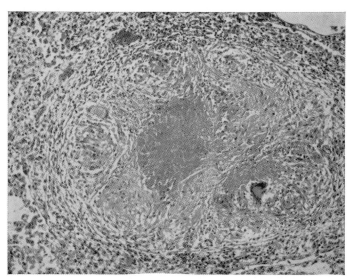

Fig. 6.1. Tubercle. Caseous center; surrounding giant cells, fibroblasts and lymphocytes. Source: Baker, Roger D. Infectious disease. In *Essential Pathology*. Baltimore: The Williams and Wilkins Co., 1961, p. 173.

In past years, when consumption of milk from tuberculous cows was common, the primary focus of infection was frequently in the throat and the lymph glands of the neck were greatly swollen, producing the condition known as scrofula. In other cases, the primary infection was in the intestine with involvement of the abdominal lymph glands. Currently, almost all primary infections are by the air-borne route and the bacilli lodge in the lungs. In childhood, most primary infections are found in the lower lobes of the lungs, while among adults these lesions generally occur in the upper third of the pulmonary organs.

The characteristic healing process of tuberculosis is laying down of fibrous tissue produced by the encircling fibroblasts. Over a long period, the area of caseation may be entirely absorbed and replaced by a solid fibrous nodule. The fibrous wall may cover a long lasting calcified nodule in which tubercle bacilli may continue to survive for many years, ready to cause new spread of infection should the host's resistance be markedly lowered.

In case the primary infection fails to heal, the characteristic process is caseation and softening. There may be direct extension of infection from this area to adjacent tissue spaces. This soft caseous material contains numerous tubercle bacilli. Continued extension of this process may lead to formation of a "cold abscess," characteristic of tuberculosis in many parts of the body. If the caseous process erodes into a bronchiole, the soft material is gradually coughed up, leaving a cavity in the lung. Such a patient is highly infectious to close contacts. Lung cavities expose blood vessels which are likely to rupture and cause the well-known pulmonary hemorrhages of tuberculous patients.

In some active areas of tuberculosis, small veins are eroded to admit tubercle bacilli into the venous circulation. Probably most of these organisms are destroyed by body defenses, but a few become lodged in various tissues where they are walled off, possibly to undergo reactivation years later. Quite likely, most of the isolated cases of tuberculosis of the kidneys, adrenals, bones, joints, and genital organs arise in this manner.

Hypersensitivity to proteins of tubercle bacilli develops shortly after infection. This sensitivity is of the cellular type. Probably the cells mostly involved are lymphocytes, the monocytes, and epithelioid types. This sensitivity is tested by tuberculin injected into the skin. The degree of tuberculin sensitivity appears to diminish with increasing age.

For many years it has been clear that infection with tuberculosis behaves differently in children than it does in adults. In children, fatal tuberculosis is usually of the acute disseminated form, resulting from generalized spread through the blood stream. An enormous enlargement of the lymph glands characterizes the disease in childhood, while the primary pulmonary focus may be quite small.

In adult-type infection, the upper areas of the

lung are most frequently affected. If the disease progresses, cavitation frequently results. In severe cases, the infectious caseous material may spread through the bronchi, causing a tuberculous bronchopneumonia. Involvement of lymph nodes is not conspicuous, generalized blood stream spread is infrequent, and death usually results from the lung disease.

In the past, the common belief was that adult-type tuberculosis is always secondary to a primary infection. It was thought to represent a reinfection disease and the differences in reaction were explained by altered immune and allergic responses. Now that opportunities for reinfection are becoming less frequent, that explanation is not quite so satisfactory. Many now believe that adult tissues react to primary infection in a different manner than is the case in childhood. This difference in behavior may be a part of the maturation process. Even so, most of the cases of active tuberculosis now being discovered in the older age groups are the result of reactivation of a quiescent primary lesion.[5]

*Morbidity and Mortality*

When Robert Koch discovered the bacillus of tuberculosis in 1882, he estimated that one-seventh of all human beings died of tuberculosis, and, in the productive middle-age group, tuberculosis was responsible for one-third of all deaths. Although tuberculosis flourished in Europe during the Middle Ages, it rose to a peak with the coming of the Industrial Revolution in the latter half of the 18th century. Esmond Long states: "The maximum morbidity from tuberculosis in England apparently occurred about 1780, when the recorded mortality rate for consumption was 1,120 per 100,000 population." This high rate soon began to decline, probably due to some improvements in living and working conditions. In London, the tuberculosis mortality rate had fallen to 716 per 100,000 by 1801 to 1810 and to about 567 per 100,000 as an average for the period 1831 to 1835.[6]

This "epidemic wave" of tuberculosis struck the American cities somewhat later, as their growth and industrialization came after independence had been achieved. In Boston, New York, and Philadelphia, evidence indicates a mortality rate for tuberculosis higher than 500 per 100,000 in 1850. As social conditions improved, a steady decline in the mortality rates began. It is believed by many students of the disease that improvements in nutrition, housing, and working conditions have been fully as effective in reducing the dimensions of the tuberculosis problem as have been all the medical and public health measures combined.

From a relatively high death rate in the United States in 1900, *i.e.,* 194.4 per 100,000, there was a continued decline until a figure of 45.8 per 100,000 had been reached in 1940. Following the introduction of effective drug therapy in the late 1940's, the death rate has fallen at a more rapid pace, reaching 22.5 in 1950, 6.1 in 1960, 4.1 in 1965, and to 2.1 in 1971.[7]

The decline in occurrence of new cases of tuberculosis in recent years has also been dramatic (see Table 6.1). In 1953, there were 84,304 new active cases of tuberculosis reported, representing 53 cases per 100,000 population in the United States, while in 1966 the number of new active cases was 47,767, or 24.4 per 100,000. These figures had fallen in 1971 to 35,217 new active cases, or a rate of 17.1 per 100,000. Provisional figures for 1972 are 32,932 new cases, or a rate of 15.8 per 100,000 of the population. Case rates for individual states ranged from a high of 41.6 in Hawaii to a low of 4.0 in Utah. The tuberculosis case rate in big cities was 31.2 per 100,000 in 1971, while the remainder of the nation had a rate of only 13.2 per 100,000. In every community the case rates are far higher among the low income groups than in the more favored segment of the population.[8] In Table 6.2, case rates for white and other races are given for the year 1971 divided by sex, age, and race.

Before the introduction of chemotherapy, mortality rates were accepted as the best index of prevalence of tuberculosis among the population. The mortality rate is now so low that this index is no longer very useful in determining the dimensions of the tuberculosis problem. The occurrence of new active cases and the use of tuberculin surveys in standardized surveys give more reliable information.

With falling mortality rates, there has been a marked shift in the age distribution of deaths. The decline in young adult rates has been more rapid than for older age groups. Female mortality rates have fallen more rapidly than the male rates and are now less than half that of the males in the United States.

Tuberculosis death rates for the non-white are

## TABLE 6.1

*New active tuberculosis cases and deaths, United States, 1953-1972*

| Year | New Active Cases | | | | Tuberculosis Deaths | | | |
| | Number | Rate | % Change | | Number | Rate | % Change | |
| | | | Number | Rate | | | Number | Rate |
|---|---|---|---|---|---|---|---|---|
| 1953 | 84,304 | 53.0 | | | 19,707 | 12.4 | | |
| 1954 | 79,775 | 49.3 | −5.4 | − 7.0 | 16,527 | 10.2 | −16.1 | −17.7 |
| 1955 | 77,368 | 46.9 | −3.0 | − 4.9 | 15,016 | 9.1 | − 9.1 | −10.8 |
| 1956 | 69,895 | 41.6 | −9.7 | −11.3 | 14,137 | 8.4 | − 5.9 | − 7.7 |
| 1957 | 67,149 | 39.2 | −3.9 | − 5.8 | 13,390 | 7.8 | − 5.3 | − 7.1 |
| 1958 | 63,534 | 36.5 | −5.4 | − 6.9 | 12,417 | 7.1 | − 7.3 | − 9.0 |
| 1959 | 57,535 | 32.5 | −9.4 | −11.0 | 11,474 | 6.5 | − 7.6 | − 8.5 |
| 1960 | 55,494 | 30.8 | −3.5 | − 5.2 | 10,866 | 6.0 | − 5.3 | − 7.7 |
| 1961 | 53,726 | 29.4 | −3.2 | − 4.5 | 9,938 | 5.4 | − 8.5 | −10.0 |
| 1962 | 53,315 | 28.7 | −0.8 | − 2.4 | 9,506 | 5.1 | − 4.3 | − 5.6 |
| 1963 | 54,042 | 28.7 | +1.4 | 0.0 | 9,311 | 4.9 | − 2.1 | − 3.9 |
| 1964 | 50,874 | 26.6 | −5.9 | − 7.3 | 8,303 | 4.3 | −10.8 | −12.2 |
| 1965 | 49,016 | 25.3 | −3.7 | − 4.9 | 7,934 | 4.1 | − 4.4 | − 4.7 |
| 1966 | 47,767 | 24.4 | −2.5 | − 3.6 | 7,625 | 3.9 | − 3.9 | − 4.9 |
| 1967 | 45,647 | 23.1 | −4.4 | − 5.3 | 6,901 | 3.5 | − 9.5 | −10.3 |
| 1968 | 42,623 | 21.3 | −6.6 | − 7.8 | 6,292 | 3.1 | − 8.8 | −11.4 |
| 1969 | 39,120 | 19.4 | −8.2 | − 8.9 | 5,567 | 2.8 | −11.5 | − 9.7 |
| 1970 | 37,137 | 18.3 | −5.1 | − 5.7 | 5,560[1] | 2.7 | − 0.1 | − 3.6 |
| 1971 | 35,217 | 17.1 | −5.2 | − 6.6 | 4,380[1] | 2.1 | −21.2 | −22.2 |
| 1972 | 32,882 | 15.8 | −6.6 | − 7.6 | 4,550[1] | 2.2 | + 3.9 | + 4.8 |

[1] Provisional. Deaths for 1970, 1971 and 1972 are based on the NCHS ten percent sample.

Source: Tuberculosis Statistics 1972: States and Cities; Center for Disease Control, Public Health Service, DHEW Publication No. (CDC) 74-8249, June, 1973 Issue.

## TABLE 6.2

*Case rates for white and other races, males and females by age,*
*United States, 1971*

| Age | Total | White | | | Other | | |
| | | Total | Male | Female | Total | Male | Female |
|---|---|---|---|---|---|---|---|
| All ages | 17.1 | 11.7 | 16.3 | 7.3 | 53.8 | 71.8 | 36.9 |
| 0 − 4 | 8.8 | 5.1 | 5.1 | 5.2 | 28.0 | 28.8 | 27.3 |
| 5 − 14 | 3.8 | 2.1 | 2.1 | 2.2 | 12.8 | 12.4 | 13.1 |
| 15 − 24 | 8.3 | 5.0 | 5.3 | 4.8 | 28.7 | 30.2 | 27.3 |
| 25 − 44 | 19.5 | 11.4 | 14.8 | 8.0 | 79.1 | 108.2 | 53.5 |
| 45 − 64 | 28.9 | 20.5 | 33.3 | 8.9 | 103.2 | 156.9 | 53.6 |
| 65+ | 35.7 | 28.6 | 46.4 | 16.1 | 107.6 | 162.3 | 61.9 |

Source: Reported Tuberculosis Data 1971, DHEW Publication No. (HSM) 73-8201, Center for Disease Control, December 1972, issue.

much higher than for the whites in each age group; both among whites and non-whites males have higher rates than females, especially in the older ages.

Infection rates, as demonstrated by the percentage of positive tuberculin tests in the population, have declined sharply as the mortality rates have fallen (see Table 6.3).

*Epidemiology*

*The Infectious Agent.* Since its discovery by Koch, the tubercle bacillus has been the subject of intensive research. Now classed as a mycobacterium or fungus-like bacterium, the tubercle bacillus has several varieties. The bovine strain chiefly infects cattle, but is a source of infection to man; the avian and mouse strains are mainly parasites of the fowl and of mice. Another strain is limited to infection of cold-blooded animals.

The tubercle bacillus grows rather readily in culture under aerobic conditions at 37°C. Mycobacterium tuberculosis is resistant to physical and chemical agents, so it is possible to treat sputum with alkali or other substances prior to inoculation of culture media to prevent overgrowth of other bacteria.

An egg yolk medium is commonly employed for primary isolation. More recently several other media have been devised to promote more rapid growth. These media consist of synthetic nutrient mixtures to which serum albumin and oleic acid has been added.

The mycobacteria are characterized by a peculiar reaction to stains. Once stained with carbolfuchsin, these bacilli are resistant to decolorization with acid-alcohol (Ziehl-Neelsen technique). This quality of acid fastness is an important distinguishing characteristic for identifying tubercle bacilli.

The guinea pig is highly susceptible to both human and bovine strains of tubercle bacillus. This animal has been used extensively both for research and for diagnostic purposes.

In culture medium, the tubercle bacillus survives for periods up to eight months. It is susceptible to direct sunlight, but in sputum it may remain viable up to 20 hr. Droplets of dried sputum adhering to dust particles may prove infectious for several days. The bacillus is resistant to ordinary chemical disinfectants. Moist heat will inactivate the organism promptly, as demonstrated by pasteurization of milk.

The surface of the tubercle bacillus is composed of a polysaccharide or lipoprotein polysaccharide which stimulates the production of antibodies when injected into animals. Probably such antibodies have little protective effect. Hypersensitivity to tuberculoprotein can be transferred from an immune animal to a non-immune one by injection of white blood cells.

Tuberculin is prepared from glycerine-peptone broth in which tubercle bacilli have been cultivated for six to eight weeks. The entire culture is boiled and then filtrated. The filtrate is concentrated in a water bath. In recent years, a purified protein derivative of tuberculin has been in general use. This material, known as PPD is standardized to contain 5 tuberculin units (TU) in 0.1 ml. of solution for intracutaneous injection.

During recent years, there has been an increasing recognition of human infections with unclassified acid-fast mycobacteria. There are four groups of organisms called atypical or unclassified mycobacteria which resemble tubercle bacilli closely in appearance, but which can be differentiated from them by cultural methods.

In some areas of the United States, infections by these atypical mycobacteria are responsible for many weakly positive tuberculin tests which are confusing to tuberculosis control officers.

In bacteriological studies of patients admitted to sanatoria for apparently typical pulmonary tuberculosis, from 1 to 10 per cent excrete atypical mycobacteria in the sputum. Some of these mycobacteria produce yellow pigment in culture when exposed to light. These are termed photochromogens. Others grow much more rapidly on artificial media than does *Mycobacterium tuberculosis*. None are pathogenic for guinea pigs. Most are resistant to the drugs employed for the treatment of tuberculosis.

*Reservoirs and Sources of Infection.* Man is the primary reservoir, but tuberculous cattle may be an important source of infection in some countries. The principal source of human infection is the respiratory secretions of active cases of pulmonary tuberculosis.

*Mode of Transmission.* Close contact with an active case of pulmonary tuberculosis usually leads to infection of contacts and often to active disease. Infection is most frequently caused by the air-borne route of breathing in infectious aerosols or contaminated dust. Most particles breathed in, on which tubercle bacilli may be carried, are too large to reach the terminal alveoli of the lungs. Droplet nuclei, the tiny dried residues from droplets expelled into the air, are small enough to be breathed deeply into the lungs and to set up the slow growth of tubercle bacilli.

Some active cases appear to be more efficient transmitters of tubercle bacilli than others. Possibly this is related to the numbers of organisms being released in the sputum and to the personal standards of hygiene of the patient. Unfortunately, in some cases, the source of infection is unaware of the nature of his own disease.

In regions where tuberculosis in dairy cattle is not well controlled, humans, usually children, may become infected through drinking contaminated milk.

*Incubation Period.* A period of four to six weeks is required from time of infection to the development of demonstrable primary lesions. Years may go by before progressive pulmonary or extrapulmonary disease is found. The first six to twelve months after primary infection are the hazardous period.

*Period of Communicability.* Some cases of chronic pulmonary tuberculosis discharge tubercle bacilli in their sputum intermittently over a long period of years. The period of communicability has been shortened in most instances by the use of drug therapy.

*Susceptibility and Resistance.* All humans are susceptible to some extent. Children under three years have highest susceptibility; those from three to 12 years have the lowest. Susceptibility is probably inherited on a genetic basis. Some families are relatively resistant; others are more susceptible than the average population. Isolated peoples whose ancestors have not been subject to infection are generally highly susceptible. Certain physiological conditions such as malnutrition, fatigue, and diabetes render persons less resistant. Resistance conferred by healed primary infections is not very effective. Tuberculosis among the older age groups is thought to be due to a breakdown of defense mechanism, *i.e.,* a relapse of earlier infection.[9]

Silicosis appears to render the lungs of miners more subject to progressive tuberculosis.

The use of cortisone in the treatment of arthritis and other chronic conditions may be harmful in reactivating quiescent foci of tuberculous infection.

*Diagnostic Procedures*

Tuberculosis is often suspected in patients consulting a physician on the basis of symptoms or because of known contact with an infectious case. A careful history of previous illnesses is helpful, but especially of recent symptoms of ill health. Frequently, a physical examination will reveal definite signs of the disease. This clinical diagnosis must then be confirmed by other methods. In many instances, the history and symptoms may be negative and even a carefully carried out physical examination may be at best inconclusive. It is in these cases that the laboratory and X-ray examinations are of especial importance.

The *tuberculin test* has become an essential procedure in the differential diagnosis of tuberculosis. Either old tuberculin (OT) or the purified protein derivative (PPD) may be used. The intracutaneous Mantoux test or one of the multipuncture tests is commonly employed. A positive skin reaction signifies that the individual has previously been infected with tubercle bacillus.

With rare exceptions, the tuberculin test is most reliable. One exception is that the individual may have become infected so recently that sufficient time has not elapsed for skin sensitivity to have developed. Another false reading may occur in the presence of far-advanced tuberculosis or of disseminated tuberculosis. In some such cases the test frequently reverts from positive to negative.

The tuberculin test is of particular value as a screening mechanism in populations with low-prevalence rates. It is also most useful in surveillance of exposed groups such as student nurses, medical students, or laboratory technicians. Few proven cases of tuberculosis fail to react to a proper tuberculin test. Those individuals with marked sensitivity to small doses of tuberculin have been shown to be more likely to have clinical illness than are the "low-grade" reactors.

X-ray examination, performed properly and interpreted by trained personnel, offers a sensitive method of discovering those with suspicious areas of pulmonary infiltration. Serial films over a period of months will demonstrate either progression or retrogression of the disease process.

There are limitations to the X-ray technique as a diagnostic tool. In many cases, it is impossible to distinguish tuberculosis from

222

other pulmonary infections with certainty. Further studies by laboratory methods are then required to determine the nature of the infection.

Once discovered, X-ray examinations at intervals are of utmost importance in following the progress of the disease.

Laboratory tests are essential to confirm a diagnosis of tuberculosis. The most important examination is to check the sputum for acid-fast bacilli. If not found on first examination, concentration of the sputum may aid in demonstrating the organisms.

The findings of this microscopic examination must be confirmed by culture or by inoculation into guinea pigs. These procedures are also indicated, if no acid-fast bacilli are found by microscopic examination of the sputum.

If sputum is not obtainable, gastric lavage may be indicated. This test is performed before fluids or food are taken in the morning. Bacilli in the stomach are the result of sputum that has

TABLE 6.3

*Tuberculin test reaction rates, school years 1965-1971 ***

| School Year | Under 1st Grade | First Grade | 7,8,9th Grades |
|---|---|---|---|
| 1965-66 | 0.4 | 0.5 | 1.5 |
| 1966-67 | 0.2 | 0.5 | 1.8 |
| 1967-68 | 0.3 | 0.4 | 1.2 |
| 1968-69 | 0.2 | 0.3 | 0.8 |
| 1969-70 | 0.2 | 0.2 | 0.7 |
| 1970-71 | | 0.2 | 0.7 |

*Percent reactors to all types of tests.

Source: Tuberculosis Programs 1971, Tuberculosis Programs Reports, November, 1972, Edition. Center for Disease Control, DHEW Publication No. (HSM) 73-8189.

TABLE 6.4

*New active tuberculosis cases among U. S. Indians and Alaska natives*

| Year | U. S. Indians[1] | | Alaska Natives | |
|---|---|---|---|---|
| | New cases | Case rate[2] | New cases | Case rate[2] |
| 1962 | 647 | 209.4 | 260 | 604.7 |
| 1963 | 596 | 192.3 | 230 | 534.9 |
| 1964 | 578 | 184.1 | 271 | 630.2 |

[1] Excluding Alaska.
[2] Per 100,000 population.

Source: *Reported Tuberculosis Data,* 1966. Public Health Service Publication 638, 1968 edition. Compiled from "Illness among Indians," reported incidence of notifiable diseases among Indian and Alaska natives, Public Health Service, Bureau of Medical Services, Division of Indian Health, September, 1965.

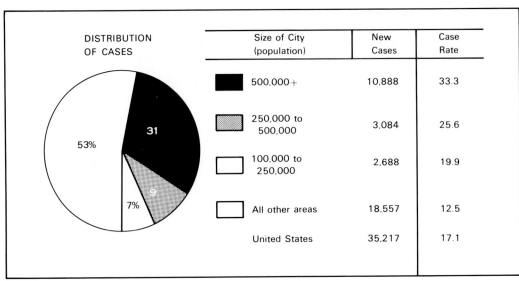

Fig. 6.2. Cases in large cities, United States, 1971. (Redrawn from Reported Tuberculosis Data 1971, Public Health Service, Center for Disease Control, DHEW Publication No. (HSM) 73-8201.)

been swallowed. The gastric contents are tested by culture or by animal inoculation.

Examination of urine for tubercle bacilli is only indicated if tuberculosis of the urogenital tract is suspected.

*Occurrence*

Tuberculosis is found in every country around the globe. In some countries with less favorable conditions, the mortality rates from tuberculosis are still quite high. In most parts of the world, mortality rates are declining steadily as the result of improved living conditions and preventive measures. Bovine tuberculosis in man is rare in Canada, the United States, Scandinavia, and The Netherlands. It is still a serious problem in some countries.[10]

Tuberculosis has been reduced among all races in the United States, but the decrease among Negroes and other races has been slower. In the last ten years incidence of new disease among whites has gone down 43 per cent, and among other races only 15 per cent. An increasing proportion of all new cases of tuberculosis is found now among Negroes and other minority races—a rise from 30 per cent in 1960 to 40 per cent in 1971. Tuberculosis case rates are also higher in the large cities than in smaller urban or rural areas (see Fig. 6.2).[11]

Tuberculosis remains a serious health problem among the American Indian and Alaskan native populations. There has been great improvement in both the new active case rates and in the death rates since 1954, when the U. S. Public Health Service was given responsibility for the operation of Indian health services (see Table 6.4).

In 1963, tuberculosis death rates were 24 per 100,000 among the Indians, excluding Alaska, and 37 per 100,000 among the Alaskan natives. During the same year, the rates were 4.9 in the United States for all races. The 1963 new active-case rates for Indians was 184 per 100,000 and for Alaskan natives, 630. The figure for the U.S. for all races was 29.

*Methods of Control*

General measures of social betterment to improve housing, nutrition, and working conditions are of prime importance. Health education of the public on the nature of the disease and of the danger of contact with active cases is highly necessary.

Many agencies participate in the tuberculosis control program; private physicians. veterinarians, public health agencies, voluntary health agencies, and state sanitoria are only some of those concerned.

Specific control measures are aimed at early diagnosis of active cases, the prevention of spread of infection, enhancing the resistance of exposed individuals, and providing effective treatment and rehabilitation of patients.

*Preventive Measures*

These include control of tuberculosis in cattle to protect the population from the threat of tuberculous milk. Bovine-type infection is said to have accounted for 20 to 40 per cent of human pulmonary tuberculosis and 60 per cent of extrapulmonary tuberculosis in Denmark and Germany before the initiation of the campaign to control the disease in cattle.[12]

The joint efforts of government veterinarians and veterinary practitioners resulted in some 424 million tuberculin tests in cattle in the United States over a 40-year period beginning around 1917. Positive reactors were slaughtered. This campaign has practically eradicated the disease in the cattle of the United States. The anti-bovine tuberculosis effort plus compulsory pasteurization of milk has removed bovine tuberculosis as a human threat in those countries where the methods are practiced.

*Immunization.* A living attenuated tubercle bacillus as a vaccine has been widely applied in many countries during recent decades. This vaccine was developed by Albert Calmette (1863-1933) and Camille Guérin (1872-1961) at the Pasteur Institutes of Lille and of Paris over a period of years beginning in 1906. The vaccine known as BCG *(Bacillus Calmette-Guerin)* is prepared from a bovine tubercle bacillus. The virulence of the strain was greatly modified by a long series of culture passages in a potato medium boiled in ox bile to which glycerine was added. After some years, this vaccine began to be used to immunize calves against tuberculosis. By 1921, the cultured bacilli was shown to be incapable of producing disease in guinea pigs and in 1922 it was first used in human infants. The vaccine was administered to these babies by mouth in three doses during the first 10 days of life. By 1928, some 50,000 French infants had received the vaccine.

Heimbeck of Norway began, in 1926, to use BCG by subcutaneous injections to immunize student nurses. Later he changed to intracutaneous inoculations.

During the 1930's, the use of BCG progressed slowly. Following World War II, the Scandinavian Red Cross Societies formed mobile teams and, with the aid of UNRRA and later WHO, a total of nearly 17 million persons was vaccinated, mostly in Europe. BCG has continued to be widely used in tuberculosis control programs, especially in the Far East. In the western Pacific Region, some 12 million children were vaccinated with BCG in 1972. High priority is also being given to BCG vaccination in Africa. During 1972, 25 WHO-assisted vaccination programs were in operation.[13]

The object of vaccination is to produce a benign primary infection that will stimulate an acquired resistance to possible subsequent infections with virulent organisms. BCG vaccine must be used only in individuals with negative tuberculin tests. A few weeks after vaccination, the tuberculin test becomes positive.

One problem with BCG has been variability between different lots of vaccine. Freshly made vaccine could be used only for short periods and had to be at icebox temperatures. Heat or sunlight quickly destroys the activity of the vaccine. To overcome these problems, vaccine is now prepared by the "freeze-drying" method. Vaccine prepared by this technique can be preserved with little deterioration for periods up to nine months in an ordinary refrigerator.

Where risk of infection is low, as is currently in most parts of the United States, the use of BCG on a mass scale is not indicated. The vaccine is a useful means of protecting tuberculin-negative individuals in certain highly exposed groups. These are: (1) household contacts of active cases; (2) persons exposed to infection in their occupations, such as medical and nursing students or medical technologists; (3) children residing in areas with a high prevalence of tuberculosis in the younger age group; (4) inmates and employees of institutions such as prisons or mental hospitals in which exposure to tuberculosis is likely to be high.

*Chemoprophylaxis.* This is defined as prevention of active disease by the use of isoniazid in therapeutic dosage over a period of one year. It now is established as an effective control measure of tuberculosis. This method is applicable to household contacts of active cases, for the protection of persons who during the previous year have converted from a tuberculin-negative to a tuberculin-positive state, for tuberculin-positive children under three years of age, and for cases of inactive tuberculosis never previously treated with antibacterial drugs.

Primary tuberculosis with lesions visible by X ray and a history of recent development of a positive tuberculin reaction is a clear indication for isoniazid prophylaxis.

Other situations in which chemoprophylaxis has been recommended are: (1) tuberculin-positive children who are suffering from severe chronic illnesses, and (2) patients with a positive tuberculin test who are to receive long-term steroid therapy.

For prophylaxis, two drugs are not necessary, Isoniazid is the recommended drug. It is cheap, easy to administer, and effective when taken by mouth. It is of low toxicity and generally well-tolerated. The recommended dose of isoniazid for prophylaxis for adults and older children is 300 mg. daily, and for young children, 8 to 10 mg. per kg. of body weight.[14] This may be given in a single dose or in divided doses. Chemoprophylaxis is usually continued for at least one year.

*Case Finding.* New cases of tuberculosis can be found through carefully planned screening programs that include tuberculin testing as a primary diagnostic tool. Positive reactors are then X rayed and, as indicated, bacteriological tests are carried out.

In areas where prevalence rates are low, case-finding surveys should be directed toward groups that are likely to show higher rates of tuberculosis than in the general population—nurses, medical students, patients, and outpatients of general and mental hospitals, selected groups of industrial workers, and residents of old people's homes. When feasible, these groups should first have tuberculin tests with X-ray examination for those reacting to tuberculin.

As tuberculosis in the United States is found more frequently in males of the older age groups, case finding must be intensified among older men. This applies especially to those in the lower socioeconomic groups, *i.e.,* alcoholics, drug addicts, prison inmates, and migrant workers.

With declining tuberculosis rates, mass chest X-ray campaigns are being abandoned by most state health departments. The approach to case finding now must be more carefully focused to meet the current situation.

A most important source of new cases of

tuberculosis is to be found in those who are exposed to active cases in the household. All such contacts should be followed for a period of years by means of tuberculin tests with chest X-ray examination at intervals on all reactors. Prophylactic treatment should be used when indicated.

Another group of persons that requires careful follow-up is made up of individuals with inactive tuberculosis. These people are always potentially liable to suffer a relapse. Periodic check-ups are strongly indicated to discover early signs of disease activity in such cases.

A tuberculin-testing program for children entering school has been found to be a fruitful method of discovering tuberculous households. Of course, it is essential that all schoolteachers and staff personnel should be frequently examined to weed out any individuals with active tuberculosis.

*Management of the Patient.* It is preferable to hospitalize all patients with active tuberculosis. Hospitalization removes the patient as a threat to his family and associates until his disease can be arrested. A period of institutional care also gives an opportunity for detailed study of the case, for establishment of the correct regime of drug therapy, and for the education of the patient about the nature of the disease and the proper precautions necessary to avoid spreading the disease to others. After a few months of sanitorium supervision, many patients can be released for home care.

Home care may be carried out under the direction of private physicians, but is more commonly directed by the staff members of the local health department. The public health nurse is particularly valuable in this program.

Prompt treatment with a combination of antituberculosis drugs is indicated. Isoniazid (INH), *para*-aminosalicylic acid (PAS), and streptomycin (SM) are the drugs of choice. Treatment should be continued for one year or more.

At the beginning of treatment, cultures of the patient's strain of tubercle bacillus must be tested against the drugs to demonstrate any evidence of resistance to the therapeutic agents. This test should be repeated at intervals, especially if there is no sign of clinical improvement.

Early in the use of these antituberculosis drugs, it was learned that the tubercle bacillus became rather rapidly resistant to the drug, if a single drug was employed. When two drugs are used in combination, the danger of drug resistance is greatly diminished. The most frequently used drug combinations are *para*-aminosalicylic acid and isoniazid, or *para*-aminosalicylic acid and streptomycin.

In addition to the three drugs mentioned, there are a number of other potent compounds that are used in the treatment of cases that fail to respond. These drugs are generally more toxic, less effective, and more expensive, and require more supervision than the three basic drugs. The "secondary" drugs include ethionamide, pyrazinamide, cycloserine, ethambutol, capreomycin, viomycin, kanamycin, and thiocarbanidin.

A valuable addition to the drugs available for the treatment of tuberculosis was discovered by Italian scientists in 1957. This drug, now being used extensively, is called rifampin. It is a semi-synthetic derivative of an antibiotic rifamycin isolated from *Streptomyces mediterrain.* A combination of rifampin and isoniazid is frequently used as the initial drug therapy of pulmonary tuberculosis.

Rifampin is also especially useful for use in cases that have relapsed following treatment with other drugs. The combination of rifampin and ethambutol has been recommended in such cases.[15]

In a few patients, thoracic surgery is still necessary to bring the pulmonary disease under control.

Supervision of patients after hospitalization through home care and outpatient clinics is of utmost importance. Patients must be made to realize that tuberculosis is a chronic relapsing disease that must be lived with throughout one's life.

*Rehabilitation*

It is often possible to return the cooperative tuberculosis patient to the occupation for which he was trained before his illness. When this is not possible or advisable, every effort should be made to restore the individual to a productive place in society and enable him to be self-supporting to whatever extent that may be possible. Occupational therapy should be begun in hospital as soon as the condition of the patient permits. It represents an integral part of the whole treatment program for each patient.

Unfortunately, some 35 per cent of the newly discovered patients in the United States are found to have advanced disease, and a considerable number of these remain totally disabled or unemployable. In general, the difficulty in rehabilitation of the tuberculous patient is directly related to the severity of his disease. At best, such rehabilitation is a complex problem requiring the coordination of medical, health, and welfare agencies of the community.[16]

# Influenza

## Introduction

Influenza is an acute infectious respiratory disease of man, commonly encountered in epidemic form. It is characterized by abrupt onset of fever, chills, headache, muscle aches, and sometimes prostration. Cough, often severe and prolonged, is a most common symptom. Usually there is pharyngitis and a running nose. Influenza is a self-limited disease, running its course with recovery in two to seven days. Complication by bronchitis and bronchopneumonia is frequent. Epidemics spread rapidly in the population with a high morbidity and low mortality. Influenza derives its importance from the high attack rates which sometimes threaten the normal functioning of a community and also from the deaths caused by pneumonia. Deaths are chiefly among the elderly and in persons debilitated by chronic disease.

Identifiable epidemic waves of influenza have been described in the medical literature as far back as the 16th century. From 1510 to 1930, at least 30 widespread epidemics and many outbreaks of lesser extent were described. During the past 75 years, pandemics occurred in 1889, 1918, 1957 and 1968. The name "influenza" was derived from the Italian phrase, *un influenza di freddo* (an influence of cold).

Epidemics, the most usual pattern of occurrence, may be local, community, or nationwide. In susceptible populations, attack rates during outbreaks may vary from 15 to 40 per cent or more. Major epidemics have a periodic tendency. Influenza A occurs in the United States at intervals of two to three years; influenza B at longer periods, usually four to six years. In temperate zones, epidemics tend to appear during winter months. In the tropics, there is no seasonal appearance. Influenza attacks swine, horses, and possibly other animals in many parts of the world.

## The Infectious Agent

Influenza is caused by a virus first isolated in London in ferrets in 1933. The virus was quickly adapted to mice, serological tests were developed, and thus investigators became able to study the nature and distribution of influenza. In 1940, a second serological type of virus was isolated from a patient. The designation of influenza A was then given to the earlier type and influenza B to the second strain. Later, 1949, a third type of virus called influenza C was discovered.

Influenza virus in the fully infectious form is predominantly a spherical particle from 80 to 120 m$\mu$ in diameter. In the center is a dense central helix, 9 to 10 m$\mu$ in diameter, consisting of ribonucleoprotein. Around the ribonucleoprotein helix is an outer envelope of lipoprotein, 7 to 10 m$\mu$ thick, which is studded with tiny spikes 8 to 10 m$\mu$ high. These spikes possess hemagglutinating activity which serves as the basis for a valuable laboratory test for the identification and typing of influenza virus (see Fig. 6.3, also Fig. 5.5).

Influenza virus grows readily in chick embryos and reaches maximum concentrations in the allantoic and amniotic fluids. The virus can be grown in primary cultures of tissues from many animal species and in human embryonic lung or kidney. Kidney cells from various species such as monkey, chick, hamster, and calf have been found to support virus multiplication.

For primary virus isolation, the chick embryo is the most susceptible host. New strains are readily isolated by inoculation of throat washings into the amniotic sac of 13- to 14-day embryos.

The mouse provides another valuable system for investigative and diagnostic studies. Intranasal instillation of virus into lightly anesthetized mice, after a few passages, produces fatal pulmonary disease. This technique does not serve for primary isolations, but is useful in studies on influenza viruses. Virus has also been adapted to hamsters.

Influenza virus displays various activities. A selective affinity for the epithelial cells of the respiratory tract is demonstrated in all susceptible species. The nasal epithelial cells are

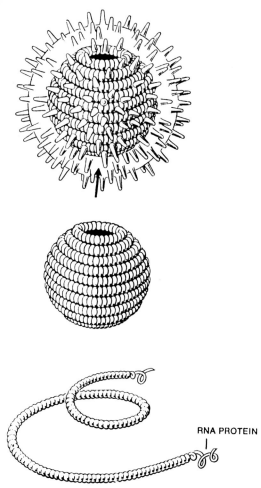

Fig. 6.3. Schematic sketch of component parts of influenza A₂ virus. *Top*, protein, lipid, and carbohydrate coat. The *arrow* indicates the lipoprotein coat of influenza virus particle. *Middle*, nucleoprotein strand core. *Bottom*, nucleoprotein strand. Source: *Influenza: Its Virology and Pathologic Significance*. Wilmington, Delaware: Pharmaceutical Division, E. I. du Pont de Nemours & Co., Inc., 1967.

RNA PROTEIN

especially vulnerable, but, with well-adapted strains, it extends to the respiratory epithelium of the trachea and bronchi.

Multiplication of virus occurs intracellularly. The ribonucleic acid component is the fundamental genetic material of the influenza virus. This material is apparently reproduced in the nucleus of the infected cell and accumulates at the cell surface. The assemblage of viral components appears to take place at this point.

Evidence indicates that the dominant antigen concerned with strain specificity and immunity is located at the surface of the virus particle.

This antigen coincides with the lipoprotein viral envelope. This lipoprotein coat seems to be important for the attachment of virus particles to susceptible cells.

Influenza viruses possess the capacity to cause agglutination of red blood cells. This hemagglutination is the result of the interaction of virus and the surface of the blood cells. After a period of time, the virus is spontaneously disassociated from the red cells. The virus so released retains its hemagglutinating capacity, but the red cells can no longer combine with virus of the same strain. This reaction is enzymatic in action, and the specific mucoprotein on the surface of the red blood cell is destroyed. Probably the same kind of reaction is involved in the attachment of influenza virus to susceptible respiratory epithelial cells.

The specific enzyme of the influenza virus has been designated either neuraminidase or sialidase because it splits both *N*-acetylneuraminic acid or sialic acid from the red cell surface. Probably several enzymes are involved. Various substances in body fluids or tissues will react with the virus and inhibit its combination with red blood cells. These inhibitors comprise a part of the natural defense system of the body. Influenza virus is classified as a member of the myxovirus group (*i.e.*, it has an affinity for mucus). In this group are several subgroups: influenza, parainfluenza, respiratory syncytial, mumps, and other viruses.

At present, human influenza viruses are divided into three immunologically distinct types. These are designated A, B, and C. Three subtypes of influenza A virus have been isolated from man: A (1934), A1 (1947), and A2 (1957). Within a period as short as 10 to 15 years, the prevailing influenza A subtype has been replaced by a new and antigenically distinct group of influenza A families. The Hong Kong strain of type A virus which appeared with the pandemic of 1968, is presently classed as a major variant of type A2 virus, not as a new subtype. With the coming of the new strain, the previously prevailing strains disappear as a recognized cause of human disease. This capacity of influenza A virus to alter its antigenic identity ensures that a supply of susceptible human hosts will never be lacking. Thus, strains related to A-type virus were responsible for A outbreaks between 1934 to 1944, and A1 viruses for A epidemics between 1947 and 1953. Since 1957, all A epidemics have been caused by A2 subtypes.

Definite variations of influenza B virus have been reported, but are less sharply distinctive than are the A subtypes. At least three subtypes of B virus have been recognized.

Type C virus appears to be antigenically homogeneous.

The serological type of influenza virus is readily determined by complement fixation with the ribonucleoprotein antigen. Within the type, the strain variation can best be demonstrated by hemagglutination tests.

Epidemics of influenza have been recognized among swine for many years. Shope, in 1931, demonstrated that the disease was produced by a combined attack of a virus and a bacillus.[17] The virus has been shown to be an influenza virus, closely related to but not identical with viruses causing human influenza. The bacillus is *Haemophilus influenzae suis.* The swine influenza virus is a distinct subtype of the influenza A group. It has never been isolated from man during epidemics.

In 1963, a widespread epidemic of influenza affected horses in the United States and Canada. A distinctive new strain of the A group was identified as the causal agent. Humans were apparently not affected.[18] However, influenza in human volunteers with horse influenza virus has been produced and ponies have been infected with the A2/Hong Kong/68 virus of human origin.[19,20]

Certain strains of living influenza viruses are toxic. This toxicity is said to be destroyed when the virus is killed by heat or formalin. However, most influenza vaccines produce some toxic reactions when injected.

Infectivity of virus preparations is lost after heating to $56°$ C. for a few minutes. The virus is readily inactivated by ultraviolet irradiation, by sonic vibration, or by numerous reagents including formaldehyde. Virus may be preserved indefinitely at $-70°$ C. The viruses may also be preserved by drying *in vacuo* or by storage in 50 per cent neutral glycerol.

*Pathogenesis and Pathology*

Concepts of pathogenesis of influenza virus are based largely on the study of infections in experimental animals. The virus exerts its primary injury on the lining epithelial cells first of the upper respiratory tract, and, as infection proceeds the lining cells of the trachea and large bronchi are severely damaged. In Burnet's view,[21] the infective process conforms to the following outline:

1. Inhalation of virus on droplet nuclei into the lung with deposition on the surface lining of small bronchioles.

2. Adsorption by specific receptor mechanisms to epithelial cells of bronchioles, possibly after ridding itself of respiratory mucus by action of virus mucinase.

3. Multiplication in epithelial cells with liberation of virus on respiratory surfaces.

4. Surface spread to adjacent cells, mainly in the direction of the ciliary movement toward the larynx.

5. Spread to other sectors of the bronchial tree, possibly by inhalation after coughing. When this spreading involves a large area of the respiratory epithelium, toxic symptoms appear.

The terminal air sacs become inflamed and many of them become lined with a hyaline membrane cutting off gaseous exchange between the inspired air and the capillary blood. Edema, hyperemia, congestion, and increased secretions are observed throughout the pulmonary tissues. Some patients die of viral pneumonia without demonstrable bacteria in the lung tissues.

However, infection with influenza virus appears to predispose the respiratory system to bacterial invasion, and complicating pneumonias due to staphylococci, streptococci, pneumococci or the *H. influenzae* bacillus are not infrequent. Such complications must be suspected if fever persists beyond the fourth to fifth day after onset.

Influenza virus rarely if ever can be demonstrated in the blood stream, except occasionally in the terminal stages of fatal cases.

*Diagnosis*

When acute febrile illnesses with an abrupt onset and three- to four-day duration occur in rapid succession without signs pointing to another disease, influenza should be suspected. The clinical diagnosis may be confirmed by laboratory procedures. The three most reliable methods are: (1) the isolation of virus from the nose and throat of the patient, (2) the demonstration of antibody rise in the serum of the patient to one of the influenza viruses and (3) demonstration of specific immunofluorescent staining of infected respiratory epithelial cells obtained by nasal washing or smear.

For virus isolation, washings from the patient's throat and nose are inoculated into the amniotic sacs of chick embryos. These are then incubated for two to four days at 32 to 35°C. and tested by hemagglutination for the presence of virus. If present, the virus can be identified promptly by the appropriate immune serum. Virus can be more readily isolated from the patient early in the course of illness.

Serological diagnosis is based on the rise of antibodies to influenza virus in the blood beginning some five to seven days after onset and reaching a peak in 12 to 14 days. Since a sizeable proportion of people possess demonstrable antibodies as a result of earlier experience with related virus strains, it is essential that two specimens of serum be obtained for comparison. One blood sample should be collected in the early acute phase of the illness, the other some two weeks later during convalescence. A significant rise of antibody of at least two-fold and preferably four-fold is usually acceptable as evidence that the recent illness was due to influenza, the type being determined by identifying the specificity of the antibodies. The hemagglutination inhibition test is the serological method most commonly employed for this diagnostic procedure.

*Epidemiology*

A characteristic feature of influenza is its occurrence in epidemics which arise abruptly and spread rapidly but irregularly over a region. The disease appears in small, local outbreaks, which quickly spread to wide areas and frequently sweep from one continent to another. Most epidemic strains of virus extend in a pandemic distribution. Influenza is most common from early autumn to late spring, but may begin or extend into the warm seasons. There is a high attack rate of influenza and a low mortality, although an excess of deaths usually occurs in the older age groups from pneumonia.

Man is the only known reservoir; discharges from the nose and throat of infected persons are the source of infection.

Mode of transmission is by direct contact, through breathing in droplet nuclei, or by contact with clothing or articles contaminated with discharges of the nose and throat of infected individuals.

The incubation period is short, usually one to three days.

The period of communicability is short, probably limited to three days from the onset of symptoms.

All people are susceptible to influenza. Infection produces immunity to the type and subtype of the infecting virus. The duration of this immunity is probably variable, but of fairly long duration. Multiple infections broaden the antigenic base of immunity. Immunization provokes serological responses specific for the subtypes included in the vaccine, with booster effects for those subtypes with which an individual had been previously infected.

Age-specific attack rates in a given epidemic reflect the past experience of various age groups in the population with strains of the prevailing subtype and the degree of exposure to infection.

Immunity after attack with the same or closely related subtypes may persist for several years, but this subject has not been adequately investigated.

The incidence of influenza cases varies from one epidemic to another. An incidence of 20 to 40 per cent was detected in surveys of the 1918 to 1919 pandemic in the United States, while in the 1957 outbreak of Asian influenza an estimate of 39 per cent incidence was estimated by the United States National Health Survey. Even higher rates of incidence were reported from other countries.

Children react differently to influenza at different ages. The infection attacks preschool children only slightly less frequently than it does those of five to eight years, and yet the younger children usually show less signs of illness than do older ones. Children of school age complain less than adults of uncomfortable symptoms. Possibly muscle pains and other symptoms of toxicity are dependent on sensitization by earlier contacts with influenza virus.

Mortality from influenza is difficult to determine. Most of the deaths occur in the very young and the very old, and the influenza carries off those debilitated by previous ill health. Statisticians usually compute mortality data as excess deaths from influenza and pneumonia, *i.e.,* in excess over the average of the five previous years (see Fig. 6.4). During the greatest of all pandemics in 1918 to 1919, it is estimated that some 20 million people around the world died as a result of influenza. An unusual feature of the mortality from influenza at that time was the great proportion of deaths in the young adult age group. No one has adequately explained this phenomenon.

Influenza is of special importance for the pregnant woman. In the 1957 epidemic of

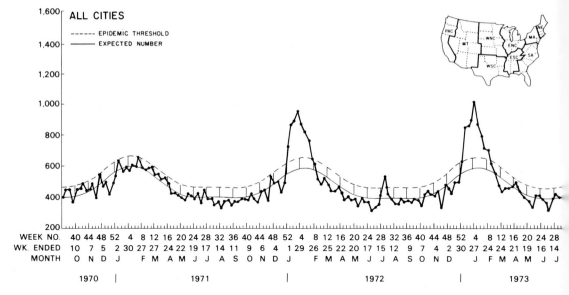

Fig. 6.4. Pneumonia-influenza deaths in 122 United States cities. Source: Center for Disease Control; Influenza–Respiratory Disease Surveillance, Report #89 1972-73, Issued February, 1974, DHEW Publication No. (CDC) 74-8207.

Asian influenza, pulmonary complications were more common in pregnancy. Some observations indicate that influenza during the first weeks of pregnancy may lead to congenital malformations of the fetus. These reports have not been fully confirmed.[22]

The highest incidence of cases in a new epidemic is usually in the 5- to 14-year age group. Incidence declines to about 25 years of age, followed by a rise in the 25- to 34-year period. After the 40th year, incidence declines to about 10 to 15 per cent.

All of the major widespread epidemics of influenza have been attributed to members of the influenza A group. Influenza B has been encountered less often in extensive, abrupt epidemics, and there tends to be a longer interval between outbreaks. Endemic and sporadic distribution appears to characterize influenza B to a considerable extent. As a virus of lower pathogenicity, its distribution is on a more continuous scale. Influenza C is also widely distributed in the population, but produces only mild upper respiratory infections with localized prevalence or only scattered sporadic cases.

It is now clear that changes in the antigenic structure of the influenza viruses are a fundamental property of the organism and have great significance in relation to epidemics. The only known habitat of influenza virus between epidemics is in the form of man-to-man transmissions, first in one part of the world and then in another. The mechanism for the evolution of a new antigenic strain of virus is unknown, nor is it understood how the new epidemic strain can replace the previous one so quickly and completely.

### Prevention and Control

At present, immunization is the only effective method of preventing influenza. The increase in frequency and speed of travel makes the application of isolation and quarantine of little effect.

The use of vaccine for protection is based on observations that recovery from influenza is accompanied by a rise of antibodies and resistance to infection with the same strain of virus. Inoculation of animals with active or inactive viruses produces an immunity. Vaccination of man produces demonstrable circulating antibody and enhances the neutralizing capacity of nasal secretions, thus providing local protection against the entry of virus.

Data accumulated over a period of some 25 years establish the prophylactic value of appropriate vaccines against epidemic influenza. The virus content must be altered at frequent intervals to ensure that the antigenic composition of the prevailing virus strains is adequately represented.

The antibody response to influenza vaccine is closely related to the quantity of antigen present in the vaccine. The virus is cultivated in the allantoic fluids of chick embryos. It is concentrated, purified, and inactivated by formalin. Vaccine is administered by subcutaneous injection.

Febrile reactions to influenza vaccine are common, especially in children. This is apparently due to the toxic effect of virus nucleoprotein. A method of treating virus suspensions with ether and then by precipitation to separate the nucleoprotein from the hemagglutinin fractions has been devised. The hemagglutinin fraction separated in this way is an effective antigen and causes little or no reaction in children. Probably vaccines will be produced by this method in the future.

Vaccine is recommended for people subjected to unusual risk of complications or death. This category includes elderly people or individuals suffering from chronic debilitating diseases. Immunization should be considered for those engaged in essential community services, such as policemen, firemen, hospital employees, and transport workers, as well as important industrial and military personnel (see Table 6.5 for suggested immunization schedule).

Vaccine should be administered well in advance of the expected influenza season. Routine immunization of whole populations is not recommended.

The effectiveness of influenza vaccine is difficult to estimate, but, if the prevailing strain is represented in the vaccine, protection may approach 75 to 80 per cent effectiveness. Duration of immunity produced by vaccine is not well-established. Annual revaccination is probably advisable for those special groups in the population for which immunization is recommended.

Attempts have been made to immunize by modified respiratory infection with live attenuated virus. This method has been studied extensively by the Russians. Apparently, it is difficult to maintain a strain with the correct amount of attenuation. Either the vaccine strain produces illness in those immunized or it is so avirulent that no immunity is produced.

Isolation and quarantine have not proved effective in stopping the spread of influenza infection. Probably mild and inapparent cases of infection are too common to make such measures of much value. Isolation of the patient may help protect him from secondary bacterial infections.

The World Health Organization has set up a global system of surveillance designed to discover new waves of influenza and to detect as early as may be possible the advent of new antigenic strains of influenza virus so that vaccines can be modified to provide protection against the new strain. Necessary throat washings and blood samples may be sent to one of 85 WHO influenza laboratories throughout the world. The World Influenza Center is located in London, England, and the International Influenza Center for the Americas is located at the Center for Disease Control, Atlanta, Georgia.

There is no known treatment for influenza.

TABLE 6.5

*Schedule for influenza vaccine*

| Patient | Dose (CCA Units)[1] | Not Previously Vaccinated | | Previously Vaccinated (Number of Doses) |
|---|---|---|---|---|
| | | Number of doses | Interval | |
| Adult, child over 10 yr. | 1000 | 1 or 2 | 2 wk. | 1 per yr. |
| Child 6 -10yr. | 500 | 1 or 2 | 2 wk. | 1 per yr. |
| Child 3 mo.-6 yr. | 100-200 | 3 | 2 wk. | 1 per yr. |

[1] Review of influenza epidemiology and antigens of strains annually is used as a basis for recommendations to the manufacturer on dose and type of virus for each year's vaccine. See package insert before use.

Source:  Report of the Committee on Infectious Diseases, 1974, American Academy of Pediatrics, Evanston, Ill.

Antibiotics are sometimes given to prevent secondary bacterial infections.

In 1964, E. I. du Pont de Nemours and Company announced that the compound amantadine hydrochloride (Symmetrel) had an inhibitory effect on influenza A, A1, and A2 strains in tissue culture, in chick embryos, and mice. Influenza C was also inhibited but not the influenza B strains. Studies on small numbers of human volunteers also gave promising results.

The drug was approved for prescription use by the U. S. Food and Drug Administration in October, 1966. Amantadine hydrochloride (Symmetrel) is not intended for use in the treatment of influenza, but only for chemoprophylaxis when the threat of influenza is present in the community.

A number of trials of amantadine for prophylaxis in influenza A2 outbreaks have been conducted in recent years. Galbraith and his associates did a controlled study among household contacts of confirmed cases in England. The incidence of clinical cases of influenza was 14.1 per cent in the control group and 3.6 per cent in the group that had received amantadine. In Finland, Oker-Blom *et al.* and in Leningrad, Smorodintsev *et al.* conducted field trials of the efficacy of amantadine as a prophylactic measure. In Finland, a protection rate of 52 per cent and in Leningrad a marked reduction of cases was found amond the treated groups. The drug was well tolerated at a daily dose of 100 mg. Only 1.14 per cent of Smorodintsev's treated group had significant complaints, mainly of sleep disturbances. The above workers recommend amantadine for prophylactic use in the face of an influenza epidemic for the elderly, those having physical disabilities, and for groups such as firemen, police, or medical workers.[23-25]

## Hemolytic Streptococcal Disease

*Introduction*

Streptococci constitute a large, heterogeneous group of bacteria. They are classified primarily by their action on blood-agar cultures. The groups of streptococci which hemolyze red blood cells and produce a completely clear zone around the colony are designated as β-hemolytic streptococci. The α-hemolytic group produces a zone of incomplete hemolysis with green discoloration. Many other streptococci are completely non-hemolytic.[26]

β-Hemolytic streptococci have been separated into 15 groups by Lancefield by identifying specific carbohydrates in the cell wall with serological tests.[27] Of these groups, only A, C, D, G, and K produce human infections and over 90 per cent of human streptococcal disease is attributable to group A organisms.

Most of the disease entities caused by Group A streptococci have been known to man for hundreds of years. Probably their history goes back to antiquity. Scarlet fever was described by the great English clinician, Thomas Sydenham (1624–1689). Certainly, septic sore throat, erysipelas, and puerperal fever were well-known for several centuries before the bacteriological age.

It was not until 1883 that the streptococcus was discovered and described by Friedrich Fehleisen. This finding was confirmed and extended by F. J. Rosenbach in 1884. H. Schottmuller, in 1903, demonstrated the hemolytic action of certain streptococci. The causative relationship of streptococci to tonsillitis and scarlet fever was demonstrated in 1895.

Understanding of streptococcal disease remained confused until research workers had isolated the various toxins and enzymes that are produced by streptococci and until further careful serological studies had demonstrated the multiplicity of types of organisms that go to make up Group A streptococci. Rebecca Lancefield of New York and Frederick Griffith of London were largely responsible for the separation of Group A streptococci into some 50 distinct types on the basis of protein components of the cell wall.

Group A streptococci causes a wide variety of diseases. The kind of disease is determined by the portal of entry and by the characteristics of the particular streptococcus involved. The more important diseases are scarlet fever, streptococcal sore throat, erysipelas, and puerperal fever. Other infections include cellulitis, mastoiditis, osteomyelitis, otitis media, peritonitis, pneumonia, septicemia, meningitis, impetigo contagiosa, and infections of wounds. All of these disease entities are different manifestations of the same infectious agent. Epidemiologically, the problems of each disease type are quite similar and the methods of control hold good generally for the group.

Two important sequelae of infections with Group A streptococci are: (1) acute glomerulonephritis, which is related to infection with certain types of Group A streptococci, and (2) rheumatic fever, which appears following repeated streptococcal infections.

Streptococcal disease appears around the globe quite commonly in the temperate zone. The organisms are also found in the tropics and there are the cause of many inapparent infections, but little frank disease.

Outbreaks of streptococcal disease occur more frequently and are generally more severe in cold, damp climates, such as the New England States, the Great Lakes region, and the Rocky Mountain area, especially during the winter months.

*The Infectious Agent*

Streptococci are more or less spherical in shape and are arranged in chains. The length of the chain varies with the medium on which the organisms are grown. Streptococci are usually non-motile. Capsule formation is not conspicuous, but does occur. Hemolytic streptococci are readily stained by the ordinary dyes. They are gram-positive. In cultures, they grow best at 37°C. On ordinary media, their growth is scanty and slow, but on media suitably enriched with blood, serum, or glucose, growth is more rapid. Even on enriched media, colonies are small. Growth will occur either under aerobic or anaerobic conditions, but is better with air. In general, pigment is not formed.

On blood agar, the ability to produce hemolysis is a differential characteristic. Edgar Todd[28] demonstrated that there are two kinds of hemolysin, O and S, one oxygen-labile but reactivated by a reduction process, the other oxygen-stable and soluble in serum.

Heating for ½ hr. at 55°C. destroys hemolytic streptococci. They are readily destroyed by the usual strengths of disinfectants. By freezing and drying, the organisms can be preserved indefinitely.[29]

The antigenic structure of hemolytic streptococcus is complex. Groups are separated by possession of specific polysaccharide antigens. Almost all organisms causing human disease belong to Group A. Within the group, types are established by demonstration of specific M proteins which are soluble in alcohol.

The streptococcal capsule is composed of a sticky mucopolysaccharide called hyaluronate. This material is not antigenic and does not produce antibodies in infected individuals. This capsular substance is probably not involved in the pathogenesis of streptococcal disease.

Beneath the capsule is a layer of carbohydrate substance in the bacterial cell wall. This material is group-specific and, on the basis of serological tests on this polysaccharide, β-hemolytic streptococci are divided into groups. Groups are designated by capital letters from A to O. Almost all human infections are caused by Group A members.

This group-specific polysaccharide is weakly antigenic in man, and antibodies against this substance appear in the blood of only a few of those infected with Group A streptococci.

Another layer of the streptococcal cell wall contains three important protein constituents. These are termed M, T, and R proteins, of which the M protein is considered the most important.[29] By serological tests on the M protein, Group A streptococci are separated into about 50 distinct types. These types are designated by numbers 1 to 50.

Virulence of Group A streptococci depends mainly on the presence of M protein which has ability to suppress phagocytosis by white blood cells. M protein is highly antigenic and stimulates type-specific antibodies which are responsible for a long enduring immunity to the particular type of streptococcus causing the infection. They are not protective against other type strains, thus permitting successive streptococcal infections in one individual with other strains. Antibodies to M protein appear slowly in the blood; sometimes several months are required for their detection. Formation of these antibodies is suppressed by early and adequate treatment with antibiotics.

The innermost layer of the cell wall is composed of a mucopeptide. This substance gives form and rigidity to the bacterium. The inhibitory action of penicillin depends upon interfering with the formation of this mucopeptide substance.

When the entire cell wall has been removed from Group A streptococci, the remainder of the organism is the protoplast. The protoplast may be identical with so-called L-forms which appear as variants of streptococci when cultured under certain conditions. These forms are penicillin-resistant. Their possible significance in infections is unknown.

Group A streptococci secrete a number of extracellular substances when grown in culture. These substances, with one exception, are antigenic and stimulate the formation of antibodies in persons infected by streptococci. The demonstration of such antibodies is indicative of recent streptococcal infection. Among the important secretory products of Group A streptococci are the following:

1. Streptolysin O hemolyzes red blood cells under anaerobic conditions. It is a potent antigenic agent and stimulates demonstrable antibodies within one week after onset of infection in 70 to 85 per cent of patients. Maximum titer of antibody is reached in three to five weeks.

2. Streptolysin S hemolyzes red blood cells in presence of oxygen. It does not produce antibodies.

3. Streptokinase liquifies fibrin clots. This substance is antigenic, but not so frequently useful an indicator of infection as antistreptolysin O.

4. Hyaluronidase breaks down hyaluronic acid.

5. Diphosphopyridine nucleotidase (DPNase) is antigenic, and determination of antibody levels in patients has been found quite valuable in rheumatic fever cases.

6. Deoxyribonuclease (DNase) is active on deoxyribonucleic acid (DNA). There are at least four distinct DNases, designated A, B, C, and D. Type B gives the best rise in antibodies and has been suggested as a useful test in studying cases of rheumatic fever.

7. Erythrogenic toxin is responsible for the skin rash of scarlet fever. It is antigenic and produces effective antibodies. The production of erythrogenic toxin may be due to the action of bacteriophage on certain strains of Group A streptococci.[29]

*Pathogenesis*

The establishment of an infection is dependent upon both bacterial and host factors. Bacterial factors are the size of the inoculum and the presence of M protein . The production of large amounts of M protein is directly related to the ability of the streptococcus to resist phagocytosis. A hyaluronic acid capsule also contributes to resistance to phagocytosis. Rapid passage of streptococci from man to man usually results in an increase of M protein and frequently in an increase of capsular substance.

As the streptococci multiply in the tissues, a great variety of extracellular products is released. These include streptolysin O, streptokinase, hyaluronidase, and other enzymes. Antibody responses to one or another of these

are useful in diagnosis. These extracellular products contribute to the pathological features of the infection. Hyaluronidase aids in the spread of the organisms through the tissues. Streptokinase breaks down fibrin to produce the characteristic thin pus of streptococcal infections. If present, the erythrogenic toxin causes the typical skin rash of scarlet fever if the individual is not immune to that toxin.

*Epidemiology*

The most common forms of streptococcal disease are upper respiratory infections, pharyngitis, and tonsillitis. Scarlet fever may be associated with these. The variation in the clinical pattern can be accounted for to a considerable extent in terms of the host. In most streptococcal illnesses in man, the clinical pattern is easily recognizable when symptoms are severe or moderately severe. Studies by culture and by testing the blood reveal that many cases are atypical and even inapparent. The streptococci isolated from such cases appear to be the same as from severe cases, so presumably variation in host resistance accounts for the differences.[29]

These illnesses occur most frequently in children from five to 15 years. In young infants less than two to three years of age, streptococcal infection tends to be a prolonged, low-grade affair with frequent suppurative complications; rheumatic fever and nephritis are rarely encountered at that age as complications. Osteomyelitis does occur as a complication. Tonsillitis and pharyngitis tend to attack older children and adults as acute, self-limited diseases followed by the non-suppurative complications. Scarlet fever occurs most commonly between three and 10 years of age; erysipelas may occur at any age; septic complications occur in both young and old.

The role of bacterial variation in human infections is difficult to interpret. During an epidemic of streptococcal disease, it has been frequently observed that a few types or sometimes a single type is predominant in the population at a given time. Continuous observation of the same population over long periods of time often show a decline in prevalence of certain types and a rise in others. The significance of these variations in type prevalence in initiating or perpetuating epidemics is not known.[29]

Some carriers appear to be more efficient

spreaders of infection than others. Children transmit streptococci more readily than adults. Nasal carriers appear to be more dangerous than those harboring the organisms only in the throat. Most infections are spread by persons in the acute phase of the disease (see Table 6.6).

*Reservoir and Source of Infection.* The oropharynx of man is the chief reservoir in acutely ill or convalescent patients and healthy carriers. The nose, throat, or purulent lesions or objects contaminated with such discharges are sources of infection. Nasal carriers are particularly likely to spread the infection.[30]

*Mode of Transmission.* Direct contact with a patient or carrier, by indirect contact with contaminated objects, or by intake of infected droplets in the patient's vicinity are the usual modes of transmission. Dust contaminated from bedclothing, handkerchiefs, or droplet nuclei discharged by coughing or sneezing may be a minor source of infection. Explosive

outbreaks of streptococcal sore throat may result from ingestion of contaminated milk or other food. Milk is usually contaminated by coming from a cow with an infected udder.[30]

*Incubation Period.* This is rarely longer than one to three days.

*Period of Communicability.* Communicability usually exists during the period of incubation and of illness, approximately 10 days. In untreated cases, communicability progressively declines in most persons up to two to three weeks. A few patients continue to discharge virulent streptococci for months. Persons with untreated complications such as draining middle ear infection may spread infection for months. Treatment with adequate doses of penicillin will eliminate probability of transmission within 24 hr.[30]

*Susceptibility and Resistance.* Susceptibility to streptococcal infections is general. Antibacterial immunity develops only against the type

TABLE 6.6

*Hemolytic streptococci transferred by nasal carriers during handshaking:*
*carrier blew nose immediately before shaking hands*

| Carrier No. | Streptococcal Type | Hemolytic Streptococci Recovered from Sterile Handkerchief into Which Carrier Blew Nose | Hemolytic Streptococci from Carrier's Hands | Hemolytic Streptococci Recovered from Recipient's Hands | |
|---|---|---|---|---|---|
| | | | | Before shaking hands | After shaking hands |
| 1 | 17 | 2,005,000 | 82,000 | 0 | 49,920 |
| 2 | 17 | 440,000,000 | 84,000 | 0 | 10,560 |
| 3 | 3 | 75,000 | 1,640,000 | 0 | > 6,000 |
| 4 | 3 | 395,000 | 94,000 | 0 | 3,960 |
| 5 | 17 | 8,960,000 | 94,000 | 0 | 2,520 |
| 6 | 3 | 45,500 | 4,000 | 0 | 920 |
| 7 | 19 | 20,000,000 | 414,000 | 0 | 720 |
| 8 | A | 2,160,000 | 86,000 | 0 | 520 |
| 9 | 19 | 1,120,000 | 160,000 | 0 | 320 |
| 10 | 3 | 500 | 122,000 | 0 | 240 |
| 11 | A | 1,600,000 | 22,000 | 0 | 80 |
| 12 | 19 | 15,000 | 2,000 | 0 | 40 |
| 13 | A | 870,000 | 2,000 | 0 | 40 |
| 14 | 3 | 500 | 11,000 | 0 | 0 |
| 15 | 17 | 3,260,000 | 42,000 | 0 | 0 |
| 16 | A | 209,000,000 | 2,000 | 0 | 0 |
| 17 | 17 | 103,000 | 3,000 | 0 | 0 |
| Average | | | 169,000 | 0 | 4,450 |

Source: Hamburger, M., Jr. Transfer of beta hemolytic streptococci by shaking hands. *Amer. J. Med.,* 2:23-25, 1947.

of Group A streptococcus by which the patient has been infected. Repeated attacks of sore throat or other streptococcal disease due to a different type of the organism are common.

Immunity to scarlet fever may be acquired through inapparent infection. Only a few types of Group A streptococcus can produce the erythrogenic toxin that is responsible for the skin rash. Immunity to this toxin develops within one week after the onset of scarlet fever and is usually permanent. Second attacks of scarlet fever with a rash are rare, but may occur because there are two immunological forms of the erythrogenic toxin.

An attack of erysipelas seems to predispose an individual to subsequent recurrences. The explanation for this phenomenon is not clear.[30]

Crowding is an important factor in streptococcal disease. Infection spreads readily in barracks, dormitories, and other such situations. Perhaps the influence of climate on streptococcal infections is largely due to the effect of crowding indoors in cold weather.

*Clinical Manifestations*

Acute infections with hemolytic streptococci are quite varied in their characteristic features. The principal ones are:

*Streptococcal Sore Throat.* The onset of symptoms is sudden. The throat becomes sore and painful in swallowing. Fever is moderately high, 38 to 40° C. The patient complains of headache, chilliness, general malaise, and loss of appetite. In patients who receive no specific treatment, the illness reaches a peak within 24 to 48 hr., and all symptoms generally disappear in about five days.

Examination shows a red, swollen throat with discrete patches of grayish-white exudate in the tonsillar area. The lymph glands at the angles of the jaws are swollen and tender.

A count of the white blood cells shows a moderate leukocytosis, which may vary from 12,000 to 20,000 white blood cells. Culture of the throat usually produces almost a pure culture of $\beta$-hemolytic streptococci in large numbers.

Many patients do not develop this full-blown set of symptoms. Frequently patients complain only of a cold, or a slight sore throat.

*Scarlet Fever.* This disease begins in a manner exactly similar to ordinary streptococcal sore throat, but in 24 to 48 hr. a generalized red skin rash appears. The rash is more marked on the neck, chest, in the folds of the axilla, elbow, and groin, and on the inner aspects of the thighs. There is a flushing of the cheeks and a zone of pallor around the mouth. The tongue is red and has the appearance of a ripe strawberry.

In short, scarlet fever is a streptococcal sore throat in which the strain of organism is capable of producing erythrogenic toxin and the patient has no antibodies to that toxin. The rash is usually a fine erythema, commonly punctate, blanching on pressure. The injection of 0.1 ml of scarlet fever antitoxin into an area where the rash is florid will be followed by blanching around the site of injection in 8 to 12 hr.

High fever, nausea, and vomiting may accompany severe infections.

Desquamation of the skin begins as a fine scaling of the face and body. It is most clearly seen at the tips of fingers and toes. Desquamation is usually completed during the second week of the illness.

Scarlet fever and streptococcal sore throat may be followed by suppurative complications such as otitis media or peritonsillar abscess. At intervals of one to four weeks, non-suppurative sequelae such as rheumatic fever or glomerulonephritis may appear.

The severity of scarlet fever varies greatly. Since just prior to 1900, its severity has been decreasing. This decline has continued to the present time. The fall in mortality during the past 30 years was accelerated by the advent of sulfonamide therapy and later by the availability of penicillin. The fatality is low in the United States, about one death for each 300 to 400 cases (see Table 6.7). Deaths were 41 in 1969.

*Erysipelas.* An acute, spreading red inflammation of the skin characterized by fever, chills, malaise, and rise in white blood cell count. Face and legs are the locations most commonly affected. The edge of the advancing inflammation is often raised.

The means by which the Group A streptococci are introduced into the skin are not clear. Usually one finds large numbers of streptococci in the nose and throat of individuals who come down with erysipelas. It may be that infection is transferred from these areas to enter the skin through small, almost invisible abrasions.

Erysipelas occurs most frequently in infants and in persons over 50 years of age. Formerly common, especially in cold climates, it is now seen infrequently. The disease is particularly severe in people suffering from debilitating disease. Fatality varies with the part of the body affected and according to associated disease.

There has been a gradual decline in mortality in the United States since 1900. The average annual mortality rate from 1900 to 1904 was 46 per 100,000. This had fallen to 22 by 1930, but declined sharply after the introduction of sulfonamide drugs and even more dramatically with the advent of penicillin. For 1970, only 12 deaths from erysipelas were reported in the United States (see Table 6.8).

TABLE 6.7

*Incidence, incidence rates, deaths, death rates, and case fatality for scarlet fever and streptococcal sore throat: United States, 1935 to 1961 (ISC codes 050, 051)*

| Period | Incidence No. | Rate | Deaths No. | Rate | Case Fatality Rate |
|---|---|---|---|---|---|
| | | | | | % |
| 1959-1961 | 988,376 | 1,835.2 | 368 | 0.7 | 0.0 |
| 1949-1951 | 235,865 | 521.1 | 1,179 | 2.6 | 0.0 |
| 1955-1959 | 1,149,679 | 1,336.9 | 957 | 1.1 | 00 |
| 1950-1954 | 543,042 | 689.3 | 1,601 | 2.1 | 0.3 |
| 1945-1949 | 583,191 | 813.5 | 3,308 | 4.7 | 0.6 |
| 1940-1944 | 791,846 | 1,184.0 | 7,878 | 11.8 | 0.9 |
| 1935-1939 | 1,126,980 | 1,749.6 | 9,094 | 4.1 | 0.8 |

Source: Dauer, C.C., Korns, R.F., and Schuman, L. M. *Infectious Diseases.* Cambridge: Harvard University Press, 1968.

TABLE 6.8

*Deaths and death rates for erysipelas: United States, 1930 to 1961 (ISC code 052)*

| Period | No. of Death | Death Rate |
|---|---|---|
| 1959-1961 | 82 | 0.2 |
| 1949-1951 | 165 | 0.4 |
| 1955-1959 | 142 | 0.1 |
| 1950-1954 | 236 | 0.3 |
| 1945-1949 | 505 | 0.7 |
| 1940-1944 | 1,580 | 2.4 |
| 1935-1939 | 5,705 | 8.9 |
| 1930-1934 | 10,753 | 17.2 |

Source: Dauer, C.C., Korns, R.F., and Schuman, L. M. *Infectious Deseases.* Cambridge: Harvard University Press, 1968.

Occurrence of rheumatic fever rarely follows erysipelas, although acute nephritis may be seen after some attacks.

*Puerperal Fever.* In newly delivered women, the raw surfaces of the uterus are highly susceptible to bacterial infections. The infectious agents include a variety of bacteria. Group A streptococci are of primary importance after full-term delivery. Other agents such as colon bacilli, anaerobic organisms, bacteroides sp., and staphylococci predominate in postabortion infections.

Puerperal fever was a devastating problem, especially in hospitals, before the era of antisepsis. Infection was carried from one woman to another by the contaminated hands of nurses, physicians, and medical students. Semmelweis, in 1847, demonstrated in Vienna that a simple procedure such as washing the hands in chlorinated lime water between examinations of patients greatly reduced the incidence of puerperal fever in hospitals. Development of sterile techniques and of stringent precautions against infection brought puerperal fever rates to a lower level. Introduction of potent antibacterial drugs and antibiotics has hastened the reduction of puerperal fever in all countries where modern obstetrical care is available.

In fatal cases of puerperal fever, death usually is due to an invasion of the blood stream by the responsible organism.

*Diagnosis of Streptococcal Infections*

Scarlet fever and erysipelas can usually be diagnosed by clinical examination. Cultures of the throat are required to make a definite diagnosis of streptococcal sore throat and pharyngitis. Before any chemotherapy is begun, swabs should be rubbed over the tonsillar and posterior pharyngeal areas. These swabs should be streaked without delay on sheep blood agar plates. After incubation for 12 hr., the numbers of hemolytic streptococci should be estimated. If only a few are observed, it is unlikely that hemolytic streptococcus is responsible for the illness. If large numbers of hemolytic streptococci are present, simple tests to determine whether the organisms belong to Group A may be carried out.

Serological tests may be run for antibody such as antistreptolysin O. A positive test is of no value in determining the diagnosis of the current attack, as from 10 to 20 days are required after the onset of illness for the antibodies to appear. It does indicate a prior Group A streptococcus infection. This information is of value in assessing possible care of rheumatic fever or acute nephritis.

*Treatment*

The prompt institution of antimicrobial treatment is important to obtain quick control of the infection, to prevent suppurative complications, to avoid non-suppurative complications, and to eliminate the possibility of transmission of infection to others. Penicillin is the drug of choice, but erythromycin is an acceptable second choice. Sulfonamides are not effective in achieving the therapeutic objectives listed above.

*Non-suppurative Complications of Streptococcal Infections*

*Acute Glomerulonephritis.* Usually the period of onset following an infection with Group A streptococcus is short, about 10 days. The onset is rather abrupt with blood in the urine, swelling of face and lower legs, pain and tenderness in the kidney region, and raised blood pressure. Death occurs occasionally in the acute stage of the illness, but complete recovery is the rule. Possibly 10 per cent of the cases progress to a chronic nephritis. Apparently, children are most likely to recover from this complication, while adults are more prone to develop the chronic form of the disease.

It is now known that strains of streptococcus types 1, 4, 12, and 49 are responsible for most of the acute nephritis cases following a primary Group A streptococcal infection. Type 12 is the most common offender. Two or three other types may also be involved. Careful studies have provided data to support the theory that acute nephritis is caused by a toxic substance acting directly on the glomeruli of the kidney. An immunological mechanism may also be involved.[31] It appears that only a small number of those infected with the nephritogenic strains of streptococci do indeed develop nephritis. Possibly an individual factor of susceptibility to this toxin, as yet unknown, may be the decisive determinant.

Once the patient is infected with a nephritogenic strain, early and adequate treatment with penicillin appears to reduce the likelihood of kidney complications. To protect contacts,

once the diagnosis of acute nephritis is made, treatment should be started to eliminate the responsible streptococcal strain from the household or from the immediate associates in military establishments. In one such outbreak in a naval installation, 147 cases of acute nephritis developed before the spread of infection was halted[32] (see Fig. 6.5).

*Rheumatic Fever.* Rheumatic fever represents a major health problem. In addition to over 14,090 deaths in the United States in 1972 (provisional figures) due to rheumatic fever and chronic rheumatic heart disease, there were thousands of patients suffering from the acute effects of the disease. Physical limitation, eventual incapacitation, and early death are the prospects facing many of these victims. Despite the declining mortality, rheumatic fever and rheumatic heart disease are still the leading causes of fatal heart disease in the 5- to 24-year age group, causing more than four times the number of deaths as tuberculosis and syphilis combined. They are still major public health problems in the United States.[33]

Rheumatic fever occurs as one of the sequelae in a small proportion of patients with Group A streptococcus upper respiratory infections.

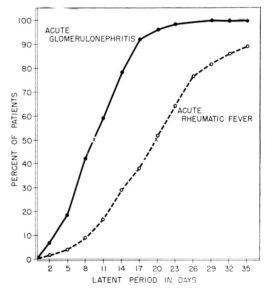

Fig. 6.5. Cumulative distribution of latent periods in acute glomerulonephritis and acute rheumatic fever. Source: Rammelcamp, C. H., Jr. Concepts of pathogenesis of glomerulonephritis derived from studies in man. In *The Streptococcus, Rheumatic Fever and Glomerulonephritis,* edited by J. W. Uhr. Baltimore: The Williams and Wilkins Co., 1964.

Sometimes the inciting infection is mild or inapparent, but it can be demonstrated by appropriate serological tests.

The important manifestations of rheumatic fever are acute inflammation of the joints, tender nodules under the skin, sometimes involvement of the nervous system causing chorea or St. Vitus's Dance, and, most serious of all, a frequently occurring inflammation of the heart which may attack one or all of the cardiac tissues. The acute attack is characterized by fever, rapid pulse, pallor, nose bleeds, painful swollen joints, abdominal and precordial pain, and skin rashes. Mild or inapparent attacks of rheumatic fever may occur, but these can also affect the heart.

The course of illness is extremely variable. Some patients recover in one week; others develop progressive heart failure and die. The joint manifestations of rheumatic fever always subside completely no matter how extensive or how severe is the arthritis. Likewise, no known impairment of the nervous system occurs, despite repeated attacks of chorea. It is only the heart that suffers irreversible damage. Carditis occurs in from 40 to 50 per cent of initial attacks of the disease.

In outbreaks of streptococcal infections, it is estimated that approximately 3 per cent of the patients who received no antibiotic therapy develop rheumatic fever. Recent studies point out that carriage of Group A streptococci which is not associated with an immune response does not cause rheumatic fever. The magnitude of the immune response to the inciting streptococcal infection appears to be an important factor, as does the duration of carriage of streptococci in the convalescent period. Strong immune responses and prolonged convalescent carriage occur with greatest frequency under epidemic conditions. Individuals who have experienced a primary attack of rheumatic fever are far more likely to develop subsequent bouts of the disease following streptococcal infections. The likelihood of serious heart damage increases also with secondary attacks.[33]

Rheumatic fever is a world-wide disease, and its frequency appears to be determined by climate and geography. The disease appears to be less frequent and milder in warm climates. The incidence of rheumatic fever is greater at high altitudes and in cold, damp climates such as New England, the Rocky Mountains, and the north and central Atlantic states. It occurs predominantly in the late winter and early spring.

Rheumatic fever occurs among all levels of society, but is more common and more severe in children from poverty-stricken homes. Crowding, poor hygiene, poor housing, malnutrition, and substandard medical care all favor the spread of streptococcal infections. Of these factors, crowding may be the most important.

Children less than five years of age develop rheumatic fever infrequently; under two years, rheumatic fever is a rarity. The greatest incidence is found between six and 15 years, with a peak at about eight years. Under ordinary circumstances, the incidence of primary attacks of rheumatic fever decreases after puberty, but experience in the military forces has demonstrated that when young adults are exposed to outbreaks of streptococcal infections the attack rates of rheumatic fever are high.

It is now generally accepted that rheumatic fever is a sequel of Group A streptococcal infection, but the pathogenesis of the disease process is still uncertain. There is a latent period following the streptococcal infection which varies from about one to three weeks. This observation has led some investigators to compare rheumatic fever to serum sickness. It is known that those who develop rheumatic fever usually demonstrate evidence of an exaggerated streptococcal antibody response. Recent studies have demonstrated that Group A streptococci and normal human heart muscle share a common antigen (cross-reactive antigen). This antigen is present in the cytoplasmic membrane of the streptococcal cell. When the sera of rheumatic patients are added to a preparation of normal human myocardium, an antigen-antibody reaction takes place along the muscle fibers. These studies suggest that rheumatic fever may be an autoimmune disease.[34,35]

Although reliable statistics on the incidence of rheumatic fever are not available, the indications are that there has been a progressive decline in both the occurrence and in the severity of the disease during the past generation. This decline is reflected in the death rates (see Table 6.9) and in the prevalence of rheumatic heart disease among school children (see Table 6.10). Additional evidence of this decrease is revealed by results of examinations of those registered for military service. In the

TABLE 6.9[1]

*Death rates from rheumatic fever and chronic heart disease per 100,000*
*population in United States, 1942-44 and 1962-64*[2]

| | Whites | | | Non-whites | | |
|---|---|---|---|---|---|---|
| | 1942-44 | 1962-64 | Per Cent Decline | 1942-44 | 1962-64 | Per Cent Decline |
| All Ages[3] | 19.1 | 8.3 | 57 | 28.1 | 7.5 | 73 |
| Under 5 | 1.2 | 0.1 | 92 | 2.8 | 0.4 | 86 |
| 5-14 | 5.2 | 0.3 | 94 | 8.9 | 1 2 | 87 |
| 15-24 | 7.4 | 1.2 | 84 | 9.5 | 3.7 | 61 |
| 25-34 | 9.8 | 3.3 | 66 | 11.8 | 6.3 | 47 |
| 25-44 | 15.8 | 8.5 | 46 | 21.9 | 10.1 | 54 |
| 45-54 | 22.7 | 17.2 | 24 | 40.0 | 13.5 | 66 |
| 55-64 | 35.7 | 27.0 | 24 | 68.0 | 17.1 | 75 |
| 65 and over | 107.9 | 30.9 | 71 | 139.2 | 17.1 | 88 |

[1] Modified from Reports of the Division of Vital Statistics, National Center for Health Statistics. *In:* Statistical Bulletin, Metropolitan Life Insurance Co., July, 1966.
[2] Data exclude New Jersey, 1962-1963.
[3] Adjusted to U.S. Census, 1940.

Source:   *Rheumatic Fever* by M. Markowitz and L. Gordis, 2nd Edition, Table 5, page 12, Volume II in the Series, *Major Problems in Clinical Pediatrics,* Consulting Editor, A. J. Schaffer, W. B. Saunders Co., Philadelphia, 1972.

TABLE 6.10

*The prevalence of rheumatic heart disease among school children: results of selected surveys*

| Location | Date | Age Group | Rate/ 1000 | Reference |
|---|---|---|---|---|
| New York City | 1920 | 6-17 | 4.3 | Halsey (1921) |
| Boston | 1926 | 6-17 | 4.5 | Robey (1927) |
| Philadelphia | 1934 | 6-18 | 5.0 | Cahan (1937) |
| Toronto | 1948-1949 | 5-15 | 1.6 | Gardiner and Keith (1951) |
| Buffalo | 1949-1952 | 5-18 | 1.8 | Mattison et al. (1953) |
| Chicago | 1959-1960 | 6-13 | 1.3 | Miller et al. (1962) |
| New York City | 1961 | 5-18 | 1.6 | Brownell and Stix (1963) |

Source:   Markowitz, M., and Kuttner, A. G. *Rheumatic Fever: Diagnosis, Management and Prevention.* Philadelphia: W. B. Saunders Co., 1965.

years 1941 to 1943, a total of 2.4 per cent of those examined were rejected as having evidence of rheumatic heart disease, while in the period 1960 to 1962 this figure had fallen to 0.88 per cent.[33]

With modern treatment, reductions in mortality have occurred at all ages. Persons who reached adulthood before antibiotics became available have not fared too well. Among the adult population an estimated number of 1,250,000 persons suffer from chronic rheumatic heart disease. The prevalence increases sharply with advancing age.[36]

*Prevention and Control.* The only specific therapy in rheumatic fever is based on the knowledge that Group A streptococcus plays an essential part in the etiology of the disease.

Penicillin is considered to be the drug of

choice for the elimination of streptococci completely before initiation of palliative treatment for the symptoms of rheumatic fever. Every patient with an acute attack should receive penicillin in amounts to maintain therapeutic levels for 10 days. If the patient is sensitive to penicillin, erythromycin may be used.

The sulfonamide drugs should not be used for the treatment of streptococcal infections. They will not eradicate the streptococcus, and therefore will not prevent rheumatic fever. However, the sulfonamides are effective in preventing reinfection and recurrences, and may be used to replace penicillin as continuous prophylaxis in rheumatic fever patients.

One of the most striking features of rheumatic fever is its tendency to recur. Before antibiotic prophylaxis was available, from 60 to 75 per cent of patients with an initial attack had one recurrence or more.[37] The recurrence rate is highest during the first three years following an initial attack. The younger the child at the time of the initial attack, the greater the likelihood of recurrences.

As soon as the initial attack of rheumatic fever has subsided, the patient should be put on prophylactic therapy. Three different antibacterial regimes have been carefully compared for the ability to prevent recurrences: (1) sulfonamide; (2) oral penicillin; and (3) penicillin by injection. Benzathine penicillin G by injection gave best results.

The duration of prophylactic treatment cannot be determined with certainty. A reasonable program appears to be for the continuation of prophylaxis without interruption at least up to the age of 18 years or for a minimum period of five years following the end of the last recognizable attack of rheumatic fever, whichever is longer.[38]

If for any reason, rheumatic fever patients cannot be maintained continuously on prophylactic treatment, every care should be taken to treat adequately any streptococcal infections that the patient may develop. This treatment, if possible, should be with penicillin and should be prolonged at full doses for 7 to 10 days.

Epidemics occurring in closed communities with a large turnover of streptococci through new arrivals can best be controlled by injections of penicillin for the total population. Less vigorous measures have not met with success.

Such epidemics are likely to occur in recruiting centers, schools, children's homes, or even large households.

Two drugs have proved valuable in controlling the symptoms of rheumatic fever, although it is not believed that they affect the damage to the heart to any great extent. Salicylates, usually in the form of aspirin, are recommended in acute cases with little or no evidence of heart damage. If a satisfactory response occurs, the drug may be discontinued after one to two weeks. If joints again become inflamed, aspirin is begun again. A dosage of 50 mg. of aspirin per pound of body weight given in six divided doses per day is considered adequate.

Patients with moderate to severe heart involvement along with their acute rheumatic symptoms should be given steroids to bring the acute manifestation of the generalized inflammatory process under control rapidly. Prednisone has been widely used for this purpose. A dose of 1 mg. per pound in four divided doses over a 24-hr. period is sufficient for most patients. This treatment is usually continued for 7 to 10 days. After discontinuation of the steroid, salicylates are begun and continued until all signs of rheumatic activity have subsided.[33] These treatment regimes must be modified to meet the particular responses of individual patients.

*Public Health Significance of Rheumatic Fever.* On account of the duration and severity of physical disability resulting from rheumatic heart disease and the expense this problem imposes upon the community, public health agencies must participate actively in the control of rheumatic fever. Everything possible should be done to decrease streptococcal disease, such as compulsory milk pasteurization, good food hygiene, and rapid control of outbreaks of streptococcal infections that may be discovered.

The finding of undiagnosed cases of rheumatic heart disease, especially among school children, is important so that these persons can be put on prophylactic drugs to prevent further heart damage. Local diagnostic clinics have proved valuable in studying suspected cases. These may be maintained by health departments or by hospitals assisted by voluntary agencies. Drugs are frequently supplied free or at low cost by public health agencies. Then public health nurses are essential to visit the families to supervise the administration of prophylactic drugs and to follow the progress of each patient.

## St. Louis Encephalitis

*Introduction*

The arthropod-borne viruses (arboviruses) at present represent about 250 immunologically distinct agents. These viruses are classified by immunological relationships. About 80 of the arboviruses are recognized as being capable of infecting man. Probably most of this group are basically parasites of arthropods and animals and are not dependent upon man for survival. The arboviruses generally produce three types of clinical illness in man: (1) fevers, such as dengue fever, usually fairly mild; (2) infection of the central nervous system or encephalitis commonly severe, with considerable fatality rates; (3) hemorrhagic fevers, also severe and frequently fatal.[39]

Among the arboviruses which affect man in continental United States during recent years St. Louis encephalitis virus is the most important. This virus causes an acute inflammatory disease of short duration that involves the brain, spinal cord, and meninges. Mild cases and inapparent infections often occur. Severe infections usually have an acute onset, high fever, stiff neck, stupor, coma, spasticity, tremors, and headache. Of the cases which show definite signs of brain involvement, about 20 per cent are fatal. The disease is more fatal among the very young and the elderly. Permanent sequelae are uncommon. When they do occur, there may be personality changes, mental deterioration, muscle weakness, or even paralysis.

*Occurrence*

The disease was first known to have occurred in 1932 in Paris, Illinois. The following year a large-scale epidemic of this "new" disease broke out in the environs of St. Louis, Missouri. The causative agent was isolated in 1933 during the St. Louis outbreak. Since then, sporadic cases, small outbreaks, and major epidemics of St. Louis encephalitis have occurred from Pennsylvania to Washington state, California, Colorado, Texas, and the lower Ohio Valley to Florida. It occurs in the summer and early autumn, typically affecting rural populations in the Far West and urban-suburban residents elsewhere in the country.

Serological surveys indicate that St. Louis virus has been present in Mexico, Panama, Colombia, Brazil, Argentina, and the West Indies. Virus has been isolated during an outbreak in Jamaica, West Indies.

*The Virus*

The St. Louis encephalitis virus is a small, spherical virus of 20 to 30 m$\mu$ in diameter. It belongs to antigenic Group B of arboviruses, being most closely related to the viruses of Japanese B encephalitis, Murray Valley encephalitis, and West Nile fever. It is sensitive to heat and readily inactivated by ether and bile salts, and has both complement-fixing and hemagglutinating antigens. The virus multiplies in chick embryos and grows well in hamster, duck, and chicken kidney cells in tissue culture. The white mouse is a suitable animal for laboratory studies. Chickens, as well as many species of birds and bats, develop an inapparent viremia upon inoculation. Such infections in nature are of considerable epidemiological significance, if the blood contains enough virus to infect mosquitoes.[40]

*Pathogenesis and Pathology*

Virus is introduced through the skin by the bite of an infected mosquito. Probably the virus is transported to the regional lymph glands where primary multiplication takes place. As the virus multiplies, it is spread throughout the body by the blood stream to other sites favorable to virus multiplication. This results in a major viremia that may endure for several days until the defense mechanism of the body becomes effective enough to overcome the circulating virus. During this viremic phase, virus enters the nervous system in a certain number of those infected. Incubation period from the time of infection to onset of symptoms varies from 5 to 15 days.

Examination of fatal cases shows a swollen, edematous brain with vascular congestion and tiny hemorrhages throughout the brain and meninges. Microscopically, there are red blood cells and lymphocytes around the blood vessels. Nerve cell damage occurs in small clusters of cells in the gray matter. Lesions are found most marked in the midbrain and brain stem, but other parts of the brain may be affected.

*Diagnosis*

Definite diagnosis can only be made by laboratory tests. Serological tests to compare antibody levels in acute and convalescent sera are most useful in patients who survive the disease. In rapidly fatal cases, virus may be isolated from the brain in tissue culture or in mice.

There is usually a mild to moderate leukocytosis. Examination of the cerebrospinal fluid shows an increase in protein and in cell count. These findings are not useful in differentiating St. Louis from the other arbovirus types of encephalitis.

Frequently, isolation of St. Louis encephalitis virus from mosquitoes in the vicinity of the patient's residence lends credence to the diagnosis.

*Prognosis*

Most of those infected by St. Louis encephalitis virus show no symptoms whatever, but do develop specific antibodies to the virus, which provide future protection. Another segment of those infected runs a mild fever for a few days and may have a few symptoms including headache and stiffness of the neck. These patients usually recover rapidly and completely within a few days. In a small percentage of persons infected, especially among the elderly, a severe illness with full-blown symptoms of encephalitis occurs. Among these, the mortality rate is high.

*Epidemiology*

Sabin[41] has theorized that members of arbovirus Group B may have evolved from a "stem" virus in the tropics. He selected the West Nile virus discovered in East Africa as the most probable progenitor of the group. Other pathogenic Group B viruses that might have evolved from West Nile are Murray Valley encephalitis of Australia, Japanese B encephalitis of the Far East, and St. Louis encephalitis of the American continent. Each of these viruses shows close antigenic relationships, but each has its own regional distribution. All are transmitted by *Culex* mosquitoes.

There is no knowledge of St. Louis encephalitis prior to 1932. Since that time, it has appeared frequently in the United States with a wide geographical distribution. The vectors of St. Louis encephalitis have varied with the area involved. *Culex tarsalis* appears to be the principal mosquito transmitter in California and other far western areas. In the central states, *Culex pipiens* and *Culex quinquefasciatus* have been frequently incriminated as the usual vectors. In the recent Florida epidemics, *Culex nigripalpus* is reported to have been responsible for spreading the virus. Other mosquitoes have been found infected with St. Louis virus, but have not been confirmed as vectors.

Most mosquitoes take a blood meal as a requisite to maturation of their eggs. Different mosquito species vary widely in their preferences for hosts. The vectors of St. Louis encephalitis exhibit a preference for feeding on domestic fowls and wild birds. The avian species in general demonstrate a marked viremia after infection with St. Louis virus, which provides an excellent source of virus to infect other mosquitoes. Birds are usually abundant in suburban areas and in populated rural districts, thus providing ample opportunity for the build-up of intensive wildlife infections with St. Louis encephalitis in the mosquito-breeding season.[42]

The mechanisms of reintroduction of St. Louis virus into an endemic area or of its maintenance there from one warm season to another are not entirely clear. It is known that adult mosquitoes do overwinter in protected locations. Virus may survive in such mosquitoes and be transmitted to susceptible birds in the following spring, thus leading to a renewed build-up of virus activity as the warm season advances.[43]

Wild-caught rodents in endemic areas show a high percentage with antibodies in their sera against St. Louis encephalitis virus. Horses also become infected, but develop no symptoms. It is not known whether these animals have any significant role in the epidemiology of the infection. Man is of little or no importance as a source of infection for mosquitoes. In highly endemic areas, adults are largely immune by reason of previous infections, so that most of the susceptible population is found among children.

In most outbreaks in the United States, cases are noted in July with the peak of the epidemic occurring in late August or September. The occurrence of cases ceases when the onset of cold weather stops the activity of mosquitoes.

During the past 10 years, sharp outbreaks

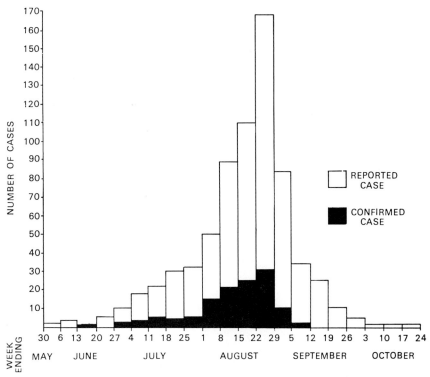

Fig. 6.6. Confirmed and reported cases of St. Louis Encephalitis by week of onset (week of admission for 35 patients with unknown time of onset), Houston, 1964. Source: Epidemic St. Louis encephalitis in Houston, 1964, a cooperative study. *J.A.M.A., 193.* 142, 1965

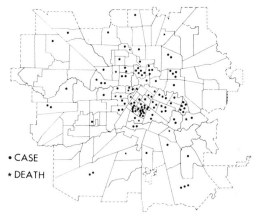

Fig. 6.7. Confirmed cases and deaths from St. Louis Encephalitis by census tract, Houston, 1964 (eight cases occurring outside city limits are excluded). Source: Epidemic St. Louis encephalitis in Houston, 1964, a cooperative study. *J.A.M.A., 193:* 142, 1965.

the first recognized cases of St. Louis encephalitis appeared in Florida in the Miami area. In 1959, 1961, and 1962, the Tampa Bay area of Florida suffered a severe outbreak. A total of 222 confirmed cases with 43 deaths occurred during the 1962 season.[44] Texas has suffered heavily from St. Louis encephalitis more recently. In 1964, there were 712 reported cases in Houston, of which 123 were confirmed by laboratory tests. Nineteen deaths were reported to have occurred. The vector was *C. quinquefasciatus*[45] (see Figs. 6.6 and 6.7).

During 1966, there were 168 cases with 20 deaths in the Dallas area, and in the same summer Corpus Christi reported 98 cases and five deaths. In the period 1967-1971 only 134 cases of St. Louis Encephalitis have been reported in the United States.[46]

*Control*

There is no effective vaccine available to protect against St. Louis encephalitis. Control of the mosquito vector is the only method of

have occurred in the Central Valley of California, the Rio Grande Valley in Texas, the lower Ohio River Valley, the Grand Junction region in Colorado, and Louisville, Kentucky. In 1958, prevention now recommended. Knowledge of the local vector is essential to plan control programs most efficiently. The usual methods of mosquito control apply: (1) elimination of potential breeding places by drainage, efficient handling of irrigation, and so on; (2) spraying of homes, outhouses, and chicken shelters with long lasting residual insecticides; (3) screening of homes; (4) the use of aircraft for area spraying of insecticides.[47]

## Histoplasmosis

*Introduction*

Histoplasmosis is a systemic disease caused by a fungus, *Histoplasma capsulatum*, of varying severity, with the primary lesion generally, if not always, in the lungs. Infection with this fungus is common; actual disease due to infection is uncommon, and the chronic progressive form of the disease is quite unusual. Histoplasmosis is recognized in five different clinical forms:

1. The asymptomatic form is recognized only by a skin test to demonstrate acquired hypersensitivity to histoplasmin. Calcified nodes in the lungs, representing healed primary lesions, may be seen in X-ray films.

2. The acute benign respiratory form varies from mild respiratory illness to temporary incapacity with weakness, fever, chest pains, and dry or productive cough. Recovery is slow. Healing may leave calcified areas in the lung demonstrable by X-ray examination.

3. The acute disseminated form shows high fever, prostration, and rapid course. It is most common in infants and young children. Liver and spleen are involved and enlarged. Without treatment, it is usually fatal.

4. The chronic disseminated form is similar to the acute disseminated form, but runs a slower course. It usually occurs in adults and may be slowly progressive over a period up to five years.

5. The progressive pulmonary form with cavitation is often confused with tuberculosis. It may persist for months or years and eventually become disseminated, and is frequently fatal unless treated vigorously.[48]

The disease was discovered in Panama in 1905 by Dr. Samuel T. Darling, who thought the organism that he found in a fatal case to be a protozoan. He gave the name, *H. capsulatum*,

to the organism. In the course of the next year, Darling found two other fatal cases caused by his new agent.[49]

The next report of histoplasmosis was by a distinguished Brazilian scientist, Dr. Henrique de Rocha-Lima, who, in 1912, studied cases of histoplasmosis in Brazil. He concluded that Darling's classification of the agent was erroneous and that it belonged to the fungus group.

In 1926, the first case of histoplasmosis was reported in the United States. Drs. William Riley and Cecil J. Watson described a case in Minneapolis that appeared at autopsy to be identical with Darling's cases.

At Vanderbilt University in 1934, Dr. W. A. DeMonbreun grew *H. capsulatum* on culture media from a fatal case of histoplasmosis. DeMonbreun worked out culture methods and described the morphology and growth characteristics of the agent. His studies included animal inoculations which proved conclusively the relationship between his organism and the disease provoked in animals.

Working almost simultaneously with DeMonbreun, G. H. Hausmann and G. R. Schenken also reported the cultivation of a fungus that proved to be *H. capsulatum*.

At this point, the general opinion was that histoplasmosis was a rare, generalized disease in the United States that was uniformly fatal.

During the 1930's, a number of studies on the epidemiology of tuberculosis in widely separated American communities revealed a high incidence of calcified nodules in the lungs of individuals whose tuberculin tests were negative. These findings began to cast doubt on the tuberculin test as an accurate indicator of previous infection with the tubercle bacillus.[50]

In 1941, the use of a filtrate of a broth culture of histoplasma as a skin test for sensitivity to the organism was recommended by Van Pernis, Benson, and Holinger.[51] This test was employed by Drs. A. Christie and J. C. Peterson, who tested a considerable group of individuals in the Nashville, Tennessee, area with this filtrate, called histoplasmin. They found a high incidence of positive histoplasmin tests in persons whose tuberculin tests were negative. These findings soon led to a nationwide project of skin testing of student nurses. In 1945 and 1946, the results of these tests were published.[52,53] The incidence of positive tests varied greatly in different areas of the United States. Equally important was the high degree of correlation shown between positive histoplasmin tests and pulmonary calcifications in persons reacting negatively to tuberculin.

As a result of these studies with histoplasmin, the existence of a widely spread benign subclinical form of histoplasmosis was established. As time went on, evidence of world-wide distribution was uncovered.

In a review of the published results of histoplasmin tests carried out in many regions of the world, Edwards and Billings found the highest reactor rates were in the central areas of the United States. There were also areas of high prevalence found in some parts of Central and South America. In Africa high rates were reported from the West Coast from Siberia to the Congo. In Southeast Asia rates up to 30 per cent positive had been found. In Europe and the Mediterranean countries only small foci of infection appear to exist.[54]

*Occurrence*

Infection is common up to 80 per cent of the population in wide areas of the Americas, Europe, Africa, and the Far East. Histoplasmin sensitivity indicating previous infection is highly prevalent in eastern and central United States, infrequent in the Rocky Mountain region. The frequency of positive skin reactors increases in endemic areas from childhood to 30 years of age. Severe disease occurs at all ages, but is more common in infants and in older adults.

*The Infectious Agent*

*H. capsulatum* is a dimorphic fungus growing as a mold in the soil and as a yeast in animal and human hosts. In cultures, a filamentous growth occurs on Sabouraud's glucose agar at room temperature. At first, the growth is cottony and white, but becomes brown in older cultures. In early cultures, the branching molds bear small, round spores. As the cultures get older, the number of round to pear-shaped spores increases. These spores develop thick walls and become covered with small finger-like spikes.

The filamentous form usually can be converted to the yeast-like form by subculturing the branching forms on blood-agar slants, which are sealed and incubated at 37°C. Conversion of the yeast phase to the filamentous form is accomplished by dropping the temperature of the yeast phase cultures from 37 to 25°C.

*H. capsulatum* is killed at 55°C. for 15 min. and by exposure to 1 or 2 per cent formalin for 24 hr.

The filtrates of culture of the filamentous phase of *H. capsulatum* may be used to detect hypersensitiveness to the organism. The cultures are grown for two to four months in a synthetic medium to produce the material called histoplasmin.

A number of animals are susceptible to histoplasmosis. Spontaneous infections have been found in dogs, cats, cattle, horses, rats, mice, and skunks. In the laboratory, studies have been carried out in mice, hamsters, guinea pigs, and dogs.

*Pathogenesis*

The natural route of infection with *H. capsulatum* is thought to be the respiratory tract. The inhaled histoplasma spore lodges in the terminal bronchioles and air sacs of the lungs. Careful studies on mice infected by inhalation indicate that the spores are first surrounded by polymorphonuclear leukocytes. These are replaced within two to three days by epithelioid and macrophage cells. The walls of the spores gradually break down and yeast-like histoplasma forms appear. By the end of one week, a considerable exudate has appeared, clogging a number of air sacs. The phagocytic cells engulf the histoplasma organisms. These inflammatory areas may be numerous, scattered throughout the lungs, if the infective dose has been large. By one month, the acute reaction has subsided. Epithelioid cells become predominant. There is neither necrosis nor fibrosis. Over a period of two to four months, the lesions gradually disappear.

In mice, the yeast form is disseminated early, about the fourth day after infection, by the blood stream to all parts of the body, setting up inflammatory foci in spleen, liver, and other organs. The animal may succumb to this acute generalized infection.

In the human, the primary infection in the lung begins as in the mouse, but proceeds on usually to necrosis. These necrotic foci become caseated and later calcified very much in the same manner as in tuberculosis. The large lymph nodes around the large bronchi and trachea also become inflamed and this process goes on to calcification. In rare cases, the infection becomes disseminated in the primary stage, going on to a severe, acute, generalized histoplasmosis which may terminate fatally. Usually, the primary infection subsides completely, leaving calcified nodules in the lungs and in the regional lymph glands. Probably organisms remain viable in the healed lesions for long periods of time.

It is not known whether reinfection plays a significant role in the causation of chronic histoplasmosis. People living in endemic areas do have abundant opportunity to become reinfected.[50]

*Clinical Manifestations*

Approximately 60 per cent of those who become infected with *H. capsulatum* recognize no symptoms due to the process. Many of these individuals show calcified nodules in the lungs and lymph glands. Others do manifest signs of illness in the primary stage.

In the primary acute form, the symptoms are of varying severity, running from a mild influenza-like illness lasting for one or two days to extremely serious bouts of pneumonia-like symptoms lasting sometimes for two months. It appears that the degree of illness depends upon the resistance of the host and the size of the infecting dose of histoplasma. The illness is characterized by cough, shortness of breath, chest pain due to pleurisy, fever, chills, muscle aches, and loss of weight. The infection may be generalized as shown by calcified areas in the spleen and by the occasional isolation of *H. capsulatum* from the urine. X-ray examination of the lungs usually shows a nodular type of reaction, but pulmonary infiltration is sometimes seen.

In many patients, the lesions resolve completely, but in others, calcification or fibrotic scarring persists. A distinctive residue of primary infection is the solitary nodule, called the histoplasmoma, which is frequently mistaken for lung cancer or tuberculosis. Severe disseminated forms of histoplasmosis are rare. Illness may be characterized by enlargement of liver and spleen, fever, anemia, and loss of weight. Pulmonary symptoms may be of little importance. This form of the disease is found most commonly among the very young or the very old. The patient may recover, may proceed to a rapidly fatal outcome, or may linger on to suffer from the chronic form of the disease. Chronic histoplasmosis may go on for years. It is usually found in adults and in individuals suffering from other diseases. The course of chronic disseminated histoplasmosis is quite varied. The bone marrow may be destroyed, producing leukemia-like symptoms. The adrenal glands are frequently severely damaged and other organs may be involved. The disease is usually fatal.

The chronic cavitary form of histoplasmosis closely resembles and is frequently mistaken for pulmonary tuberculosis. The diagnosis must be made by isolation of *H. capsulatum* from the sputum. In cases in which no tubercle bacillus can be found, serological tests may indicate histoplasmosis.[48,55]

*Epidemiology*

Histoplasmosis is not a contagious disease in terms of being spread from person to person or from animals to humans. It is considered to be a disease of nature, peculiarly localized in certain regions and spread to humans by inhalation of spores of the fungus in dust from contaminated soil. The incubation period in reports of groups with a known exposure time is from 5 to 18 days.

Fungi are known to produce spores in profuse quantities during their growth phases. These spores are extremely persistent organisms and resistant to heat or drying. They are viable for long periods of time.

The mycelial phase of *H. capsulatum* is also highly resistant to drying, heat, and other unfavorable factors in the environment.

In 1949, Emmons isolated *H. capsulatum* from soil around a rodent burrow under a chicken coop.[56] A few years later, Zeidberg[57] called attention to the frequency of isolation of the organism from soil taken from chicken yards or around chicken houses. No naturally infected chickens have been found, and the chicken is not susceptible to progressive experimental infection. All the known evidence points to the soil as the reservoir of the fungus.

For many years, it has been known that persons get peculiar fevers from exploring certain caves. Sometimes whole groups of cave explorers come down almost simultaneously with the fever, now recognized as histoplasmosis. Histoplasma organisms have been repeatedly isolated from soil collected from cave floors. It is thought that the fungus grows in the soil enriched by the droppings of birds or bats in these locations.

Other outbreaks of histoplasmosis have been discovered among children who play in parks where starlings roost in the trees in large numbers.

From currently available evidence, it appears that the droppings of chickens, pigeons, other birds, and bats provide an enrichment of the soil in climatic areas favorable to growth of *H. capsulatum* that enable it to flourish. Infections of man and other animals are dead-end routes for the parasite and have no, or only a slight, importance in its life cycle.[58]

The Center for Disease Control in Atlanta, Georgia, began a cooperative study of fungal diseases in 1958. The states are cooperating. Histoplasmosis has accounted for the largest number of cases (937) in the study through 1971. Reported deaths have averaged about 64 each year in the period 1965-1969.

An illuminating outbreak of histoplasmosis occurred in a junior high school in Delaware, Ohio, in 1970. As an "Earth Day" activity students decided to clean up the school's courtyard, an old roosting place for starlings and blackbirds. The raking and sweeping stirred up clouds of dust containing masses of histoplasma spores. The entire school building was contaminated with courtyard air through the forced air ventilation system with intakes in the courtyard. Three hundred and eighty-four (40 per cent) of the exposed students became ill and probably an equal number had subclinical infections.[59]

The reasons for the peculiar geographical distribution of *H. capsulatum* are not understood[60] (see Fig. (6.8). It may be related to soil conditions, as well as climatic factors. A similarly sharply demarcated geographical distribution has been found for *Coccidioides immitis,* another fungus disease, in California and the Southwest.

*Diagnosis*

Isolation and identification of the fungus in culture are the most convincing methods of diagnosis. In primary cases, sputum and urine should be cultured. In disseminated forms, blood, bone marrow, lymph gland or liver tissue obtained by biopsy, urine, sputum, cerebrospinal fluid may be positive for histoplasma.

In addition to cultures, inoculation of mice with human material is a valuable method for isolation of the organisms.

Conversion of the skin test from negative to positive and a rise in complement-fixing antibodies may give support to the clinical diag-

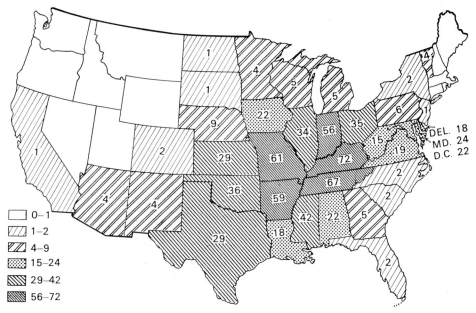

Fig. 6.8. Provisional estimates of the percentage of U. S. Navy recruits infected with histoplasma among lifetime residents of each state. Source: Edwards, P. Q. and Palmer, C. E. Nationwide histoplasmin sensitivity and histoplasma infection. *Public Health Rep.,* 78: 241-259, 1963.

nosis. In some cases both the skin test and the antibody test are negative in the presence of severe histoplasmosis. Careful microscopic examination of properly stained tissue sections may show fungal forms characteristic of histoplasma and give additional support to the diagnosis.

*Treatment*

In benign primary lung lesions, bed rest, a good diet, and general supportive treatment may be all that is required to restore the individual to health. In disseminated and severe cases, antifungal agents should be employed. Amphotericin B is considered to be the most active agent now available. It is given intravenously in dilute form over a period of 6 hr. In seriously ill patients, the drug is given daily. As treatment progresses, three times per week is usually adequate. Some patients experience rather severe side effects, and the treatment sometimes has to be discontinued. On the whole, results have been favorable, better in the disseminated form than in the chronic cavity cases.[61]

A newer polypeptide drug, Saramycetin X-5079C, has been introduced for treatment of histoplasmosis in humans. It is administered daily by the subcutaneous route. This drug is well tolerated.[62] It appears to be effective in some patients in whom amphotericin B has failed.

Surgery has been beneficial in a few cases with localized pulmonary diseases. This is carried out after a period of chemotherapy.

*Prognosis*

Except in the localized outbreaks in which large numbers of organisms are inhaled, acute primary histoplasmosis is almost always a benign infection. The infection threatens life in less than one in 1000 infections.

Severe disseminated disease is fatal in 80 to 90 per cent of the cases and the chronic cavitary form in 30 per cent of cases without specific chemotherapy. Adequate treatment has reduced these fatalities.

*Control*

There are no effective methods to control the spread of histoplasma infection. As yet no safe and effective vaccine has been developed.

Education of the public as to the dangers involved in cleaning chicken coops and pigeon roosts and in stirring up dust in caves that serve as bat or bird shelters is warranted, but not likely to be an effective deterrent. Attempts to discover effective antifungal chemicals to sterilize the soil in such infected spots are being pushed.

## DEGENERATIVE DISEASES

### Cerebrovascular Disease

*Introduction*

Vascular lesions of the central nervous system rank third in the United States among all causes of death. In 1972, there were 210,050 deaths from stroke, representing a death rate of 100.9 per 100,000 of the United States population (estimated figures). Almost 40,000 of the deaths from stroke were of persons under 65 years of age but, to a great extent, stroke is a disease of the aged.

Unlike heart disease and cancer, stroke attacks females more often than males in the United States (107.9 to 96.3 per 100,000 in 1967).

Non-white females have the highest stroke death rate. The mortality rates for non-white men and women for 1966 under 65 years of age were 47.6 and 45 per 100,000, whereas they were only 19.4 and 15.0 for white males and females of this age. The highest stroke rates occur in the southeastern states and the lowest in the southwestern and mountain regions.

It is estimated that at least 2 million persons now alive in the United States have suffered a stroke. About eight out of every 10 stroke victims survive the acute phase of the attack. Many live for years afterward, but usually in a seriously disabled state. Stroke victims make up 16 per cent of the patients in skilled nursing homes.[63] Stroke is a disease of the elderly—about three-fourths of all deaths due to strokes are reported in individuals of 70 years of age or older.

For many years, stroke has been a badly neglected disease. A mounting interest during recent years has begun to change the outlook for stroke patients. The disease is now considered neither inevitable nor irremediable. Many stroke attacks can be forseen. Some three of four patients with occlusive stroke have symptoms that forewarn of a disabling attack.

Some of the warning signs are brief occurrences of loss of speech, weakness of limbs, and staggering or loss of consciousness. In some of these patients, surgery to improve the blood flow to the brain may prevent stroke. The use of anticoagulant drugs might be beneficial in other such persons.

Much too little has been learned about restoration of function to stroke patients by rehabilitation procedures. Such programs, if started early enough and carried through, can make the difference between total dependence and self-sufficiency for many patients.

Perhaps more hopeful is the intensive research program now being undertaken in dozens of centers to determine means to prevent the underlying deterioration of the cerebrovascular system that leads to stroke and to develop more effective methods of therapy.

In general, strokes may be divided into three main types: (1) occlusion of a cerebral vessel by a thrombus or clotting of blood; (2) occlusion of a cerebral vessel by an embolus, a fragment of a clot broken off in the heart or vessels of the neck, thus plugging up the vessel in the brain; and (3) rupture of a cerebral vessel due to high blood pressure or a flaw in the vessel wall resulting in a pouching out to form a sac or aneurysm.

For general discussion, cerebrovascular disease can be divided into two groups: those producing ischemic cerebral infarction (tissue injury due to lack of blood), and those due to hemorrhage into the brain. In a series of 966 patients from Bellevue Hospital reported by McDowell,[64] 88 per cent of the patients had cerebral infarction while only 12 per cent were diagnosed as intracerebral hemorrhage. Of the infarctions, about one in eight was due to emboli.

*Pathogenesis*

The underlying pathological processes that lead to stroke have been summarized as follows:[64]

1. Severe atherosclerotic cerebrovascular disease involving the arteries in the neck, at the base of the brain, and in the brain that nourish the nervous tissue. This arterial disease may affect persons with normal or high blood pressure and may or may not be complicated by thrombosis.

2. Hypertensive intracerebral hemorrhage secondary to fibrinoid degeneration of small arteries or arterioles that weaken the walls of the vessels causing the formation of small aneurysms.

3. Embolic cerebrovascular disease, secondary to old rheumatic heart disease, or atherosclerotic disease of the coronary arteries of the heart or atherosclerotic thrombosis in major arteries, supplying the brain with fragments breaking off to form emboli.

4. Ruptured saccular aneurysms usually producing subarachnoid hemorrhage.

Atheromatous vascular disease begins early in life. It is a silent process until the middle years, when signs of disease of heart, brain, or lower extremities may appear. Portmortem studies show that from 80 to 90 per cent of all patients in older age groups examined at autopsy have significant atheromatous disease. A considerable proportion of people have anomalies in the arteries supplying the brain. These anomalous arteries appear to increase the chance of stroke in those also having atheromatous disease.

Other factors related to the occurrence of strokes are diabetes and high blood pressure. These two conditions can be detected in at least two-thirds of patients who develop overt cerebrovascular disease. Either diabetes or hypertension in an individual tends to bring on cerebral attacks earlier and the process proceeds more rapidly.

Inflammatory conditions in the cerebral arteries are another cause of cerebral accidents. Inflammation causes thickening of arterial walls, reducing the blood-carrying capacity. Syphilis was a common cause of such arterial disease in years past, but is less frequent now that adequate treatment is available. Rarely, bacteria are the cause of inflammation of the arteries. Generalized disease of the collagen tissues may affect the cerebral vessels.

Cerebral emboli may occur even with a normal arterial system. In persons under 50 years of age, rheumatic heart disease is the most common source of these emboli which break off from the heart valves and plug up small arteries in the brain causing death of tissues, *i.e.,* an infarction. Other sources of emboli in the brain are pulmonary infections and atheromatous plaques in the major arteries between heart and brain.

Alterations in blood-clotting time are thought to play some role in the blocking of cerebral vessels. Hypercoagulability has been described in some patients with cerebral infarctions.

The brain tissue is highly sensitive to its

oxygen supply. When oxygen deprivation occurs, irreversible and extensive damage to nerve cells may be expected after 3 to 10 min. A variable amount of swelling or edema accompanies cerebral infarction. If this swelling is extensive enough, it may prove fatal.

*Classification of Strokes*

Strokes are classified on the basis of the anatomical site of the lesion and on the time sequence of the symptoms. In relation to time, several types of attack occur.

The transient attack or incipient stroke includes short episodes of brain dysfunction due to cerebrovascular disease. The episodes are fleeting 5- to 30-min. attacks that leave no permanent disabilities. It is believed this form of "little stroke" is due to a temporary lack of blood or ischemia in the brain area affected, perhaps due to a spasm of the arterial wall.

A more serious condition is progressive stroke found in patients who develop increasing neurological dysfunction due to cerebral ischemia for periods of minutes, hours, or rarely, for days. This evolving stroke is characterized by the gradual development of paralysis and sensory losses over a period of hours.

A stroke may be designated as completed in patients showing no further progression in neurological dysfunction or in those whose earlier brain damage has begun to improve.

The artery affected determines the characteristic set of symptoms. For example, infarctions in the brain stem produce a wide variety of symptoms including dizziness, double vision, difficulty in swallowing, and clumsiness. When the middle cerebral artery is occluded, infarction occurs in the lateral portion of the cerebrum and produces muscle weakness and sensory loss of the opposite side of the body, mainly in the face, arm, and hand. The distribution and severity of these symptoms are quite variable.

Examination of the patient usually reveals evidence of vascular disease at other sites. About one-fifth of patients give a history of a previous attack of coronary artery disease. Twenty per cent of the patients have diabetes, and over one-half of them have serious hypertension. A few report occlusive disease of arteries of the legs.

Laboratory examinations may reveal blood in the cerebrospinal fluid. If much blood is present, the finding is indicative of intracerebral

hemorrhages. Spinal puncture must be undertaken with caution, as the intracranial pressure may be high and damage to vital centers results.

X-ray examination of the skull is useful to discover signs of fracture or head injury.

The electroencephalogram (EEG) may be useful in distinguishing the type and location of the brain injury.

Cerebral angiography has two main values for studying patients with cerebrovascular disease. First, it helps to rule out such conditions as brain tumor or subdural hemorrhage which can be relieved by surgery. The second important value of angiography is to demonstrate clearly the site, extent, and incidence of arterial obstructions that might be improved by surgery. This diagnostic procedure is somewhat hazardous and must not be undertaken lightly.

*Course and Prognosis*

Some improvement in function usually follows almost every infarction of the brain. When function improves rapidly after the onset, the chance for recovery is good. A slow return of recovery over a period of weeks indicates a less favorable outlook. With large infarctions, the patient may get steadily worse because of edema and swelling of the brain.

About 20 to 25 per cent of patients with cerebral infarction die in the first attack. The mortality rate rises sharply with age; nearly half of the patients 70 years and over die in the first attack.

*Intracranial Hemorrhage*

Hemorrhage accounts for about 10 per cent of all cerebral vascular accidents. The physician can only suspect the diagnosis which must be confirmed by finding blood in the cerebrospinal fluid or by demonstration of a blood clot at surgery. Bleeding may (1) take place from vessels on the surface of the brain and be limited to the space beneath the arachnoid membranes (subarachnoid hemorrhage); (2) take place from surface vessels with intracerebral extension injuring proximal brain tissue by the force of the hemorrhage; (3) take place from ruptured vessels within the substance of the brain or intracerebral hemorrhage; and (4) extend through brain tissue to the ventricles or subarachnoid space, causing signs and symptoms of both intracerebral and subarachnoid hemorrhages.

Most intracranial hemorrhages are from ruptured arteries, although veins may also bleed. The usual rupture is through a small aneurysm which probably develops in congenitally defective arteries. Most of these small aneurysms develop in arteries at the base of the brain. Such hemorrhages are more frequent in hypertensive patients.

In atheromatous patients with hypertension, there is often a degeneration of cerebral arteries, especially of the middle cerebral artery which has been designated as "the artery of cerebral hemorrhage."

Leukemia, thrombocytopenia, and long periods of anticoagulant drugs all predispose to intracranial bleeding.

Subarachnoid hemorrhage may cause rapid rise in intracranial pressure and a fatal outcome. Moreover, the blood, as it deteriorates, acts as an inrritant, causing symptoms and tissue damage. The onset of violent headache is sudden. The headache is generalized and may spread to the neck and back area. The patient may also experience dizziness, vomiting, stupor, and loss of consciousness. If bleeding is minor, consciousness may be regained in a few hours; if extensive, the patient may remain in coma until death ensues.

Subarachnoid hemorrhage is serious, with a mortality rate of about 45 per cent.

### Treatment

In the acute phase, the objectives of treatment are to preserve life, limit brain damage, lessen disability, and prevent recurrence. Maintenance of adequate respiratory function is essential. In comatose patients, tracheotomy may be necessary for this purpose. Fluid and electrolyte balance should be preserved. During the first one or two days, fluids may have to be given intravenously. Food may have to be given through a nasogastric tube. Catheterization may be necessary to prevent distention of the urinary bladder. Enemas are indicated, if bowel movements do not occur naturally.

Care of the skin is of great importance to prevent pressure sores.

If headache is severe, codeine or other drugs may be required for relief. Sedation may be necessary in hyperactive or delirious patients.

Reserpine or other antihypertensive drugs should be used to reduce excessively high blood pressure.

Physical therapy should be started within a few days after stroke to prevent development of contractures. If muscle spasticity develops, hot packs to promote relaxation may be of value.

The use of anticoagulants is not indicated in the acute phase of most stroke cases. Some physicians do advocate their use in selected cases, and the subject is still under investigation. Surgery in the acute state of stroke has been disappointing in the results yielded.

When the critical condition of the patient has passed and he has recovered consciousness. an evaluation of his status should be untertaken. If the patient has been in bed for any length of time, a series of disabilities may be expected. These are: (1) loss of mobility, (2) loss of muscle strength and coordination, (3) circulatory weakness, (4) metabolic disturbances, (5) deterioration of urinary function, (6) respiratory inadequacy, (7) skin ulcerations, and (8) intellectual and emotional disturbances.[65] In addition, there may be defects in vision and in speech. If the patient has multiple impairments, arrangements for care in a rehabilitation center are preferable.

### Rehabilitation

The aim of rehabilitation programs is to retrain the remaining functions for maximum effectiveness. The program begins by increasing the patient's tolerance to sitting and standing. Daily active and passive exercises of weakened extremities are carried out. Sometimes leg braces are required. One of the main goals of rehabilitation is to get the patient walking again. At the same time, he should be trained to develop new skills with the affected arm. Speech therapy is helpful to those with mild to moderate dysphasia. Occupational therapy and vocational rehabilitation are important.[66] Emotional disturbances are common among stroke victims. Frequently consultations with competent psychiatrists and psychologists are helpful in correcting the underlying emotional problems. To give the patient a hopeful outlook on his condition is of real importance in promoting his recovery.

Usually the maximum effect in restoring the patient's functions is achieved in six to eight months, but occasional patients continue to show gains up to 24 months.

Rehabilitation is begun and continued in the hospital, but must be continued in a nursing home, in the patient's home, or, in the case of patients with multiple impairments, in special rehabilitation centers. Visiting nurses, public health nurses, and various categories of rehabilitation personnel are available for home care in many communities. Outpatient rehabilitation facilities are being developed in many urban areas.

It is recognized that there are numerous communities in the United States in which rehabilitation facilities are unavailable or entirely inadequate. More and more public health departments are undertaking the responsibility to discover patients who need such services and to arrange that these services should be made available to them.

In North Carolina a Comprehensive Stroke Program has been organized to increase the opportunities for the stroke patient to receive early, high quality, and continued care. Over 915,000 people reside in the 19 counties included in the stroke program. Each county public health agency is involved in follow-up care of patients. Twenty-two hospitals and 9 nursing homes are enrolled in the program. The 1005 personnel have received special training in problems of stroke patients.[67]

*Epidemiology*

A number of epidemiological investigations have been undertaken on cerebrovascular diseases in recent years. Although data are still rather scarce, there appears to be general agreement that the incidence rate of stroke in the United States is around 1.5 per 1000 of population per year. The rate is generally negligible prior to age 45 years and rises steeply with age thereafter. For persons below 85 years, the rates were slightly higher in men than women. Above 85 years, the rate was considerably higher in women.[68]

Apparently the key to the stroke problem is the closely intertwining conditions of hypertension and atherosclerotic disease. A better understanding of stroke depends upon research on these basic pathological processes.

Studies to date point out certain risk factors that predispose to cerebrovascular disease. These include a hereditary tendency to stroke that runs in some families. Other factors are hypertension, diabetes, high blood cholesterol levels, overweight, heavy cigarette smoking, and abnormal electrocardiogram readings. Screening

for these abnormalities makes it possible to identify stroke victims before they actually have an attack.[64]

A study during a two-year period, 1969-1971, of women between 15 and 44 years of age with stroke, compared to a control group matched for age, race, and residence, showed a considerable increase in the incidence of strokes due to thrombosis of cerebral vessels among the women using oral contraceptives. There was a smaller increase of stroke due to hemorrhage in the brain among the women taking oral contraceptives. Indications are that the risk of thrombotic stroke is related to the estrogen content of oral contraceptives.[69]

*Prevention*

It is not certain whether it is possible to reverse the tendency toward cerebrovascular disease among the high risk group. Control of blood pressure through antihypertensive drugs, lowering the blood cholesterol level by dietary regimes, an active program of physical exercise, control of diabetes by diet and insulin, giving up smoking, and leading a nonstressful life may prevent or at least postpone stroke attacks.

In the prevention of recurrent attacks in persons with transient ischemia, or who have recovered from cerebral infarction, two methods have been used extensively: (1) anticoagulation therapy, and (2) surgical correction of arterial obstruction. Good results have been claimed for both methods, but carefully controlled series of patients have not yet been evaluated.[70]

## Coronary Heart Disease

*Introduction*

Cerebrovascular disease, coronary heart disease, and hypertensive disease are so closely related and their etiologies are intertwined in such a complex manner that it is difficult to consider one apart from the other. While the fundamental pathology of the arterial diseases may be almost identical, epidemiological differences set them apart. Cerebrovascular disease has been commonly recognized for a long time in the western world; on the other hand, deaths from coronary heart disease were rarely diagnosed at the beginning of the 20th century, but have occurred with great frequency during the past three to four decades. There is a much higher attack rate of coronary disease among men in comparison with women which is not seen in cerebrovascular disease. There are also striking differences in international figures; for example, cerebral hemorrhage is common in Japan, but coronary disease is not.[71]

Atherosclerosis is the result of focal accumulation of certain fatty proteins in the form of plaques in the inner lining of the larger and medium-sized arteries (see Fig. 6.9). The fatty compounds involved include cholesterol, cholesterol esters, phospholipids, and neutral fat. Other biological materials are also deposited in these plaques such as carbohydrates, blood, blood products, calcium, and fibrin. As deposition of materials in the inner arterial walls continues over the years, the arterial lumen is diminished and blood flow to vital tissues is reduced. Complete blocking of an artery usually results from a secondary process superimposed upon the underlying atherosclerosis. Most occlusions result either from hemorrhage into a sclerotic plaque or the formation of a thrombus or blood clot. Arteries in any part of the body may be affected. The symptoms that result from insufficiency of blood supply depend upon which organs are involved. When the brain is deprived of adequate blood, the symptoms are usually those of cerebral deterioration. Stroke is the most dramatic manifestation of arterial disease affecting the brain (see Figs. 6.10 and 6.11).

When atherosclerosis affects the coronary arteries, the heart muscle, or myocardium, may have its normal blood supply greatly reduced (see Fig. 6.12). If this ischemia of heart muscle occurs suddenly, the muscle fibers can no longer survive in the area affected. This is termed a cardiac infarction. If a large branch of the coronary arterial system is thus blocked by thrombus or embolus, the resultant muscle damage may be the cause of sudden death. Intermittent narrowing of the coronary arteries may cause a temporary acute pain known as angina pectoris. The pain of angina pectoris appears in paroxysms, rather suddenly. It may be mild or moderately severe, but seldom of the intensity that characterizes myocardial infarction. Anginal pain usually subsides within 1 to 5 min. Most patients with angina pectoris experience pain only occasionally, during some unusual exertion or emotional strain. The pain is most often located over the area of the heart, but may also radiate to the left shoulder and

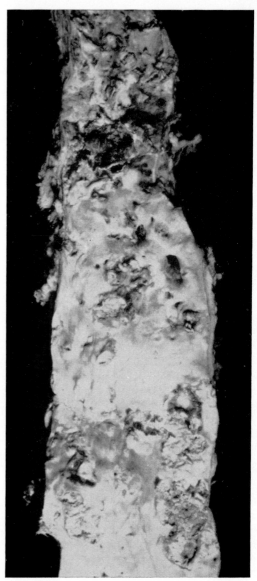

Fig. 6.9. Atherosclerosis of the aorta. The irregular plaques contain much lipid. The glint of the cholesterol crystals is just visible in the photograph. From an obese, hypertensive man of 65 years who died of acute myocardial infarction. The atherosclerosis of the aorta is therefore, an incidental finding at autopsy. Source: Baker, Roger D. Local metabolic, histochemical and nutritional lesions. In *Essential Pathology*. Baltimore: The Williams and Wilkins Co., 1961, p. 45.

arm. Relief of pain may occur spontaneously with rest or rapidly after administration of nitroglycerin.

The pain of angina pectoris is generally considered to arise from the heart muscle and not in the diseased coronary arteries. The essential condition is too little oxygen supplied to the muscle as a result of coronary narrowing. Myocardial infarction is quite likely to occur in angina pectoris patients or they may develop heart failure as an eventual result of repeated injuries to heart muscle.

In early stages of angina pectoris, electrocardiograms may be normal. Diagnosis can be made by the history and the relief of pain by nitroglycerine.[72]

Most coronary infarctions are associated with sudden, intense pain in the heart area that is unremitting. About one-fifth of all cardiac infarctions occur without major symptoms and are usually diagnosed only by electrocardio-

grams and laboratory tests for myocardial necrosis.

Some persons suffer from coronary insufficiency that produces neither clear-cut infarctions nor definite bouts of angina pectoris (see Fig. 6.13). Pain may be persistent, relieved partially, if at all, by coronary vasodilator drugs. Transient electrocardiographic changes may be observed, but not the definite infarction tracings. Serious irregularities of rhythm, congestive heart failure, and death may result.

*Pathogenesis*

An increased risk of death from arteriosclerotic heart disease has been associated with obesity, hypertension, high serum cholesterol, high intake of saturated fats in the diet, cigarette smoking, lack of exercise, and stressful living situations. Persons with diabetes, gout, familial hypercholesterolemia, familial hyperlipemia, or a strong family history of premature coronary disease are regarded as having a high risk of dying from heart disease.

It would appear that arteriosclerotic heart disease has a multiple causation; preventive measures are now directed mainly toward a modification of diet in an effort to reduce blood cholesterol levels and at increasing physical exercise.[73]

Atherosclerosis, by itself, reduces blood flow, but rarely causes a complete occlusion of an artery (see Fig. 6.14). This reduction of blood supply stimulates a dilation of nearby blood vessels, setting up a collateral circulation, which may provide adequate blood to the affected area if the diseased artery should later become occluded. If the occlusion occurs suddenly,

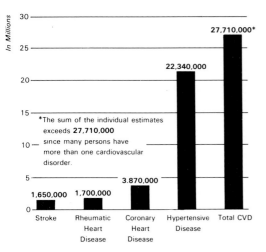

Fig. 6.10. Estimated prevalence of the major cardiovascular diseases, United States, 1971. (Redrawn from *Heart Facts–1974*. The American Heart Association, New York, 1974.)

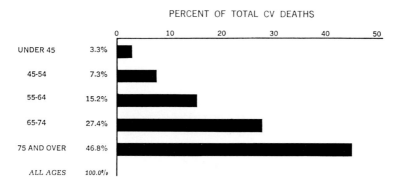

Fig. 6.11. Percentage breakdown of total cardiovascular deaths by age group, 1962. Source: *Cardiovascular Diseases in the U. S.: Facts and Figures.* New York: American Heart Association, 1965.

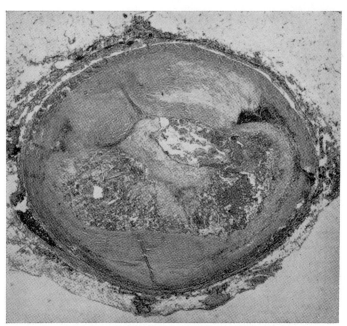

Fig. 6.12. Coronary arteriosclerosis, hemorrhage into atheroma and thrombosis. From a hypertensive white man of 57 years who died suddenly while in conference. At autopsy, hypertrophied heart, severe atherosclerosis of coronaries. Hemorrhage into the wall several weeks previously is indicated by the hemosiderin in upper right segment of artery; recent hemorrhage below. Thrombus in lumen, of several days duration. Source: Baker, Roger D. The cardiovascular system. In *Essential Pathology*. Baltimore: The Williams and Wilkins Co., 1961, p. 324.

however, time is lacking for the development of a collateral blood supply and an infarction of the muscle results.

Following a large cardiac infarction, if the patient survives, the damaged muscle is gradually replaced by scar tissue (see Fig. 6.15). This scar tissue in the heart wall represents a weakened area that may rupture leading to sudden death at some future date. Small infarctions may heal completely and are not incompatible with many years of active life.

*Occurrence*

Mortality from coronary heart disease varies widely in its distribution around the world. The frequency is low in Japan, Italy, and Yugoslavia and among the black population in South Africa. Rates are high in the United States, England, Netherlands, Finland, among the white population of South Africa, and among Japanese and Italians living in the United States.[36]

A National Health Survey report[74] covering the period of 1960 to 1962 estimates that, among adults aged 18 to 79 years in the United States, 3.1 million had definite coronary heart disease and 2.4 million others had suspected coronary heart disease. More than 1.5 million had definite angina pectoris and more than 2.3 million had suspect angina pectoris. A total of 1.4 million had experienced myocardial infarction.

Only 8 per cent of individuals with clinically manifest coronary heart disease are found under 45 years of age, but, in general, up to 75 years, prevalence increases strictly with age (see Fig. 6.16). By 65 to 74 years of age, 15.4 per cent of all persons have some form of coronary heart disease.

It is estimated that arteriosclerotic heart disease develops in 1 per cent of the population annually. The average middle-aged male has one chance in five of developing arteriosclerotic heart disease before he is 65, and one chance in 15 of dying from it.[75] Deaths from arteriosclerotic heart disease, including coronary disease, have continued to increase in the United States (see Table 6.11).

Six hundred and seventy-five thousand deaths from coronary heart disease were reported in the United States in 1971 (provisional figures).

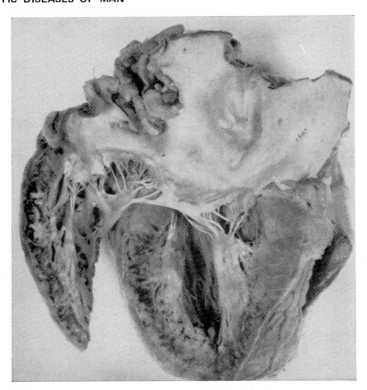

Fig. 6.13. Ischemic necrosis of the left ventricle of the heart due to obstruction of the coronary artery (recent myocardial infarct). The lesion is softer than normal, and mottled yellow and red. From a woman of 60 years with severe, continuing, substernal pain, vomiting and leukocytosis, beginning 10 days before death. The white scarring of the large papillary muscle is an earlier infarct. Source: Baker, Roger D. Necrosis. In *Essential Pathology*. Baltimore: The Williams and Wilkins Co., 1961, p. 31.

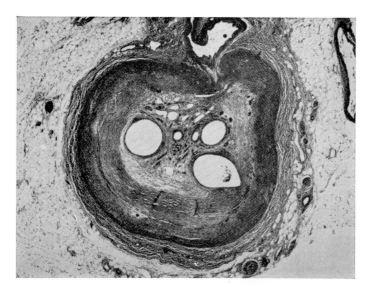

Fig. 6.14. Recanalized thrombus of artery. New channels are seen in the organized thrombus of many years duration. The vessel also has much arteriosclerosis with fibrous thickening of the intima. Source: Baker, Roger D. Fluid and blood vascular disturbances. In *Essential Pathology*. Baltimore: The Williams and Wilkins Co., 1961, p. 85.

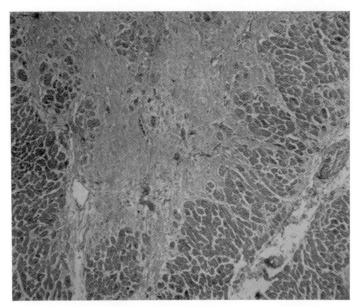

Fig. 6.15. Myocardial scar of healed infarct. Source: Baker, Roger D. The cardiovascular system. In *Essential Pathology*. Baltimore: The Williams and Wilkins Co., 1961, p. 330.

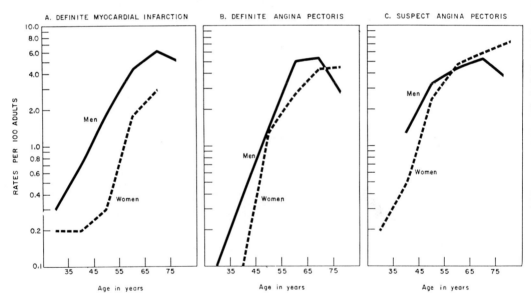

Fig. 6.16. *A,* prevalence of definite myocardial infarction in adults, by sex, and age. *B,* prevalence of definite angina pectoris in adults, by sex and age. *C,* prevalence of suspect angina pectoria in adults, by sex and age. Source: *Coronary Heart Disease in Adults, U. S., 1960-1962,* Public Health Service Publication 1000, series 11, no. 10. Washington, D. C.: National Center for Health Statistics, 1965.

This is more than a third of all deaths for that year (34.1 per cent). In younger age groups (25-44 years) most deaths from this disease are among males. Then the rate of increase among males begins to slow. The rate of increase for white females is nearly constant throughout the age range 25 to 84 years.[36]

*Diagnosis*

There are no effective screening tests for early atherosclerosis. Diagnosis is only made after the appearance of a typical manifestation of the underlying disease process. Arteriosclerotic heart disease is often detected on the basis of the occurrence of angina pectoris. In asymptomatic persons, electrocardiographic evidence of myocardial hypoxia or of a prior small myocardial infarction may lead to the diagnosis. An exercise tolerance test with the electrocardiogram showing any changes due to exercise may reveal signs of coronary insufficiency. Definite myocardial infarction is diagnosed by symptoms and is confirmed by electrocardiogram and by demonstration of elevation of serum glutamic oxaloacetic transaminase (SGOT), lactic dehydrogenase (LDH), or serum creatinine phosphokinase (CPK).

Even with the aid of these confirmatory tests, postmortem examinations reveal a substantial number of incorrect clinical diagnoses.[76]

*Treatment*

While not definitely established, there are suggestions that atherosclerosis may be a reversible process. The levels of blood cholesterol and lipids are responsive to a reduction of intake of cholesterol and saturated fat. Other major coronary risk factors, hypertension, diabetes, overweight, cigarette smoking, and physical inactivity, are subject to control by modification of living patterns and by medical supervision.[77]

Attacks of angina pectoris respond as a rule to rest and coronary vasodilators. Sedatives or tranquilizers are helpful in some cases. Surgical procedures to improve coronary circulation are recommended by some advocates, but have not been generally accepted.

Treatment of acute myocardial infarction is carried out whenever possible in special intensive care units. Rest, narcotics for pain, anticoagulants (unless contraindicated), oxygen, and sedatives are used. Electrical and mechanical devices to regulate cardiac arrhythmias and to maintain heart action are used as indicated. Digitalis may be required in event of congestive heart failure.

*Prognosis*

During the acute attack, the outcome is often unpredictable because of possible fatal complications which usually occur in the first few days. The first 24 hr. are the most hazardous as there is constantly a threat of sudden death from cardiac arrest, arrhythmias, shock, or pulmonary edema. If the symptoms subside, as the days go by, the prognosis becomes more favorable.

The outlook for patients with coronary heart disease is variable. In general, patients experience slow progression of symptoms of ischemia and eventually succumb to myocardial infarction or congestive heart failure.

The overall mortality in the first attack of myocardial infarction is around 30 per cent; with subsequent attacks, the percentage increases. Of those patients who survive one month after acute myocardial infarctions, nearly one-half survive five years; of those who recover from symptoms completely, 85 per cent are alive after five years.[75]

*Rehabilitation*

As soon as acute symptoms of myocardial infarction have subsided, measures to restore

TABLE 6.11

*Mortality and prevalence figures for rheumatic, hypertensive, and ischemic heart disease: United States, 1969*

| Heart Diseases | Deaths | Prevalence |
|---|---|---|
| Rheumatic heart disease | 15,432 | 1,670,000 |
| Hypertensive heart disease | 24,712 | 21,790,000 |
| Ischemic heart disease | 669,829 | 4,040,000 |

Source:  Table C, page 6, National Center for Health Statistics: Vital Statistics of the United States, 1969, Vol. II, DHEW Publication No. (HSM) 72-1101, Health Services and Mental Health Administration, Washington, D.C., U.S. Govt. Printing Office, 1972.

the patient to active life should be initiated. The physician is responsible for determining the rate at which the patient can undertake physical activity. The patient is usually kept in bed for two to six weeks. As soon as shock has cleared up, free movement in bed is encouraged. Simple exercises with feet and legs to promote venous return are helpful. The use of a bedside commode may be allowed. Use of a chair, meals out of bed, and standing by the bed may be permitted within two weeks after onset of illness. Careful evaluation of the cardiac status and work capacity is necessary in planning rehabilitation following convalescence from the cardiac attack. Special centers with a well-rounded staff representing all of the necessary specialties are most useful in caring for the convalescent experience in cardiac patients.

About 50 per cent of employed patients are able to return to work. In some cases the work load has to be modified to fit the capacity of the convalescent individual.

*Prevention*

Epidemiological studies have demonstrated that atherosclerosis, the basic pathological process responsible for coronary heart disease, almost certainly depends upon environmental factors that are susceptible to change. Research is required to clarify the fundamental causes of atherosclerosis and to point out methods of preventing the disease and its thrombotic complications.

The investigations to date indicate that high serum cholesterol is a high risk factor for coronary heart disease. These levels occur in individuals who habitually eat diets high in calories, total fat, saturated fat, and cholesterol. Modifications of this diet to reduce total calories, to decrease fat consumption, and to increase unsaturated fats in relation to total fat in the diet are recommended. In many persons, such a diet will reduce body weight and lower the serum cholesterol level. The smoking of cigarettes should be reduced or stopped. Perhaps the most important aspect of prevention is the adoption of a physically active living regime. Periodic medical check-ups to detect hypertension or diabetes in the early stages are advisable.

In a recent study, 92 high school students were selected because they combined high blood levels of cholesterol, phospholipids, triglycerides, uric acid, glucose, elevated blood pressure, and relatively high body mass. Examination of the fathers of these students so selected revealed three-quarters with a history of coronary disease or with high blood pressure. This method of early identification of men in the middle-age group with high susceptibility to coronary disease may offer a promising screening device to discover high risk individuals.[78]

Evidence indicates that such a protective regime does lower the risk of clinically manifest coronary heart disease in those who follow the course over a period of years.[73] So far, the data on these preventive measures are limited in quantity. Health education to stimulate the public to modify its ways of life have so far met with only partial success.

To save life, coronary intensive care units should be developed in all major hospitals staffed by specially trained personnel and provided with the essential special equipment.

## IATROGENIC DISEASE

### Introduction

New techniques and new substances are introduced in medicine so rapidly that adequate testing of all of them would paralyze progress. Attempts to control new drugs point up this problem. In 1962, a new Food and Drug Act came into effect in the United States, greatly increasing the regulatory powers of the Food and Drug Administration. In January, 1963, the Administration issued a set of regulations instructing pharmaceutical manufacturers to submit detailed reports of all drugs currently in the course of being tested on human beings in the United States. Within 6 months, about 2500 reports had been submitted, each containing hundreds of pages of data. Sixty physicians were assigned to the review of these reports, each being responsible for evaluating more than 40 new drugs.[79] In the period between 1940 and 1971, almost 900 new single chemical entities were introduced to the United States market. A "single entity" is a unique compound in terms of chemical structure. It may be used as an active ingredient in a number of different pharmaceutical products.[80]

It has been estimated that only 20 out of every 3000 compounds tested by pharmaceutical companies are sufficiently active and nontoxic to permit human trials. Of these 20, only one is released for general clinical use. Only a very few of these released drugs produce unexpected responses in man. But some 3 per cent of drugs that pass all tests cause serious adverse reactions in man. These reactions are usually rare occurrences, developing no more than once in several thousand patients who are treated with the drug.[81,82]

Although tests on laboratory animals protect against most serious toxic reactions, such testing has definite limitations. It would be helpful to choose animals which resemble man in the way they handle the drug being tested. To choose the most appropriate animals for pharmacological examination of new drugs, information is required which can only be obtained by early tests of the drug on man. A few carefully planned, clinical pharmacological experiments on man are needed early in the development of a drug.

Recent experience with new drugs suggests that close surveillance of each new compound should be maintained for one to three years after its release. During this surveillance period, physicians should be encouraged to keep patients receiving the new drug under observation and to report unexpected effects to the Food and Drug Administration. Use of a drug in from 1000 to 5000 patients will supply enough information to exclude all but the rarest drug reactions. The very rare reaction can only be uncovered from groups as large as 150,000 patients. It was necessary to use Phenacetin for 75 years before it became suspect as a cause of renal disease, 30 years to realize that amidopyrine caused agranulocytosis, and 10 years to demonstrate that tetracyclines disturb bone development. This is good evidence that physicians do not quickly discover what they are not looking for.[82] Unfortunately, the theoretical basis of toxicology is not sufficiently developed to permit the prevention of all accidents by safety regulations, no matter how diligent are those who try to apply them. Indeed, it is the very nature of a drug to be toxic. Most drugs are utilized because they do have a valuable repressive action on some vital metabolic process in the body. This very toxicity is the most characteristic and useful property of the drug. Still the dosage of the drug must be such as to render the toxic property a selective one.[83,84]

The adverse responses to drugs may be due

to: (1) intolerance, (2) idiosyncrasy, (3) allergy, or (4) drug interactions. In a brief account of the subject, it is impossible to even touch upon all aspects of the problem. The conclusion of the Second International Pharmacology Congress which met in Prague in 1963 was that it must be recognized that laboratory tests cannot completely eliminate the risk involved in taking of drugs. Accidents due to toxic reactions in man will continue to occur as long as drugs are used.[85]

## Inherited Drug Intolerance

One of the most bizarre drug reactions is demonstrated by the relationship of barbiturates and other drugs to porphyria. This disease is a hereditary abnormality of porphyrin metabolism. It is inherited as a dominant trait, and the sexes are equally affected. Among the white settlers of South Africa, the disease is found in about three per 1000 of the population. Incidence is lower in others parts of the world. In those affected, the skin is more than usually subject to injuries on the exposed portions of the body. Wounds heal slowly. Excessive pigmentation of the face and hands is common. The taking of certain drugs triggers acute attacks in these people, characterized by abdominal pain, emotional disturbances, and even paralyses. The resulting mortality from these attacks is from 25 to 50 per cent. The drugs chiefly responsible for setting off these acute episodes of porphyria are the barbiturates, sulfonamides, and, sometimes, general anesthetics. Acute attacks that are not fatal usually clear up completely, although muscle weakness and nervous effects may persist for months. Thus, the porphyric gene, essentially harmless by itself, becomes lethal when the bearer encounters modern medicines.

Another illustration of a hereditary drug idiosyncrasy is the hemolytic effect of the antimalarial drug, primaquine, and some other drugs in an occasional individual. The peculiar reaction to primaquine depends on a hereditary biochemical deficiency of the red blood cells. Investigations revealed that the defect of the red cells was due to a deficiency in the amount of the enzyme, glucose 6-phosphate dehydrogenase.

The hereditary deficiency is particularly common among Negroes (8 to 10 per cent in the United States) and among Mediterranean peoples. It is inherited as a sex-linked trait, and occurs more commonly among males. Female carriers have two populations of red blood cells, those with normal enzyme activity and those markedly deficient.

The red blood cells that are deficient in glucose 6-phosphate dehydrogenase are apparently susceptible to injury by certain drugs, so that they are removed from circulation by the normal tissue mechanisms. This disorder is the underlying mechanism for most hemolytic anemias that are related to drugs. In addition to primaquine, other antimalarial drugs such as pamaquine, sulfonamides, and some antipyretics as acetanilide, acetophenetidin, and aspirin in large doses have been associated with hemolytic anemia in subjects with glucose 6-phosphate dehydrogenase deficiency.[86]

A third type of genetic abnormality has some significance in causing abnormal reactions to drugs. This condition results from a deficiency of pseudocholinesterase. The function of this enzyme is not definitely known, but it is found in the plasma, liver, and other organs in considerable quantities. Certain individuals have low levels of this enzyme, and it has been established that this deficiency is inherited as an autosomal recessive trait. Individuals with this deficiency are markedly sensitive to the muscle-relaxing drug, Suxamethonium. Ordinarily, this drug has a very short action, and it is used along with general anesthetics in certain surgical procedures. In patients deficient in pseudocholinesterase, the action of the drug is greatly prolonged, persisting for 2 to 3 hr. instead of a few minutes.[86]

Isoniazid was introduced in the treatment of tuberculosis in 1952. When taken by mouth, it is rapidly absorbed. The maximum blood level is attained within about 2 hr. after administration. A large portion of the drug is acetylated in the liver and excreted in the urine in the acetylated form. The metabolism of isoniazid in each individual in remarkably constant, but there is considerable variation between individuals in the fraction of the drug which is acetylated. There are two classes of people: (1) those who acetylate isoniazid efficiently; and (2) those who are slow inactivators of the drug. This ability to inactivate isoniazid rapidly is dependent on the presence of a specific enzyme. The distribution of this enzyme appears to be on a genetic basis. About 50 per cent of the population of the United States are

estimated to be slow inactivators. Fortunately, this genetic defect does not seriously affect the efficacy of isoniazid as a therapeutic agent for tuberculosis.[87]

It seems probable that other hitherto undiscovered examples may be found of persons whose genetically determined response to a given drug makes them more susceptible in the action of that drug.

**Thalidomide Episode**

During the past 15 years, a great deal of attention has been focused on the effects of drugs given to women in pregnancy on the health of the developing embryo or fetus. There is substantial evidence to indicate that in the early weeks of embryonic development vulnerability to injurious agents is greatest. It has been demonstrated that chemicals with a molecular weight less than 600 can readily penetrate the blood vessels of the placenta and thus reach the fetal circulation.[88]

The most dramatic episode in the history of adverse drug effects arose through the use of thalidomide as a tranquilizing agent for pregnant women. This drug was produced in Germany under the name "Contergan"; in England, as "Distaval"; Canada and the United States, as "Kevadon." It was not released in the United States by the Food and Drug Administration for general use.

Apparently, thalidomide as used widely for sedative purposes was considered to be a safe and highly satisfactory drug. Beginning in 1959, a few cases of infants born with congenital malformations began to be reported. These malformations were different from those commonly seen. The bones in the arms and legs were defective or absent. The term "phocomelia" (seal-like extremities) was applied to these deformities. Other abnormalities affected the eyes, nose, heart, and other organs. As use of the drug spread, the numbers of infants with phocomelia increased. By 1961, it became apparent to investigators that use of thalidomide during the early weeks of pregnancy was associated with the causation of the deformities. The drug was withdrawn from the market shortly afterward.

Another report[89] gives much interesting data on the rapid increase in usage of thalidomide in Germany and other countries (see Table 6.12). According to Dr. Widukind Lenz of the

Hamburg Institute of Human Genetics, it is difficult to estimate the total number of thalidomide victims. A figure of 7000 cases of congenital abnormalities is a good approximation of the total. The incidence of malformations of the thalidomide type in the various countries that have been investigated is roughly proportional to the known sales of the drug (see Table 6.13).

The Health Ministry of West Germany has recently made a thorough check of the incidence of thalidomide malformations that occurred in Germany between 1958 and 1962.[90] The figure given in this report is 2625 defective babies, a considerably lower number than previously estimated. The Ministry's study states that about 1000 of the deformed children will have to use artificial limbs, while 100 must stay under constant medical supervision for life.

It is significant that thalidomide was discovered as a teratogenic agent because of the frequency and severity of the defects that it caused. Dr. F. O. Kelsey of the United States Food and Drug Administration[91] estimated that 30 out of every 50 women who took thalidomide in the early weeks of pregnancy gave birth to defective offspring. Lenz stated that in Germany he knew of no well-documented case where a woman had taken the drug during the sensitive phase of pregnancy without damage to the embryo.[92]

The critical period of fetal susceptibility in man is estimated to be approximately three to

TABLE 6.12

*Sales and samples of thalidomide in western Germany*

| Year | Amount Distributed |
|------|--------------------|
| | $kg.^1$ |
| 1957 | 33 |
| 1958 | 728 |
| 1959 | 3,800 |
| 1960 | 14,480 |
| 1961 | 11,060 |
| (up to August) | |

[1] A total of 1000 kg. equals 1 trillion mg., which equals 20 million teratogenic doses.

Source: Lenz, W. Malformations caused by drugs in pregnancy. *Amer. J. Dis. Child. 112:* 99-106, 1966.

TABLE 6.13

*Sale of thalidomide and incidence of thalidomide cases*

| Countries | Sale | Thalidomide Cases |
|-----------|------|-------------------|
| | *kg.* | |
| Austria | 207 | 8 |
| Belgium | 258 | 26 |
| Great Britain | 5,769 | 349 |
| Netherlands | 140 | 25 |
| Norway | 60 | 11 |
| Portugal | 37 | 2 |
| Switzerland | 113 | 6 |
| West Germany | 30,099 | 5,000 |
| United States | 25? | 10 + 7[1] |
| | (2,500,000 tablets) | |

[1] Thalidomide obtained from foreign sources.

Source: Lenz, W. Malformations caused by drugs in pregnancy. *Amer. J. Dis. Child., 112:* 99-106, 1966.

10 weeks after conception occurs. Rapid cell proliferation is evidently related to high sensitivity to chemical teratogens. In addition to thalidomide, several other drugs are thought to cause fetal damage. Aminopterin and progestins are especially risky. Streptomycin is known to cause deafness in the developing fetus.[84]

Probably other drugs cause less obvious and less frequent injury to the human embryo and escape notice of the attending physicians.

### Reactions to Chloramphenicol

One of the most controversial drugs on the market during recent years has been chloramphenicol. Parke, Davis and Company of Detroit gave a grant to Dr. Paul Buckholder of Yale University to search for new soil organisms which might produce a useful, new antibiotic. In 1948, an organism, *Streptomyces venezuelae,* was sent to Parke, Davis and Company. From this organism, Chloromycetin was obtained. Shortly thereafter chloramphenicol was synthesized and replaced Chloromycetin. This product was the first broadspectrum antibiotic introduced into medicinal use. It was also the first antibiotic to be completely synthesized in the laboratory and is still the only antibiotic which is industrially produced by chemical synthesis rather than by fermentation.[93]

In 1949, the year after its introduction, sales of the antibiotic amounted to $9,293,000. In 1950, sales rose to $28,260,000; and in 1951, to $52,410,000. Then the fortunes of chloramphenicol had a setback, when in 1952 it was reported that the antibiotic had caused a number of cases of aplastic anemia. Sales dropped by 94 per cent between March and September, but still totaled $47,000,000. In the following year and in 1954, sales were less than $26,000,000, and Parke, Davis and Company closed the special plant that it had built for the production of chloramphenicol.

The drug continued to be popular in many parts of the world, and some use of it continued in the United States. Chloramphenicol soon experienced a return to favor. Its sales rose to $35,000,000 in 1955 and to $53,000,000 in 1957. This amazing acceptance for widespread use after such a setback is perhaps unique in the history of chemotherapy.[94]

Chloramphenicol inhibits the growth of most bacteria, of rickettsiae, and of organisms of the psittacosis group. It is predominantly a bacteriostatic agent. Inhibition of protein biosynthesis is the means by which chloramphenicol affects the growth of microorganisms. Chloramphenicol is the only drug that has proved highly effective in the treatment of *Salmonella typhosa* infections (typhoid fever). It is not so uniformly effective against other types of salmonella infections. The antibiotic has also been recommended as especially effective in the treatment of serious infections with *Haemophilus influenzae* (influenza bacillus).

Chloramphenicol is rapidly absorbed from the gastrointestinal tract. After a single dose, the maximum blood concentration is reached within 2 hr. The drug passes readily into the cerebral spinal fluid and in appreciable quantity in the bile. It is broken down by the liver into inactive fractions and excreted in the urine.

The most serious toxic effect associated with its use was aplastic anemia. Other types of blood dyscrasia were also reported, but not so commonly as aplastic anemia. There appear to be two types of toxic effect on the bone marrow. One type has a rapid onset and occurs during treatment with the antibiotic. It is related to the dosage of the drug. The bone marrow is not destroyed. Certain changes occur in the blood cells that disappear upon discontinuance of treatment. The other type has a late onset from two weeks to five months and is not always related to the amount of drug administered but produces an aplastic anemia that is frequently fatal. While chloramphenicol is the most frequent single cause of drug-induced aplastic anemia, the actual incidence is in the order of one in 200,000 of those who receive the drug. The incidence of this severe complication is higher in women than men. Age apparently has little influence.[95]

In spite of these reports of rare but extremely serious reactions to chloramphenicol, physicians continue to order it for their patients with undiminished zeal. Parke, Davis and Company is said to produce 7½ tons of the antibiotic annually. Two recent reports indicate that the seriously adverse reactions are continuing. The Committee on Safety of Drugs of the British Medical Association observed in 1967 that "during the past two years, 24 fatal cases of blood dyscrasia following administration of chloramphenicol have been reported." This represents 80 per cent of all fatal blood dyscrasias in patients treated with antibiotics.[96] The Committee further reports that 1 million prescriptions for chloramphenicol had been written in Britain during 1964 to 1965. The Committee recommended that physicians use chloramphenicol only for typhoid fever, other serious salmonella infections, and infections in which no other antibiotic will serve.

A report of 408 cases in patients treated with chloramphenicol that have come to the notice of the American Medical Association's Registry of Blood Dyscrasias has appeared.[97] These cases had either been reported to the Registry or accounts of them had been published in the medical literature. These dyscrasias range from mild reversible blood changes to fatal aplastic anemia. No explanation for the occasional case of bone marrow injury by chloramphenicol is now known, but there appears to be an abnormal susceptibility in some individuals due to a biochemical defect that may be inherited. Best estimates that there is one case of serious bone marrow toxicity in each 100,000 patients treated with chloramphenicol.[97]

*Aplastic Anemia*

Ehrlich gave this name in 1888 to a well-defined type of blood disorder. Other names that have been suggested are primary refractory anemia, aregenerative anemia, and anemia of bone marrow failure. All elements of the bone marrow may be involved, so that there is a general deficiency of all types of blood cells or pancytopenia or there may be a failure to produce certain types of blood elements. The clinical course depends upon which blood elements are involved. If the white blood cells or the blood platelets are suppressed, infections or hemorrhagic manifestations may shorten life. Some patients can be kept alive and active for many years.[98]

*Causation*

About half of the cases in ordinary civilian life develop without any ascertainable cause. They are classed as idiopathic. In addition, there are rare cases in children, probably based on hereditary causation. In the remaining patients, a variety of known agents may cause severe injury to the bone marrow. Exposure to ionizing radiation is well-established as a threat to the blood-forming tissues.

Agents responsible for causing aplastic anemia may be divided into two categories: (1) those that regularly damage the bone marrow, if a sufficient dose is given (among these are radiations from nuclear explosions, X rays, radium, radioactive isotopes, benzene, and agents used in the therapy of malignant tumors); (2) those compounds that are occasionally associated with bone marrow failure. Some of these agents have been reported to be responsible for 20 to 100 cases or more, for example, chloramphenicol, sulfonamides, quinacrine, phenylbutazone, gold preparations, and other drugs. Other compounds have been only occasionally suspected. This is a large list, increasing each year.

Chloramphenicol is the agent most frequently associated with aplastic anemia since 1952. It is suspected that compounds containing the benzene ring are particularly likely to be injurious to the bone marrow. These organic compounds are used so commonly in current society that everyone frequently has some contact with them.

*Incidence*

Idiopathic aplastic anemia occurs only rarely. It may occur at any age, but more commonly affects young adults.

The incidence of cases associated with noxious agents varies with the exposure of each population group. The two atomic bomb explosions in Japan are said to have caused thousands of cases of aplastic anemia. Of the patients who receive therapeutic doses of chloramphenicol, it is estimated that one of every 20,000 to 30,000 develops the disease.[98]

*Clinical Manifestations*

The onset may be abrupt following severe radiation exposure or large doses of drugs to control cancer. In other cases, the symptoms tend to appear insidiously. The type of reaction depends on the severity of the anemia and the extent to which the various blood elements are involved. As a result of anemia, weakness and fatigue are the prominent symptoms. As the blood count falls, headache, shortness of breath, fever, and excessive pounding of the heart are troublesome. If there is a severe fall in the white blood cell count, infections may appear. Pneumonia, abscesses, and urinary infections as well as other types of bacterial invasions are likely to occur. With a low blood platelet count, hemorrhages can be expected. The patients become quite pale. With increasing anemia, the heart becomes enlarged.

*Diagnosis*

Examinations of the blood should be complete and thorough. The red blood cells are usually fairly normal in appearance, although there may be a slight irregularity in shape and size. The degree of anemia is variable, but may be severe. The white blood cell count and the blood platelet count may be normal or severely diminished.

The bone marrow should also be examined. Aspiration of marrow from the sternum is usually a safe procedure. The bone marrow sometimes shows a marked aplasia as a result of the action of the causative agent.

Studies on utilization of iron are sometimes done. These reveal a slow turnover of iron in the plasma and poor utilization of iron for synthesis of hemoglobin.

The most difficult differentiation to be made is from some early forms of leukemia.

*Treatment*

Stop any continuing exposure to the noxious agent. Transfusions of blood are of value in maintaining the patient's strength. General supportive care is highly important. In occasional cases, the removal of the spleen is advisable. The patient is warned to refrain from the use of organic compounds such as hair dyes, pesticides, plant sprays, and all drugs except those recommended by the physician.

Transfusions should be kept to the minimum necessary to support the patient's strength. Repeated transfusions result in damage resulting from excess of iron building up in the system and from sensitizations to minor blood groups, white blood cells, or platelets.

The spleen should be removed if it becomes enlarged and if there is evidence that it is destroying red blood cells faster than is normal. This is demonstrated if the count of red blood cells falls very rapidly after transfusion.

*Prognosis*

Spontaneous remissions occur rarely. Those most likely to survive are cases with mild damage to the bone marrow and with mild

effects on the circulating blood. Some patients do recover slowly over a period of years.

Death occurs usually as a result of infection or from hemorrhage. The outlook is poor, therefore, when there is marked leukopenia and a low platelet count. If there are good levels of white blood cells and platelets, patients may survive in reasonable comfort for several years. Roughly 50 per cent of such patients were alive after one year, and 25 per cent at the end of three years. Removal of the spleen tends to improve the figures considerably.

## Incidence of Iatrogenic Mishaps

Two reports from university-connected hospitals in recent years have expressed concern about the increasing incidence of ill health due to severe reactions to drugs and to other therapeutic or diagnostic procedures. Barr[99] pointed out that, during a period in which approximately 1000 patients were admitted to a large general hospital, more than 50 patients were found to be suffering from major toxic reactions and accidents consequent to treatment or diagnostic measures.

Schimmel,[100] in a study of over 1000 patients admitted to a university hospital over an 8-month period, found that about 20 per cent of the patients experienced some adverse reaction to treatment or other procedures ordered by their physicians. Eleven per cent of the patients suffered moderate to severe reactions. About one of each 10 patients had their hospital stay increased by at least one day on account of these reactions.

Drugs are capable of upsetting the physiological balance of the body. Prolonged therapy with antibiotics, steroids, or immunity suppressing drugs diminish the resistance of the body to pathogenic agents. Infection with yeasts or various types of bacteria are common and difficult to control. Approximately 3 per cent of those discharged from hospitals are reported to have acquired such secondary infections, many with agents that have become drug resistant.[101]

As more new drugs are introduced and as diagnostic procedures become more complex, one can expect the number of these unfavorable reactions to continue to increase.[102,103]

In addition to adverse reactions to drug therapy, many other forms of iatrogenic disease occur. Among these may be listed the transmission of syphilis, malaria, or hepatitis through blood transfusions. Of these, hepatitis is by far more common.

Approximately 1 per cent of apparently healthy blood donors are carriers of the virus of hepatitis. Use of their blood as whole blood, plasma, or fibrinogen will produce hepatitis in susceptible recipients. Equally dangerous in the transmission of this infection is the use of contaminated syringes or needles, either in groups being immunized or among drug addicts. Also hepatitis has resulted from use of supposedly normal human serum in the preparation of vaccines. The episode of the contaminated yellow fever vaccine in World War II is the best known such incident. Many thousands of United States servicemen contracted serum hepatitis from their protective inoculations against yellow fever.

## GENETIC DEFECTS

### Phenylketonuria

*Introduction*

The discovery that one form of mental retardation is related to a hereditary biochemical abnormality gave an immense impulse to research. It was particularly encouraging to those concerned with preventive medicine when it became evident that specific changes in the diet of children born with phenylketonuria might prevent in some children the development of severe mental, motor, and psychological retardations.

Phenylketonuria (PKU) was first recognized by a Norwegian physician, Dr. A. Fölling. A mother had brought her retarded children to the doctor to seek an explanation of their condition. She had noted a musty odor of the children's urine. Dr. Fölling discovered that the children's urine turned green upon the addition of ferric chloride. He isolated a substance from the urine which proved to be phenylpyruvic acid. Fölling reported in 1934 a series of 10 patients who excreted phenylpyruvic acid and were mentally defective.[104]

Within a few years, it became known that PKU was a hereditary condition transmitted through a single autosomal recessive gene. On the average, one out of four children from two heterozygous parents has both defective genes and PKU results. Both sexes are affected with equal frequency. The disease is more frequent in children of European stock, particularly in Scandinavian families. It is rare among Negroes or Semitic peoples.

It was shown that large amounts of phenylalanine accumulate in the bodies of PKU children. This is due to the inability of the body to oxidize phenylalanine to tyrosine. In 1953, G. A. Jervis demonstrated that the defect was due to inactivity of the enzyme, phenylalanine hydroxylase, in the liver.[105]

*Occurrence*

It is estimated that in the United States the incidence of PKU in the general population is between 5 and 10 per 100,000. In Northern Europe, the incidence has been calculated to be somewhat higher.

The concentration of mental retardation cases into institutions and the possibility of effective treatment has stimulated the finding of new cases. These factors have made PKU the best known of the rare hereditary diseases.

The life span of PKU patients is commonly curtailed. About half die by the age of 20 years, and three-quarters of PKU victims fail to survive more than 30 years. Thus, in surveys, most cases are discovered among children.

*Clinical Features*

The disability becomes manifest during the first weeks after birth. At this stage, it is discovered by biochemical tests that demonstrate greatly increased amounts of phenylalanine in the blood plasma and the presence of phenylpyruvic acid in the urine. After six months of age, mental retardation is evident. Neurological abnormalities may appear. There may be changes in the pigmentation of the hair and skin.

The time for development stages, that is, for sitting, walking, and talking, is usually delayed. The appearance of the first teeth may be delayed several months. Children with PKU are often below standard height and weight for their ages. The adults are smaller than the average size.

The large majority of adult cases are severely retarded mentally. Some 65 per cent are classified as idiots, 30 per cent as imbeciles, and some 3 per cent in the moron category.[106] Usually, progressive deterioration of the mind continues during the first five or six years of life, when a plateau is reached.

Epileptic attacks occur in about 25 per cent of PKU patients. Such attacks may begin early in infancy, but often decrease in frequency with increasing age. Other neurological disturbances may include spasticity of muscles, tremors, and involuntary jerking movements. The gait is stiff with short, jerky steps. This has been described as a "stumbling gait."

This physical appearance is somewhat characteristic. About two-thirds of the patients have blond hair, blue eyes, and a lightly pigmented skin. Eczema and other skin abnormalities are common, possibly due to lack of protective pigmentation in the skin.

A peculiar odor is given off by some patients, described as "musty" or "mousy." It is probably due to decomposition products in the sweat and in the urine. It is found especially in children who do not control their passage of urine.

### Nature of the Metabolic Defect

Phenylalanine is an essential amino acid and makes up about 5 per cent of the protein portion of the usual diet. It is normally converted to tyrosine in the liver by action of a specific enzyme, phenylalanine hydroxylase. Because of the genetic defect, this enzyme is not produced in the body or is produced in an inactive form. As a consequence of this metabolic block, phenylalanine accumulates in the body. Instead of the normal level of 1 to 3 mg. per 100 ml. in the blood, in PKU patients it may rise to 20 to 60 mg. per 100 ml. This great increase in phenylalanine acts as a toxic inhibitor of other important enzyme systems in the body. Probably the excess of phenylalanine in the blood inhibits the uptake of other essential amino acids by the central nervous system. It is likely that compounds may be synthesized in the brain from phenylalanine that are injurious to the nervous tissues. PKU appears to be the result of many disturbances in the brain metabolism rather than of a single metabolic change. Some of these disorders produce chronic and irreversible effects, manifested by a lowered intelligence quotient. Others may cause less severe and reversible symptoms.[107]

As biochemical investigations have become more precise, children with high levels of phenylalanine in the blood but who are not true PKU cases have been discovered. It now appears that some of these children with elevated plasma phenylalanine are atypical cases of PKU and others have quite different causes of phenylalanemia.[108] Some of these children have a delayed maturation of phenylalanine transaminase; others have delayed maturation of p-hydroxyphenylpyruvic acid oxidase; a few have high plasma levels of phenylalanine for unknown reasons. In the present state of knowledge, it is difficult to determine the best course of treatment for these atypical cases.

### Diagnosis

Recognition of the disease depends upon laboratory procedures. Demonstration of phenylpyruvic acid in the urine is the most frequently used procedure. A presumptive test may be done by adding a few drops of 5 per cent solution of ferric chloride to a small amount of recently voided urine. A green color, lasting for a few minutes, indicates a positive test. Some drugs may cause a false reading. Another test is done by mixing equal volumes of urine and a 0.1 per cent solution of dinitrophenylhydrazine in 2 N hydrochloric acid. In a positive test, the mixture becomes turbid and a yellow precipitate forms.

The diagnosis must be confirmed by the demonstration of a high level of phenylalanine in the blood. The normal level of phenylalanine in the blood is from 1 to 3 mg. per 100 ml. In PKU patients, the levels range from 20 to 60 mg. per 100 ml.

### Treatment

The only method of treatment now available that promises to reduce the likelihood of brain damage in PKU patients is a diet designed to lower the plasma phenylalanine. An adequate diet very low in phenylalanine usually causes a prompt lowering of the level of phenylalanine in the blood and a disappearance of phenylpyruvic acid from the urine. Balanced diets are available commercially consisting of protein, hydrolyzed to remove phenylalanine, together with fat, carbohydrate, minerals, and vitamins. It is recommended that the blood level of phenylalanine be maintained between 3 and 6 mg. per 100 ml. A small amount of phenylalanine is necessary to the body since it is an essential amino acid.

The dietary treatment of PKU should be started as early as possible, preferably within the first six months of life. Many physicians advocate treating all PKU patients discovered under three years of age with the low phenylalanine diet. Some even feel that PKU children of any age deserve a trial of dietary therapy for about one year. Probably it is not worthwhile to treat older children who already show severe mental retardation. There is need to follow the dietary regime carefully and to check the blood phenylalanine and tyrosine levels.

The age at which treatment can safely be stopped is still uncertain. Some physicians recommend a transition period from the strict phenylalanine-reduced diet to a mixed diet of low protein content be tried at the age of eight years or soon thereafter. Others feel that the dietary therapy should be stopped earlier.

Experience to date indicates that adequate treatment begun before impairment occurs will prevent or ameliorate the development of the expected mental retardation. It must be admitted that some PKU patients, despite early diagnosis and good dietetic control, do poorly. There are others who do relatively well intellectually on no treatment at all.[108] These observations point up the inadequacy of current knowledge about the treatment of PKU.

*Public Health Aspects*

Preventive measures are largely confined to genetic counsel of parents who already have one affected child. Progress has been made in setting up biochemical tests to select prospective parents of PKU children, but experience is too limited and the significance of current tests is too uncertain to attempt genetic counseling for individuals at the present time.

The more promising approach now is the discovery of PKU patients early with the purpose of instituting proper dietary treatment. A few states have laws making it obligatory to test all newborn infants for evidence of PKU. A few days after the baby has begun feeding, a drop of blood is obtained on filter paper from a heel puncture. The blood is tested for inhibition of growth of special bacterial strains which require phenylpyruvic acid for growth. This test is remarkably simple and is well adapted for mass screening of children. The urine test can

be carried out after the infant is about four weeks of age. The blood test should be performed before the mother and child are released from the hospital.[109,110]

In some communities, mass screening tests have been undertaken. This is a rather laborious procedure to detect a disease as rare as PKU. Surveys of all children in public institutions should be carried out as a function of public health agencies.

In 1962, the State Health Department of Massachusetts began to screen newborn infants for evidence of phenylketonuria. Each year from 85,000 to 90,000 infants are tested. Since the beginning of the program 981,361 have been tested (1973) and 67 infants found with PKU or 1:15,000.[111]

To maintain an adequate service for PKU patients, expert pediatric consultation facilities for diagnosis and treatment are required. A competent laboratory to conduct diagnostic tests and to provide necessary information to control diet therapy must be available for close cooperation.

A registry of PKU cases for the community should be carefully maintained. This is important for a number of reasons, one being to control excess phenylalanine blood levels in PKU females during pregnancy. High blood levels of phenylalanine in the pregnant woman can damage the brain of the fetus.

Much interest has developed in methods to diagnose genetic and congenital abnormalities in the prenatal stage. By introducing a needle into the amniotic sac in the early weeks of pregnancy, fluid can be removed for biochemical tests. Cells of fetal origin can also be obtained for studies on chromosome patterns.[112]

## NEOPLASTIC DISEASE

### Hodgkin's Disease

*Introduction*

Dr. Thomas Hodgkin, a distinguished English pathologist, gave a clear-cut description of seven cases of the disease that bears his name in 1832. The patients all suffered from a slowly wasting disease characterized by an enlargement of the lymph glands and a fatal termination. Forty years passed before giant cells were described in the diseased lymph glands. It was

1902 before Dorothy Reed at Johns Hopkins Hospital described these cells more clearly. These cells, now known as Sternberg-Reed cells, are regarded as characteristic of the disease.

The lymph node enlargement comes on insidiously. It is painless and may be localized to one group of nodes. Eventually the involvement becomes more generalized. Fever is a common symptom. This led early students of the disease to believe that it was due to an infectious agent. Other symptoms depend upon the extent of pressure on vital organs by the enlarged glands. The cause of the disease is unknown. It is now classified with the malignant tumors. Treatment of Hodgkin's disease has improved in recent years and has extended the period of survival considerably. However, the disease still frequently terminates fatally.

There are a number of other conditions affecting lymph nodes, spleen, and other organs that resemble Hodgkin's disease closely in many of its aspects. They include lymphoma and lymphosarcoma. The differentiation of these disorders is difficult and frequently impossible without careful study of biopsy material. The course of the disease over a period of months or years serves also as a distinguishing factor.

### Causation

The cause of Hodgkin's disease is unknown. The disease has a world-wide distribution. It appears to be unrelated to occupation or social status. Men are affected twice as often as women. The peak frequency is around the third decade of life. More than 60 instances of familial Hodgkin's disease have been reported. The disease has occurred at the same time in twins, in husbands and wives, and in mother and baby. However, the evidence so far indicates that heredity plays a small and possibly only an indirect role in the causation of Hodgkin's disease.

There has been disagreement about the fundamental nature of Hodgkin's disease. It appears to fall almost midway between an inflammatory process and a form of malignant neoplasm. The disease has never been successfully transmitted to animals, nor has there been any convincing evidence that any specific microbial agent is regularly associated with the diseased tissue. Many pathologists consider it to be, along with lymphoma and lymphosarcoma, a neoplasm. Now that viruses are known to cause a number of different neoplasms in

animals, more attention is being given to the search for possible virus agents as the cause of Hodgkin's disease. A cogent argument for a neoplastic basis comes from the infiltrative character of the disease in the late stages.

There is some evidence that one case of Hodgkin's disease is sometimes associated with another, especially among younger people, thus indicating a possible infectious origin of the disease. In a two-county study in New York State, Vianna and Polan followed each high school in which a case of Hodgkin's had been diagnosed in either a student or teacher. Control schools were selected in the same or adjacent townships. Five of the eight high schools with at least one case diagnosed between 1960 through 1964 had additional cases in the period 1965 through 1969. In the control schools no cases were discovered in either period. These results are consistent with the possibility that a transmissible agent may be involved.[113]

### Incidence

Hodgkin's disease occurs among all peoples, but appears more frequently in the white races. The American Cancer Society estimates that there will be 3700 deaths in 1974 from Hodgkin's disease in the United States. Of these, it is estimated that 2200 will be among males and 1500 in females.[114] A total of 6900 new cases was predicted for 1974.

The greatest number of cases occurs among young adults from 20 to 39 years of age, but, during the seventh and eighth decades, there is another peak of occurrence. There appears to be a slow increase in deaths from Hodgkin's disease during recent decades. In 1921, the death rate in the United States was 0.7 per 100,000 population; in 1951, 1.7; and in 1965 the rate was 1.8 per 100,000. In 1973, the rate remained about the same.

### Pathology

Early in the disease, the lymph nodes are firm and usually discrete. Microscopic examination of these glands may show only a great increase of lymphocytes and occasional large Sternberg-Reed cells. These giant cells have large nuclei that may be either single or multiple. The chromatin network is prominent in these nuclei. The protoplasm may appear granular or show vacuoles or fatty granules. These cells are found characteristically in Hodgkin's disease.

TABLE 6.14

*Staging of Hodgkin's disease*

| Stage | Symptom Involvement |
|---|---|
| I | Disease localized to one anatomical region (most common presenting finding is enlarged group of nodes on one or the other side of the neck) |
| II | Disease limited to two areas |
| III | Disease on both sides of the diaphragm but limited to involvement of nodes, spleen and Waldeyer's ring |
| IV | Involvement of bone marrow; parenchyma of lung, liver, and bone |
| Subclasses | |
| A | Presence of systemic symptoms otherwise unexplained |
| B | Absence of systemic symptoms otherwise unexplained (most important symptoms unexplained other than by Hodgkin's disease itself include fever, night sweats, pruritus, and weight loss exceeding 10% of the body weight) |

Source: Perry, S. (Moderator). Hodgkin's disease: combined clinical staff conference at the National Institutes of Health. *Ann. Intern. Med., 67:* 424–442, 1967.

who have suffered recurrences after the maximum tolerable dosage of irradiation. In 1966, Karnofsky[118] reported that 65 per cent of the patients with Hodgkin's disease will present with disease above and below the diaphragm or in various viscera, described as Stage III or IV. Of the remaining, Stage I and II patients, approximately 60 per cent of the patients with Stage II will have no recurrences or will have recurrences that can be managed by X ray. On the other hand, by 10 years, as many as 20 per cent of the patients with Stage I and 50 per cent of patients with Stage II will have evidence of dissemination during some phase of their illness. In the treatment of these patients, as well as of the patients who present primarily with disseminated disease, chemotherapy has a major role. Nitrogen mustard is the compound used most commonly. The drug is given intravenously in an infusion of normal saline and 5 per cent glucose in water. The dose of nitrogen mustard is usually 0.4 mg. per kg. of body weight given in divided doses on successive days.

The effects of nitrogen mustard are often dramatic. Fever may disappear and enlarged glands, spleen, or areas of infiltration may return to normal or apparently so. Remissions may last for periods up to one year.

Nitrogen mustard is toxic for the bone marrow. The white blood cell count may drop to a 1000 or less per cubic millimeter and the blood platelets to a low level. These abnormalities usually last only about 10 to 14 days.[119]

As courses of treatment with nitrogen mustard are repeated, the period of remission becomes shorter, getting down to six to 12 weeks. Eventually the drug becomes ineffective.

Triethylene melamine acts in a manner similar to nitrogen mustard, but is not as satisfactory. It has the advantage of oral administration. The bone marrow is also affected by this drug.

In hope of extending survival rate, several studies have been recently reported in which a combination of antineoplastic drugs were employed simultaneously. Best results were obtained using the recommended schedule of the National Cancer Institute. During a 24-week period six courses of intensive therapy were given. The drugs used were nitrogen mustard, vincristine sulfate, a plant alkaloid, procarbazine hydrochloride, and prednisone. It is believed that combining radiotherapy with a combination of drugs will secure long range remission and probably cures in a good percentage of early cases of Hodgkin's disease[120] (see Table 6.15).

Corticosteroids are helpful in some cases to improve constitutional symptoms. Usually they are employed for short periods.

TABLE 6.15

*Chemotherapy drugs for the treatment of Hodgkin's disease: clinically proved agents*

| Name | Type | Route and Usual Doses | Side Effects |
|------|------|----------------------|--------------|
| Nitrogen mustard | Alkylating agent | Intravenously 0.4mg./kg.single dose or divided 2–4 daily doses | Nausea vomiting; bone marrow depression |
| Chlorambucil | Alkylating agent | Orally 0.1–0.2 mg./kg.daily | Bone marrow depression sometimes delayed after last dose |
| Cyclophosphamide | Alkylating agent | Intravenously 40 mg./kg. single dose or divided doses or 10–15 mg./kg. weekly Orally 2–3 mg./kg. | Nausea, vomiting; alopecia; bone marrow depression; hemmorhagic cystitis |
| Vinblastine | Metaphase inhibitor | Intravenously 0.1–0.3 mg./kg. weekly | Bone marrow depression; peripheral neuropathy, ileus |

Source:   Perry, S. (Moderator). Hodgkin's disease: combined clinical staff conference at the National Institutes of Health. *Amm. Intern. Med., 67:* 424–442, 1967.

General support care includes blood transfusions and antibiotic drugs when indicated.

The outlook for patients with Hodgkin's disease has improved, but is still grave. It is hopeful that some cases do respond to treatment with highly satisfactory results.

## DISEASES OF OBSCURE CAUSATION

### Diabetes Mellitus

*Introduction*

Diabetes is a constitutional, chronic metabolic disorder characterized by high blood sugar levels and excretion of sugar in the urine. The disease usually develops in subjects with a hereditary predisposition. It is associated with partial or relative insulin insufficiency. In its fully developed form, the characteristic symptoms are weakness, lassitude, loss of weight, or, in children, a failure to grow, and ketosis and acidosis. The disease is dangerous not only for its acute derangements of the body's chemistry, which may lead to fatal acidosis, but also its long continuance produces secondary abnormalities of the small arteries which may ultimately cause kidney failure, blindness, neuritis, hypertension, and other unpleasant effects.

Diabetes has been known for at least 2000 years. The Greeks noted the loss of weight and the excessive urination. They gave it the name "diabetes," which means to siphon off. The presence of sugar in the urine was discovered by taste somewhat later, hence the term "mellitus," which means honey.

Late in the 19th century, experimenters produced the disease in dogs by excising the pancreas. It was not until 1921 that Banting and Best, in Toronto, produced a pancreatic extract capable of keeping alive dogs from whom the pancreas had been removed. In a purified form, this extract was shown to be efficacious in the treatment of human diabetics. It was given the name "insulin." For a time it was believed that diabetes resulted from a simple failure of the pancreas to produce sufficient quantities of insulin. Subsequent investigations have shown that many physiological factors are involved, endocrine, immunological, and chemical.[121]

*Abnormal Physiology*

The disturbance of the carbohydrate metabolism is the most obvious aspect of diabetes. In the intestinal tract, the carbohydrates taken in with food are broken down to form glucose, fructose, and galactose. These are absorbed into the blood system and are stored in the liver. Almost all of the sugar utilized in the body is in the form of glucose.

In normal individuals, the concentration of glucose in the blood is maintained within rather narrow limits, usually between 50 and 150 mg. per 100 ml. The movement of glucose through cell membranes is expedited by insulin in the case of certain tissues, including skeletal and heart muscle and fat. Other tissues, such as the nervous system, testicles, and ovaries, appear to be uninfluenced by insulin. Once within the cell, glucose is broken down by enzyme action. Hexokinase is the enzyme involved in most tissues, but the liver has a second enzyme, glucokinase. The activity of hexokinase is not influenced by food intake, insulin, or exercise. Glucokinase becomes more active as concentrations of glucose rise in the blood, thus increasing glucose storage in the liver and tending to restore blood levels to normal.

In the fasting subject, the liver is the only important source of the required glucose. The glucose stored in the liver in the form of glycogen is released as glucose by the action of phosphorylase. This enzyme is activated by glucagon, a hormone released by certain cells of the pancreas in response to the stimulus of a lowered blood sugar. Other adjustments reduce the utilization of glucose. The production of insulin is diminished. Hormone from the pituitary gland reduces absorption of glucose by muscles.

When glucose enters the blood stream rapidly as a result of eating carbohydrate, the liver quickly ceases secreting glucose and begins to take it up for storage. Insulin begins to appear to speed up the utilization of glucose. The amount of fatty acids in the blood is reduced. Free fatty acids tend to hinder the entrance of glucose into muscle cells. As a result of these adjustments, the blood glucose level soon falls to fasting levels.

Glucose is readily converted to fat by action of the liver and the fat cells of the body. This conversion of glucose to fatty acids is greatly inhibited in the absence of insulin. The fats produced may be utilized as a source of energy or may be stored to increase the adipose tissues of the body. Factors that increase movement of glucose into fat cells, such as insulin and high blood sugar, tend to reduce the mobilization of fatty acids, whereas factors that lower glucose utilization by the fat cell, such as pituitary hormone or insulin deficiency, tend to increase the mobilization of fat.

The proteins of the body are formed from amino acids absorbed from the digestive tract, but also to some extent from fragments supplied by the breakdown of carbohydrates and fatty acids. As proteins break down, the amino acids released are reused to form new proteins, but, when protein synthesis is proceeding slowly, the free amino acids may be transformed into carbohydrates and fatty acids.

Consequently, when carbohydrate utilization is inhibited in diabetes, protein breakdown is increased and may create a protein deficiency. This situation is corrected when the diabetes is brought under control by insulin therapy.

Insulin is a protein hormone of highly complex nature. It is secreted by the $\beta$-cells of the islets of Langerhans of the pancreas in response to a rise in the concentration of blood glucose above a figure of about 70 to 80 mg. per 100 ml. As it is released, insulin enters the portal vein and goes directly to the liver cells and on to the general blood stream.

In normal man, approximately 4 units of insulin can be extracted from 1 gm. of pancreas. This would indicate that upward of 200 units of insulin may be stored in the appropriate pancreatic cells at one time. Probably this insulin is stored in a modified form to decrease the threat of a sudden release of such a large amount of active hormone.[121]

Little is known of the mechanisms by which insulin acts. It seems certain that it increases the permeability of some cells to glucose. In addition, it stimulates the formation of new proteins in the muscles. Probably the principal actions of insulin in the body are: promotion of fat synthesis, growth, glycogen synthesis, and lowering the blood glucose level.[122]

Insulin is not effective when given by mouth. When given subcutaneously, insulin is used up fairly rapidly, requiring repeated injections during the day. Preparations of crystalline insulin that are absorbed slowly are available and are generally used in treating diabetics.

Insulin, a powerful hormone, is a protein usually made from a combination of beef and pork pancreas material. Some insulins are prepared from pure beef or pure pork tissues. Various modifications of insulin production have been introduced by commercial laboratories. Regular insulin was found to be more stable at a neutral pH. Later it was found that neutral insulin mixed with protamine and zinc had a long enduring action when injected into the body. Thus the number of daily doses of the hormone could be reduced. Other modifications of insulin to adapt the product to the requirements of individual patients have been made available.

Recently, accurate methods to measure insulin in the blood have been discovered. These methods show that the concentration of glucose in the blood is not the only stimulus for insulin release by the pancreas. The response to intravenous glucose was only 30 to 40 per cent of that produced by glucose administered by mouth.

It has also been shown that certain amino acids are capable of stimulating release of pancreatic insulin.

In diabetics, glucose appears to enter cells with difficulty; the liver fails to reduce its glucose output; the concentration of glucose in the blood rises and begins to be eliminated by the kidney tubules into the urine. The failure of glucose to enter the fat cells results in a rise of fatty acids in the blood. Reduced protein synthesis interferes with release of fat by liver cells, so that fat accumulates in the liver. As a result of these metabolic disturbances, fatty acids increase in the blood and ultimately cause a severe form of acidosis.

The high level of glucose in the blood and other body fluids causes an imbalance of osmotic pressure across cell membranes. This is adjusted by movement of water from the cells. This excess of water promotes the secretion of large amounts of urine, thus depleting the body of water in excess of the loss of salt. This causes an intense thirst, a characteristic symptom of severe diabetes.

The loss of glucose in the urine may reach 500 gm. per day. The severe water depletion and the electrolyte changes may produce coma in some diabetics.

Diabetic acidosis is the most feared complication of the disease, and may prove rapidly fatal. However, more important as a cause of disability are the abnormal changes that occur over a period of time to the blood vessels. Diabetics commonly develop atherosclerosis earlier and in a more severe form than do other persons. This is especially true of poorly controlled cases. Probably the atherosclerosis is a result of the high cholesterol and other fatty substances in the blood.

Before the discovery of insulin almost half (48 per cent) of the diabetics died in coma. This figure has now dropped to 1.2 per cent. Most diabetics now die of the complications of the disease, deterioration of kidneys, arteries or changes in the nervous system. With insulin it is easy to keep the average diabetic patient alive for a long period of years, but little is known about how to prevent the serious complications that occur so frequently among diabetics.

Diabetic disease of small arteries is a different process. The lining membrane of the small vessels becomes thickened by excessive deposition of collagen and mucoprotein substances. The effects of this arterial disease are especially important in the kidney, retina, skin, and nervous system. The mechanism of this vascular damage is not understood. In some patients it may appear in the prediabetic stage before the disturbance of carbohydrate metabolism has become manifest. A third change in the blood vessels of diabetics involves the capillaries. This lesion especially affects the kidneys, eyes, and skin. The basic alteration is a thickening of the basement membrane in the capillary wall. The vascular changes in diabetes are probably responsible for many of the characteristic pathological and clinical manifestations of the disease.

Another serious aspect of diabetes is that certain infections appear to be aggravated in diabetic patients. Tuberculosis and staphylococcal infections of the skin are more difficult to control. Kidney infections that are ordinarily controlled with ease may present severe problems.

Neurological disturbances are also common as complications of diabetes. Neuritis with pain may occur in the arms and legs. This may be accompanied by weakness and wasting of muscles in the extremities.

*Etiology*

In a small percentage of cases, a ready explanation of diabetes can be found. The disease in those whose islets of Langerhans have been destroyed in the pancreas by surgery, inflammation, or other causes is readily explained. In other individuals the disease may be caused by excessive hormone therapy. Perhaps this factor merely hastens development of diabetes in persons with a predisposition to the disease.

Juvenile diabetes has a number of aspects that differ from the condition among adults and there may be a difference in causation. It is known that in juveniles the insulin content of the pancreas may be very low indeed, while, in those whose disease appeared in adulthood, the pancreatic insulin content may be normal. Whatever may be the explanation, it appears clear that in diabetes the requirement for insulin is greatly increased. In the early stages of the disease, the pancreatic cells may be able to increase insulin output sufficiently to meet the demand. As time goes on, the organ gradually may "wear out." A great deal of research has been done and many have theorized as to possible mechanisms of the diabetic defect. As yet no acceptable evidence as to the causation of diabetes has been produced.

Recently, special studies on the β-cells in the pancreas have shown some decrease in total cell mass, some diminution in cell size, or some abnormality in cell appearance. This is particularly true in the juvenile form of diabetes.[123]

Another possible explanation of insulin deficiency is that the β-cells might synthesize an incomplete or abnormal form of insulin or that there might be a defect in the mechanism for releasing insulin stored in the β-cells. Insulin deficiency might result from an abnormality in the system for transporting the hormone to the body tissues. This might occur from excess insulin-binding or insulin-neutralizing proteins or from inappropriate insulin destruction. Deficiency might also occur if there is an inadequate interaction between insulin and the responsive tissues.

Any form of physical stress may unmask or aggravate diabetes. Emotional stress may act in the same way. Other factors may be hyperthyroidism, prolonged therapy with adrenocortical steroids, obesity, or repeated pregnancies. Certain drugs are thought to have diabetagenic effects. Among these are the thiazide diuretics.

The high familial incidence of diabetes suggests a genetic causation. Identical twins also have a high degree of concordance in developing diabetes. Those who have studied the matter consider that genetic inheritance as a simple autosomal recessive characteristic fits the known distribution of diabetes best. Three genotypes appear possible: DD (non-diabetic); dD (normal, but a carrier of the diabetic gene); and dd (susceptible to diabetes). The last group is likely to develop diabetes, given the proper environmental factors. Other investigators believe this simple inheritance pattern does not fit observed data, and that there must be a multifactorial or multigenic mechanism.[124] It is certain that children of diabetic parents often do develop diabetes.

*Clinical Course*

The earliest stage of the disease is prediabetes. This stage represents the time from conception to the earliest recognizable abnormality of the carbohydrate tolerance test. Some vascular changes suggestive of the diabetic state have been found in these genetically prediabetic individuals. It is believed that early abnormalities of insulin metabolism have been observed in this stage.

The next stage of diabetes is called the subclinical phase. In this stage the fasting blood sugar level and the glucose tolerance test are normal. Diabetes may be suspected because of evidence of insufficient functional reserve in the insulin-producing cells of the pancreas. An example is a woman who develops sugar in the urine during pregnancy which clears up after delivery. A high percentage of these women progress to diabetes in after years.

The third stage of diabetes is latent disease. The glucose tolerance test is the most sensitive means for detecting latent asymptomatic diabetes. The ability to lower the blood glucose levels within a normal time period is impaired, but no clinically significant abnormality of carbohydrate metabolism is ordinarily apparent. It is believed that abnormalities in the blood vessels may have developed long before diabetes has become clinically manifest.

The clinical stage of diabetes appears when clear-cut symptoms of the disease can be observed. This phase of diabetes clearly may have developed over a long period of years, and indeed represents an advanced stage of the disease process. The onset of diabetes is slow, and the first intimation of a patient having the disease may be the incidental finding of sugar in a routine urine examination. In others, the symptoms of diabetes present themselves unmistakably, thirst, hunger, increased urine secretion, and loss of weight. As the disease progresses, nocturia may be troublesome. In more severe cases, weakness and a feeling of ill health may develop. Later, acidosis produces shortness of breath, nausea, and vomiting. Loss of water from the tissues may produce shock, marked acidosis, and coma. These symptoms may unfold slowly over a period of years or, as happens to some individuals, the course of the disease may progress all too rapidly leading to fatal coma.[125]

*Prevalence*

Diabetes ranks eighth among the leading causes of death in the United States. It accounts for over 37,000 deaths annually. In addition to the 2.4 million known diabetics, there are estimated to be over 1.6 million persons who have diabetes unknown to themselves.[126] Since the introduction of insulin in 1922, the duration of life after diagnosis of diabetes has increased 3-fold. Advances in dietary treatment, the therapy of infections, and the care of surgical complications have also helped to extend the life expectancy of diabetics. During the period 1964 to 1965, an estimated 1.3 per cent of the civilian, non-institutional population of the United States were reported to be diabetic. About 58 per cent of these persons were female. Prevalence of diabetes did not differ by geographical area. Prevalence increased by age with a peak at 65 to 74 year group. Two-thirds of the diabetics were over 55 years of age. There were relatively few juvenile diabetics; only 5 per cent of the diabetic population was under age 25. The rates of disability were roughly three times higher for diabetics than for the total population. The data on which these figures were based were collected as part of the 1964 to 1965 Health Interview Survey[126] (see Table 6.16 and Fig. 6.18).

### Treatment

Diabetes is not a curable disease in the present state of our knowledge. The objectives of treatment are to prevent acidosis and the symptoms that arise from high blood glucose levels. The prevention of the complications of diabetes are also important.

The available methods for treating diabetics include diet, insulin, exercise, and the oral hypoglycemic drugs. The progress of treatment is determined by testing the urine for sugar and the blood for glucose levels. A careful watch must be maintained for complications and on the state of the patient's nutrition.

Diet is important in reducing the weight of obese patients. The sugar content of the diet should be lowered. It is important to maintain regularity of eating habits and of meal size to keep insulin dosage in proper adjustment. Otherwise, emphasis on diet has diminished in the care of diabetics.

Two types of oral hypoglycemic agents are available for trial in those whom diet alone did not bring under control. The sulfonylurea group is thought to stimulate the pancreas to greater production of insulin or to release insulin that has been bound to other tissues. Several drugs of this group are available and differ in the duration of their action and in their toxicity. Tolbutamide is least dangerous and shortest in action. Treatment is effective in from 50 to 75 per cent of patients with adult-type diabetes. It is not satisfactory in juvenile diabetes or in patients with a tendency to develop acidosis. Other longer acting drugs of the sulfonylurea group sometimes are effective if tolbutamide is unsatisfactory.

Other hypoglycemic drugs belong to the

TABLE 6.16

*Prevalence of diabetes, by sex, age, and ratio of females to males: United States, July, 1964 to June, 1965*

| | Prevalence per 1000 Population | | | |
|---|---|---|---|---|
| Age | Both sexes | Male | Female | Ratio of females to males |
| yr. | | | | |
| All ages | 12.2 | 10.5 | 13.8 | 1.4 |
| Under 25 | 1.3 | 1.2 | 1.3 | 1.1 |
| 25-44 | 6.2 | 6.2 | 6.2 | 1.1 |
| 45-54 | 17.8 | 15.4 | 20.0 | 1.4 |
| 55-64 | 36.9 | 32.0 | 41.4 | 1.4 |
| 65-74 | 54.5 | 47.1 | 60.6 | 1.6 |
| 75+ | 49.2 | 47.0 | 50.8 | 1.5 |

Source:   National Center for Health Statistics. *Characteristics of Persons with Diabetes, U.S. 1964-1965*, Public Health Service Publication 1000, series 10, no. 40, 1967.

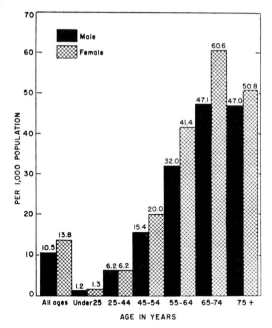

Fig. 6.18. Number of diabetics per 1,000 population by sex and age. Source: *Characteristics of Persons with Diabetes, U. S. 1964-1965.* Public Health Service Publication 1000, series 10, no. 40. Washington, D. C.: National Center for Health Statistics, 1967.

biguanide group. The most commonly used is phenformin. The mechanism of action of phenformin is not known, but it has some role in the release of insulin. This drug may cause nausea, vomiting, drowsiness, and weakness. It is best to begin with a small dose and gradually increase the dosage to a tolerance level. Again, this group of drugs is not suitable to treat diabetics prone to develop acidosis or to maintain diabetics about to undergo serious surgery or who are suffering from complications of diabetes.

Those patients whose diabetes is not controlled by diet or by oral drugs must rely on insulin. The dosage of insulin must be determined by trial and error, starting with a small dose 10 to 20 units and increasing every few days by 2 to 4 units until control can be attained. Some experiment with each individual is necessary to determine the dosage and to learn whether short-acting or intermediate-acting insulin is required. Once a regular regime has been set, the actual control of therapy must be the responsibility of the patient or of the parent in childhood cases. The patient must clearly understand the relationship of insulin to meals. He must learn to administer his own insulin safely. It is important that he know the

effect of exercise on carbohydrate metabolism. Following vigorous exercise, the dose of the hypoglycemic drug must be reduced or additional carbohydrate eaten. He must be taught the importance of care of the skin and to recognize the signs of developing acidosis and hypoglycemia. Finally, it is recommended that each diabetic carry an identification emblem stating that he has diabetes.

*Emergency Complications*

Severe acidosis is a dangerous result of failure to control diabetes. The patient should be transferred to a hospital for treatment if possible. Intravenous insulin should be given without delay. Blood is drawn to determine glucose, sodium, potassium chloride, bicarbonate, and acetone. Restoration of fluids by intravenous route should be started without delay. A solution of 0.45 per cent saline with 2.5 per cent fructose is recommended. The laboratory tests on the blood will determine the patient's requirements for salts. Sodium bicarbonate should be added to the fluid in severely acidotic cases. Insulin will have to be continued for several hours depending on the patient's response. As the blood glucose drops, insulin can be reduced.

A fairly common result of premature atherosclerosis is diabetic gangrene of the toes and feet due to occlusion of the blood supply. Sometimes surgery on the arteries to improve blood flow may help, but amputation is a frequent recourse to relieve the condition.

Hypoglycemic attacks or insulin shock results from overdosage of insulin or of oral drugs. Usually the condition is heralded by sweating, palpitation, hunger, and nervousness. If mild, the eating of sweets or drinking orange juice may relieve the symptoms. In severe cases, unconsciousness occurs so that intravenous glucose must be given to bring the patient back. Repeated attacks of hypoglycemia may damage the brain.[125]

*Surgery in the Diabetic*

Surgery, unless of an emergency nature, should not be undertaken in patients whose diabetes is not under control. On the day of operation, the patient should receive intravenously 100 gm. of glucose to which an adequate amount of insulin has been added. This may have to be repeated until the patient can resume oral feeding.

Diabetes adds an extra risk to surgery and

patients must be carefully observed and treated, especially if signs of infection occur.

### Diabetes in Pregnancy

Younger patients with no signs of atherosclerosis or other vascular disease do well in pregnancy. The risks of the fetus are much higher than among normal women. Because of the heavy fetal losses near the end of pregnancy, premature delivery is frequently induced. The birth weight of these babies is usually high, largely due to fluid retention. The newborns should be handled with all of the precautions shown to premature infants.

In severe diabetics, pregnancy apparently speeds up the disease process. It is unwise for such patients to attempt the pregnant state.

### Prognosis

Although life expectancy has been extended considerably by the modern treatment of diabetics, the vascular complications tend to progress slowly even in well-controlled cases. Diabetics usually succumb to kidney failure, stroke, or coronary heart disease or vascular disease of the extremities or a combination of complications within 15 years of the beginning of treatment. A few individuals go along for long periods with little evidence of these complications. Unfortunately, control of diabetes does not appear to affect the progress of vascular deterioration.

### Prevention

No effective measures for the prevention of diabetes are known. The only controllable factor known to be associated with the occurrence of diabetes is obesity. It is by no means established that weight reduction lowers the risk of developing diabetes, but it is known that weight reduction in obese diabetics is sometimes sufficient to control the disease.

From the public health point of view the detection of diabetes in the early stages appears to offer the best hope of preventing some diabetic complications and of prolonging life expectancy by instituting adequate treatment. The discovery of diabetes early in pregnancy may increase the likelihood of getting a live baby. Mass screen tests for blood glucose levels can be carried out in large numbers. A few drops of blood are taken from the fingertip in a capillary tube and tested in the laboratory.

Those individuals with higher than normal blood glucose levels are sent to the physicians for definitive tests to determine whether the person is a diabetic.

Since heredity is involved in the development of diabetes, it is inadvisable for diabetics to marry one another. Should they do so, the children should avoid obesity and have periodic examinations for the presence of sugar in the urine and for high blood sugar levels.

## Emphysema

### Introduction

Emphysema is the most common cause of pulmonary disability. According to estimates, several million individuals in the United States are living restricted lives on account of this chronic disease of the lungs. Emphysema is the basic problem in most patients past the age of 40 who suffer from cough, wheezing, and shortness of breath.[127]

Chronic bronchitis and pulmonary emphysema are frequently associated. Obstruction of the bronchi from bronchitis and the pathological changes of pulmonary emphysema can cause a similar clinical picture. Chronic bronchitis is characterized by an excessive secretion of mucus from the bronchi, resulting in a cough with sputum, in the absence of any other demonstrable lung disease. Patients with bronchitis may maintain clear air passages or show the effects of obstruction of air flow from the small bronchioles to the air sacs. The definition of pulmonary emphysema involves pathological changes in the air sacs beyond the termination of the smallest bronchioles. The normal lung tissue becomes overinflated, the normal air sacs being replaced by larger spaces of variable size. As a result of the changes, the pulmonary vascular bed is diminished, thus reducing the capacity of the blood to exchange gases with the inspired air. Chronic bronchitis and emphysema coexist in many patients. It is difficult in these patients to determine the relative contribution each disease makes separately to the overall obstruction of air flow.

### Occurrence

As a result of survey in the United States, it is estimated that at least 3 per cent of all persons over 40 years of age have evidence of chronic obstructive disease of the lungs. There were 14,897 workers in 1963 who were declared by the Social Security Administration to be totally and permanently disabled because of emphysema.[128] The variation from state to state in the mortality and disability rates for chronic respiratory disease is small, except for a higher frequency in Arizona. The extremely high rate in Arizona is probably due to migration of patients from other states seeking the benefits of the desert climate.

Mortality trends from emphysema without mention of bronchitis are rising progressively. The death rates were 0.8 per 100,000 in 1950, 5.2 per 100,000 in 1960, and 10.6 in 1967. The rates are much higher for men than for women (see Figure 6.19). The number of deaths attributed to emphysema is about twice the number reported as dying of tuberculosis. In 1971, deaths attributed to emphysema (without mention of bronchitis) were 22,420 (provisional); of these the large majority were men.[129]

Chronic bronchitis and emphysema are more common in Great Britain than in the United States. The distribution of cases in Britain is much higher in urban than in rural areas, possibly on account of the heavy air pollution of the cities.

*Pathogenesis and Pathology*

There is no recognized single, primary cause of emphysema. The disease most commonly follows recurrent or chronic infection and obstruction of the bronchioles such as is found in chronic bronchitis, bronchial asthma, or asthmatic bronchitis.[75] About two-thirds of

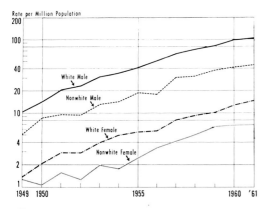

Fig. 6.19. Death rates for emphysema. Source: Dauer, C. C., Korns, R. F., and Schuman, L. M. *Infectious Diseases.* Cambridge, Massachusetts: Harvard University Press, 1968.

emphysema patients have previously had bouts of coughing with expectoration.

More than 90 per cent of emphysematous patients are heavy smokers.[130] Air pollution may also cause or aggravate emphysema. Conditions that cause extensive scarring of the lungs, such as silicosis or tuberculosis, are frequently complicated by development of emphysema.

The disease is far more common in men than in women. The reasons for this sex difference in attack rates are unknown. Emphysema increases in prevalence and severity with advancing age. There is some evidence that emphysema occurs more often among relatives of cases than in unrelated control groups. Such environmental factors as cigarette smoking, however, appear to be of more importance in the causation of the disease.

In emphysema, the total lung capacity may be increased, so that the lung contains more air than normal during full inspiration. There is an increased resistance to air flow, particularly during expiration. The greater resistance to air movement in chronic bronchitis and emphysema is caused by a narrowing of the lumen of the bronchi by mucus or by swelling of the epithelial lining. This partial blockage of respiration results in greater work in breathing, which in turn calls for more oxygen for the muscles.[131]

*Clinical Manifestations*

Chronic bronchitis and pulmonary emphysema frequently begin with cough as the first symptom. Following acute upper respiratory infections, the sputum may become purulent and episodes of wheezing and difficult breathing may occur. Gradually shortness of breath on exertion begins. This becomes progressively worse. Considerable loss of weight may ensue. The rate of progress of the disease is variable. In some, the respiratory failure moves rapidly, but in other cases, the disease moves slowly over a period of years. Most patients eventually die from heart failure. Pneumonia is also a frequent complication.

*Diagnosis*

The patient's history usually gives a strong indication of the diagnosis. Physical examination and X ray of the chest may be helpful. Tests of lung function, that is, lung volume and expiratory air flow, are important. Determination of the levels of oxygen and carbon dioxide in the blood are revealing in understanding the severity of the disease. Examination of the sputum to determine the volume and pus content is useful, as well as bacteriological studies to learn the nature of the infecting agents.

## Prognosis

The long-term outlook for the patient is poor. The course of the disease varies considerably from a rapidly fatal outcome in two to three years after a diagnosis is made up to years of reasonably active life. Treatment and rehabilitative measures can decrease disability and prolong life in up to 50 per cent of patients.

Signs pointing to a poor prognosis include persistently low blood oxygen levels and high levels of carbon dioxide. Enlargement of the heart and heart failure are other unfavorable developments.

## Treatment

Treatment is essentially palliative. It has not been found possible to reverse the disease process by use of drugs or other measures. Treatment should be directed toward improvement of the bronchitis. Antimicrobial therapy should be based on cultures of the sputum. Such treatment is of special importance during an acute flare-up of bronchitis. Either penicillin intramuscularly or a broad spectrum antibiotic may be used. Dosage should be adequate and therapy maintained for three to four weeks.

Bronchodilators may be helpful to some patients. Such drugs with liquefying agents may be given by nebulizers. Oxygen is administered when indicated to relieve hypoxia. If heart failure occurs, heart stimulants are required. In severe respiratory difficulty, a tracheotomy may be necessary to improve the patient's breathing.

All irritants to the respiratory tract should be avoided, especially the smoking of tobacco.

## Rehabilitation

Limitation of activity often leads to retirement from regular work. Many patients become excessively anxious and mental depression is not infrequent. An important aspect of treatment is relief of the anxiety that goes with shortness of breath. Breathing exercises may be helpful. In some communities, pulmonary rehabilitation centers are in operation with special equipment and trained physiotherapists in charge.

## Prevention

In the present state of knowledge, the smoking of cigarettes appears to be by far the most important factor in the etiology of bronchitis and emphysema. Air pollution and probably some occupational exposures also are unfavorable factors for large numbers of people. A drastic reduction in cigarette smoking and an effective campaign to control air pollution are certainly strongly indicated (see Fig. 6.20).

There are suggestions that genetic, socioeconomic, geographical, and climatic influences have had some importance in the causation of emphysema. Knowledge is limited, and extensive research programs to clarify the basic mechanisms of injury to the lungs are sorely needed. Investigation of the epidemiology and natural history of chronic bronchitis and emphysema through long-term studies in several communities may also be valuable.

There is a general lack of services, programs, and facilities for patient care. Pulmonary function laboratories, respiratory care units, and home care and rehabilitation programs should be made more widely available.

## REFERENCES

1. *Cecil-Loeb Textbook of Medicine*, Ed. 13, edited by P. M. Beeson and W. McDermott. Philadelphia: W. B. Saunders Co., 1971.
2. Bretoneau, P-F. *Des Inflammations Spéciales du Tissu Muqueux et an Particular de la Diphthérite, on Inflammation Pelliculaire, Connue Sous le Nom de Croup, d'Angine Malique, d'Angine Gangrenouse.* Paris: Crevot, 1826.
3. Burke, R. M. *An Historical Chronology of Tuberculosis*, Ed. 2. Springfield, Illinois: Charles C. Thomas, Publisher, 1955.
4. Florey, H. W. In *General Pathology*, Ed. 4, edited by H. W. Florey, London: Lloyd-Luke, 1970.
5. Hetherington, H. W., and Eshleman, F. W. *Tuberculosis: Prevention and Control*, Ed. 4. New York: G. P. Putnam's Sons, 1958.
6. Long, E. R. The decline of tuberculosis, with special reference to its generalized form. *Bull. Hist. Med., 8:* 819-843, 1940.
7. Center for Disease Control. *Reported Tuberculosis DAta, 1971.* DHEW Publication, No (HSM) 73-8201. December 1972 issue.
8. Center for Disease Control. *Morbidity and Mor-*

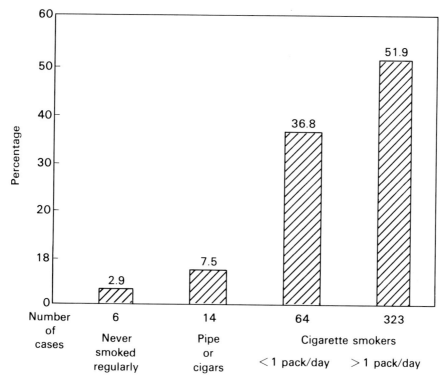

Fig. 6.20. Age-standardized percentage distribution of whole lung sections of males with moderate to far-advanced emphysema (score 3-9) by smoking category Source: Auerbach, O., E. C. Hammond, L. Garfinkel and C. Benante, *Relation of Smoking and Age to Emphysema—Whole Lung Section Study, New Engl. J. Med., 286:* 853-857 April 20, 1972. As reproduced in *Health Consequences of Smoking,* Public Health Service (HSMHA), January, 1973.

*tality Weekly Report.* Annual Supplement Summary, 1972. Vol. 21, No. 53, p. 12, July, 1973.

9. Lurie, M. G. *Resistance to Tuberculosis: Experimental Studies in Native and Acquired Defensive Mechanisms.* Cambridge, Massachusetts: Harvard University Press, 1964.

10. Waksman, S. A. *The Conquest of Tuberculosis.* Berkeley and Los Angeles: University of California Press, 1964.

11. *Tuberculosis Statistics: States and Cities, 1972.* Public Health Service, Center for Disease Control. DHEW Publication No. (CDC) 74-8249. June 1973 issue.

12. Schwabe, C. W. *Veterinary Medicine and Human Health,* Ed. 2. Baltimore: The Williams and Wilkins Co., 1969.

13. The Work of WHO, 1972. *Annual Report of the Director-General to WHO Assembly and to the United Nations.* WHO, Geneva, 1973.

14. *Report of the Committee on Infectious Diseases, 1974,* Ed. 17. American Academy of Pediatrics, Evanston, Illinois.

15. Rifampin—A valuable drug for use in the treatment of tuberculosis. Special Issue by various authors. *Chest: 61:* 517-598, 1972.

16. Myers, J. A. *Tuberculosis: A Half Century of Study and Conquest.* St. Louis: Green, 1970.

17. Shope, R. E. Swine influenza; experimental transmission and pathology. *J. Exp. Med., 54:* 349-359, 1931.

18. *Viral and Mycoplasmal Infections of the Respiratory Tract,* edited by V. Knight. Philadelphia: Lea & Febiger, 1973.

19. Todd, J. D., Lief, F. S., and Cohen, D. Experimental infection of ponies with the Hong Kong variant of human influenza virus. *Amer. J. Epidem., 92:* 330-336, 1970.

20. Conch, R. B., *et al.* Production of the influenza syndrome in man with equine influenza virus. *Nature, 224:* 512-514, 1969.

21. Burnet, F. M. *Principles of Animal Virology,* Ed. 2, New York: Academic Press, 1960.

22. Stuart-Harris, C. H. *Influenza and Other Virus Infections of the Respiratory Tract.* Baltimore: The Williams and Wilkins Co., 1965.

23. Oker-Blom, N., Hovi, T., Leinikki, P., Palosuo, J., Pettersson, R., and Suni, J. Protection of men from natural infection with influenza A2 (Hong Kong) virus by amantadine: a controlled field trial. *Brit. Med. J., iii:* 676-678, 1970.

24. Smorodintsev, A. A., *et al.* The prophylactic effectiveness of amantadine hydrochloride in an epidemic of Hong Kong influenza in Leningrad in 1969. *Bull. WHO 42: 865-873, 1970.*

25. Galbraith, A. W., Oxford, J. S., Schill, G. S., and Watson, G. I. Protective effect of 1-Adamantanamine hydrochloride on influenza A2 infections in the family environment. *Lancet II,* 15 Nov., 1026-1028, 1969.

26. Stollerman, G. H. Streptococcal diseases. In *Cecil-Loeb Textbook of Medicine,* Ed. 13, edited by P. B. Beeson and W. McDermott Philadelphia: W. B. Saunders Co., 1971.

27. Lancefield, R. C. A serological differentiation of human and other groups of hemolytic streptococci. *J. Exp. Med., 57:* 571-595, 1933.

28. Todd, E. W. Streptolysins of various groups and types of haemolytic streptococci; serological investigation. *J. Hyg. (Camb.), 39:* 1-11, 1939.

29. Wannamaker, L. W., and Matsen, J. M. *Streptococci and Streptococcal Diseases—Recognition, Understanding, and Management.* New York: Academic Press, 1972.

30. *Control of Communicable Diseases in Man,* edited by A. S. Benenson, Ed. 11 New York: American Public Health Association, 1970.

31. Rammelcamp, C. H. Concepts of pathogenesis of glomerulonephritis derived from studies in man. In *The Streptococcus, Rheumatic Fever and Glomerulonephritis,* edited by J. W. Uhr. Baltimore: The Williams and Wilkins Co., 1964.

32. Stetson, C. A., Jr., Rammelcamp, C. H., Krause, R. M., Kohen, R. J., and Perry, W. D. Epidemic acute nephritis: studies on etiology, natural history and prevention. *Medicine (Balto.)), 34:* 431-450, 1955.

33. Markowitz, M. and Gordis, L. G. *Rheumatic Fever, Ed 2, Vol. II. Major Problems in Clinical Pediatrics.* A. J. Schaffer, consulting editor. Philadelphia: W. B. Saunders Co., 1972.

34. Stollerman, G. H. The epidemiology of primary and secondary rheumatic fever. In *The Streptococcus, Rheumatic Fever and Glomerulonephritis,* edited by J. W. Uhr. Baltimore: The Williams and Wilkins Co., 1964.

35. Kaplan, M. H. Immunological relation of streptococcal and tissue antigens. I. Properties of an antigen in certain strains of group A streptococci exhibiting an immunological cross reaction with human heart tissue. *J. Immunol., 90:* 595-606, 1963.

36. Moriyama, I. M. Krueger, D. E., and Stamler, J. *Cardiovascular Diseases in the United States.* Cambridge, Massachusetts: Harvard University Press, 1971.

37. Roth, I. R., Ling, C., and Whittemore, A. Heart disease in children. A rheumatic group. I. Certain aspects of the age at onset and of recurrences in 488 cases of juvenile rheumatism ushered in by major clinical manifestations. *Amer. Heart J., 13:* 36-60, 1937.

38. WHO, Expert Committee. *Prevention of Rheumatic Fever.* WHO Techn. Rep. Ser. No. 342, 1966.

39. Theiler, M., and Downs, W. G. *The Arthropod-Borne Viruses of Vertebrates.* New Haven Yale University Press, 1973.

40. Clarke, D. H., and Casals, J. Arboviruses: group B. in *Viral and Rickettsial Infections of Man,* Ed. 4 edited by F. L. Horsfall and I. Tamm. Philadelphia: J. B. Lippincott, 1965.

41. Sabin, A. B. Survey of knowledge and problems in field of anthropod-borne virus infections. *Arch. Ges. Virusforsch., 9:* 1-10, 1959.

42. Reeves, W. C. Ecology of mosquitoes in relation to arboviruses. *Ann. Rev. Entom., 10:* 25-46, 1965.

43. Reeves, W. C., and Hammon, W. McD. *Epidemiology of the Arthropod-borne Viral Encephalitides in Kern County, California, 1943-1952.* Berkeley: University of California Press, 1962.

44. Bond, J. O., Quick, D. T., Witte, J. J., and Oard, H. C. The 1962 epidemic of St. Louis encephalitis in Florida. 1. Epidemiologic observations. *Amer. J. Epidem., 81:* 392-404, 1965.

45. A cooperative study: epidemic St. Louis encephalitis in Houston, 1964. *J.A.M.A., 193:* 139-146, 1965.

46. *Neurotropic Viral Diseases—Surveillance.* Center for Disease Control. Annual Encephalitis Summary—1971. DHEW Publication, No. (CDC) 74-8252, July, 1973.

47. Peavy, J. E., Dewlett, A. J., Metzger, W. R., and Bagby, J. Epidemiological and aerial spray control of arthropod-borne viral encephalitis in Texas. *Amer. J. Public Health, 57:* 2111-2116, 1967.

48. Furcolow, M. L. Clinical types of histoplasmosis. In *Histoplasmosis,* edited by H. C. Sweany. Springfield, Illinois: Charles C Thomas, Publisher, 1960.

49. Darling, S. T. Protozoan general infection producing pseudotubercles in lungs and focal necrosis in liver, spleen and lymph nodes. *J. A. M. A., 46:* 1283-1285, 1906.

50. *Histoplasmosis,* edited by H. C. Sweany. Springfield, Illinois: Charles C Thomas, Publisher, 1960.

51. Van Pernis, P. A., Benson, M. E., and Holinger, P. H. Specific cutaneous reactions with histoplasmosis: preliminary report of another case. *J.A.M.A., 117:* 436-437, 1941.

52. Palmer, C. E. Non-tuberculous pulmonary calcification and sensitivity to histoplasmin. *Public Health Rep., 60:* 513-520, 1945.

53. Palmer, C. E. Geographic differences in sensitivity to histoplasmin among student nurses. *Public Health Rep., 61:* 475-487, 1946.

54. Edwards, P. Q., and Billings, E. L. Worldwide pattern of skin sensitivity to histoplasmin. *Amer. J. Trop. Med. & Hyg., 20:* 288-319, 1971.

55. Utz, J. P. The mycoses. In *Cecil-Loeb Textbook of Medicine, Ed. 13,* edited by P. B. Beeson and W. McDermott. Philadelphia: W. B. Saunders Co., 1971.

56. Emmons, C. W. Isolation of histoplasma capsulatum from soil. *Public Health Rep., 64:* 892-896, 1949.

57. Zeidberg, L. D., Ajello, L., Dillon, A., and Runyun, L. C. Isolation of histoplasma capsulatum from soil. *Amer. J. Public*

*Health, 42:* 930-935, 1952.

58. Furcolow, M. L. Epidemiology of histoplasmosis. In *Histoplasmosis,* edited by H. C. Sweany. Springfield, Illinois: Charles C Thomas, Publisher, 1960.

59. *Mycoses Surveillance.* Center for Disease Control, Atlanta, Georgia. DHEW Publication No. (CDC) 74-8250, July, 1973.

60. Edwards, P. Q., and Palmer, C. E. Nationwide histoplasmin sensitivity and histoplasma infection. *Public Health Rep., 78:* 241-259, 1963.

61. Baum, G. L., Larkin, J. C., and Sutliff, W. D. Follow-up of patients with chronic pulmonary histoplasmosis treated with amphotericin B. *Chest, 58:* 562-565, 1970.

62. Witorsch, P., Andriote, V. T., Emmons, C. W., and Utz, J. P. The polypeptide antifungal agent (X-5079C): further studies in 39 patients. *Amer. Rev. Resp. Dis., 93:* 876-888, 1966.

63. President's Commission on Heart Disease,Cancer and Stroke. *A National Program to Conquer Heart Disease, Cancer and Stroke,* Vol. I. Washington, D.C.: Government Printing Office, 1964.

64. McDowell, F. H. Cerebrovascular diseases. In *Cecil-Loeb Texbook of Medicine,* Ed. 13, edited by P. B. Beeson and W. McDermott. Philadelphia: W. B. Saunders Co., 1971.

65. Kottke, F. J. The specialist's role in continuing care of the stroke patient. In *Proceedings of the National Stroke Congress, October 29-31, 1964,* Chicago, Illinois, edited by R. E. De Forest. Springfield, Illinois: Charles C Thomas, Publisher, 1966.

66. *Cerebrovascular Diseases: Prevention, Treatment and Rehabilitation.* Report of a WHO Meeting. WHO Tech. Rep. Series #469 WHO Geneva, 1971.

67. Truscott, B. L. Establishment of community stroke programs. Development of the North Carolina Stroke program. *Amer. J. Public Health. 61:* 2449-2454, December, 1971.

68. Kurtzke, J. F. *Epidemiology of Cerebrovascular Disease,* New York; Springer-Verlag, 1969.

69. Oral contraception and increased risk of cerebral ischemia or thrombosis. Collaborative group for the study of stroke in young women. *N. Engl. J. Med. 288:* 871-878. April 26, 1973.

70. Siekert, R. G., Millikan, C. H., and Whisnant, J. P. Anticoagulant therapy in intermittent cerebrovascular insufficiency. *J.A.M.A., 176:* 19-22, 1961.

71. Morris, J. N. *The Uses of Epidemiology,* Ed. 2. Baltimore: The Williams and Wilkins Co., 1964.

72. Killip, T. Ischemic heart disease. In *Cecil-Loeb Textbook of Medicine,* Ed. 13, edited by P. B. Beeson and W. McDermott. Philadelphia: W. B. Saunders Co., 1971.

73. Raab, W. *Prevention of Ischemic Heart Disease* Springfield, Illinois: Charles C Thomas, Publisher, 1966.

74. *Coronary Heart Disease in Adults: United States 1960-62.* Public Health Service Publication 1000, series 11, No. 10, Washington, D.C.: National Center for Health Statistics, 1965.

75. Blum, H. L., and Keranen, G. M. *Control of Chronic Disease in Man.* New York: American Public Health Association, 1966.

76. Robb-Smith, A. H. T. *The Enigma of Coronary Heart Disease.* Chicago: Year Book Medical Publishers, Inc., 1967.

77. *Diet and Heart Disease.* New York: American Heart Association, 1965.

78. Ibrahim, M. A., Pinsky, W., Kohn, R. M., Binette, P. J., and Winkelstein, W. Coronary heart disease: screening by familial aggregation. *Arch. Envir. Health. (Chicago), 16:* 235-240, 1968.

79. Dubos, R. *Man Adapting.* New Haven: Yale University Press, 1965.

80. *Fact Book-Prescription Drug Industry.* Washington, D.C.: Pharmaceutical Manufacturer's Association, 1972.

81. Ciba Pharmaceutical Company. Drug searchers draw on the best of two worlds. *Med. World News, 6:* 46-52, 164-167, 1965.

82. Modell, W. Chairman's closing remarks. In *Ciba Foundation Symposium: Drug Responses in Man,* edited by G. E. W. Wolstenholme and R. Porter. Boston: Little, Brown and Co., 1967.

83. *Drug-Induced Diseases* Vol. 3, edited by L. Meyler and H. M. Peck. New York: Excerpta Medica Foundation, 1968.

84. *Drug-Induced Diseases,* Vol. 4, edited by L. Meyler and H. M. Peck. Amsterdam: Excerpta Medica, 1972.

85. Wintrobe, M. M. The therapeutic millenium and its price. In *Drugs in Our Society,* edited by P. Talalay. Baltimore: The Johns Hopkins Press, 1964.

86. Beutler, E. Glucose 6-phosphate dehydrogenase deficiency. In *The Metabolic Basis of Inherited Disease,* Ed. 3, edited by J. B. Stanbury, J. B. Wyngaarden, and D. S. Fredrickson. New York: The Blakiston Division, McGraw-Hill Book Co., 1972.

87. Lehmann, H., and Liddell, J. The cholinesterase variants. In *The Metabolic Basis of Inherited Disease,* Ed. 3, edited by J. B. Stanbury, J. B. Wyngaarden, and D. S. Frederickson, New York: The Blakiston Division, McGraw-Hill Book Co., 1972.

88. Spain, D. M. *The Complications of Modern Medical Practices.* New York: Grune and Stratton, 1963.

89. Lenz, W. Malformations caused by drugs in pregnancy. *Amer. J. Dis. Child., 112:* 99-106, 1966.

90. News Report. Hosp. Trib. 2: 6,2, 1968.

91. Kelsey, F. O. Events after thalidomide. *J. Dent. Res., 46:* 1201-1205, 1967.

92. Lenz, W. Epidemiology of congenital malformations. In *Evaluation and Mechanisms of Drug Toxicity,* edited by J. J. Burns. *Ann. N.Y. Acad. Sci., 123:* 228-236, 1965.

93. Hahn, F. E. Chloramphenicol. In *Antibiotics. Vol. 1. Mechanisms of Action,* edited by D. Gottlieb and P. D. Shaw. New York: Springer-Verlag, 1967.

94. Davies, W. *The Pharmaceutical Industry.* Oxford:

Pergamon Press, 1967.

95. Yunis, A. A., and Bloomberg, G. R. Chloramphenicol toxicity: clinical features and pathogenesis. *Progr. Hematol., 4::* 138-159, 1964.

96. British Medical Association. Report of Committee on Safety of Drugs. *Brit. Med. J., 1:* 484, 1967.

97. Best, W. R. Chloramphenicol: associated blood dyscrasias. *J.A.M.A., 201:* 181-188, 1967.

98. Moore, C. V. Anemia of bone marrow failure. In *Cecil-Loeb Textbook of Medicine,* Ed. 13, edited by P. B. Beeson and W. McDermott. Philadelphia: W. B. Saunders Co., 1971.

99. Barr, D. P. Hazards of modern diagnosis and therapy. The price we pay. *J.A.M.A., 159:* 1452-1456, 1955.

100. Schimmel, E. M. The Physician as pathogen (editorial). *J. Chronic Dis., 16: 1-4, 1963.*

101. *National Nosocomial Infectious Study.* Center for Disease Control 3rd quarter, 1972. Issued August, 1973. DHEW Publication No. (CDC) 74-8257.

102. *Drugs in our Society,* edited by P. Talalay. Baltimore: The Johns Hopkins Press, 1964.

103. *Disease of Medical Progress,* Ed. 2, edited by R. H. Moser. Springfield, Illinois: Charles C Thomas, Publisher, 1964.

104. Knox, W. E. Phenylketonuria. In *The Metabolic Basis of Inherited Disease,* Ed. 3, edited by J. B. Stanbury, J. B. Wyngaarden, and D. S. Frederickson. New York: The Blakiston Division, McGraw-Hill Book Co., 1972.

105. Jervis, G. A. Phenylpyruvic oligophrenia: deficiency of phenylalanine oxidizing system. *Proc. Soc. Exp. Biol. Med., 82:* 514-515, 1953.

106. Scriber, C. R. Inborn errors of amino acid metabolism. In *Cecil-Loeb Textbook of Medicine,* Ed. 13, edited by P. B. Beeson and W. McDermott. Philadelphia: W. B. Saunders, Co., 1971.

107. Frimpter, G. W. Aminoacidurias due to inherited disorders of metabolism. N. Engl. J. Med., 289: 835-841, 1973.

108. Auerbach, V. H., DiGeorge, A. M., and Carpenter, G. G. Phenylalanemia. In *Amino Acid Metabolism and Genetic Variation,* edited by W. L. Nyhan. New York The Blakiston Division, McGraw-Hill Book Co., 1967.

109. *Genetic Disorders: Prevention, Treatment and Rehabilitation.* Report of WHO Scientific Group. WHO Tech. Rep. Series No. 497, Geneva, 1972.

110. Jervis, G. A. Phenylketonuria. In *Amino Acid Metabolism and Genetic Variation,* edited by W. L. Nyhan. New York: The Blakiston Division, McGraw-Hill Book Co., 1967.

111. Newborn Screening for Metabolic Disorders. Massachusetts Department of Public Health. *N. Engl. J. Med., 288:* 1299-1300, 1973.

112. Milunsky, A. *The Prenatal Diagnosis of Hereditary Disorders.* Springfield, Illinois: Charles C Thomas, Publisher, 1973.

113. Vianna, N. J., and Polan, A. K. Epidemiologic evidence for transmission of Hodgkins disease. *N. Engl. J. Med., 289:* 499-502, Sept. 6, 1973.

114. *Cancer Facts and Figures.* New York: American Cancer Society, 1973.

115. Lukes, R. J., and Butler, J. J. The pathology and nomenclature of Hodgkin's disease. *Cancer Res., 26:* 1063-1081, 1966.

116. Ultman, J. E., Cunningham, J. K., and Gellhorn, A. The clinical picture of Hodgkin's disease. *Cancer Res., 26:* 1047-1060, 1966.

117. Perry, S. (Moderator). Hodgkin's disease: combined clinical staff conference at the National Institutes of Health. *Ann. Intern. Med., 67:* 424-442, 1967.

118. Karnofsky, D. A. The staging of Hodgkin's disease. *Cancer Res., 26:* 1090-1094, 1966.

119. Moore, C. V. Conditions primarily affecting lymph nodes. In *Cecil-Loeb Textbook of Medicine,* Ed. 13, edited by P. B. Beeson and W. McDermott. Philadelphia: W. B. Saunders Co., 1971.

120. Stutzman, L., and Glidewell, O. Multiple chemotherapeutic agents for Hodgkin's disease. *J.A.M.A., 225:* 1202-1211, 1973.

121. Renold, A. E., Stauffacher, W., and Cahill, G. F. Diabetes mellitus. In *The Metabolic Basis for Inherited Disease,* Ed. 3, edited by J. B. Stanbury, J. B. Wyngaarden, and D. S. Frederickson. New York: The Blakiston Division, McGraw-Hill Book Co., 1972.

122. Wright, P. H., Ashmore, J., and Malaisse, W. J. Biochemical disorders in human disease. In *Diabetes Mellitus and Hypoglycemia,* edited by R.H.S. Thompson and I.D.P. Wooten. New York: Academic Press, 1970.

123. *Diabetes Mellitus,* Ed. 7 (Rev. 2) Indianapolis, Indiana: Lilly Research Laboratories, 1973.

124. Neel, J. V., Fajans, S. S., Conn, J. W., and Davidson, R. T. The evaluation of genetic factors in selected illustrative diseases: diabetes mellitus. In *Genetics and Epidemiology of Chronic Diseases,* edited by J. V. Neel, M. W. Shaw, and W. J. Schull. Public Health Service Publication 1163. Washington, D.C.: United States Public Health Service, 1965.

125. Bondy, P. K. Diabetes mellitus. In *Cecil-Loeb Textbook of Medicine,* Ed. 13, edited by P. B. Beeson and W. McDermott. Philadelphia: W. B. Saunders Co., 1971.

126. *Characteristics of Persons with Diabetes, United States, July, 1964-June, 1965.* Public Health Service Publication 1000, series 10, No. 40. Washington, D.C.: National Center for Health Statistics, 1967.

127. Farber, S. M., and Wilson, R. H. L. Chronic obstructive emphysema. *Clin. Symposia, 20:* 35-69, 1968.

128. Report of the Task Force on Chronic Bronchitis and Emphysema, Princeton, New Jersey, October 16-20, 1966. *Bull. Nat. Tuberc. Assn.,* May, 1967.

129. *Prevalence of Selected Chronic Respiratory Conditions—United States, 1970.* National Center for Health Statistics, Series 10-No. 84. DHEW Publication, No. (HRA) 74-1511, Sept. 1973.

130. *The Health Consequences of Smoking.* A Public Health Service Review, 1973, Public Health

Service Publication 1696. Washington, D.C.: United States Public Health Service, 1973.

131. Howell, J.B.L. Airway Obstruction. *Cecil-Loeb* *Textbook of Medicine,* Ed. 13, edited by P. B. Beeson and W. McDermott. Philadelphia: W. B. Saunders Co., 1971.

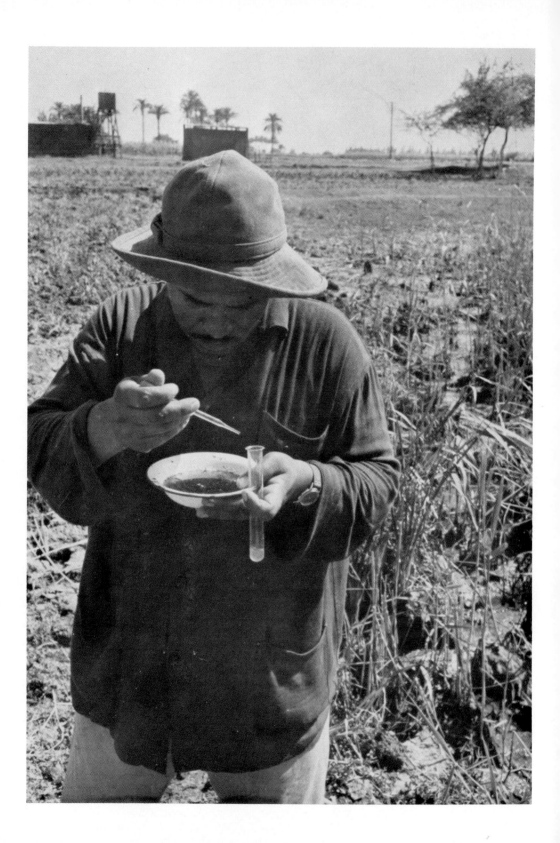

# 7

# Methods of disease control

In all countries that have adopted the Western ways of life, especially of course the United States, the emphasis is on controlling disease rather than on living more wisely. In fact, the general assumption throughout the world is that health cannot be achieved, or maintained, without vaccines, drugs, pesticides, genetic guidance, and the general availability of medical and surgical services.

RENE DUBOS, Man Adapting*

Effective measures for disease control, as outlined in Chapter 1, grew from efforts to combat the terrible epidemics of the Middle Ages and of modern times. Quarantine was developed in Venice to prevent importation of plague. Forced isolation in segregated institutions was widely practiced in Europe to control leprosy. Inoculation with smallpox infection, as developed in the Far East, and later vaccination with cowpox virus was widely introduced to prevent serious effects of smallpox epidemics. These and many less effective measures were desperately attempted to give some measure of protection against the dreaded epidemic diseases.

In the 19th century, cholera scourged Europe and America repeatedly. The fear of this fatal disease led to the beginnings of modern public health measures. The idea became widely prevalent that filth, crowding, poor housing, and uncleanliness in general were productive of ill health and indeed of epidemic disease. In England, the movement to clean up towns and cities by introducing adequate water supplies, of removing human wastes, and of improving housing quickly began to give favorable results. Cholera and typhoid fever soon largely disappeared from urban areas that had become "sanitated."

Shortly thereafter the investigations of Pasteur, Koch, and a host of other bacteriologists provided a scientific basis for the control of infectious diseases. In addition to sanitation,

a wide variety of other and more specific measures were developed to combat disease. In the pages that follow, an account of the methods that have been found effective in control of disease is stated briefly.

In discussing specific measures of disease control, it must always be borne in mind that certain broad aspects of human life are sometimes of overriding importance in the determination of the rise and decline of epidemic disease in any population. Such catastrophic influences as war, economic depression, unemployment, or crop failures that result in a decline of living standards, malnutrition, crowding, and stressful situations affect the disease pattern of a people adversely. Tuberculosis and syphilis are two important examples of human diseases that are particularly sensitive to such social and environmental adversities.

As described in Chapter 2, there are many levels at which health agencies are active in the promotion of disease control. The World Health Organization (WHO) maintains surveillance for the important epidemic diseases and gives timely notice to all governments of dangerous situations that arise. In addition, WHO is conducting several wide-scale disease control operations in countries requiring assistance. Thus, campaigns against smallpox, tuberculosis, malaria, and yaws are going forward vigorously. WHO, through its expert committees and its numerous publications, is performing a valuable service in dissemination of information and in coordination of national planning for mutual disease control activities.

National health agencies have responsibility for the prevention of the importation, as far as may be possible, of communicable disease from abroad. In the United States, the Federal Government has wide powers and responsibilities for disease control. During the past 40 years or more, the activities of Federal agencies in this field have been steadily increasing (see Chapter 2). State agencies have direct responsibility for the health of their citizens. To a considerable extent, this responsibility is passed on to local health departments, where services

* © Yale University Press, New Haven, 1965.

289

to individuals are largely centered.

In every community, large or small, individual practitioners of medicine, dentistry, nursing, veterinary medicine, pharmacy, and other professional people carry out a tremendous service in protecting the health of the people. Also, at all levels, voluntary health agencies are keenly interested in the promotion of programs for disease control, in educating the public on protective health measures, and in soliciting public support for official health activities.

A full knowledge of the factors responsible for the maintenance and transmission of a disease is of the greatest importance in discovering the most favorable points of attack. Frequently a number of possibly effective methods of control may be available. The choice of method will then depend upon such considerations as relative cost, relative effectiveness, and relative acceptability of methods on the part of the public. For example, malaria may be approached by mass treatment of populations to prevent mosquitoes from becoming infected, by larviciding methods, and by house spraying with pesticides to reduce the population density of the mosquito vector. Screening of homes also affords some protection from mosquito bites.

In controlling diseases, much can be done for the public by health agencies in the way of protecting food and water supplies, controlling insect carriers, in surveillance of epidemic infections, and in reducing air pollution. More and more, it becomes necessary for parents to take steps to protect their children and for individuals to take personal action to seek immunization or to improve the conditions of personal hygiene. This points up the increasing importance of health education to provide the public with timely, reliable, and interesting health information and advice.

## CONTROLLING THE SAFETY OF THE ENVIRONMENT

The more people are crowded together, the more urgent is the necessity for sanitary control. This basic health fact was well understood in earlier civilizations, as witnessed by drains and aqueducts found among ruins of ancient cities.

The United States population has passed the 208 million mark. Seven of every 10 Americans now live in cities, and this proportion is steadily increasing. In providing for this rising popula-

tion, water has become the number one natural resource problem. The United States is not running out of water, but there is a limit to the developable dependable water supply. If this limited supply is to be adequate for all needs, the same waters must be used over and over. The supply is relatively fixed; the demand is rapidly increasing.

### Water Purification

The problems of water pollution have been accentuated by the speed of growth of the population and of industry, as well as by changing technologies and new agricultural practices. Four major sources of water pollution are now recognized: sewage, industrial wastes, land drainage, and recreational uses of reservoirs, lakes, etc. The characteristics of sewage are changing. Organic chemicals of industrial origin are especially difficult to handle. In addition to the usual wastes from industry, new and more troublesome materials are being encountered. These include radioactive wastes and a wide range of complex substances from chemical industries. Hot wastes that increase stream temperature and hinder the biological purification process of streams are common. Land drainage, including urban runoff, is an important source of pollution. Agricultural drainage brings a variety of pesticides to the streams. Irrigation return flow is of limited use due to a heavy content of inorganic salts leached from the soil. Increasing recreational use of impounded waters introduces other sources of pollution. The wastes from motor craft and from toxic chemicals used to destroy water plants or insects are only some of the possible sources of pollution.[1]

Public water supplies come from such varied sources as streams, lakes, deep wells, and springs. Surface waters do not usually have as high a chemical content as do waters from deep wells and springs. However, waters from the latter sources tend to have less bacterial contaminants than do surface waters. Surface waters, therefore, should probably always be subjected to filtration through sand and chlorination.

The problems of ensuring a pure water supply and of safe disposal of human excreta are intimately linked. It is difficult to have one without the other. Before good water practices came into general use, almost every city experienced epidemics of water-borne disease annually. In 1900, outbreaks of typhoid fever were so common in cities as to be regarded almost as an unavoidable human experience. This much feared disease has become rare in the United States (see Table 7.1). As of 1973, there was an estimated total of 30,000 to 40,000 public water systems in the United States serving a population of approximately 144 million.

A field study conducted by the Federal Government in 1969-70 indicated that 5.4 per cent of all Americans are served impure drinking water from an estimated 5000 community water systems, mostly in smaller communities. In addition, some 20 million people are today without running water and are hauling water from suspect sources. Another 30 million use water from individual sources, such as wells or springs, many of which are not adequately protected against contamination.

In the decade 1961-70, there were 130 known or reported outbreaks of illness from contaminated water. Twenty persons died and an estimated 46,000 people became ill. Probably many outbreaks went unreported.

The safety of community water supplies is supervised constantly by the appropriate health departments. Tests are performed in the laboratory at regular intervals to check the quality of the water and to discover any signs of pollution. Both chemical and bacteriological tests are used. The total number of bacteria is estimated. High bacterial counts indicate pollution with organic material. Presence of coliform bacilli indicates probable contamination with fecal matter. The higher the coliform count, the greater is the probability of dangerous contamination.

Congress, realizing the increasing urgency of the matter, enacted the Water Pollution Control Act of 1948. This Act directed the U.S. Public Health Service to develop programs for the solution of water pollution problems in cooperation with the states, interstate agencies, municipalities, and industries. This Act was strengthened by the Federal Water Pollution Control Act Amendments of 1956 which provided grants for research, investigation, training of personnel, control programs, and construction of treatment works. In 1965, Congress further amended the law to create a Federal Water Pollution Control Administration and to increase funds for research, development and for construction of sewage treatment works. The Administration was required to establish criteria for water quality. Under the President's Reorganization Plan No. 2 of 1966, this Water Administration, except for responsibilities relating to health, was transferred from the Department of Health, Education, and Welfare to the Department of the Interior. The sum of $3.55 billion was provided for expenditure over a 5-year period to construct sewage treatment facilities and to clean up interstate river basins.[2]

The Federal Water Pollution Control Act of 1972 defines two goals: (1) by July 1983, water clean enough for swimming and other recreational use, and for the propagation of fish, shellfish, and wildlife; and (2) by 1985, an end to discharges of any pollutants whatsoever into public waters.

TABLE 7.1

*Waterborne disease outbreaks 1971-72, by etiology and type of water system*

| | Municipal | | Semi-Public | | Individual | | Total | |
|---|---|---|---|---|---|---|---|---|
| | Outbreaks | Cases | Outbreaks | Cases | Outbreaks | Cases | Outbreaks | Cases |
| Gastroenteritis | 8 | 4025 | 14 | 1590 | | | 22 | 5615 |
| Infectious hepatitis | 4 | 80 | 4 | 175 | 3 | 11 | 11 | 266 |
| S. sonnei | 1 | 187 | 5 | 427 | | | 6 | 614 |
| Giardiasis | | | 3 | 112 | | | 3 | 112 |
| Chemical poisoning | 1 | 41 | 2 | 161 | | | 3 | 202 |
| Salmonellosis | | | | | 1 | 3 | 1 | 3 |
| Typhoid | | | | | 1 | 5 | 1 | 5 |
| Total | 14 | 4333 | 28 | 2465 | 5 | 19 | 47 | 6817 |

Source:   Center for Disease Control, Foodborne Outbreaks, Annual Summary, 1972, November, 1973, DHEW Publication No. (CDC) 74-8185.

Current water purification plants provide a solution to the pollution problems of a generation ago. Then their main function was to remove suspended particulate matter and to destroy microorganisms that might cause disease. These functions are now being carried out efficiently, but even modern plants do not remove dissolved impurities effectively. To improve taste and odor, if objectionable, carbon is usually applied, but this method is not always effective. Further research is badly needed on a number of problems, such as improved separation of suspended solids, better removal of dissolved substances, and disinfection. Chlorine is not effective, in the concentrations generally used, against some viruses or the cysts of pathogenic amoeba. Presumptive tests to detect the presence and to identify toxic chemicals are also needed.

## Waste Disposal

In rural areas where water carriage of human excreta is not possible, the simplest arrangement for safe disposal of such refuse is some type of privy or chemical toilet. If a running water supply is available, household cesspools or septic tanks are commonly used. In towns and cities, a community sewerage system is generally employed. On account of the large amounts of water that sewage contains, the most frequent method of disposal of the effluent is in a body of water. As the undesirability of dumping raw sewage into streams or lakes is apparent, the practice of treating sewage at collection points has become more general. The reasons for this are to prevent the pollution of water supplies, bathing places, and food products such as fish, clams, and oysters. Proper sewage treatment also diminishes bad odors, reduces the fouling of streams, and even is economically sound as a result of the salvaging of commercially valuable products.

Since 1900, the number of communities served by sewerage systems has increased in the United States from 950 to over 13,000. Over 7500 of the towns and cities now have sewage treatment plants which serve some 63 per cent of the population. Even so, the degree of urban pollution has increased due to growth of population, wearing out of older plants, failure to construct needed facilities, increased use of sewers by industry, and greater production of sewage in the home by use of garbage disposal units, electric clothes washers, and more bathrooms. It is predicted that municipal sewage loads will increase nearly 4-fold over the next 50 years.

Table 7.2 shows the growth in sewered population and the increase in urban sewage pollution if the present rate of treatment plant construction is maintained. The data shown in this table indicate that the amount of pollution reaching the water courses in 1970 and 1980 will be substantially the same as at present. This problem is illustrated by the situation in Chicago. Although Chicago has a good modern treatment system, every day the city pours into the Illinois waterway an effluent equivalent to the sewage from 1 million people and containing solid wastes in suspension or in solution equal to 1800 tons.

The methods of sewage treatment now in use have been improved little during the past 40 years. They are proving entirely inadequate already for the large metropolitan areas. New processes of treatment that will remove much more of the pollutants are urgently required.

Responsibility for providing adequate water of a dependable quality and for the safe disposal of human wastes rests with the Division of Sanitary Engineering usually included in the State Health Department. The Federal agencies are responsible only for water used in interstate carriers such as trains, ships, buses, and airplanes. The national government, however, has been active for many years in research work in the fundamental problems involved and in the preparation of criteria for safe standards of water.

Solid wastes are increasingly difficult to dispose of satisfactorily. In the past this type of waste consisted mainly of garbage and ashes. At present, towns and cities are confronted with growing volumes of industrial waste, demolition refuse, old appliances, non-returnable containers, as well as hazardous materials from laboratories and hospitals. Landfills and burning programs cannot meet the problem. The 165 million tons of such solid waste matter of 1966 is estimated to reach 260 million tons in a decade. The 7.7 million automobiles discarded in 1970 may double or triple before the year 2000. The effects on health of the inefficient methods of solid waste disposal are

TABLE 7.2

*Growth of sewered population in the United States from 1900*
*with projected estimates to 1980*

Population Served by Sewers and Sewage Treatment (1900—1980)

| Year | Sewered Population | Served by Treatment | Discharging Raw Sewage | Population Equivalent Discharged |
|------|------|------|------|------|
| | | *millions* | | |
| 1900 | 24.5 | 1.0 | 23.5 | 24.0 |
| 1920 | 47.5 | 9.5 | 38.0 | 40.0 |
| 1935 | 69.5 | 28.5 | 41.0 | 51.0 |
| 1950 | 80.0 | 54.0 | 26.0 | 60.0 |
| 1960 | 105.0 | 80.0 | 25.0 | 75.0 |
| 1970 | (145.0) | $(130.0)^1$ | $(15.0)^1$ | $(76.0)^1$ |
| | | $(110.0)^2$ | $(35.0)^2$ | $(84.0)^2$ |
| 1980 | (210.0) | $(210.0)^3$ | $(None)^3$ | $(74.0)^3$ |
| | | $(140.0)^4$ | $(70.0)^4$ | $(150.0)^4$ |

[1] Assumes that progress toward secondary treatment for all municipal wastes by 1980 will be made; a *per capita* population equivalent (P.E.) of 1.6; and 80 per cent removal of P.E. by secondary treatment.

[2] Same as footnote [1] present rate of sewage treatment construction will continue.

[3] Assumes that all sewered population will be served by secondary sewage treatment by 1980; a *per capita* population equivalent (P.E.) of 1.75; and 80 per cent removal of P.E. by secondary treatment.

[4] Same as footnote [3] except assumes present rate of sewage treatment construction will continue.

Source:     *Report of Committee on Environmental Health Problems,* Public Health Service Publication 908, 1962. Data originally were taken or extrapolated from 'Modern Sewage Disposal," Federation of Sewage Works Association, 1938; 1957 Inventory of Municipal and Industrial Waste Facilities, United States Public Health Service; and unpublished data from Basic Data Branch, Division of Water Supply and Pollution Control, United States Public Health Service.

as yet unknown. It does appear urgent that basic studies on improvement of disposal methods be undertaken at once.[3]

## Air Pollution

Pollution of the air has always occurred in urban areas, especially in those using coal for heating and industrial purposes. The seriousness of the problem has steadily grown during this century with the expansion of industry, of power production, and by the introduction of internal combustion engines for transportation. As of 1972, there were over 86.4 million automobiles and trucks in use in the United States consuming some 97,547 million gallons of fuel annually.[4] It is estimated that the number of motor vehicles will rise to 125 million or more by 1980 (see Table 7.3).

The use of coal for energy requirements in homes, businesses, and industries is now the equivalent of 495 million tons per year. The rise of nuclear energy to produce power is growing. In 1966, about 55 per cent of new generating capacity ordered was based on nuclear power.[5] As of 1975, nuclear power provides only about 3.2 per cent of the energy input of the nation. By 1985, the figure is expected to rise to about 10 per cent.[4] The use of oil and gas for domestic and industrial purposes continues to expand. For example, consumption of natural gas rose in the United States from 6026 billion cubic feet in 1950 to 22,493 billion cubic feet in 1971.

These sources of pollutants and many others are responsible for the masses of inorganic and organic gases and particulate matter being constantly discharged into the atmosphere. The main inorganic gases are carbon dioxide and monoxide, sulfur dioxide, some hydrogen sulfide, and nitric oxide and dioxide. The organic gases come mostly from oil refineries, automobile exhausts, dry cleaning establishments, garages, and service stations. Some of these substances in the presence of sunlight combine with other gases to form what is known as "smog."

Particulate matter in the air may consist of dusts, fumes, fogs, carbon, tar, fly ash, mists, and some metallic oxides. Pollen accounts for about 20 per cent, and industrial dirt and ash for another 13 per cent. Many other pollutants make up the remainder.

The extent of air pollution in an area does not depend exclusively upon the discharge of pollutants into the atmosphere. Topographic and meteorological factors may determine whether a serious pollution situation will develop. In general, wind, rain, atmospheric stability, and topographical features govern the average distribution of air contaminants in a particular locality. Cities situated in natural bowls or valleys are especially likely to experience episodes of severe air pollution. Rain or snow tends to remove contaminating matter from the atmosphere. Wind disperses the pollutants and causes their dilution. The relation of day to night temperatures sometimes determines the formation of inversion layers with the lowest layer coolest. This stagnation of air movement traps any discharged contaminants and keeps them near the ground.

Aside from the heavy economic losses from air pollution and the undesirable aesthetic impressions, there is evidence that human health is adversely affected. These effects vary from irritation of eyes, nose, and throat to serious complications among individuals with chronic debilitating conditions. Investigations indicate that air pollution as it now exists in many American cities contributes to the incidence and the severity of acute respiratory

TABLE 7.3

*U. S. motor vehicle registration*

| Year | Passenger Cars | Buses | Trucks | Total[1] |
|------|----------------|-------|--------|----------|
| 1963 | 69,055,000 | 298,000 | 13,360,000 | 82,714,000 |
| 1964 | 71,983,000 | 305,000 | 14,013,000 | 86,301,000 |
| 1965[2] | 75,261,000 | 314,000 | 14,795,000 | 90,370,000 |
| 1965[2] | 74,913,000 | 155,000 | 14,035,000 | 89,103,000 |
| 1966[3] | 78,315,000 | 15,864,000 | | 94,179,000 |

| | | Projections | | |
|------|----------------|-------|--------|----------|
| | | *million* | | |
| 1975 | 95–115 | 20–25 | | 115–135 |
| 1980 | 105–135 | 20–30 | | 125–150 |

[1] Privately owned vehicles only.
[2] Preliminary estimate.
[3] Figures may not add precisely to totals because of rounding.
Source:   *The Automobile and Air Pollution: A Program for Progress,* Part II. United States Department of Commerce, December, 1967. Privately and public owned vehicles, excluding military vehicles. Bureau of Public Roads data, cited in 1969 Automobile Facts and Figures, p. 19 (all figures rounded to the nearest thousand).

conditions, chronic bronchitis, pulmonary emphysema, and asthma. Probably the increasing occurrence of lung cancer is at least partly caused by air pollution. Certainly, lung cancer occurs with a higher frequency among city populations than it does in rural areas.[6]

Numbers of acute instances of air pollution have occurred from 1930 onward that have served to create a public apprehension and to produce a demand for control programs. These occurred in the Meuse Valley, Belgium, in 1930; in Donora, Pennsylvania, in 1948; and in London, England, in 1952. In each of these instances, unusual weather conditions led to an excessive accumulation of air pollutants. There were several points in common in these three widely separated occurrences: each lasted only a few days; in each the symptoms produced were apparently due to a chemical irritation of the exposed membranous body surfaces; and in each case the fatalities that occurred were generally among people with pre-existing cardiorespiratory diseases. The potential danger of such acute occurrences was made clear by the discovery that London suffered 4000 excess deaths during the 7-day period of severe air pollution; *i.e.*, 4000 more people died during that week than had died in the corresponding week of the years immediately preceding.

Public concern over air pollution led various cities to enact ordinances for smoke abatement. Notably, Pittsburgh and St. Louis have brought about commendable improvements in that regard. Among the states, California in 1947 produced comprehensive legislation. The Federal Government passed the Air Pollution Control Act of 1955 providing for research support and technical assistance in smoke abatement. The Clean Air Act of 1963 provides that the Secretary of Health, Education, and Welfare may recommend to state and local air pollution agencies standards of air quality necessary to protect the health of the public. It also authorized the Secretary to call a national conference on air pollution. Grants-in-aid were also provided for state and local control programs. The Secretary was authorized in the Amendments of 1965 to prescribe emission standards for new motor vehicles. By executive order in 1966, all Federal agencies were directed to control air pollutants from their own facilities.

Air pollution control should seek to diminish harmful and obnoxious materials in the community's atmosphere to safe and acceptable levels. To accomplish this purpose, programs must be established at local, district, state and interstate levels. As of mid-1967, control activities were being undertaken in nine interstate areas, including a 17-county area of New York and New Jersey surrounding New York City, and the counties of Maryland and northern Virginia including the District of Columbia.

Many states have enacted their own air pollution laws, setting up control programs and authorizing the creation of local control districts. Each control agency must determine the sources of air pollution in its own area by area-wide sampling. Laboratory facilities must be made available for these determinations.

Several sources of pollution are common to all communities. Open burning is such a source. All control programs attempt to regulate this type of nuisance. Dusts arising from sand and gravel plants, from road and other construction work, and from drilling, crushing, and milling stone are generally common in urban areas. Emissions from all types of industrial plants are usually susceptible to some form of control. Incineration of waste products is widely practiced. Control officers can usually suggest alternate methods for waste disposal.

It is generally admitted that the worst offender in polluting the air in America is the internal combustion engine. To deal with this problem, Congress has authorized the Secretary of Health, Education, and Welfare to establish national standards for the control of emissions from new motor vehicles. These standards call for a reduction in hydrocarbon and carbon monoxide emissions from the exhaust pipe, as well as a 100 per cent reduction of hydrocarbons from the crankcase. Other measures to control evaporations from the gas tanks and carburetors have been on cars since 1970. It is hoped that the new control devices will signficantly reduce air pollution coming from motor vehicles.

Although this control program for new motor vehicles is necessary and desirable, in reality the old cars now in use represent the major source of emissions. The problems of controlling vehicles now in use on a national basis may well prove insurmountable.

A big step forward came with the passage of the Clean Air Act of 1970 setting up the Environmental Protection Agency. This Act was soon followed by the Water Pollution Control Act of 1972, the Environmental Pesticide Control Act of 1972, the Marine Protection, Research and Sanctuaries Act of 1972, and the Environmental Protection Act of 1973.

The Environmental Protection Agency has developed a strong program to reduce air and water pollution, to control pesticides, to abate noise, to dispose of solid waste, to protect wildlife, and to regulate ocean dumping.[7]

### Safety of Food

Food is a frequent source of human illness. The disease-producing substances that are food-borne may cause illness by infection, by toxins accumulating as a result of the growth of certain organisms in the food, or by chemical poisons which occur naturally in the food or which are introduced accidentally in food handling. Most instances of food-borne disease can be prevented if food is properly processed and preserved, if it is prepared under sanitary conditions, if food that should be cooked is adequately cooked, and if food is served promptly or maintained under proper conditions to ensure its safety. It is a major responsibility of health departments to safeguard food processing, handling, and preparation for serving to the public. Because a great proportion of food is prepared and eaten in private homes, the education of the public on safe food hygiene is of major importance.

The cooking of food goes back far into man's early cultural heritage. This process renders many food items edible which would otherwise be inedible, but more importantly it serves to destroy harmful microorganisms and their products, thus protecting the health of the consumer. Indeed, the cooking of food is possibly the single most important measure for the protection of human health.

#### Meat Supplies

According to *Statistical Abstracts* of the United States, approximately 36,999 million pounds of meat were produced for the market in this country in 1972. In the same year, the *per capita* consumption of chicken was estimated to be 42.9 pounds, of turkey 8.9 pounds, and of fish 11.4 pounds. Obviously the task of ensuring the safety of these important food supplies is a gigantic one.

For many years programs of the Federal Government carried on by the Bureau of Animal Industry of the Department of Agriculture have been aimed at control and eradication of the more important diseases of livestock. Many state and local governments have joined in these programs. Two eradication campaigns have been particularly successful: these were compaigns to combat tuberculosis and brucellosis, two animal diseases that commonly affect humans.

The Federal meat inspection program applies to all processing plants that send meat or meat products into interstate commerce. Congress enacted a law in 1968 requiring all states to apply the Federal standards for meat inspection to plants processing meat for intrastate consumption. According to Schwabe,[8] veterinarians assocated with this Federal service inspect for disease approximately 91 per cent of the animals which pass each year through the major public stockyards in the United States. Animals with manifest disease are condemned as unfit for human consumption. The most common causes of rejection are tuberculosis, anthrax, hog cholera, pneumonia, and tapeworm cysts. The principal hazard of meat that comes from healthy animals and that has been properly handled and refrigerated stems from the encysted larvae of tapeworms and other helminths. Adequate cooking of meat will kill such larvae and render the meat entirely safe.

#### Shellfish

Shellfish, such as oysters, clams, and mussels, are favorite items of the American diet. These articles of seafood are harvested in shallow, mildly saline waters near the mouths of rivers or in bay areas. Pollution of the water by sewage results in pollution of the shellfish. The U.S. Public Health Service together with the appropriate state agencies has developed a system of certifying shipments of shellfish taken from waters approved as safe from contamination. The plants for processing and shipping of shellfish must be approved and are subject to frequent inspection by health agencies. Even with such precautions in effect, shellfish have been incriminated as carriers of viral hepatitis and other diseases. The eating of uncooked shellfish is probably always a risk.

Along the California coast epidemics of mussel poisoning have been reported from May to October. This poisoning is thought to be a result of the plankton upon which the mussels feed. Commercial operators test their products for the toxin, so most of the outbreaks are confined to small scale mussel collectors. Occasionally, similar toxic effects are associated with the eating of fish. These are also related to the diet of the fish and are seasonal in occurrence.

*Milk Hygiene*

Milk and milk products occupy a high place in the diet of Americans. Since it is customary to consume milk without cooking, it has often in the past served as a source of disease. Milk is a favorable medium for bacterial growth. As it comes in close contact with people in the course of production and distribution, there are numerous opportunities for contamination with disease-producing agents.

Occasionally the cow may be the source of infection of the milk. Bovine tuberculosis, brucellosis, and streptococcal infection of the udder are some of the diseases that may readily affect dairy cattle and contaminate the milk. Milk may also be contaminated by contact with unclean containers.

In the past, milk-borne epidemics were all too common. According to the U. S. Public Health Service, 974 such outbreaks occurred in the United States between 1923 and 1946. Typhoid fever, scarlet fever, and food poisonings (gastroenteritis) were the most common among the epidemic diseases.

A great deal has been accomplished toward the development of disease-free dairy herds and the maintenance of rigid standards of sanitation in milking sheds and processing plants. Experience has demonstrated that the safety of community milk supplies can only be secured through the pasteurization process. Two methods of pasteurization are employed: (1) a holding process by which milk is kept at 142 to 145° F. for a period of 30 min., or (2) the flash method in which milk is heated to 160° F. for 15 sec. Pasteurization does not kill all bacteria in milk, but it does destroy all disease-producing microorganisms that are known to be milk-borne. If properly carried out, pasteurization ensures that the milk delivered to the consumer is safe. It is essential that the householder or other user care for the milk properly until it is consumed. This requires refrigeration continuously to prevent growth of bacteria that are still in the milk or that may be introduced after the container is opened. About 90 per cent of milk consumed in the United States is pasteurized.

Ice cream, cream, butter, and some cheeses may be sources of milk-borne infection. The milk from which such products are prepared should be pasteurized.

*Food Handling*

On the national level, the Food and Drug Administration (FDA) works along with industries to improve food plant sanitation. Food found by inspectors to be unfit for human use is either destroyed or diverted to non-food usage. A few plants avoid compliance with regulations and their owners are brought into court. The Food and Drug Administration has also been active in establishing allowable standards for pesticide residues in foods and in the regulation of the use of chemical additives by food industries.

About 1700 intentional food additives are now used in the food-processing industry as well as a variety of carriers, diluents, sticking agents, propellants, and other substances. Several hundred chemicals are used in producing food-packaging materials which may be absorbed by food products. Some 100 pesticides are employed in food production, traces of which may be retained in packaged food products. The benefits of most of these chemicals probably outweigh the slight hazard to human health. Constant vigilance is required to avoid the introduction of noxious chemicals into food products.[9,10]

Food may be contaminated in the process of storage, in distribution, and in preparation of meals. The sanitary inspectors of local health departments are charged with inspecting such operations to ensure that the sanitary rules and regulations are being observed properly.

Health examination of food handlers has been abandoned by most health agencies. By and large, such procedures are not worth the effort and expense. One difficulty in supervising the health of restaurant personnel is the large turnover of such employees. This applies especially to dishwashers, bus boys, and similar lower grade personnel.

More emphasis is placed on sanitation of the premises, on the education of all food handlers as to personal hygiene and proper methods of food processing, on availability of effective refrigeration for preserving food, and on proper washing of utensils, crockery, and glassware.

All public eating places are inspected regularly by trained health department staff members and, if sanitary regulations are being ignored, the permit to operate is revoked.

*Food Poisoning*

Unfortunately, outbreaks of acute food poisoning continue to occur rather frequently. In 1972, 301 outbreaks of foodborne illness, with 14,559 cases, were reported in the United States.[11] It is estimated that such outbreaks were probably 10 to 20 times higher than were reported. In many instances, only one household was involved in the outbreak, but large banquets, church dinners, club picnics—in fact, any large gathering where food is served—are frequently the source of outbreaks. In such situations, food is prepared well in advance and is often allowed to stand without adequate refrigeration or recooking before being served. These conditions permit bacterial growth which may cause illness in those consuming the food.

Two types of food poisoning are common:

1. The microorganism grows in the food, producing a powerful toxin, which, if ingested, makes an individual very ill. Botulism is a well-known condition of this kind. Toxins produced by *Clostridium botulinum* occur in improperly processed foods kept under anerobic conditions and eaten without subsequent adequate cooking. Most botulism cases in the United States are caused by home-canned vegetables, olives, or mushrooms. In Europe, most cases result from sausages, smoked meat, or fish.

Symptoms usually appear within 12 to 36 hr., rarely several days after the consumption of the contaminated food. The intoxication may prove fatal if a large amount of the toxin is eaten. The toxin attacks the nervous system and the patient usually dies of respiratory or heart failure within a few days. These bacilli inhabit the intestinal tract of animals and the soil becomes contaminated by animal excreta. Botulism can be prevented by heating the food to be preserved sufficiently to kill the spores of the botulinus bacilli. Fortunately, botulism is becoming rather rare.

Staphylococcal poisoning is also due to an intoxication by the powerful toxin produced by some strains of that organism. The source of contamination in most instances is human. Staphylococci may be introduced to food from purulent discharges from an infected hand or from nasal secretions, as many individuals are healthy carriers of the organism. The toxic materials build up in quantity as the cocci multiply in suitable foods. Pastries, custards, salads, sandwiches, and meat products are some of the articles of food commonly involved.

The interval between intake of food and the onset of symptoms is usually 2 to 4 hr. Onset is abrupt with severe nausea, crampy pain in the abdomen, vomiting, severe diarrhea, and prostration. Almost always the victim recovers.

Staphylococcal poisoning is widespread and relatively frequent. Proper refrigeration of prepared food to avoid bacterial growth is the best preventive measure. Food left over should be promptly returned to refrigeration. Persons with boils or other skin infections should be excluded from the food preparation process.

2. Salmonellosis is an infection usually acquired from eating contaminated food. The reservoir of the salmonella group of organisms is domestic and wild animals including pet turtles and chicks. Man may also be a carrier. There is a total of approximately 800 serological types of salmonellae. Some are frequently identified as agents of human disease, but all are potential pathogens. The source of infection is feces of animals and of infected persons. Eggs and egg products, meat and meat products, and poultry are the most common sources of human infection.[12]

Epidemics are usually traced to foods such as meat pies, raw sausages, lightly cooked foods containing egg material, or foods contaminated with rodent excreta. An infected food handler may also transmit infection.

In general, the period of incubation is 12 to 24 hr. after ingestion of contaminated food. The onset is sudden. The most common symptoms are those of gastroenteritis. Fever, abdominal pain, vomiting, and diarrhea are usually experienced. Death from salmonellosis is rare. The illness lasts for only a few days, but the convalescent individual may continue to shed organisms in the stools for two to three weeks.

To prevent this form of food poisoning, all meat products should be thoroughly cooked. Contamination of kitchen work areas by raw meat or poultry should be avoided. Egg products should be pasteurized or cooked. Prepared foods should be refrigerated unless served promptly.

Salmonellosis is a world-wide problem. Its occurrence is common. Small outbreaks in households frequently occur. Large epidemics are well known in hospitals, nursing homes, and other institutions (see Table 7.4).

*Chemical Food Poisoning*

Two forms of food poisoning have been reported from time to time by the National Center for Disease Control. One is known as the "red-tide" related illness. This appears on both the East and West Coasts and is due to an unusual abundance of a marine flagellate (*Gymnodinium breve* on the Florida Coast) in the offshore waters. Human illness is caused by the consumption of shellfish that have ingested large amounts of these flagellates. Symptoms are both neurological and gastrointestinal. Paralysis and death may result.

Another type of poisoning results from eating certain fish which have been improperly refrigerated. These fish are of the perciform group, suborder *Scombroidei*, (tuna, bonita, skipjack, mackeral, and albacore) and the condition is known as scombroid fish poisoning. Bacterial growth in the bodies of these improperly refrigerated fish cause a reduction of histidine of the tissues to histamine and saurine. Shortly after eating the toxic fish, symptoms appear with headache, hives, abdominal cramps, and diarrhea. Victims usually recover within a few hours.

Food may become accidentally contaminated with poisonous chemicals. Arsenic, fluorides, lead, nitrates, and cyanide-containing silver polishes are some of the common chemicals that have produced poisoning through food. Usually symptoms appear very quickly after the food is consumed.

Prevention of chemical food poisoning depends on good household practice. Potential poisons must never be stored where they can come in contact with food.

## CONTROL OF DISEASE VECTORS

### Insects

A number of man's most dangerous diseases are insect-borne. Malaria, yellow fever, typhus fever, plague, spotted fevers, dengue, filariases, and African sleeping sickness are only the most prominent among a long list of infections transmitted by the bite of insects. Other diseases such as typhoid fever, dysentery, and food poisoning may be spread by flies, cockroaches, and other arthropods through direct contamination of food by contact.

Insect vectors of disease belong to a number of genera and many species. Lice, flies, gnats, mosquitoes, fleas, ticks, and mites are the most

TABLE 7.4

*Confirmed foodborne outbreaks and cases by bacterial etiology, 1971-1972*

| | 1971 | | | | 1972 | | | |
|---|---|---|---|---|---|---|---|---|
| | Outbreaks | | Cases | | Outbreaks | | Cases | |
| | No. | % | No. | % | No. | % | No. | % |
| B. cereus | 0 | 0.0 | 0 | 0.0 | 0 | 0.0 | 0 | 0.0 |
| C. botulinum | 6 | 6.4 | 15 | 0.4 | 4 | 2.9 | 24 | 0.4 |
| C. perfringens | 3 | 3.2 | 106 | 2.7 | 9 | 6.6 | 973 | 16.2 |
| E. coli | 1 | 1.1 | 387 | 9.7 | 0 | 0.0 | 0 | 0.0 |
| Salmonella | 28 | 29.8 | 729 | 18.3 | 36 | 26.5 | 1880 | 31.4 |
| Shigella | 6 | 6.4 | 806 | 20.3 | 3 | 2.2 | 86 | 1.4 |
| Staphylococcus | 26 | 27.7 | 930 | 23.4 | 34 | 25.0 | 1948 | 32.5 |
| Group A streptococcus | 1 | 1.1 | 498 | 12.5 | 1 | 0.7 | 35 | 0.6 |
| Group D streptococcus | 0 | 0.0 | 0 | 0.0 | 1 | 0.7 | 50 | 0.8 |
| V. parahaemolyticus | 3 | 3.2 | 370 | 9.3 | 6 | 4.4 | 701 | 11.7 |
| Alkalescens dispar | 0 | 0.0 | 0 | 0.0 | 1 | 0.7 | 39 | 0.7 |
| Subtotal | 74 | 78.7 | 3841 | 96.6 | 95 | 69.9 | 5736 | 95.7 |

Source:   Center for Disease Control, Foodborne Outbreaks, Annual Summary, 1972, November, 1973, DHEW Publication No. (CDC) 74-8185.

important transmitters of disease. Each genus and indeed each species of vector frequently has characteristic biological relationships with the disease-producing agent. Each vector has its characteristic biological cycles and growth patterns. These factors must all be considered in planning control programs. Extensive knowledge of the disease vector's habitat, life cycle, breeding seasons, and susceptibility to various measures is required for successful planning of vector control. Medical entomologists have accumulated valuable knowledge and experience in this field over the past 50 years. Since the early years of this century, measures directed against insect vectors have become more widely practiced as a method of disease control. Such campaigns were intensified during and after World War II with the advent of dichlorodiphenyltrichlorethane (DDT) and other powerful pesticides (see Reference 13, Parts I and IV).

Many methods of combatting insects have been used with more or less success. WHO[14] lists such methods as mechanical, physical, biological, and chemical measures. Under mechanical methods may be listed: (1) maintaining cleanliness of housekeeping, of clothing, and, around warehouses,—maintaining proper sewage and waste disposal; (2) screening of residences, dormitories, barracks, and all places where food is stored, prepared, or served; and (3) trapping to reduce insect population. The reproduction rates of these creatures are so high that such methods are at best inadequate. (4) Mechanical destruction—the old-fashioned flyswatter is known to all. Mechanical destruction by machines which free stored grains and seeds of weevils and other pests by passing them through blowers has been successful.

Physical control measures include the following: (1) Heat—most insects die if kept at 60° C. (140° F.) for 5 to 10 min. Hot water, steam, or hot air may be used. Clothing can be rid of lice by laundering in hot water or by heating with hot air. (2) Cold—all insect activity is inhibited at 5° C. (40° F.), but some species can survive for long periods at this temperature. (3) Asphyxiants—insects are sensitive to deprivation of oxygen. Methods of storing grain in low oxygen storage bins have been used with satisfactory results. Oils and other sprays that clog up the respiratory spiracles of insects have some use in control work. (4) Dehydrants—insects are protected from drying by the tough

cuticles covering their bodies. Some mineral dusts are known to damage this cuticle and cause death to the insect through desiccation. A preparation made with silica aerogels has been found effective against cockroaches and fleas. (5) Electrocution—electrified grids have been used to control flies, midges, and moths, especially around resort areas. (6) Radioactivity—in general, insects are less sensitive to radioactivity than are higher animals. Large does of γ-rays are necessary to destroy insects. In insect control, sterility of males may be produced, however, by exposure to radioactive rays. These sterile males reduce reproduction of the species in nature.

Biological measures are relatively untried in large scale control campaigns. Perhaps they hold great promise for future development. Two methods are being considered: (1) Sterilization procedures—as mentioned above the release of males sterilized by radioactive materials. This method has been used with success in Florida and Curaçao to eradicate the screw worm fly. This method is not generally applicable against all pests. Apparently the main difficulty is in the density of insect populations. The method can probably succeed against species with sparse populations. Chemosterilants that render both males and females sterile have been tested on a small scale. Unfortunately, these substances are highly toxic for higher animals and must be used with great care. Geneticists are experimenting with the release of insects known to have harmful genes as a method of control. This proposal has not attained the level of practical testing. (2) Control by parasites and predators—this method has met most success against agricultural pests. A search is being made for similar enemies of insects influencing public health.

Chemical insecticides have been known to man for a long time. The action of pyrethrum was apparently discovered by the Persians. Nicotine as tobacco dust or infusion has been known to Europeans since the 18th century. More recently, the development of the huge chemical industries in Europe and America has made many by-products available for testing as pesticides. The chemicals available for vector control purposes can be classed as petroleum, arsenicals, chlorinated hydrocarbons, organophosphorus compounds, carbonates, and synthetic pyrethroids. The material used should be highly effective against the vector but present no hazard to man or other animals when properly applied. One synthetic organic compound, DDT, has opened a new era of insect control. Other chlorinated hydrocarbons and a variety of organophosphorous and carbamate compounds have followed. Many of these compounds have been used extensively. Two important difficulties have arisen: the development of resistant insect strains, and the increasing likelihood of toxic effects of insecticides on man, his livestock, and wild life in general.

Insecticides may be stomach poisons (which must be eaten), contact poisons (which require contact with the cuticle), and fumigants (which enter the insect's respiratory system). Stomach poisons are applied in agriculture by spraying or dusting vegetation. To combat insects that suck plant juices, the poison is introduced by absorption into the sap. These insecticides have a systemic action. Some studies have been done on protecting livestock by systemic poisons, but this method is now employed to a very limited extent. Solid or powder poisons are used against cockroaches and, to some extent, against mosquito larvae. Poison baits are useful against nuisance insects such as earwigs, crickets, or ants, and to control flies in stables.

Stomach poisons may be inorganic chemicals such as the salts of mercury, arsenic, or a number of fluorine compounds. Acetoarsenite of copper, an insoluble compound known as Paris green, was widely used to destroy mosquito larvae in earlier years. Few organic compounds are efficient stomach poisons. The chlorinated cyclodienes and organophosphorus compounds have been found useful.

Contact poisons may either be applied for an immediate kill or for long, continued, residual action. Pyrethrum insecticides produced from the flower heads of *Chrysanthemum cinerariifolium* or synthetic allethrin are frequently employed for quick knockdown and kill of insects. Such insecticides can be used for freeing airplanes of pests or for fogging of buildings or small outdoor areas for picnics.

The insecticidal properties of DDT were discovered in Switzerland in 1939. It is toxic to almost all insects, although it is relatively harmless to mammals. Dichlorodiphenyltrichlorethane has a low solubility in water, but dissolves easily in many organic solvents. The action of DDT is upon the sensory nerves of the insect. The cuticle is penetrated easily upon contact.

Many other synthetic contact insecticides have been discovered. Of these, $\gamma$-benzene hexachloride (BHC) is chemically stable and highly effective against almost all arthropods. Its toxic action is probably also effective on the nervous system. The organophosphorus compounds, such as parathion, are highly lethal to insects, but are dangerously toxic to higher mammals.

DDT has been so widely used that it has spread over most of the world. There is some evidence that DDT is carcinogenic in mice, so there is a movement to restrict or prohibit its use. Two other insecticides have been tried in its place because of their long-term residual effect for indoor application. These are Propoxur and Fenitrothion.

Repellents are being increasingly used by workmen exposed to nuisance insects, by picnickers or others on holiday, and by military units on field maneuvers. Against flying insects, repellents are usually applied to the exposed skin. Each application is effective at most for a few hours. To protect against crawling pests, the repellent is applied to the clothing, mainly around the openings—cuffs, trouser bottoms, and socks. In most cases synthetic repellents are now in use.

The development of resistance by insects to insecticides has become a serious problem. Beginning with resistant flies in 1947, over 100 species have developed resistance; about 70 of these have importance for public health. It appears that as an insecticide is applied to an insect population the more susceptible individuals die off, leaving those more tolerant of the poison to survive and breed a new population. Emergence of resistant strains, then, is a selective process based on pre-existing genetic types.

To avoid the promotion of resistant strains, insecticides should not be used regularly on a broad scale unless the objective is of real importance.[15]

*Mosquito Control (see Reference 13, Part VI)*

Probably more campaigns have been conducted against mosquitoes than against any other arthropod. Shortly after the U. S. Army Commission proved in 1901 that yellow fever is transmitted by a mosquito, a control campaign based on this knowledge was successfully undertaken in Havana, Cuba, and a few years later in Panama. Antimosquito efforts to control malaria were begun about the same time.

Mosquitoes have four distinct stages in their life history: egg, larva, pupa, and adult. The first three stages occur in water. The adult is a flying insect feeding on blood of vertebrates or upon plant juices. A blood meal is necessary for the female to maturate her eggs (see Fig. 7.1).

Mosquitoes lay their eggs either on the surface of water, as in the case of anophelines which are the vectors of malaria; on the sides of tree holes or containers just above the water-line, as do many *Aedes* mosquitoes including *Aedes aegypti,* the transmitter of yellow fever; or on the surface of the ground, as do other species of *Aedes.* All eggs require contact with water for hatching, but the eggs of some species can survive in the dried stage for three to four

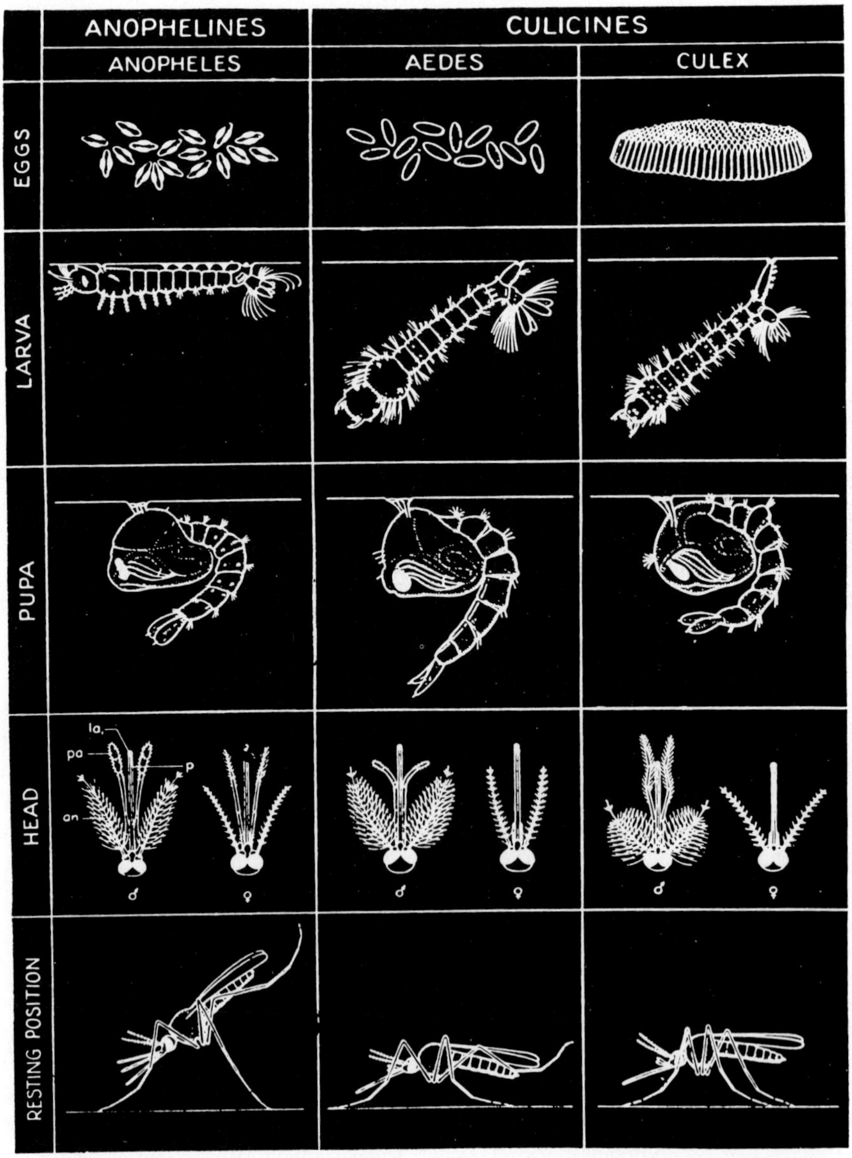

Fig. 7.1. Schematic representation of some characteristic points of differentiation of Anopheline and Culicine mosquitoes. *an.,* antenna; *la.,* labella; *p.,* proboscis; *pa.,* palp. Source: Belding, D. L. *Textbook of Clinical Parasitology,* Ed. 3. New York: Appleton-Century-Crofts Inc., 1952, p. 859.

years.

The larval and pupal stages of all mosquitoes are in water. There are four larval stages or instars. The larvae and pupae are active and come to the water's surface frequently to get air.

The whole developmental cycle of the mosquito from egg to adulthood requires from about four to 10 days depending upon the temperature. A mosquito's natural life probably is about four to five months under favorable conditions. Some species overwinter as adults, *e.g.,* anophelines; others, in the egg stage, such as *Aedes.*

Each mosquito species has its own peculiar preferences as to breeding places, resting places, times for feeding, and vertebrates preferred for its blood meals. Exact information on these points is of great importance in planning a successful control program.

Long-term control measures depend upon depriving the particular mosquito of water for breeding purposes. This involves such procedures as filling and draining, the use of tide gates in salt marshes, good irrigation practices, and the proper control of impounded waters. Ponds should be constructed with steep, clean shorelines and with marginal vegetation controlled. To reduce populations of domestic mosquitoes, all artificial water containers must be removed. These include tin cans, old automobile tires, sagging gutters, and numerous other water containers. Cisterns, water barrels, and similar containers must be screened to prevent access to egg-laying mosquitoes.

Larva-eating fish such as gambusia are frequently used to keep down mosquito breeding in water tanks, garden pools, and marshes.

Larviciding with stomach poisons or contact poisons is widely practiced. Dusts, granular pellets, wettable powders, emulsions, and oil solutions are used. DDT, BHC, lindane, chlordane, and dieldrin are effective as larvicidal agents.

Control of adult mosquitoes is attempted by screening, bed nets, protective clothing, repellents, space spraying for quick kill of adults, and residual spraying of residences and outhouses for prolonged control.

Under special circumstances, complete eradication of a mosquito species has been undertaken. The campaign in northeast Brazil against the African mosquito, *Anopheles gambiae,* a highly dangerous transmitter of malaria, was a triumph in the history of vector control. This mosquito was introduced to the coast of Brazil from West Africa about 1930. Over the next few years this anopheline spread up the river valleys over a wide area causing devastating epidemics of malaria. In cooperation with the Brazilian government, the Rockefeller Foundation undertook to wipe out this invader. In a whirlwind campaign during 1939 to 1940, *A. gambiae* was eradicated.[16]

Shortly thereafter during World War II, *A. gambiae* invaded the valley of the Nile in upper Egypt. The government of Egypt, in collaboration with the Rockefeller Foundation, using similar tactics, again eradicated this efficient carrier of malaria.

A more difficult mosquito eradication campaign was begun on the islands of Sardinia in 1946. For hundreds of years this island had the reputation of being the most malarious part of Italy. It is a little more than 9000 square miles in area. The vector of malaria in Sardinia is *Anopheles labranchiae,* which breeds in slow moving streams, isolated pockets of water, and ground pools, but can apparently breed in almost any collection of water. Both residual spraying and larviciding operations were carried on extensively. Hundreds of tons of DDT and thousands of tons of fuel oil were consumed. Many miles of drainage ditches were constructed. By 1950, *A. labranchiae* was reduced drastically and malaria declined rapidly. It appears that malaria can be completely controlled by such a campaign, but that it is not possible to destroy the vector completely with the currently available techniques.[17]

Another and more ambitious eradication campaign is now under way in the Americas against *Aedes aegypti,* the transmitter of yellow fever and dengue. Beginning during the 1930's, Brazil, Bolivia, and other contiguous countries have achieved great progress. As of October, 1967, 38 governments have been completely successful in eradication of *A. aegypti.* The United States began its campaign in 1964 and made substantial progress in the seven southern states in which *A. aegypti* were found. Unfortunately, as an economy measure the Federal Government withdrew its support of the program in 1968, and as could be expected *Aedes aegypti* have increased in previously infested areas. The same has occurred in a number of Latin American and Caribbean countries. The density of *Aedes aegypti* was sufficient to support two wide-spread epidemics of dengue fever in the American tropics in 1963-64 and in 1968-69. This has caused anxiety lest yellow fever should again appear in the region as an urban disease.[18,19]

For some years, Dichlorvos has been used as the preferred insecticide for use in airplanes employed in international travel. Dichlorvos vapor (DDVP) is released throughout the aircraft for a period of 30 minutes during flight. The passengers are unaware of the procedure, but it achieves effective control of mosquitoes.

Other compounds for airplane disinfection are being tried. These are in the synergized pyrethrins and pyrethroid group.[20]

*Tick Control (see Reference 13, Part X)*

Smith and Kilbourne demonstrated in the period 1889 to 1893 that the cattle tick was the vector of Texas cattle fever. Ricketts in 1902 to 1906 discovered that the wood tick, *Dermacentor andersoni*, transmits Rocky Mountain spotted fever. Later it was learned that two other ticks were responsible for transmission of Rocky Mountain spotted fever in the eastern states. Subsequent studies have shown that ticks can carry tularemia, Colorado tick fever, relapsing fever, and Q fever. Ticks are also responsible for spreading several virus infections. An acute form of ascending paralysis may also result from the bite of certain ticks.

Eggs are deposited on the ground. Females of some species lay as many as 18,000 eggs. Eggs hatch in two weeks to several months depending on temperature, humidity, and other environmental factors. Larvae require a blood meal to molt. They may survive for long periods if no food supply is located. The nymph also must have a blood meal to develop. Some species of ticks have only one host. Others can feed on multiple hosts and thus have more favorable prospects for survival. Some genera of ticks require several nymphal stages before reaching adulthood. Hard ticks have only one nymphal stage.

Unlike mosquitoes, both male and female ticks require blood meals before copulation. Many ticks require one or two years to complete their life cycles, but may take longer under unfavorable circumstances. Unfed hard ticks can endure frigid winter weather in sheltered retreats. They spend much of their lives on the ground or on vegetation waiting for

suitable hosts to approach. Such ticks are usually found in areas of scrub bush, especially along paths. Some one-host species spend most of their lives on their animal hosts.

Ticks may transmit disease mechanically through infected mouth parts in the course of interrupted feedings. In addition, ticks serve as reservoirs of viruses, rickettsiae, spirochetes, bacteria, and protozoa. These disease agents are transmitted from infected adults through the egg to the following larval, nymphal, and adult stages. This mechanism maintains the disease-producing organisms in one locality for long periods of time.

Repellents for ticks should be applied to clothing. Indalone, diethyl toluamide, dimethyl carbate, and benzyl benzoate provide good protection for about one week. Clothing should be thoroughly washed and retreated at weekly intervals.

Dogs and cats may be treated with rotenone or malathion. The pets' living area and bedding must also be treated. Dips and sprays of insecticide are recommended for controlling ticks on horses, cattle, sheep, and goats.

Area control of ticks can be obtained by the application of dust, suspension, or emulsion of insecticides such as DDT, chlordane, and dieldrin at rates of one to two pounds of actual insecticide per acre. If large areas are to be treated, airplane dusting may be the best method.

*Louse Control (see Reference 13, Part VIII)*

Lice transmit epidemic typhus fever, trench fever (prevalent among the soldiers in World War I), and spirochetes of relapsing fever. Frequent bites by lice may cause a severe irritation of the skin. There are three kinds of human lice: the head louse, the body louse, and the pubic or crab louse. The female head louse lays its eggs on the hairs of the head near the scalp. The egg case is strongly attached and remains fixed after hatching. These are called nits. There are three nymphal stages. Feeding on the host's blood occurs twice daily. After the third molt, the nymph reaches the adult stage.

The life cycle of the body louse is very similar except that the egg is fastened to fibers in the clothing especially along the seams of the undergarment.

The crab louse belongs to a different genus. It

too fastens its eggs to hairs. For some unknown reason, it prefers the pubic area. There are three larval stages leading to adulthood.

Lice are transmitted from person to person by intimate contact. Children sometimes get head lice in school. Body lice may be acquired from bedding or furniture of low-grade lodging houses.

Reinfestation is the greatest difficulty in control of lice. The family may be the infested group. With the body louse, a number of people living in unsanitary conditions such as jails, refugee camps, or bums on skid row may be the unit of infection.

To control the head louse, an emulsifiable concentrate containing 1 per cent BHC in alcohol is diluted with water for application to the roots of the hair. Other products are equally effective. Dusts containing 10 per cent DDT or 1 per cent BHC are applied to underclothing and inner garments to control the body louse. An application gives protection for about three weeks. Similar treatment applied to the pubic area will also control the crab louse.

*Flea Control (see Reference 13, Part VII)*

Fleas are known to be vectors of bubonic plague and of murine typhus fever. Persons bitten by fleas may have severe skin irritations and become ill with allergic reactions.

In the adult stage, fleas take periodic blood meals from animals. Nearly always each species of flea has one warm-blooded host upon which it prefers to feed. Fleas will feed readily on other hosts when hungry. Some fleas spend most of their time on the host hiding in its fur; others remain for the most part in the nest or sleeping quarters of the host. Females lay their eggs rather indiscriminately on the fur of the host or in the sleeping place. The newly hatched larvae are tiny, white, legless grubs. The larvae feed on miscellaneous organic matter such as food crumbs, feces, or other materials. There are three larval stages. After the last stage, they spin silken cocoons in which to pupate. The pupa may remain in the cocoon for an indefinite time and emerge only when a new host comes near.

The tropical rat flea, *Xenopsylla cheopis,* and other fleas are the principal vectors of murine typhus and plague. In typhus, infected fleas excrete rickettsiae in their feces and contami-

nate the bite wounds with infected feces. Inhalation of dried infective feces may account for some infections. In plague, bacilli grow in the flea's proventriculus and stomach, causing obstruction. These "blocked" fleas become very hungry and try to feed again and again. Infectious material is regurgitated, thus infecting the tiny wounds caused by the bites.

Irritations from flea bites are most likely to be due to fleas from cats and dogs in the household. The animals should be dusted with an insecticide powder. Five per cent DDT, 0.5 per cent BHC, or 5 per cent malathion are effective for dogs. Pyrethrins are safer for cats which lick their fur. The sleeping area of the animals must be cleaned and treated.

To control rat fleas, one should rid the community of rats. Insecticides are also used to advantage in rodent burrows and runways (see Fig. 7.2).

*Mite Control (see Reference 13, Part IX)*

In large areas of eastern Asia, mites of the genus *Trombicula* are transmitters of a rickettsial disease called scrub typhus. These mites only attack a single vertebrate host during their life cycle; this meal takes place in the larval stage. The females lay their eggs in the soil. The larvae soon after hatching climb up on any available vegetation to seek an opportunity for a feeding. After its meal, the larvae drops back to the soil to develop into the nymphal stage and then into the adult stage. The nymphs and adults appear to feed on the eggs and young of other arthropods.

Repellents on the socks and trousers afford protection for about two weeks. Other forms of control are generally not feasible.

Another genus of mites afflicts man by burrowing into the skin. *Sarcoptes scabiei* is the cause of scabies or "the itch" in man. This infection is not common in advanced countries, except in times of social upheaval. The mature female mite burrows in the horny layer of the skin between the fingers, in the axillary folds, the belt line, the external genitalia, and other areas. Itching is intense. Eggs are laid in the burrows in the skin. There is a larval and a nymphal stage. Both stages are passed on or in the skin.

The infestation is controlled by an application of 20 to 25 per cent emulsion of benzyl benzoate or 1 per cent benzene hexachloride

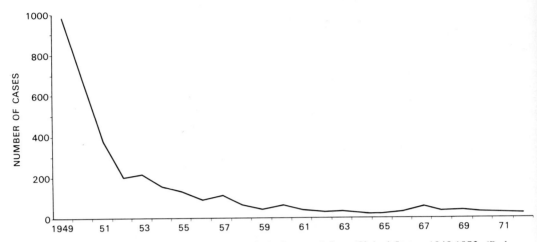

Fig. 7.2. Typhus fever, flea-borne (endemic, murine)–Reported Cases, United States, 1949-1972. (Redrawn from National Center for Disease Control, Morbidity and Mortality Weekly Report, Annual Supplement 1972, Released July 1973. DHEW Publication No. (CDC) 74-8241.)

ointment to the whole body. The next day a bath should be taken and a change made to fresh clothing and bed linen. In a few cases, a second treatment is required after an interval of seven to 10 days.

### Fly Control (see Reference 13, Part V)

The house fly is world-wide in distribution, and in all lands lives in close association with man. Flies require a moist, fermenting, or putrifying material for their breeding-animal excreta, decaying vegetable matter, dead animal remains, or garbage will serve. During a single day a fly may lay 100 to 150 eggs. This may be repeated four or five times during her lifetime. The eggs hatch in from 8 to 48 hr. The larvae appear as maggots and pass through three larval stages. A pupal stage precedes emergence as an adult fly.

The primary food of the adult is carbohydrate which the female requires for egg production. Sources of sugar are found in human dwellings.

Houseflies transmit disease to humans through mechanical contamination of food supplies. In general, intestinal infections are most commonly transmitted.

Houseflies are combatted by screening of homes, by careful handling of food, by swatting and trapping, by good sanitation to reduce breeding places, by larvicides, by poison baits, and by space spraying.

Other flies are vectors of serious diseases in the tropics and subtropics. In Africa, the tsetse fly, *Glossina,* of which there are several species, transmits sleeping sickness. The agent of this dread disease is a trypanosome. The tsetse flies breed in bush country along streams. Some measure of control is achieved by clearing away the bush around villages and by ground spraying with residual insecticides.

Another troublesome fever is carried by sandflies, *Phlebotomus,* and other types. These blood-sucking midges are difficult to control, but the use of repellents and insecticide sprays around homes helps to give protection. Sandfly fever, or 3-day fever, is particularly prevelant around the Mediterranean and eastward to Burma and China.

Other species of *Phlebotomus* transmit Oroya fever, now known as bartonellosis in Peru, Ecuador, and Colombia. Cutaneous leishmaniasis, a disease of the tropical belts of both the Old and New Worlds is also transmitted by sandflies. This ulcerating skin disease is caused by a flagellate protozoan.

Finally, an African disease introduced to a few localities in the New World probably with the slave trade is onchocerciasis caused by a tiny nematode worm. This infection causes little in the way of symptoms unless the worms reach the eye. In this case, blindness is the frequent result. The filarial worm is transmitted by small black flies of the genus *Simulium.* These flies breed in swift running streams. Some degree of control can be achieved through the use of repellents and insecticides.

## Rodents

Rodents are reservoirs of a number of infectious diseases of which plague, murine typhus, rate bite fever, leptospirosis, trichinosis, rickettsial pox, and salmonellosis are of particular interest in the United States. There are many species of rodents, but there are some that follow man to all parts of the world. These are the common house mouse, *Mus musculus;* the roof rat, *Rattus rattus;* and the Norway or brown rat, *Rattus norwegicus.*. Rats were, until recently, found commonly on all ships and so were transported to all parts of the world by sea.

Rats tend to remain within a limited area or home range for long periods of time unless there are radical changes of environment to cause transfer to a new home. In urban areas, this range may be as small as 100 to 150 feet. Rats will eat almost any edible article, but grains are their preferred foods. Roof rats prefer fruits.

Rats reproduce at all seasons; the number of pregnancies of a female per year varies from four to eight. The average number of weanlings of the Norway rat is about seven, so the average female rat may wean about 20 rats per year. The number of rats in a community is difficult to estimate, but in 1950 it was calculated that in New York City there was one rat for each 35 people, and in Baltimore (1955) one rat for eight people.[21]

The limitation of rat populations is controlled by available food and harborage. Populations become stationary at a level determined by environmental factors. Reduction in numbers by trapping, poisoning, and other measures rarely succeeds in effecting a permanent reduction in population. Actually such reductions provide favorable conditions for new population growths.

Effective control of rats must be based on reduction of food supplies and of harborage. To accomplish these objectives, alteration in sanitary conditions must be made. Buildings, especially commercial structures, must be repaired to make them rat-proof. Doors must be tightly fitted with the lower parts covered with metal to prevent rats gnawing through. Doors must be kept closed. Basement windows should be screened with heavy wire mesh. Ventilators, skylights, unused chimneys, and openings around water, sewer, gas, steam pipes, and electric cables should be stopped. Foundation walls should be laid without a break around the whole building and should extend no less than 18 inches beneath the soil surface. Rat-proofing principles must be carried out in all new construction.[22]

Favorite rat refuges in cities are markets, slaughterhouses, provision stores, warehouses, bakeryshops, candy factories, garbage dumps, residences, and vacant lots. All garbage and wastes should be placed in well-covered cans. Sanitary land fills are now generally used to cover up garbage and organic waste materials.

Trapping and poisoning are useful to reduce rat populations. Bacon, fish heads, grains, and fruit are generally good baits. Either snap traps or cage traps may be tried. For poisoning, red squill is sometimes used.

Rodenticides that may be used with relative safety are: red squill, norbormide, and zinc phosphide. Other compounds such as sodium fluoroacetate, fluoroacetamide, and strychnine should be used only with maximum precautions. Sometimes rodenticides are now considered too dangerous for use. These are arsenic trioxide, thallium sulfate, ANTU, and gophacide.[23] All poisons require that precautions be taken to prevent the poisoning of pets or of humans.

Fumigation is used to kill rats in enclosed structures such as ships and suitable buildings. Sulfur dioxide, hydrocyanic acid gas, or carbon monoxide may be used.

The common house mouse is more of a nuisance and a destroyer of food than it is of importance as a carrier of disease. Again, the methods that are effective for rat control are usually useful in ridding homes of mice.

Some wild rodents are known to be reservoirs of pathogenic agents, as, for example, the ground squirrel in sylvatic plague in western states. Control of such wild populations is not regarded as a feasible health measure.

Animals other than rodents sometimes transmit diseases directly to man. Rabies is a well-established example. The rabies virus infects man by contamination of skin abrasions or bite wounds with the saliva of a rabid animal. Dogs and cats are the most frequent sources of human rabies. Foxes, skunks, coyotes, and bats are also transmitters of rabies to man. Man's best protection against rabies is the immunization of dogs and cats, which should then be licensed; elimination of stray animals;

and avoidance as far as possible of wild animals that may be exhibiting unusual behavior patterns.

## IMMUNIZATION

It has long been known that one attack of several of the common diseases confers protection on individuals, so that they are resistant to subsequent exposures to the same disease. Our ancestors knew this to be true in the case of smallpox, yellow fever, and measles. After Edward Jenner successfully introduced immunization against smallpox by the use of cowpox vaccine, there was hope that other severe diseases might be prevented through similar measures. Pasteur was deeply interested in this possibility some three-quarters of a century later and developed vaccines against anthrax, chicken cholera, and rabies.

All of Pasteur's vaccines were produced with live, attenuated organisms. Theobald Smith and D. E. Salmon introduced in the United States between 1884 and 1886 a safer type of vaccine for hog cholera made from heat-killed cultures of the hog cholera bacillus.

A number of able investigators undertook studies of the mechanisms of immunity. Two schools of thought grew up. One group attributed protection wholly to the blood and tissue fluids. Following infection, it is possible to demonstrate protective bodies or antibodies in the serum that react specifically with the disease agent. The other group thought that immunity depended upon the action of certain cells in the body. These cells, white blood cells, engulf the bacteria and destroy them. They became known as phagocytes, or eating cells. It is now believed that both of these concepts of resistance to infection are valid. Today, in addition to the actions of antibodies and phagocytes, other mechanisms of resisting the invasions of pathogenic agents are recognized (see Chapter 5).

By 1890, it became known that the most dangerous effects of diphtheria infection result from the powerful toxin released by the diphtheria bacillus in the tissues. Studies on this toxin soon demonstrated that if animals were inoculated with small doses they could quickly develop a tolerance to large inoculations of toxin. In other words, antitoxins had been produced in the serum. This serum, when injected into children with diphtheria, rapidly counteracted the toxic effects of the disease and proved to be a great lifesaver. Continued study revealed that children could be immunized against diphtheria by a small dose of a carefully balanced preparation of toxin and antitoxin. A good many years later, it was discovered that toxin treated by formalin to destroy toxicity still retained its ability to produce antitoxin upon inoculation into an animal. This treated toxin is known as toxoid or a toxin-like substance. Thus, the underlying principles of artificial immunizing agents had all become known within 50 years after Pasteur's pioneering investigations. Many additional vaccines have been produced both for the protection of animals and humans, but all are based on these fundamental discoveries.

### Active Immunization

Immunization has proved to be the most effective means of controlling many communicable diseases. Not only does immunization provide protection to individuals, but it reduces the number of susceptibles in a community, thus building up the herd immunity, making the maintenance of the infection chain more difficult. Indeed, in the case of smallpox and measles in which man is the only known reservoir of the viruses, eradication of the disease entities can presumably be accomplished through immunization of a large enough portion of the world's population.

All known living agents of human disease contain proteins or polysaccharides, or both, and so are potentially good antigens. Thus, theoretically, it is possible to produce vaccines for all of them that would be capable of stimulating antibody production upon injection into a susceptible individual. Numerous more or less effective vaccines have been produced. In some, living organisms have been employed; in others, the antigen is introduced by a suspension of killed organisms. In still other diseases, modified exotoxins or chemical fractions of organisms are used to provide the desired antigenic stimulus. Living organisms probably are the most effective immunizing agents, but are also potentially the most dangerous.

On primary immunization, the antibody response is generally slow. Before any definite rise in antibodies in the serum can be demonstrated, 10 to 14 days are usually required. Subsequent or "booster" injections of the same vaccine evoke a rapid antibody response. This booster action, which may result from either exposure to the infectious agent in nature or by injection of a booster dose of vaccine, is of great importance for the maintenance of a long enduring immunity to most diseases. As the prevention of infectious diseases has become more generally successful, opportunities for a booster effect from repeated natural exposures to infected individuals become less frequent. The necessity for a long-term follow-up program of immunization for each individual becomes more urgent.

As the number of effective vaccines against common diseases increases, pressures grow to combine as many immunizing agents as possible into one package and thus reduce the number of injections an individual must receive. This demand necessitates further purification of antigenic material from each organism. This concentration of antigen mass tends to decrease unfavorable reactions to the vaccine and perhaps to enhance its immunizing potency.

*Primary Immunization of Infants*

Current recommended practice in the United States[24] is to immunize all infants against diphtheria, pertussis, and tetanus with an initial course of three intramuscular injections of combined antigens containing alum-precipitated, aluminum hydroxide or aluminum phosphate-adsorbed diphtheria and tetanus toxoids, and pertussis vaccine. This immunization should be started at two months of age. Intervals between injections should be not more than three months. A fourth dose of the triple antigen is recommended about 12 months following the third dose (see Tables 7.5 and 7.6).

TABLE 7.5

*Recommended schedule for active immunization of normal infants and children*

| 2 mo. | DTP[1] | TOPV[2] |
|---|---|---|
| 4 mo. | DTP | TOPV |
| 6 mo. | DTP | TOPV |
| 1 yr. | Measles[3] | Tuberculin Test[4] |
|  | Rubella[3] | Mumps[3] |
| 1½ yr. | DTP | TOPV |
| 4–6 yr. | DTP | TOPV |
| 14–16 yr. | Td[5] | and thereafter every 10 years |

[1] DTP—diphtheria and tetanus toxoids combined with pertussis vaccine.
[2] TOPV—trivalent oral poliovirus vaccine. This recommendation is suitable for breast-fed as well as bottle-fed infants.
[3] May be given at 1 year as measles-rubella or measles-mumps-rubella combined vaccines.
[4] Frequency of repeated tuberculin tests depends on risk of exposure of the child and on the prevalence of tuberculosis in the population group. The initial test should be at the time of, or preceding, the measles immunization.
[5] Td—combined tetanus and diphtheria toxoids (adult type) for those more than 6 years of age in contrast to diphtheria and tetanus (DT) which contains a larger amount of diphtheria antigen. *Tetanus toxoid at time of injury:* For clean, minor wounds, no booster dose is needed by a fully immunized child unless more than 10 years have elapsed since the last dose. For contaminated wounds, a booster dose should be given if more than 5 years have elapsed since the last dose. **Storage of Vaccines.** Because biologics are of varying stability, the manufacturers' recommendations for optimal storage conditions (*e.g.,* temperature, light) should be carefully followed. Failure to observe these precautions may significantly reduce the potency and effectiveness of the vaccines.
Source:  Report of the Committee on Infectious Diseases, Ed. 17, 1974. American Academy of Pediatrics, Evanston, Ill.

TABLE 7.6

*Primary immunization for children not immunized in infancy[1]*

### 1 through 5 Years of Age

| | |
|---|---|
| First visit | DTP, TOPV, Tuberculin Test |
| 1 mo. later | Measles, Rubella, Mumps |
| 2 mo. later | DTP, TOPV |
| 4 mo. later | DTP, TOPV |
| 6 to 12 m. later or preschool | DTP, TOPV |
| Age, 14—16 yr. | Td—continue every 10 yr. |

### 6 Years of Age and Over

| | |
|---|---|
| First visit | Td, TOPV, Tuberculin Test |
| 1 mo. later | Measles, Rubella, Mumps |
| 2 mo. later | Td, TOPV |
| 6 to 12 mo. later | Td, TOPV |
| Age, 14—16 yr. | Td—continue every 10 years |

[1] Physicians may choose to alter the sequence of these schedules if specific infections are prevalent at the time. For example, measles vaccine might be given on the first visit if an epidemic is underway in the community.

Source: Report of the Committee on Infectious Diseases, Ed. 17, 1974. American Academy of Pediatrics, Evanston, Ill.

The triple antigens combined with adjuvants are preferred to fluid or plain mixtures of vaccine. The fluid vaccines do establish immunity more rapidly and such a pertussin vaccine should be used if there is a local outbreak of pertussis in the community. Immunization with the fluid vaccine should be followed by injections of the triple vaccine to complete protection against diphtheria and tetanus.

Some physicians prefer the fluid vaccines for the combined immunization against diphtheria, tetanus, and pertussis. For routine use, four injections of 1 ml. each are usually given; the first three at monthly intervals beginning at two to three months of age, and the fourth at about 15 months of age.

All infants should receive poliovaccine along with the triple antigen. Oral poliovirus vaccine is regarded as the preferable product for prevention of poliomyelitis in children. Three doses of poliovaccine are given with intervals of about two months between doses. A booster dose of trivalent poliovaccine is recommended one year after the third dose, and another booster of the trivalent vaccine upon entrance to school at the sixth year.

Most public health officials now consider that routine smallpox vaccination is no longer necessary in the United States. It is recom-

mended for medical and hospital personnel and for travelers to endemic countries. Of course, should a case of smallpox be introduced into the country all potential contacts should be immediately vaccinated.[25]

All infants should receive measles vaccine by the end of the first year of life. Live attenuated measles virus vaccine is recommended. Either the Schwartz strain or Attenuvax vaccines are generally used. These are grown in chick embryo cells until satisfactorily attenuated. Mild symptoms including a faint skin rash may be encountered in from 10 to 20 per cent of the children receiving the vaccine. These symptoms clear up as a rule in from five to 10 days.

Measles vaccine may be combined with rubella and mumps vaccines and so administered at the same time usually at one year of age. Rubella vaccine is also a live attenuated virus grown in avian or mammalian cells. A single dose produces antibodies in approximately 95 per cent of the children inoculated. One to two per cent of those receiving vaccine develop transient pains and swellings of the joints. Since the vaccine was introduced in 1969, more than 40 million children have been immunized. The vaccine against mumps was introduced in 1967. It consists of a live attenuated strain of mumps virus grown in chick embryo cells. Ordinarily no reaction to this vaccine is noted. The immunity produced is of long duration, possibly for life.

Children who received their full primary immunizations in infancy should be given one injection of the triple antigens (DPT and TOPV) at one and a half years of age, thus assuring a relatively high level of immunity up to school age and also upon entering school, usually at the sixth year. At 14 to 16 years of age, children should receive one injection of the adult type of tetanus and diphtheria toxoids. This type of antigen produces fewer reactions in older children and adults than does the triple antigen.

For children not immunized in infancy, those up to six years of age should receive the triple antigens. Over the sixth year, single antigens or a combination of diphtheria and tetanus toxoids is preferred. This choice is based on the greater frequency of febrile reactions to DPT in the older children. Oral poliovaccine, measles, rubella, and mumps vaccines should be given to this group of children.

### Recall Immunization

For children who have completed their primary immunizations against diphtheria, whooping cough, tetanus, and poliomyelitis, resistance can be boosted by a single recall dose of the indicated antigen. In the case of whooping cough, such a recall injection is indicated for children up to six years of age following intimate exposure or during the presence of an epidemic, provided that the child has not had a routine injection in the past year. Plain (non-absorbed) pertussis vaccine, 0.5 ml., is the agent of choice.

Children exposed to diphtheria who are six years or younger should receive 0.5 ml. of diphtheria toxoid. For older children and adults, the purified "adult type" of diphtheria toxoid is recommended.

In the case of injuries that might produce tetanus, i.e., puncture wounds, dog bites, and encrusted abrasions, an injection of 0.5 ml. of tetanus toxoid is indicated. If the previous immunization history is uncertain or unknown and the wound is one likely to produce tetanus, tetanus immune serum should be administered (see "Passive Immunization").

If an individual is exposed to smallpox, immediate vaccination or revaccination is strongly advised.

Should poliomyelitis appear in a community, all age groups from two months up should receive oral poliovaccine. If the virus type is identified, the corresponding monovalent poliovaccine is preferable. If the prevalent virus type is unknown, the trivalent vaccine should be used.

### Mumps

A live attenuated mumps vaccine has been licensed for use in the United States within the past few years. The virus used was the Jeryl-Lynn strain. Attenuation was achieved by passage through embryonated hens' eggs and in chick embryo cell culture. The vaccine is prepared from virus grown in culture. The vaccine has been tested in thousands of children and a few adults. Almost no reactions to the vaccine have been noted. Over 90 per cent of the susceptibles vaccinated showed antibody response. No transmission of virus to susceptible contacts has been noted. Protection against mumps has been demonstrated up to six years after inoculation of vaccine.[26]

If mumps vaccine is to be given in early childhood, it should be combined with measles and rubella which are usually administered at one year of age. If not given in infancy, mumps immunization should be directed primarily toward susceptible children approaching puberty, adolescents, and young adults, especially males who have no history of mumps.

Immunization against mumps should also be considered among children in closed populations such as institutions.

### Influenza

Immunization against influenza has been subjected to numerous careful trials during the past 30 years. The vaccine is prepared from virus grown in the allantoic cavity of embryonated hens' eggs. It is usually employed as a fluid preparation containing several different virus strains. The chief difficulty encountered with the product of effective influenza vaccine is the antigenic variations in the virus. Experience so far indicates that a new antigen strain of type A virus evolves at intervals of eight to 10 years. Vaccine effective against the previous strain of virus gives little or no protection against the new strains.

There seems no question that an influenza vaccine of adequate potency containing at least one of the antigenic components closely matching the prevailing strain of virus will give protection, at least for a number of months, following injection. Unfortunately, the polyvalent vaccine ordinarily employed gives a considerable number of untoward reactions in young children. In the past few years, improvements in vaccine production have reduced the incidence of postvaccinal reactions considerably. Since children are a major source of influenza infection throughout a community, widespread use of vaccine, especially in children of school age, might reduce the spread of virus. Therefore, a much wider use of the vaccine among children will probably be made in the future.

Adults and children over ten years are usually given two doses of vaccine with an interval of two weeks between. Children between six and 10 years are given the same schedule, but vaccine with less influenza virus is used. Children from three months to six years are given three doses of vaccine at 2-week intervals but with a lower virus dose (see Table 7.7).

Influenza vaccine is recommended only for people having unusual risk of complications or death. It may be considered for those engaged in essential public service, such as policemen, firemen, and hospital and transport workers, as well as for those in strategic industries or military service. Persons of all ages who suffer from chronic debilitating diseases and children with heart disease, chronic pulmonary disease, chronic metabolic disease, or chronic kidney disease should receive the vaccine. Vaccine should be administered well in advance of the expected influenza season.

*Rabies*

Although evidence of the effectiveness of postexposure vaccine prophylaxis of rabies is not too complete, it seems sufficient to justify continuation of its use. In the United States, two types of vaccine are commonly used: (1) the Semple vaccine, an inactivated phenolized rabbit brain tissue virus preparation; and (2) an inactivated virus vaccine produced from rabies virus grown in duck embryos. The usual course of treatment with both vaccines is one injection per day for 14 days; in severe or multiple bites, for 21 days. The vaccine is given in the deep subcutaneous tissues, usually on the abdomen, thighs, or lower back. The lower frequency of central nervous system reaction with duck embryo vaccine (DEV) makes it preferable to the Semple type vaccine (see Table 7.8).

Acute local reactions to the vaccine do occur, but are usually not serious. In the late injections of the series, delayed sensitivity reactions with swelling, redness, and pain may develop. Allergic reactions causing serious neurological reactions with paralytic effects have

TABLE 7.7

*Schedule for influenza vaccine*

| Patient | Dose (CCA Units)[1] | Not Previously Vaccinated | | Previously Vaccinated (Number of Doses) |
|---|---|---|---|---|
| | | Number of doses | Interval | |
| Adult, child over 10 yr. | 1,000 | 1 or 2 | 2 wk. | 1 per yr. |
| Child 6–10 yr. | 500 | 1 or 2 | 2 wk. | 1 per yr. |
| Child 3 mo.–6 yr. | 100–200 | 3 | 2 wk. | 1 per yr. |

[1] Review of influenza epidemiology and antigens of strains annually is used as a basis for recommendations to the manufacturer on dose and type of virus for each year's vaccine. See package insert before use.
Source: Report of the Committee on Infectious Diseases, Ed. 17, 1974. American Academy of Pediatrics, Evanston, Ill.

TABLE 7.8

*A. Local treatment of wounds involving possible exposure to rabies*

## 1. Recommended in all exposures

a. First-aid treatment

Since elimination of rabies virus at the site of infection by chemical or physical means is the most effective mechanism of protection, immediate washing and flushing with soap and water, detergent, or water alone is imperative (recommended procedure in all bite wounds including those unrelated to possible exposure to rabies). Then apply either 40 to 70 per cent alcohol, tincture or aqueous solutions of iodine, or 0.1 per cent quaternary ammonium compounds. Where soap has been used to clean wounds, all traces of it should be removed before the application of quaternary ammonium compounds because soap neutralizes the activity of such compounds.

b. Treatment by or under direction of a physician

    (1) Treat as above (a) and then:

    (2) apply antirabies serum by careful instillation in the depth of the wound and by infiltration around the wound;

    (3) postpone suturing of wound; if suturing is necessary use antiserum locally as stated above;

    (4) where indicated, institute antitetanus procedures and administer antibiotics and drugs to control infections other than rabies.

*B. Specific systemic treatment*

| Nature of exposure | Status of biting animal irrespective of previous vaccination | | Recommended treatment |
| | At time of exposure | During 10 days[1] | |
| --- | --- | --- | --- |
| 1. Contact, but no lesions; indirect contact; no contact | Rabid | — | None |
| 2. Licks of the skin; scratches or abrasions; minor bites (covered areas of arms, trunk, and legs) | (a) Suspected as rabid[2] | Healthy | Start vaccine. Stop treatment if animal remains healthy for 5 days[1,3] |
| | | Rabid | Start vaccine; administer serum upon positive diagnosis and complete the course of vaccine |
| | (b) Rabid; wild animal,[4] or animal unavailable for observation | | Serum + vaccine |
| 3. Licks of mucosa; major bites (multiple or on face, head, finger, or neck) | Suspect[2] or rabid domestic or wild[4] animal, or animal unavailable for observation | | Serum + vaccine. Stop treatment if animal remains healthy for 5 days[1,3] |

[1] Observation period in this chart applies only to dogs and cats.
[2] All unprovoked bites in endemic areas should be considered suspect unless proved negative by laboratory examination (brain FA).
[3] Or if its brain is found negative by FA examination.
[4] In general, exposure to rodents and rabbits seldom, if ever, requires specific antirabies treatment.
Source: WHO Expert Committee on Rabies, Sixth Report, Technical Report Series No. 523, WHO, Geneva, 1973.

been reported to occur very infrequently, probably one in 2000 persons treatment. Such serious reactions have occurred much less frequently with the duck embryo vaccine.

All bites by rabid wild animals and severe bites by any rabid animals around the head and neck are especially dangerous[2 7] (see Table 7.9). The time required for rabies to develop in such cases is shorter than it is from bites on other parts of the body, so there is less time to build up a protective immunity for the individual. A potent immune serum has been prepared in horses for use to supplement the vaccine in such patients (see discussion under "Passive Immunization")[2 8] It should be emphasized that prompt cleaning of the bite wound or scratch of the rabid animal is a most important aspect of rabies prevention. Soap or detergent solution may be used with plenty of water.

For certain high risk groups, it is recommended that prophylactic or pre-exposure rabies immunization be given. Such groups include veterinarians and animal hospital employees, rabies control personnel, research laboratory personnel, Peace Corps members, and others who may have unusual exposure risks. Duck embryo vaccine is now most generally used for this purpose. Two subcutaneous injections of 1 ml. of the vaccine one month apart followed by a third inoculation six to seven months later should be given. If the immunized individual is bitten later by a rabid animal he should receive a course of five daily doses of vaccine, followed by a booster dose 20 days after the last injection.

Intensive research efforts are being made to perfect a safer and more effective vaccine against rabies. Virus grown in tissue culture purified by fluorocarbon extraction to reduce nerve tissue, concentrated and inactivated, seems to offer the best possibility.

In Mexico and other Latin American countries, vampire bats are vectors of rabies for both humans and domestic animals, especially cattle and horses. Attempts have been made to control the vampire bat population by dynamiting the caves where they roost. A method of controlling the bats by topical application of an anticoagulant has also been tried.[2 9]

In the United States, the skunk has been the most frequent animal in wildlife to infect humans.

Incidence of rabies in humans can be greatly reduced by immunization of domestic dogs and cats.

In South America, the rabies vaccine most commonly used is produced by use of suckling mouse brain. Since 1966, approximately 2 million persons have been vaccinated. It is claimed that while post-vaccinal neuroparalytic

Table 7.9
*Animal susceptibility to rabies infection[1]*

| Susceptibility | | | |
|---|---|---|---|
| Extremely high | High | Moderate | Low |
| Foxes | Hamsters | Dogs | Opossums |
| Coyotes | Skunks | Sheep,[2] goats,[2] and horses[2] | |
| Jackals[2] and wolves[2] | Raccoons | Nonhuman primates | |
| Kangaroo rats | Domestic cats | | |
| Cotton rats | Bats | | |
| Common field voles | Bobcats | | |
| | Mongooses[2] and Viverridae[2] | | |
| | Guineapigs | | |
| | Other rodents | | |
| | Rabbits | | |
| | Cattle | | |

[1] Based unless otherwise indicated on the intramuscularly inoculated dose required to infect at least 50 per cent of the animals.
[2] Epidemiological evidence only.
Source:  WHO Expert Committee on Rabies, Sixth Report, Technical Report Series No. 523, WHO, Geneva, 1973.

accidents have occurred infrequently, they are less common than is encountered with other vaccines.

In 1973, a safe vaccine for puppies and kittens was licensed in the United States. This vaccine is also prepared in the brains of suckling mice.

## BCG

There are a number of useful vaccines that are not routinely employed in the United States. Under special circumstances, these vaccines may be valuable, and in some countries they are applied widely and regularly. Perhaps the most important of these vaccines is the one prepared with *Bacillus Calmette-Guerin* (BCG) for use against tuberculosis. After years of investigation, Calmette and Guerin at the Pasteur Institute in Lille, obtained a bovine strain of tubercle bacillus with a low and relatively fixed degree of virulence. Since this vaccine was introduced in 1921, many millions of people have been inoculated with it. The BCG vaccine is harmless when properly prepared and correctly administered. The weight of evidence indicates that BCG provides about 75 to 80 per cent protection against clinical tuberculosis in tuberculin-negative individuals subject to a significant risk of infection. All who have tested the vaccine do not agree with such favorable results. A study recently completed in Puerto Rico reports only a 29 per cent reduction in tuberculosis among tuberculin negative groups of children. The intradermal route of administration is most generally employed. In the United States, where there is a low incidence of tuberculosis, BCG should be reserved for those individuals at greater than usual risk. This would include children who live in households with adults suffering from active tuberculosis, students of medicine and nursing and perhaps other clinic and hospital personnel, and, finally, children, and young adults about to move to areas of the world where tuberculosis rates are high. Consideration should also be given to the use of BCG to assist in the control of tuberculosis in urban ghetto areas where prevalence of the disease is high. It must be emphasized that BCG can only be given to persons with a negative tuberculin test, *i.e.*, to those who have not previously been infected with tuberculosis. Therefore, BCG should not be given to individuals whose tuberculin test is already positive nor should it be given to persons with agammaglobulinemia, skin infections, fresh smallpox vaccinations, nor to those with other open skin injuries.[30,31]

## Typhoid-Paratyphoid Fevers

Typhoid fever vaccine has been in use for over half a century, but few well-controlled studies on its efficacy have yet been reported. Three types of vaccine are available: (1) heat-killed phenol preserved; (2) alcohol-killed; and (3) acetone-killed acetone dried vaccine. It is now believed that an acetone vaccine is superior. In the United States, immunization against typhoid fever is indicated as follows: exposure to a carrier in a household, outbreaks of the disease in the community, and travel to areas where typhoid is endemic.

Adults and children 10 years and over should receive two doses of 0.5 ml. injected subcutaneously four or more weeks apart; or three doses at weekly intervals. Children from six months to 10 years are given smaller doses (0.25 ml.) with the same intervals. Recall doses every one to three years are recommended if there is continued exposure.[32]

## Yellow Fever

Immunization against yellow fever is not needed in the United States except for personnel in virus research laboratories where yellow fever virus may be in use for investigations. All persons who expect to travel or to reside in endemic areas are strongly urged to take the vaccine (see Tables 7.10 and 7.11). The vaccine in use in the Americas is the 17D strain of living attenuated yellow fever vaccine virus prepared from infected chick embryos. A single subcutaneous injection of vaccine containing viable virus is effective. Antibodies appear in the blood seven to 10 days after vaccination and persist for at least 17 years, probably much longer. Yellow fever immunization is available in this country only at certain centers designated by the U.S. Government.

## Cholera

Vaccination against cholera is thought to provide some protection that endures for a period no longer than six months. The vaccine generally used is prepared of phenol or formalin killed cholera vibrios. Two doses are

TABLE 7.10

*Reported jungle yellow fever cases and deaths, South America,*
*1971–1972*

|  | 1971 | | 1972 | |
|---|---|---|---|---|
| Country | Cases | Deaths | Cases | Deaths |
| Bolivia | 8 | 5 | 9 | 0 |
| Brazil | 11 | 9 | 12 | 7 |
| Colombia | 9 | 7 | 3 | 3 |
| Peru | 0 | 0 | 7 | 7 |
| Surinam | 0 | 0 | 1 | 1 |
| Venezuela | 0 | 0 | 22 | 22 |
| Total | 28 | 21 | 54 | 40 |

TABLE 7.11

*Reported yellow fever cases and deaths, Africa, 1971–1972*

|  | 1971 | | 1972 | |
|---|---|---|---|---|
| Country | Cases | Deaths | Cases | Deaths |
| Angola | 65[1] | 42 | 0 | 0 |
| Cameroon | 0 | 0 | 2 | 2 |
| Ghana | 0 | 0 | 4 | 4 |
| Zaire | 2 | 2 | 0 | 0 |
| Total | 67 | 44 | 6 | 6 |

[1] Includes suspected cases.

Source:   National Center for Disease Control, Morbidity and Mortality Report, Vol. 22: No. 39, page 326, September 29, 1973.

recommended with an interval of at least 7 days between injections. Booster doses are required at 6-month intervals. Immunization against cholera is advised only for those subjected to unusual or continued risk. Cholera immunization is required for travel through some countries.

*Plague Vaccine*

Well-controlled data on the effectiveness of plague vaccine are not available. Nevertheless, the observations reported indicate that both types of plague vaccine—the killed and the live attenuated strains—do provide a certain degree of protection against the disease. Protection by repeated injections of the killed vaccine for individuals doing research on plague in the field or in the laboratory and for others who are subject to unusual risk is probably indicated. The living plague bacillus vaccine has been used for widespread active immunization of native populations in the face of plague outbreaks. A single dose of the live vaccine is required.

Many other vaccines to combat a variety of diseases have been prepared. In Russia, vaccines against brucellosis, tularemia, and tick-borne spring-summer encephalitis have been used widely with satisfactory results. Vaccines against rickettsial diseases have been produced using infected chick embryo yolk sac as the source of antigen. These vaccines have been effective in protecting against Rocky Mountain spotted fever and typhus fever, but have been used only on a small scale.

*Immunization Advised for Foreign Travel*

Before going abroad, and especially when going to tropical regions, several immunization or reimmunization procedures are generally indicated. For those who have never had a particular immunization, the complete "initial series" of doses is necessary. For those who have completed a particular immunization in the past, a single booster injection will be sufficient. If time permits, the immunizations should be spaced out, but, if necessary, several immunizations can be given on successive days.[33]

The immunization regulations vary considerably from one country to another. The United States Public Health Service publishes a pamphlet, "So You're going Abroad! Health Hints for Travellers" (Public Health Service Publication 748A), which is revised from time to time. This bulletin may be purchased from the Superintendent of Documents, Government Printing Office, Washington, D.C., at a small cost.

All persons going to tropical areas should be vaccinated against smallpox and against typhoid fever. Persons under 50 years of age should be immunized against poliomyelitis since the risks of acquiring that infection are considerable in tropical countries. All children should be adequately protected against diphtheria, whooping cough, and tetanus. Adults are well advised to bring their immunity to diphtheria and tetanus up to effective levels.[34,35]

Some diseases have a limited geographical distribution. Persons traveling to regions where these diseases are known to be prevalent should receive the appropriate vaccines. Yellow fever vaccination is recommended for all going to Central and South America and to tropical Africa, and is required by some Asian countries if the traveler passes through a yellow fever area enroute to the East. Visitors to India and Pakistan and to neighboring areas of Southeast Asia should be immunized against cholera. Plague vaccine is available, but not usually indicated except for areas in which known cases of plague exist or where exposure is highly probable.

Infectious hepatitis due to a virus infection is a real hazard in most tropical areas. In recent years, considerable protection has been provided to travelers to these areas by a prophylactic injection of immune globulin. A dose of 5 ml. will give protection for approximately six months.

In the United States, all vaccinations except for yellow fever may be given by private physicians. Yellow fever vaccine is given in centers designated by the U.S. Public Health Service.

Vaccinations should be recorded in the official form, "International Certificate of Vaccination." This can be obtained at passport offices.

## Passive Immunization

The use of immune serum for providing temporary protection against infection began some 75 years ago when diphtheria antitoxin was introduced into clinical medicine. The obvious success of antitoxin in combating diphtheria led to the development of other immune sera for use in preventing other diseases. Some of these have been effective, but with others the results have been at best equivocal. Probably this disparity in results may depend upon differences in disease pathogenicity. Another factor is that high antibody titers can be obtained against some microorganisms, but satisfactory titers for other agents are difficult or impossible to achieve.

A major feature of passive immunization is its rapid effectivity after injection of the serum into the body. In contrast, active immunization requires more time to develop, probably a minimum of several days. The use of passive immunization is mainly an emergency measure, when it is too late to provide protection by active immunization, or for situations in which active immunization is not practical.

Passive immunity may be produced by use of human serum from recovered cases, pooled immune globulin fraction of sera from healthy blood donors, or artificially produced immune sera produced in animals or in human volunteers—either the whole serum or a concentrated globulin fraction may be used.[36]

Protection provided by passive immunization is of short duration. Human serum or immune globulin has two advantages: (1) the duration of protection is longer, and (2) almost no undesirable reactions occur after its use. Foreign sera, usually taken from rabbits or horses, may produce severe serum sickness about one week after being injected into the body. There has been a steady shift, during the past 20 years, toward use of human sera rather than the sera of animals for passive immunization. In some instances, however, this has not been possible.[37]

Passive immunization is recommended in the following situations:

### Diphtheria

For exposed susceptible children who cannot be kept under daily surveillance, an intramuscular injection of diphtheria antitoxin varying from 1000 to 10,000 units in accordance with body weight is given at the same time as a dose of toxoid.

### Pertussis

Intimately exposed infants under two years of age who have not been immunized should receive chemoprophylaxis in the form of erythromycin for 10 days after contact is broken. Immune serum has proved to be unreliable in protecting such exposed children.

### Measles

An effort to prevent measles in exposed susceptible individuals of all ages is worthwhile, especially for infants under three years of age, individuals suffering from chronic illnesses, and children in institutions. Children previously unimmunized should receive live measles vaccine and a dose of 0.04 ml. per kg. of immune serum globulin (ISG) at separate sites to be followed by a second dose of live virus vaccine in eight or more weeks.

If the exposed susceptible child is known to have leukemia or immunodeficiency, a dose of 20 to 30 ml. ISG should be given immediately.

### Tetanus

For individuals who are injured and who have no definite history of immunization against tetanus, the human immune globulin is the preferred agent for passive immunization. The immune serum globulin should be given intramuscularly with a part of the dose infiltrated around the wound. A dose of 3000 to 6000 units is recommended. Active immunization with tetanus toxoid should be started at the same time. The injection should be made at a different site. Tetanus antitoxin (horse serum) may be given if human immune globulin is not available. Tests for sensitivity to horse serum must be carried out.

### Infectious Hepatitis

The best evidence now available indicates that infectious hepatitis is contracted only after fairly intimate exposure. When exposure is definite, protection should be provided to exposed susceptibles by an injection of immune serum globulin (human). The recommended dose for household exposure is 0.02 ml. per kg. of body weight given intramuscularly within one week after exposure. For intensive exposure such as may be encountered in mental institutions, a larger dose of 0.06 ml. per kg. is advisable. If the exposure continues, the dose should be repeated once after five to six months.

For travelers to areas of the world where infectious hepatitis is endemic, the tropics especially, considerable protection can be obtained by an injection of 5.0 ml. of immune serum globulin. For persons remaining in high risk areas longer than six months, a second injection of 5.0 ml. is indicated at the end of the 6-month period.

### Rubella (German Measles)

The incidence and severity of congenital malformations occurring in infants whose mothers contracted rubella during the first trimester of pregnancy have impelled physicians to attempt to prevent rubella through the use of immune serum globulin for those women who have been exposed to rubella in the early stages of pregnancy. Available evidence indicates that ISG may modify or suppress the clinical manifestations of rubella without preventing infection. Infants with congenital rubella have been born to women who have been given ISG soon after exposure.

When pregnant women are exposed to rubella, the blood should be tested to determine whether or not the woman is immune. The hemagglutination-inhibition test is usually employed. If she is immune, no concern need be felt. If she is not immune, the physician may recommend ISG for those who would not consider therapeutic abortion.

### Vaccinia (Cowpox) Virus and Smallpox

Vaccinia immune globulin (human) (VIG) injected by the intramuscular route will prevent or modify smallpox, if given within 24 hr. after exposure. This same product may be used in the treatment of accidental infections of the eye with vaccinia or in other severe infections with vaccinia virus. Another valuable use for VIG is in young children suffering from eczema who have been exposed to vaccinated household members, in children who have suffered severe burns during the course of smallpox vaccination, or in eczematous children who are required to have smallpox vaccination prior to travel abroad. The dose for prophylaxis is 0.3 ml. per kg., and the dose for treatment of complications of vaccination is 0.6 ml. per kg. by the intramuscular route. Information as to availability of VIG is listed in the Report of the Committee on Infectious Diseases, American Academy of Pediatrics, 1974.

*Rabies*

During recent years, the use of rabies antiserum in addition to vaccine in the postexposure prophylaxis of rabies has been widely accepted. Antirabies serum should be given as early as possible after exposure to individuals who have suffered multiple bites and bites around the face, head, neck, and fingers or to those bitten by rabid wild animals. The dose recommended is 1000 units per 40 pounds of weight up to 6000 units. If the bite is located so as to make it feasible, serum should be infiltrated around the bite area. Unless the biting animal is proved to be free of rabies, the full 14 doses of vaccine should be administered. In addition, subsequent doses of vaccine, preferably not produced from nervous tissue, should be given 10 and 20 days after completion of the regular vaccine series. Antirabies serum is produced in horses, so all precautions required in the injection of foreign serum must be observed. Rabies immune globulin of human origin is now being prepared. Presumably this product will be available commercially in the not too distant future.

## Immunizations: Precautions and Contraindications

No discussion of immunization methods in the control of disease can be regarded as complete without a consideration of their safety and public acceptability. All immunization procedures are known to have produced at least occasional unpleasant reactions, and some are reported to have been responsible, although very rarely, for fatal reactions. One must therefore balance the gains with the possible losses to be expected.[38]

The following paragraphs are taken from the *Report of the Committee on the Control of Infectious Diseases,* American Academy of Pediatrics:

*Precautions*

1. Needles and syringes must be sterilized before each injection. The use of one syringe with change of needle between injections is not considered safe. Sterilization should be carried out by autoclaving at a temperature of 121° C (250° F) for a period of 15 minutes at 15 pounds pressure. An appropriate indicator or control should be employed. Dry heat for two hours at 170° C or boiling for 30 minutes are acceptable if precautions are taken to assure that the desired time and temperature are attained. The use of sterilized disposable needles and plastic syringes is recommended.

2. The skin should be clean and should be swabbed with an antiseptic solution such as 2 per cent tr. iodine which is allowed to dry and then removed with 70 per cent alcohol. Acetone or ether or no treatment is preferred by many preceding smallpox vaccination.

3. The rubber stopper of the antigen container should be disinfected (as in 2. above).

4. "Depot" antigens combined with adjuvants (potassium alum, aluminum phosphate and aluminum hydroxide) are injected intramuscularly.

5. Antigens without adjuvants (fluid toxoids and suspended vaccines) are injected intramuscularly but may be given subcutaneously or, in special cases, intracutaneously.

6. Only well infants should be injected.

7. Acetylsalicylic acid, 65 mg. (1 grain) per year of age, up to 0.6 gm. (10 grains). may be given 2-8 hours after injection.

8. When an infant is brought for a second injection, the parent should be questioned concerning the occurrence of fever, somnolence, or unusual reactions following the previous injection. If these are reported, the volume of the next injection may need to be decreased. If a convulsion or severe reaction is reported, no further injection of pertussis vaccine should be given. Other inoculations should be completed with single antigens only, beginning with fractional doses to test tolerance (*e.g.*, 0.05 to 0.01 ml). Phenobarbital in appropriate doses may be useful in addition to acetylsalicylic acid in some instances.

*Contraindications*

1. Any acute respiratory disease or other active infection is reason for deferring an injection. Prolonging the interval between injections does not interfere with the final im-

munity.

2. The presence of cerebral damage in an infant is an indication for delay in starting immunization procedures. Severe febrile reactions, with or without convulsions, may be encountered. In such infants, active immunization procedures should not be initiated until after one year of age. Single antigens rather than the usual multiple antigens are recommended and fractional doses should be employed.

3. During an outbreak of poliomyelitis, inoculation with multiple "depot" antigens should be deferred. When an outbreak of diphtheria, pertussis, typhoid or smallpox occurs simultaneously with poliomyelitis, the appropriate specific antigen should not be deferred. Fluid antigen rather than "depot" antigen should be used. Oral poliovaccine may be given during a poliomyelitis outbreak.

4. Infants with eczema, impetigo, or other forms of dermatitis, should not be vaccinated against smallpox because of the danger of eczema vaccinatum. Eczema vaccinatum is produced by direct skin contact with the virus. Siblings of infants with eczema or dermatitis should not be vaccinated against smallpox because of the danger of cross infection. An exception may be made when it is possible to separate the child to be vaccinated from sibling with eczema or dermatitis. Separation of the children in different rooms of the same household is not adequate; they must live in separate buildings and remain apart until the vaccination scab falls off.

5. Children receiving cortico-steroid therapy or other immuno-depressants (antimetabolites, irradiation, alkylating agents) may have diminished antibody response to active immunization procedures. In patients on *short term* therapy, immunizing injections should be deferred until treatment is discontinued. Children on *long term* therapy should not receive certain live vaccines (smallpox, measles, BCG) but may receive killed vaccines during treatment, followed by an extra dose of killed or living vaccine one month or more after therapy is discontinued.

6. Specific contraindications to the use of measles, rubella, and mumps live attenuated vaccines are pregnancy; leukemia; lymphoma or other generalized malignancy; diseases in which cell mediated immunity is impaired; immunodepressive therapy (steroids, irradiation, antimetabolites, alkylating agents); severe febrile illness; or recent administration of immune serum globulin, plasma, or blood.

Products prepared for immunization may produce troublesome reactions either through inherent characteristics or through faulty production or administration.

## Progress in Disease Control by Immunization

### Diphtheria

Since 1921, diphtheria cases and deaths in the United States have fallen steadily. The total of 152 cases reported in 1972 is the lowest so far on record. This figure contrasts sharply with the 206,939 cases recorded in 1921 and the 18,675 cases in 1945 (see Fig. 7.3). However, the decline of diphtheria was broken in 1970 when 442 cases were reported in the U. S. Most of these cases occurred in southern states where the percentage of immunized children is somewhat lower than in other regions of the country.

Immunization against diphtheria has never proved to be 100 per cent effective. Cases occur among inoculated individuals and yet reports from many different countries tell of marked reductions in diphtheria attack rates in vaccinated as compared to neighboring or intermingled unvaccinated population groups. Following immunization, protection wanes unless it is sustained by periodic booster injections of toxoid at intervals of three to five years. Such a program of booster doses will probably have to be maintained in those areas where the incidence of the natural disease has become so low that it no longer provides the population with the recurring antigenic stimulus formerly obtained through natural exposures.

### Pertussis

Reported cases of pertussis and death from the disease have fallen steadily in the United States in recent years. In the past, over 70 per cent of deaths have occurred among children under one year of age. With a good vaccine preparation about 75 to 80 per cent protection can be expected. Only 13 deaths from pertussis were reported in the United States in 1969. (see Fig. 7.4.).

Recently, outbreaks of pertussis have been reported among teenagers and adults who had been immunized in infancy. The pertussis vaccine produces sharp reactions in older children and adults, so there is no effective method that can be recommended at present for recall injections to maintain immunity induced in early infancy.

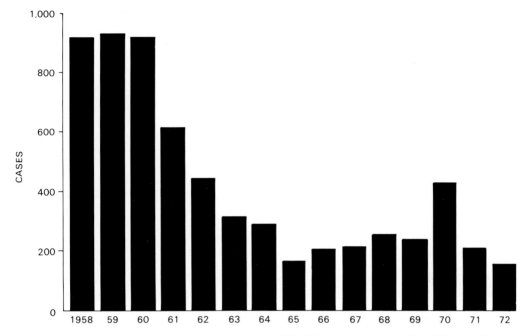

Fig. 7.3. Diphtheria—reported cases, United States, 1958-1972. (Redrawn from Morbidity and Mortality Weekly Report Summary 1972. Vol. 21: No. 53, p. 44, Center for Disease Control, Public Health Service, July 1973.)

### Tetanus

The incidence of tetanus has declined slowly despite the extensive use of immunization. Tetanus cases occur in all regions of the United States but are reported more frequently from the southern states (see Fig. 7.5). Tetanus in newborn infants is now a rarity outside of the South. In the 1968-69 period, 328 cases of tetanus were reported in the United States with a case-fatality ratio of 61.3 per cent. Tetanus attack rates were five times as high in Negroes and other minority racial groups as among whites. The states of the lower South continued to lead the nation in incidence. No documented cases of tetanus were reported among fully immunized persons.[39] In 1972, 128 cases of tetanus were recorded. Over half of all cases occur among adults. Probably most of these adults had never received tetanus immunization or had been given an inadequate series of inoculations.

Tetanus is a very severe disease with an overall fatality rate of 61 per cent in the United States. Among the infants and old age groups, the fatality rate is greater than 75 per cent. Puncture wounds and lacerations accounted for about 60 per cent of the reported cases of tetanus. No wound or obvious source of infection could be found in a few of the tetanus cases.

In World War II, the incidence of tetanus was less than one per 200,000 injuries or wounds. Tetanus toxoid is regarded as one of the most effective known immunizing agents, and reactions of any consequence are rare.

### Poliomyelitis

Following the introduction of inactivated poliovaccine in 1955, poliomyelitis incidence fell precipitously. The live attenuated poliomyelitis vaccine came into use shortly afterward and has largely replaced the inactivated vaccine. Only 31 cases of poliomyelitis, of which 29 were paralytic, were reported in the United States in 1972. The majority of paralytic polio cases occur in young adults and in preschool-age children. An occasional case was due to travel abroad to areas where poliomyelitis is still prevalent.

In 1971, one case appeared to result from the vaccine itself. This case was in a five-month old infant who became ill 13 days after receiving monovalent type 3 vaccine. In addition, there were six cases that occurred in family or close contacts of recent vaccinees. These are termed "contact vaccine associated cases" (see Fig. 7.6).

Most of the poliomyelitis cases give a history of no immunization or only a partial immunization.[40]

Recent experience points up the necessity for persistent, continuous vaccination programs with poliovaccine aimed particularly at the lower socio-economic preschool population.

## Eradication of Disease Through Immunization

*Measles*

Measles spreads by direct contact from person to person without intermediate hosts or other non-human reservoirs. It has a striking potentiality for rapid spread among susceptibles. Immunity to measles is of long duration; probably it is lifelong following an attack in childhood. Most of the susceptibles are concentrated in childhood groups. So far, experience with the measles virus indicates that only one strain exists. In other words, it is antigenically stable. This constancy of the measles virus in nature has permitted development of live attenuated virus vaccines which produce an uniform immunity not unlike that following an attack of natural measles. The availability of these vaccines provides the means not only to control but to eradicate the disease.

Careful studies on the epidemiology of measles indicate that epidemics of measles occur as a direct function of the proportion of susceptibles in the population and the closeness of contact. In large cities, epidemics tend to recur every two to three years. It is estimated that prior to major epidemics of measles, the proportion of the population under 15 years of age susceptible to measles ranges from 45 to 50 per cent. At the end of the epidemic, this proportion has fallen only to 30 to 35 per cent. In essence, this signifies that measles epidemics do not occur when 65 to 70 per cent of the population is immune to the disease. From the standpoint of eradicating measles, it is important that transmission of the disease ceases when the population immunity reaches a level which is considerably below 100 per cent.

Beginning in 1962, immunization of children against measles has become more widespread in the United States each year. By 1964 to 1965, definite decreases in the incidence of reported cases of measles were obvious. As experience in the use of the measles vaccine increased,

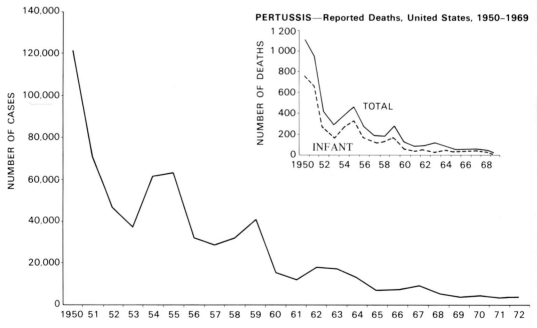

Fig. 7.4. Pertussis–reported cases, United States, 1950-1972. (Redrawn from Center for Disease Control, Morbidity and Mortality Weekly Report–Annual Supplement, 1972. DHEW Publication No. (CDC) 74-8241, July 1973.)

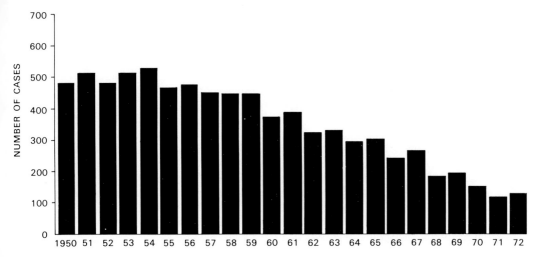

Fig. 7.5. Tetanus–reported cases, United States, 1950-1972. (Redrawn from Center for Disease Control, Morbidity and Mortality Weekly Report–Annual Supplement, 1972. DHEW Publication No. (CDC) 74-8241, July, 1973.)

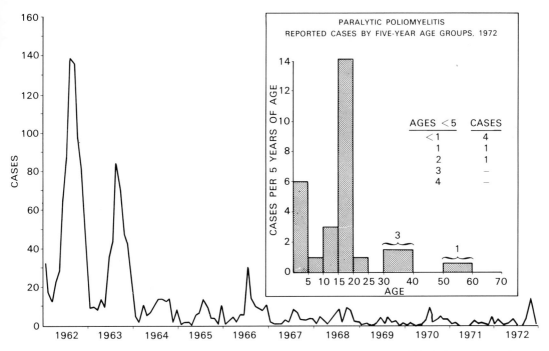

Fig. 7.6. Paralytic poliomyelitis–reported cases by month, United States, 1962-1972. (Redrawn from Morbidity and Mortality Weekly Report Summary 1972. Vol. 21: No. 53, p. 44, Center for Disease Control, Public Health Service, July 1973.)

epidemiologists began to think in terms of eradication of the disease from the United States. President Johnson and the Surgeon General of the Public Health Service called for eradication of measles by the end of 1967. This date, however, proved to be somewhat premature.

The program outlined by the Center for Disease Control of Atlanta, Georgia, for the eradication campaign is:[27]

1. Routine immunization of infants at about one year of age.

2. Immunization of all susceptible children on entry to school or kindergarten, nursery school, and day care homes.

3. Surveillance—intensive efforts must be made to obtain reporting to health agencies of all cases of measles that do occur. Sample surveys to determine the status of immunity to measles in the community will be helpful in guiding health authorities to problem areas.

4. Epidemic control—immediate action should be taken to verify the diagnosis and to trace the source of infection. All susceptible contacts must be immunized or inoculated with immune globulin. Intensification of the vaccination campaign in the surrounding areas is indicated.

The total number of measles cases reported in the United States for 1966 was 204,136. Through intensive efforts to apply the new vaccine, this number had fallen to 22,231 in 1968. Unfortunately, measles cases began to increase again reaching 75,290 in 1971, but falling to 32,275 in 1972 (see Fig. 7.7).

In addition to an increase in cases, there was a sharp rise in deaths and complications of measles. Encephalitis occurs in about one case per 1000 and one child in three with measles encephalitis is left retarded. Death occurs in one of every 2000 to 3000 cases of measles.

The typical measles patient today is three years old, poor, non-white, and lives in a large city. The 1970 United States Immunization Survey showed that only 41 per cent of children one to four years old in urban poverty areas had been immunized against measles.[41]

One difficulty in the widespread application of measles vaccine has been the relatively high price of this product. This obstacle has largely been removed by the provisions of the National Vaccination Assistance Act (1962) which, since 1966, has included the measles vaccine along with the other immunizing agents supplied by the Federal Government for use among children whose families could not otherwise afford the cost of immunization. Unfortunately, this support was withdrawn in 1969.

*Smallpox*

Smallpox is still a prevalent disease in many parts of the world. Under the leadership of the World Health Organization, programs for eradication of this disease are being undertaken in a number of countries. Because of the inherent difficulties in administering the vaccine widely in many undeveloped regions, it appears likely that complete eradication of smallpox on a world-wide basis is many years away.

Each year, several focal outbreaks of smallpox have occurred in western European countries, introduced by supposedly adequately vaccinated travelers from endemic areas. Notably, transmission of the disease has occurred most frequently among hospital employees and patients.

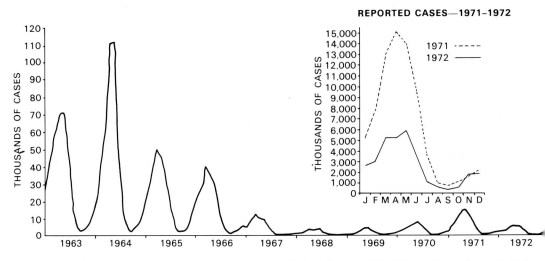

Fig. 7.7. Measles (rubeola)—reported cases by month, United States, 1963-1972. (Redrawn from Morbidity and Mortality Weekly Report Annual Supplement, Summary 1972. Vol. 21: No. 53, p. 44. Center for Disease Control, Public Health Service, July 1973.)

The principal barrier against an outbreak of smallpox due to importation from abroad is a well-vaccinated population. No indigenous case of smallpox has been reported in the United States since 1949. It would appear that the disease has been eradicated from the national territory. However, an occasional case of smallpox may evade the quarantine authorities and be introduced to a partially susceptible population. Surveys of immunization levels undertaken by the Center for Disease Control a few years ago in four widely separated areas of the country revealed that less than 20 per cent of the populations surveyed had been vaccinated against smallpox during the previous four years. With so many susceptible or partially susceptible persons in the country, the introduction of an infectious case of smallpox from abroad poses a definite threat. The best protection for the United States would be the successful extension of the world-wide immunization program.

In 1967, the World Health Organization stated that 131,000 cases of smallpox were reported from 42 countries, 30 of which were considered endemic for the disease. The actual number of cases was estimated at 2.5 million. In that year WHO initiated its world-wide eradication campaign against smallpox. In the six years since the vaccination campaign began the number of endemic countries has been reduced to six, although, in 1972, outbreaks were recorded in ten countries due to importation into their smallpox-free areas.

A potent and stable freeze-dried vaccine became available for the WHO eradication campaign. It is believed that smallpox may disappear from the earth if this campaign continues to be pushed vigorously.[42]

## ISOLATION AND QUARANTINE

Until a few decades ago, isolation and quarantine were measures frequently employed by health officers to control the spread of communicable disease among the population. As other means of control were discovered and as the natural history of some diseases became clearer, these measures declined in popularity and are used much less frequently.

"Isolation" means separation of infected persons from other persons during the period of communicability. This must be done under such conditions as will prevent the direct or indirect spread of the infectious agent from the infected person to others who are susceptible or who may spread the agent to other people. Isolation may also be applied to animals, for example, dogs suspected of being rabid. Isolation of sick individuals also protects the patient, possibly in a weakened state, from exposure to secondary infection in other people during the period of illness.

To carry out the necessary techniques of isolation, one should know the portals of exit of the infecting agent and the usual mode of entry to a new host. In case of streptococcal infections, particular attention must be given to safe disposal of secretions of the mouth, nose, and throat, while in intestinal infections attention is focused on urine and feces.

Isolation may be of little use in preventing the spread of some communicable diseases, including poliomyelitis or mosquito-borne encephalitis. Strict isolation in cases of smallpox for the entire period of communicability is of real importance, and is required and enforced by official health agencies.

Probably isolation accomplishes little in such diseases as influenza, mumps, measles, and chickenpox. Such patients should be kept from school and at home during the period of communicability. The attending physician advises a modified system of isolation for these diseases to meet different circumstances, and its duration is usually left to his discretion.

Quarantine is the limitation of freedom of movement of well persons or animals who have been exposed to a communicable disease for a period of time equal to the longest usual incubation period of the disease, in such manner as to prevent effective contact with those who have not been exposed. Quarantine may have different degrees of completeness, depending upon the circumstances.

1. Complete quarantine limits freedom of movement of the person or persons concerned so that they are not in contact with others.

2. Modified quarantine is a selective, partial limitation of movement of persons or animals. Children may be kept from school; contacts may be stopped from handling food; military personnel may be confined to the post or to quarters.

3. Personal surveillance is the practice of close observation of contacts in order to discover signs of illness or infection promptly. Movements of such persons are not restricted.

The Center for Disease Control in Atlanta, Georgia, has responsibility for enforcing laws and regulations designed to prevent the introduction and spread of epidemic diseases from other countries. Medical inspections are made on board ships, at ports of entry, and at international airports. By international agreement, the quarantinable diseases are smallpox, yellow fever, cholera, plague, louse-borne typhus, and relapsing fever. The Department of Agriculture has responsibility for enforcing the foreign-quarantine regulations relating to plant and animal diseases.

## PROPHYLACTIC VITAMINS AND MINERALS

The 20th century has brought great advances in the knowledge of the relation of diet to health. Such authoritative agencies as the Food and Nutrition Board of the National Research Council in Washington and the Food and Agriculture Organization of the United Nations have provided recommended dietary allowances which are revised periodically in the light of new information as it becomes available. The public in all advanced countries is exposed to intensive educational campaigns from early childhood to promote good dietary practices. Public health agencies all concentrate their efforts to improve the nutritional status, especially of mothers and infants. All of these activities have been productive of better nutrition, but still the results leave much to be desired. The relation of diet to the onset of degenerative diseases has not been adequately clarified. High cholesterol levels in the blood may be of importance in the development of atherosclerosis, but there appear to be other important factors in this process that are not well understood. Obesity clearly leads to increased mortality rates from a number of diseases, and yet one-third of American men from 50 to 59 years are 20 per cent overweight or more.

Men who are overweight, who lead a sedentary life, and whose blood cholesterol is elevated are thought to be in danger of attacks of coronary heart disease. In recent years, a number of long-term studies to observe the effect of placing such men on modified fat diets, to reduce their weight, and to lower blood cholesterol levels have been undertaken. This combined effort to control weight and to manage dietary intake appears to produce encouraging results in reducing coronary attacks and in prolonging life.[43]

In spite of the high dietary levels prevailing in all advanced countries, there are large groups of the population which are especially vulnerable to nutritional deficiencies. Many of the lower social and economic groups lack the funds required to obtain the necessities for healthy existence. Frequently, nutrition does not have high priority in their family budgets. Ignorance of good nutritional practices is also likely to be prevalent among these people.

Another population group which may be particularly vulnerable to malnutrition includes elderly men and women. Many old people are living on inadequate incomes and many dwell alone and have little interest in preparing regular meals. Others suffer from physical, emotional, and mental disabilities which interfere with normal living patterns. Lack of adequate dentures handicaps many individuals in securing balanced diets. Poor absorption of nutrients from the digestive tract in some aged people may make dietary supplements advisable. Individuals with chronic, debilitating diseases and those who have undergone major surgical procedures must be closely observed to ensure that proper nutritional balance is maintained.

Physiological stress periods impose increased demands for certain nutrients. Infants and rapidly growing children have such requirements. Cow's milk is used more frequently for infants than is human milk in the United States. Water and sugar are usually added to cow's milk to obtain a formula more nearly like that of human milk. Since both cow's milk and human milk are low in Vitamin D and iron, the diet of the infant should be supplemented with these nutrients. Vitamin C is provided by adding orange juice to the diet. The trend in the United States has been to add solid foods to the diet at an early stage, usually at the third month. These foods should provide sufficient iron to meet the infant's requirements.

Pregnancy and lactation are other periods of physiological stress. Nutritional requirements are somewhat increased to provide for the developing fetal tissues and for other requirements. Apparently the woman's body adapts itself to the new situation, so that the need for additional nutrients is minimized. Adequate supplies of protein and of iron are of particular importance.

In highly developed countries, the great

majority of women can safely go through pregnancy without dietary supplements, but with women on marginal diets and in countries with low nutritional standards supplementation is advisable. Lactation frequently causes malnutrition in women on poor diets. Protein and calcium in particular should be increased in the nursing mother's diet. It is advisable also to supplement her intake of Vitamin A and the water-soluble Vitamin B group to ensure that the nursing infant receives adequate amounts of these vitamins in the milk.

Patients with extensive burns or who have undergone major surgery or have suffered severe injuries have need of additional protein in their diets. This is due to the increased protein destruction and also to some extent to lowered food intake.[44]

As a prophylactic measure, the addition of specific nutrients to food supplies has shown great promise. A definite limitation to this measure is that it is not readily applicable where most needed, i.e., in underdeveloped countries where food is produced and consumed locally and handled in small quantities. Enrichment of foods has been undertaken with success where manufacturing and processing facilities are conducted on a large scale.

Examples of this method are the addition of thiamine to rice in the Far East to prevent beriberi; the use of niacin to enrich cornmeal in Yugoslavia and in the southern United States to combat pellagra; and the improvement of incomplete protein diets by addition of fish flour, skimmed milk powders, and yeast or purified amino acid preparations in Central America. Probably such measures will be employed with increasing frequency as the food supplies of the world continue to grow less adequate to meet minimum demands of a rising population.[45]

In the American food industry, enrichment of various foods is frequently practiced. Vitamin A is added to milk, margarine, vegetable oils, and some cheeses, and Vitamin D is added to milk, margarine, enriched breakfast cereals, bread, cornmeal, and grits. Niacin, riboflavin, and thiamine are added to breakfast cereals, enriched flour, cornmeal, grits, macaroni, and noodle products. Calcium and iron salts are frequently included in these same food substances.

Two other important health programs are the addition of iodides to table salt to prevent goiter and the inclusion of fluorides in drinking water to reduce the incidence of dental caries.

Iodine is an essential nutrient for the normal metabolism of the thyroid gland and for the synthesis of the thyroid hormone. If iodine is not available to the body in sufficient amounts, the thyroid gland becomes prominent and a goiterous condition develops. In certain regions of the world, goiter is exceedingly common. This is thought to be due to iodine-deficient soil. Most of these goiter areas had been subject to flooding or to intense glacier activity, so that iodine had been removed from the soil and carried down to the sea.

Rates of thyroid enlargement increase with age. In males, they decline after puberty; in females, the rates fall after about age 20. In later years, goiter may occur during pregnancy or at the menopause, periods when iodine demand is enhanced. Other causes of goiter are the eating of large quantities of cabbage as a dietary staple, increased excretion of iodine, and other less common conditions.

In the United States, the Northwest and the region around the Great Lakes have the highest goiter rates. Other goiter belts are located in high mountain regions such as the Alps, the Pyrenees, and the Himalayas. Endemic goiter is indeed a world-wide problem which is found on every continent in almost every country.

Heavily iodized salt was used for a time in Austria, France, and Italy during the 19th century, but was abandoned because of some adverse reactions, possibly due to overdosage. Iodine was again taken up as a goiter preventive around 1920 in several cities of the United States. Experiments with iodine in the drinking water were tried, but given up as more costly than the use of iodized salt.

Michigan began the first state-wide program of using iodized salt for its population. A survey there in 1923 to 1924 revealed that 38.6 per cent of the school children had enlargement of the thyroid. By 1951, this percentage had fallen to 1.4 per cent.[46]

In cool climates, potassium iodide is usually the compound of choice for inclusion in salt, but in hot moist regions the more stable potassium iodate is used. An interesting modification of the program is the use of intramuscular injections of iodized oil in New Guinea. Almost no salt is added to food in this area of severe endemic goiter. A single injection of iodized oil controls iodine deficiency for about two to three years.

Iodized salt does not prevent the occurrence

of all goiters, but it does ensure a great reduction in the incidence of this disfiguring disease. The World Health Organization is attempting to persuade more countries to undertake the program.

It has long been known that an excess of fluorine in drinking water causes mottling of the dental enamel. Studies in regions with high fluorine content in the water revealed that the incidence of dental caries is markedly diminished in comparison with areas of low fluorine content in the water. It is now generally agreed that a small amount of fluorine is necessary for the building up of healthy bones and teeth.

Carefully controlled studies have established that if fluorine is present in drinking water at a concentration of 1 p.p.m., the incidence of dental caries in children is low. In natural waters, the concentration of fluorine is found to vary from 0.1 to 8.0 p.p.m.

Beginning in 1945, long-term experiments which demonstrated that additions of small amounts of fluorides to the community water supplies were harmless were carried out in Newburgh and Kingston, New York; in Brantford and Stratford, Ontario; and in Grand Rapids and Muskegon, Michigan. The incidence of dental caries was sharply reduced among children who began to drink the fluoridated water early in life. The controlled fluoridation served as well as natural fluorides in inhibiting caries of teeth. Teeth that had erupted before the addition of fluorides to the water were not protected against caries. The annual cost of maintaining optimal fluoride levels in the community water supply ranges from $0.04 to $0.14 per person. Experience so far indicates strongly that controlled water fluoridation at levels between 0.7 to 1.3 p.p.m. is a safe and practicable method that can be expected to reduce dental caries and subsequent loss of teeth from dental caries by approximately 60 per cent.

As with many new public health measures, a certain amount of highly vocal opposition has arisen in opposition to water fluoridation. This opposition has prevented the adoption of the measure by many American communities. Late in 1969, almost 83 million people were using communal waters containing 0.7 p.p.m. or more fluoride. Of these, some 74.5 million were in communities where the water had been fluoridated at the level of 1.0 p.p.m. The others had access to water in which the natural concentration of fluoride was at least 0.7 p.p.m.[47]

In communities that have rejected this measure to combat dental caries, individuals may take fluoride tablets to provide for their personal protection. A daily supplement of 0.5 mg. of fluoride during the first three years of life and 1.0 mg. of fluoride thereafter will provide preventive action equivalent to that of fluoridated drinking water. The difficulty with this method is the failure of human beings to follow faithfully a daily regime of taking tablets.

Another method of preventing dental caries is the application of fluoride solutions to the teeth. The solutions frequently used are 2 per cent sodium fluoride or 8 to 16 per cent stannous fluoride. The teeth must be cleaned and dried prior to application. The treatment is applied four times over a 7- to 14-day period. The effectiveness lasts from two to three years. Usually fluoride is applied at age three and again at about the seventh year of age. In communities in which water fluoridation is practiced, topical application of fluoride is not indicated.

For several years, toothpaste including sodium fluoride has been on the market. In 1964, the American Dental Association reviewed the results of tests carried out with such toothpastes and concluded that they may be of significant value in preventing dental caries, if applied regularly and properly.

## MEDICATIONS

Very few drugs with any specific activity against disease were discovered before the present century. The ancients learned through empirical methods that antimony is effective in the treatment of schistosomiasis. The Greeks treated round worms with an extract of wormwood, now known as santonin. North American Indians used chenopodium oil for the same purpose. In Rome, the extract of the male fern (aspidium) was often employed to combat intestinal worm infections. Because of the toxicity of these substances and the frequently poor condition of the patient, these drugs were hazardous. Early in the 16th century, Paracelsus (1493-1541) introduced salts of mercury for the treatment of syphilis which was then sweeping across Europe in an epidemic form.

The discovery of the New World brought to

Europe at least two drugs of great merit. The more important of these was cinchona bark. The Indians of Peru were familiar with its action in relieving symptoms in certain forms of fever. A Jesuit priest was cured of his fever by a friendly Indian chief and soon demonstrated the virtues of "the bark" to others among the Spanish colonists. The name cinchona is derived from that of the Viceroy of Peru, the Count of Chinchon. A supply of the cinchona bark reached Europe about 1633 and soon became popular as a treatment for intermittent fevers, which we now know were caused by malaria. For about two centuries, the bark was employed in medicine as a powder, extract, or infusion. In 1820, P. J. Pelletier (1784-1841) and J. B. Caventou (1788-1842) isolated the alkaloid, quinine, from cinchona bark. The use of this alkaloid gradually replaced the cruder preparations.

Shortly after the introduction of cinchona bark to Europe, another specific plant substance was brought from Brazil. This drug, ipecac, which is derived from the dried root of *Cephaelis ipecacuanha* plants of Brazil, had long been used by the natives for the treatment of diarrheas. Wilhelm Piso (1611-1678) of Leiden, who accompanied the Count von Nassau to Brazil as personal physician during the years 1637 to 1644, is said to have brought ipecac back to Europe. Its use in Europe appears to be largely due to a Dutch physician Hadrianus Helvetius (1685-1755), who tried it successfully in cases of dysentery. Having cured the Dauphin of France, Helvetius sold the remedy to Louis XIV, whereupon its use in the treatment of diarrheal disease became common.

Pelletier, the discoverer of quinine, attempted to extract the specific agent from ipecac in 1817. He apparently succeeded in obtaining a mixture of active principles, but it remained for J. L. Bardsley (1801-1876) to obtain emetine from ipecac in a pure state and to use it for the treatment of diarrheas and dysenteries in 1829.

Little further progress in chemotherapy was made until the end of the 19th century. The beginning of the great advances in this important field of medicine quickly followed the discoveries of the living organisms that cause infectious disease. Once the organism could be brought into the laboratory and a suitable experimental animal became available, advances in the knowledge of chemotherapy often came quickly. Another highly significant factor in the advance of chemotherapy was the spectacular rise of the chemical industry in Europe and, soon afterward, in America. Many new compounds appeared for testing. The chemists also developed great skill in producing variations of any compounds that gave indications of future usefulness.

In Germany, Paul Ehrlich (1854-1915) began studies on aniline dyes. He found that such dyes reacted differently with one living tissue than with another. This suggested to Ehrlich that some substances might be taken up selectively by parasites rather than by normal body tissues. Possibly one might destroy the disease agent in this way without damaging the host. Working with a trypanosome in mice and rats, Ehrlich did find a dye, trypan red, which killed the parasites with doses that were harmless to the animal host. This drug was not useful, however, in treating human diseases. Ehrlich was led to study arsenicals by the work of other German workers who discovered that Atoxyl (sodium arsanilate) was effective in the treatment of human trypanosomiasis. Unfortunately, the effective dose of Atoxyl was too near the toxic level and overdosage could cause blindness. Working with great persistence, Ehrlich tested a great many arsenical compounds in the treatment of experimental syphilis in rabbits. Finally, Compound 606, Salvarsan, was found to be highly effective in clearing up syphilitic infections both in rabbits and in humans. This was a great triumph for rational medicine and gave an enormous stimulus to the study of chemistry in medicine. Salvarsan came into extensive use in the treatment of syphilis in 1909, and, together with other less toxic arsenicals and with bismuth, remained the generally accepted treatment until it was displaced by penicillin in 1943.

In the years following Ehrlich's great contributions, progress in chemotherapy was slow. A few specific drugs were introduced: suramin (1920) for the treatment of trypanosomal infections, Neostibosan (1919) for leishmaniasis, and plasmoquine (1926) and Atabrin (quinacrine) (1930) for malaria. Finally, in 1932, came a hopeful discovery in the treatment of bacterial diseases. Gerhard Domagk (1895-1964), of Germany, published his studies on the therapeutic value of Prontosil and Prontosil Rubrum in bacterial infections, especially those caused by the hemolytic streptococcus. Investigations by a group at the Pasteur

Institute of Paris soon made clear that the active component of Prontosil is a sulfanilamide. Derivatives of sulfanilamide, or sulfa drugs, revolutionized the therapy of pneumonia, meningitis, gonorrhea, and many other infections. The sulfone group of drugs is derived from this source. These compounds are now used in the treatment of leprosy.[48]

The sulfonamides are produced by chemical synthesis. More than 5000 sulfonamides have been so produced. Several of these have valuable uses in fields of medicine other than the field of infectious diseases.

Before the practicing physician had fully digested the potentialities of the sulfa drugs, a dazzling new prospect broke into view. Alexander Fleming (1881-1955), in London, found a mold spreading on the media in a Petri dish which he saw was inhibiting the growth of his culture of staphylococci. Instead of discarding the plate in disgust, as many a bacteriologist had previously done, Fleming began to grow the mold and to test a filtrate of the liquid medium that he had used. This filtrate inhibited the growth of staphylococci as well as many other bacteria. The mold was recognized as *Penicillium notatum,* so the name penicillin was given to the antibiotic substance that it produced. Little interest was demonstrated in Fleming's report which appeared in 1929.

In 1938, Howard Florey (1898-1968), a pathologist, and Ernst B. Chain (1906-    ), a chemist, jointly initiated a study of antibacterial substances produced by microorganisms. Penicillin was one of the first to be investigated. By crude methods in the laboratory sufficient amounts of penicillin were produced to carry out tests in animals. Preliminary trials *in vitro* and in animals showed great promise for penicillin as a therapeutic agent. Despite all obstacles, enough penicillin was accumulated by 1941 to treat five persons desperately ill with staphylococcal and streptococcal infections resistant to other therapy. The results were most encouraging. Expansion of the program demanded increased facilities for production of the antibiotic. Because of wartime restrictions, these facilities were not available in Britain. Florey and other members of his group visited Washington in 1941 to solicit the interest of the U. S. government in this project. So successful was the visit that a vast research program was launched in which laboratories of the government, of universities, and of industry worked in cooperation. During 1942, sufficient amounts of penicillin were produced to permit large scale clinical trials, which soon confirmed the great potentialities of the antibiotic. Coming in the middle of World War II, penicillin proved a great boon in the treatment of wounds. In 1943, the efficacy of penicillin in the treatment of syphilis was proclaimed. Although penicillin has been of the greatest utility in the treatment of infections, there were some diseases for which it was not effective, for example, tuberculosis, typhoid fever, and malaria.

Scientists began an intensive search for other antibiotics and, within a few years, several extremely valuable agents were discovered which were efficacious in treating a wider range of bacteria than penicillin. The first was Streptomycin (1944), isolated from a soil organism, *Streptomyces griseus,* by Selman A. Waksman at Rutgers University. Streptomycin showed great activity against the bacilli of tuberculosis and plague. In 1947, chloramphenicol was produced from an organism, *Streptomyces venezuelae,* in a soil sample from Venezuela. One year later came the first of the tetracycline antibiotics. These two antibiotics, chloramphenicol and tetracycline, have a broad spectrum of activity. They are especially valuable in the treatment of rickettsial infections and chloramphenicol is effective against typhoid fever. Both can be taken by mouth.

All of the early antibiotics were developed from living organisms. Chemists, however, quickly earned to synthesize new ones and to produce purified products and modifications of those already in use.[49]

As with insecticides, difficulties soon arose as strains of microorganisms developed that are resistant to a given antibiotic. Some organisms, such as staphylococci, appear to have a greater capacity to develop resistant strains than do others. Fortunately, new antibiotic agents have come along to provide for effective therapy in most infectious diseases (see table 7.12).

### Chemotherapy of Virus Infections

In the field of virus diseases, progress toward discovery of effective therapeutic agents has been slow. In infections with the psittacosis-lymphogranuloma venereum-trachoma group of agents the tetracyclines are usually employed with satisfactory results. This group of agents, although frequently classified with the viruses, is probably more closely related to the rickettsiae.

TABLE 7.12

*Events of importance in development of antimicrobial chemotherapy*

| Year | Compound | Discoverer | Pathogen or Disease |
|------|----------|------------|---------------------|
| 1633 | Cinchona bark | Calancha | Malaria |
| 1820 | Quinine | Pelletier | Malaria |
| 1905 | Atoxyl | Thomas | Trypanosomiasis |
| 1907 | Benzopurpurin dyes | Ehrlich (P.) | Trypanosomiasis |
|      | Arsphenamine | Ehrlich (P.) | Syphilis |
| 1924 | Plasmoquine | Bayer group | Malaria |
| 1932 | Sulfonamides (Prontosil) | Domagk | Pneumococcus |
| 1929, 1938 | Penicillin | Fleming, Florey, Chain | Gram-positive bacteria, syphilis |
| 1944 | Streptomycin | Waksman | Tuberculosis |
| 1945 | Isoniazid | Chorine | Tuberculosis |
| 1947 | Chloramphenicol | Ehrlich (J.) | Gram-negative bacteria |
| 1948 | Tetracyclines (Aureomycin) | Duggar | Broad spectrum of bacteria |
| 1952 | Erythromycin | McGuire | Broad spectrum of bacteria |
| 1959 | Synthetic penicillins | Batchelor | Resistant staphylococci |
| 1962 | $\beta$-Isatin thiosemicarbazone | Bauer, Sadler | Smallpox |

Source: Busch, H., and Lane, M. *Chemotherapy: An Introductory Text.* Chicago: Year Book Medical Publishers, Inc., 1967.

Signs of progress have recently been reported in a few other viral infections. Amantadine hydrochloride (Symmetrel) inhibits influenza infections in tissue culture, in chicks, and in mice. This was discovered in an industrial screening program for antiviral substances in 1964. This antiviral agent is useful in preventing illness in persons exposed to respiratory infection during an epidemic confirmed to be due to an A2 strain of influenza virus. It is used in persons over one year of age for whom an attack of influenza would be a grave risk. Although the manufacturer recommends amantadine only for prophylaxis, the drug may have therapeutic value if given promptly after the first symptoms have appeared.

A number of field trials of amantadine in the presence of outbreaks of A2 influenza have been reported, the most extensive of which was by Smorodintsev *et al.* in Leningrad. It was concluded that amantadine gave good protection to a high percentage of the treated group.[50]

The compound, 5-iododeoxyuridine, which is referred to as IDU or IUDR, has been found useful in treating keratitis caused by the Herpes simplex virus. It is applied in solution, topically.[51] In severe cases of infection with Herpes simplex virus or in cases of severe Herpes zoster, two drugs have a marked therapeutic effect. These are adenine arabinoside (Ara A) and cytosine arabinoside (Ara C). As these

drugs are dangerous, their use must be confined to severely ill patients.[51]

Another substance of real potential usefulness in the prevention of smallpox is isatin B-thiosemicarbazone (Methisazone) which was tested during 1963 in India. It was shown that this drug suppressed infection among 1101 contacts of smallpox with only three mild cases developing. Among 1126 untreated contact controls, there were 78 cases of smallpox with 12 deaths. Methisazone has been used successfully in the treatment of patients with generalized infections with vaccinia virus following smallpox vaccinations.

### Specific Treatment of Bacterial Diseases

Until the demonstration of the value of sulfonamides by Domagk in 1935 in the therapy of bacterial infections, this group of diseases had been notoriously difficult to treat. With the advent of antibiotics in 1940, there has been a plethora of chemotherapeutic agents for diseases caused by bacteria. In Table 7.13 are listed drugs of first and second choice for a number of the more common bacterial agents of disease.

Unfortunately, some of the important bacterial agents have developed resistance to antimicrobial drugs. This has been especially true of staphylococci, tubercle bacillus, meningococci, and more recently the typhoid bacillus. In early

1972, an outbreak of typhoid fever was reported in Mexico. The bacilli isolated in this epidemic were found to be highly resistant to chloramphenicol. Since then drug-resistant typhoid bacilli have been discovered in small outbreaks in the United States. Amphicillin has been suggested as the best drug to use in typhoid in place of chloramphenicol.

Physicians often use a combination of antimicrobial drugs in an attempt to avoid or postpone this development of drug resistance on the part of bacteria.

Soon after the discovery of streptomycin in 1944, Lehman reported that *para*-aminosalicylic acid is also useful in the treatment of tuberculosis.[52] Within a very few years, in 1952, there came another even more effective drug which revolutionized the treatment of tuberculosis. This compound, isoniazid, has a high degree of efficacy against the tubercle bacillus, good penetration into caseous foci, activity against intracellular organisms, and low toxicity, and it is easy to administer. The chief difficulty with isoniazid is the rapidity with which the tuberculosis bacillus develops resistance to its action. Isoniazid in moderate doses is well tolerated by patients who can be maintained on it for the long periods required in the therapy of tuberculosis.[53]

Unfortunately, the numbers of strains of tubercle bacillus that are resistant to the three primary antituberculosis drugs are increasing. There are a number of drugs less satisfactory because of poorer activity against the tubercle bacillus or because of their greater toxicity for the patient. One of these drugs or more may be employed in case of necessity.

A new antibiotic, rifampin, derived from *Streptomyces mediterranei* by Italian scientists, has proved to be valuable for the treatment of tuberculosis. Rifampin is a valuable drug with isoniazid for the primary treatment of cases but is especially useful in the treatment of patients whose disease has relapsed.

Experience has taught that when two drugs are administered simultaneously in the early stages of treatment there appears to be little likelihood of the bacillus becoming drug resistant.

## Antifungal Drugs

Little progress was made in discovering effective drugs for the treatment of systemic

TABLE 7.13

*Chemotherapeutic agents most likely effective in common bacterial infections*

| Bacterial Species | Drug of First Choice | Drug of Second Choice |
|---|---|---|
| Aerobacter | Kanamycin | Tetracycline, streptomycin |
| Bacterioides | Tetracycline | Ampicillin, chloramphenicol |
| Brucella | Tetracycline | Chloramphenicol |
| Cl. tetani | Penicillin G | Cephalosporin, erythromycin |
| Diplococcus pneumoniae | Penicillin G | Erythromycin, cephalosporin |
| Francisella tularensis | Streptomycin | Tetracycline |
| Hemophilus influenzae | Ampicillin | Tetracycline, cephalosporin |
| Klebsiella pneumoniae | Cephalosporin | Kanamycin, polymyxin, chloramphenicol |
| Neisseria gonorrhoeae | Penicillin G | Erythromycin, tetracycline |
| Neisseria meningitidis | Penicillin G | Sulfonamide, tetracycline |
| Proteus mirabilis | Ampicillin | Kanamycin, cephalosporin |
|    other species | Kanamycin | Tetracycline |
| Psudomonas aeruginosa | Polymyxin | Gentamicin |
| Salmonella | Chloramphenicol | Ampicillin |
| Shigella | Ampicillin | Tetracycline |
| Staphylococcus aureus | | |
|    Penicillinase-producing | Penicillinase-resistant penicillins | Cephalosporin, erythromycin, lincomycin, vancomycin |
|    Non-penicillinase-producing | Penicillin G | Semi-synthetic penicillins |
| Streptococcus pyogenes, groups A, B, C and G | Penicillin G | Cephalosporin, erythromycin |
| Treponema pallidum | Penicillin G | Erythromycin, tetracycline |

Source: *Pharmacy and Therapeutics,* A. Grollman and E. F. Grollman, Ed. 7, p. 562. Philadelphia: Lea and Febiger, 1970.

mycoses until the era of sulfa compounds and antibiotics. For one thing, serious mycotic infections were regarded as relatively rare until the last 25 years. The increase in such diseases may be a result of increased foreign travel, especially by military units, the widespread use of broad spectrum antibiotics, and the introduction of corticoids and anticancer drugs. Any agent that weakens the body's normal immunological defenses enhances the possibility of the development of a severe mycotic infection.

Four drugs are now available for use in the therapy of mycotic disorders. Nystatin (Mycostatin) was isolated in 1950 from a soil actinomycete.[54] Studies in animals demonstrated that the antibiotic was effective against a variety of fungal infections. The toxicity of nystatin has limited its usefulness mostly to topical application. Nystatin can also be tolerated after oral administration, and is so used in association with broad spectrum antibiotics to prevent overgrowth of mycotic agents. Its principal use is in the treatment of cutaneous or ophthalmic fungal infections.

Amphotericin A and B were produced from a strain, *Streptomyces nodosus,* found in a soil sample from Venezuela.[55] Amphotericin B proved to be the more potent drug against mycoses. Taken orally, amphotericin B is not very effective. Given intravenously, the drug provides the best available treatment for a number of systemic mycoses including histoplasmosis, cryptococcosis, coccidioidomycosis, blastomycosis, candidiasis and mucormycosis. It is also effective for treating leishmaniasis, an important protozoan disease of the tropics. Intravenous treatments must be given every two or three days and may be required over a prolonged period. Hospitalization is advisable. This antibiotic cannot be used without great caution and intravenous use is justified only in patients with spreading systemic infections.

Amphotericin B is sometimes used topically in place of nystatin.

In 1959, griseofulvin was introduced in the United States for the treatment of cutaneous fungal infections. This antibiotic had been isolated some years previously in England,[56] as a product of *Penicillium griseofulvin dierckx.* Synthesis of the drug has not proved economical. It is now produced by fermentation of a strain of *Penicillium patulum.* Griseofulvin is effective for the treatment of all types of ringworm. About one month is required for successful clearing of skin infections, but infections of the nails may not be cured for several months. Oral administration of the drug is recommended. It is tolerated well by most individuals, but a few do experience unpleasant reactions.

Iodides are generally used with success against sporotrichosis, a relatively rare fungal ulceration of the skin. If iodides are not effective, amphotericin B should be tried.

In the treatment of tinea pedis (athlete's foot) undecylenic acid ointment usually gives good results.

## Chemotherapy of Protozoal Diseases[57]

As pointed out in the introductory paragraphs of this chapter, some effective treatments for protozoal diseases were known to the ancients. Some improvements have been made in the chemotherapy of this important group of human afflictions during the past 50 years, but currently available drugs are not very satisfactory (see Table 7.14).

Amebiasis is probably the most frequent protozoal disease in the United States. The large intestine is the primary site of infection. The amebae often cause an acute dysentery with profuse blood and mucus in the stools, or a chronic diarrhea. Infection may be spread by the blood stream to the liver, lung, or brain, resulting in abscess formation.

Drug therapy for amebiasis is directed toward the elimination of the causative agent, *Entamoeba histolytica,* from the infected individual. The organism commonly infects the wall of the intestine and the liver. Carbarsone, diodoquin, and the antibiotic paromomycin act primarily on organisms in the intestinal lumen. These are contact amebicides.

Tetracycline and other broad spectrum antibiotics act indirectly on the amebae free in the intestine or invading the intestinal wall by modifying the intestinal flora necessary for survival of the amebae.

Emetine and chloroquine act against amebae principally in the intestinal wall and liver. Chloroquine acts mainly on amebiasis of the liver.

Metronidazole (Flaggl) has recently been introduced as a drug for the treatment of amebiasis. It is unique in that it acts against amebae at all the sites where these are commonly found. It has established itself as a most useful amebicide.

Malaria continues to be of great importance

TABLE 7.14

*Protozoal diseases and their therapy*

| Disease | Agent | Drugs of Choice |
|---|---|---|
| Amebiasis | | 1. Tetracycline, bacitracin, paromomycin |
| Enteric | *Entamoeba histolytica* | 2. Carbarsone, glycobiarsol |
| | | 3. Diiodohydroxyquin, iodochlorhydroxyquin |
| | | 4. Chloroquine |
| Systemic | *Entamoeba histolytica* | 1. Chloroquine |
| | | 2. Emetine |
| Malaria | *Plasmodium* species | 1. Chloroquine |
| | | 2. Primaquine |
| | | 3. Pyrimethamine |
| | | 4. Chloroguanide |
| Trypanosomiasis | *Trypanosoma gambiense* | Suramin |
| | | Melarsen compounds |
| | *Trypanosoma rhode-siense* | Tryparsamide |
| | | Pentamidine |
| Coccidiosis | *Isospora belli* | Sulfonamides, prevention of reinfection |
| | *Isospora hominis* | |
| Trichomoniasis | *Trichomonas hominis* | 1. Acetarsone, 8-hydroxyquinolines |
| | | 2. Nitrothiazoles |
| Leishmaniasis | | |
| Kala-azar | *Leishmania donovani* | Sodium stibogluconate |
| Oriental sore (cutaneous leishmaniasis) | *Leishmania tropica* | Sodium stibogluconate |
| American (mucocutaneous leishmaniasis) | *Leishmania brasiliensis* | Sodium stibogluconate |
| Giardiasis | *Giardia lamblia* | Chloroquine |
| Balantidiasis | *Balantidium coli* | Diiodohydroxyquin, Carbarsone, tetracycline |
| Toxoplasmosis | *Toxoplasma gondii* | Pyrimethamine, sulfonamides |
| Chagas' disease | *Trypanosoma cruzi* | Intracellular, none; |
| | | Peripheral, primaquine |

Source:   Busch, H., and Lane, M. *Chemotherapy: An Introductory Textbook.* Chicago: Year Book Medical Publishers, Inc., 1967.

in the tropics and subtropics as a cause of ill health and of death. Indigenous malaria in the United States had disappeared, but malaria has been reintroduced frequently in recent years by returning servicemen or other world travelers (see Table 7.15).

Malaria is still a serious problem in 60 countries with a population of over 400 million people particularly in tropical Africa and Asia. The World Health Organization has undertaken a campaign to eradicate malaria. This control campaign has met with marked success in some countries, but in many undeveloped nations lack of trained personnel and other difficulties have impeded progress.

There are four different malaria parasites known to cause illness in man. These are: *Plasmodium malariae, Plasmodium vivax, Plasmodium falciparum,* and *Plasmodium ovale. P. vivax* accounts for almost 90 per cent of the total cases of malaria, whereas *P. falciparum* causes some 90 per cent of malarial deaths.

Although the malarial infections caused by *P. vivax, P. malariae,* and *P. ovale* vary somewhat in their courses, the life cycles of these parasites are similar and the same principles are involved in their treatment. *P. falciparum,* although causing a more serious form of malaria, is more amenable to treatment since the parasite has a simpler life cycle.

The infected anopheline mosquito, when feeding, introduces sporozoites with its saliva. These sporozoites invade cells in the liver of man and develop into primary fixed tissue forms. As these fixed tissue forms develop, another parasitic form, the merozoite, is released into the blood stream and, in turn, invades the red blood cells. In the red blood cell, the parasite continues its evolution. The cycle varies in time from 42 to 72 hrs., depending upon the type of plasmodium. When the parasite matures, the red cell bursts, releasing great numbers of new merozoites, which, in turn, invade other red blood cells. If sufficient numbers of parasites are formed, chills and fever occur.

After a few such cycles in the blood, the sexual forms or gametocytes are produced in some red blood cells. These are the forms that infect the mosquito when it feeds on the blood of a malaria patient. Eventually, the cycle is completed in the mosquito and sporozoites migrate to the salivary glands.

In infections caused by *P. vivax, P. malariae,* and *P. ovale,* some of the merozoites released from red blood cells enter other liver cells to set up new fixed tissue forms. In *P. falciparum* the repetition of the liver phase does not occur. These forms may release other merozoites months later and are the source of relapses in apparently cured patients.

Antimalarial drugs are active against different stages of the life cycle of the parasite. Causal prophylactic drugs act against the primary fixed tissue forms in the liver cells and prevent the invasion of the red blood cells. Suppressive drugs inhibit the development of the merozoites in the blood and can cure *P. falciparum* infections, since no secondary fixed tissue forms develop to cause relapses. Curative drugs for *P. vivax, P. malariae,* and *P. ovale* act on the secondary fixed tissue forms. These must be given in association with suppressive drugs. Some drugs also act against the sexual forms of the parasite, gametocytes, to prevent infection of mosquitoes.

During and after World War II, supplies of cinchona bark were greatly reduced by the Japanese conquests in the Far East. A vast program of research was undertaken in Britain and America to discover new effective antimalarial drugs. This research is still underway on a reduced scale.

Cinchona, and its derivative, quinine, were the first effective antimalarials. Quinine attacks the asexual forms of plasmodia in the red blood cells. It is therefore a suppressive drug. Quinine has been largely replaced by less toxic and more effective drugs. Recently, it has been used against *P. falciparum* cases that have become resistant to the newer drugs.

Quinacrine or atabrine, a synthetic compound, acts in a manner similar to quinine. This drug was widely used during World War II as a prophylactic. Prolonged use produced a yellowing of the skin. Quinacrine has also been largely replaced by other compounds.

The 4-aminoquinolines, amodiaquine (Camo-

TABLE 7.15

*Military and civilian malaria cases, United States, 1959–1972*[1]

| Year | Military | Civilian | Total |
|------|---------|----------|-------|
| 1959 | 12 | 38 | 50 |
| 1960 | 21 | 41 | 62 |
| 1961 | 45 | 37 | 82 |
| 1962 | 75 | 40 | 115 |
| 1963 | 58 | 90 | 148 |
| 1964 | 52 | 119 | 171 |
| 1965 | 51 | 105 | 156 |
| 1966[2] | 621 | 143 | 764 |
| 1967[2] | 2699 | 158 | 2857 |
| 1968[2] | 2567 | 131 | 2698 |
| 1969[2] | 3914 | 145 | 4059 |
| 1970[2] | 4094 | 151 | 4245 |
| 1971[2] | 2970 | 202 | 3172 |
| 1972 | 442 | 146 | 588 |

[1] Onset of illness in the United States and Puerto Rico.
[2] Figures for these years have been updated to include cases reported after the publication of previous annual summaries.
Source:   Malaria Surveillance, Annual Summary 1972, National Center for Disease Control, Issued September, 1973, DHEW Publication No. (CDC) 74-8259.

quin), chloroquine (Aralen), and hydroxychlor-oquine (Plaquenil) serve well as suppressive and curative drugs. Their action is against the parasites in the red blood cells. Primaquine, an 8-aminoquinoline, is usually also given to destroy the secondary fixed tissue forms.

Pyrimethamine (Daraprim), a folic acid antagonist, has a broad spectrum of action. It is effective both for the suppression and for the treatment of malaria. Its action is somewhat slower than that of the 4-aminoquinolines.

When an acute attack of falciparum malaria occurs in an individual who has been in an area where malaria parasites have become drug-resistant (Brazil, Colombia, Southeast Asia) or has transfusion malaria, the patient is treated with a combination of quinine sulfate and pyrimethamine (Daraprim) or with the same drug with dapsone, a sulfone derivative.[58]

Of the other protozoal diseases of man, probably trypanosomiasis is the most important. The African sleeping sickness caused by *T. gambiense* or *T. rhodesiense* and Chagas' disease of South America caused by *T. cruzi* are responsible for much ill health in their respective areas of prevalence.

In the early stages of trypanosomiasis, suramin, a dye derivative, given intravenously or intramuscularly, is effective. The drug does not enter the cerebrospinal fluid.

Tryparsamide does penetrate to the cerebrospinal fluid and is thus effective after the parasites have invaded the central nervous system. Adverse effects of the drug, especially optic atrophy, may curtail its use for individual patients.

Melarsoprol appears to be the most useful drug in the late stages of African trypanosomiasis.

Other arsenic compounds of the Melarsen group have proved useful in treatment of advanced cases of sleeping sickness. It would appear that really satisfactory drugs for this serious disease have not yet been found. Clinical trials in South America have shown promise for nifurtimox, a nitrofuran derivative, in the acute cases of Chagas' disease (American trypanosomiasis).

### Treatment of Helminth Diseases[57]

Perhaps the most significant human disease resulting from a worm is schistosomiasis which occurs in the tropical and subtropical belts around the world. The adult worms, known as blood flukes, live in the veins of the host. There are three known species of this parasite: (1) *Schistosoma mansoni* and (2) *Schistosoma japonicum* which give rise primarily to intestinal manifestations; and (3) *Schistosoma haematobium*, which attacks the urinary bladder. The eggs of the schistosomes leave the body with the urine or feces. The egg hatches in water and the larvae invade the tissues of suitable fresh water snails. After several weeks, free-swimming larvae emerge from the snail and are capable of penetrating the skin of humans working, wading, or swimming in the water. The larvae get into the blood stream, are carried to blood vessels of the liver where they grow to maturity, and then migrate to the veins of the abdominal cavity. Eggs are deposited in the walls of small veins. By process of necrosis of tissues, they enter the bladder or bowels.

For treatment of *S. mansoni* and *S. haematobium*, stibophen (Fuadin) given intramuscularly is used; tartar emetic is more effective, but must be given intravenously. For *S. japonicum*, tartar emetic intravenously is essential.

A number of new drugs not containing antimony have been tried. Niridazole (ambilhar) given by mouth has given good results in parts of Africa.[59]

Filariasis is a mosquito-borne disease caused by a tiny nematode, *Wuchereria bancrofti*. It occurs in the West Indies, Central America, South America, India, southeast Asia, and most islands of the South Pacific. Another form is caused by *Brugia malayi* in India, southeast Asia, and China. The larvae, or microfilaria, frequently cause blockage of lymph channels with a resulting swelling of the limbs or genitalia called elephantiasis, the characteristic late effect of the disease.

Diethylcarbamazine (Hetrazan) taken orally for 10 to 12 days causes rapid disappearance of microfilaria from the blood, but does not destroy the adult female worm; the microfilariae usually reappear in a few months. Sodium thiacetarsamide (caparsolate sodium) clears up the larvae more slowly, but they do not return. The action of this drug is apparently against the adult worm (see Table 7.16).

Hookworm, which used to be a serious disease of the American South, still occurs commonly in the unsanitary tropical regions of the world. *Necator americanus* is the prevailing species of West Africa, the West Indies, and

TABLE 7.16

*Commonly used drugs in helminthic infestations*

| Disease | Worm | Drugs |
|---------|------|-------|
| Ancylostomiasis (hookworm) | *Ancylostoma duodenale* <br> *Necator americanus* | Bephenium <br> Tetrachlorethylene <br> Dithiazanine |
| Ascariasis | *Ascaris lumbricoides* | Piperazine <br> Dithiazanine <br> Diethylcarbamazine |
| Enterobiasis (oxyuriasis or pinworm) | *Enterobius vermicularis* | Pyrvinium <br> Piperazine |
| Strongyloidiasis | *Strongyloides stercoralis* | Dithiazanine |
| Trichuriasis (whipworm) | *Trichuris trichiura* | Dithiazanine <br> Bephenium |
| Cestodiasis (tapeworm) | *Hymenolepis nana* <br> *Diphyllobothrium latum* <br> *Taenia saginata* <br> *Taenia solium* | Quinacrine <br> Dichlorophen <br> Niclosamide |
| Schistosomiasis (bilharziasis) | *Schistosoma mansoni* <br> *Schistosoma hematobium* <br> *Schistosoma japonicum* | Stibophen <br> Stibophen <br> Tartar emetic |
| Filariasis | *Wuchereria bancrofti* <br> *Onchocerca volvulus* <br> *Loa loa* | Diethylcarbamazine <br> Diethylcarbamazine <br> Diethylcarbamazine |
| Fluke infestations | *Clonorchis sinensis* <br> *Fasciolopsis buski* <br> *Fasciola hepatica* <br> *Paragonimus westermani* | Chloroquine <br> Tetrachlorethylene <br> Emetine <br> Emetine |

Source:   Busch H. and Lane, M. *Chemotherapy: An Introductory Textbook.* Chicago: Year Book Medical Publishers, Inc., 1967.

parts of the Americas; *Ancylostoma duodenale* prevails in Mediterranean areas and many other regions. Eggs are deposited in the feces and hatch in the soil. The larvae penetrate the human skin, usually of the foot, enter the lymphatics, get into the blood stream, and then into the lungs, migrate up the trachea, are swallowed, and attach themselves to the wall of the small intestine, where they develop to adulthood in about five weeks. Hookworm is the cause of a chronic anemia which is a debilitating condition.

Several drugs are effective in the treatment of hookworm. These are tetrachlorethyline, or hexylresorcinol, and a newer compound, be-phenium (Alcopar), a quaternary ammonium derivative. A new drug, pyrantel pamoate, not yet approved by the FDA, has been recommended.

The common roundworm infection of the intestinal tract, ascariasis, is best treated by piperazine. Frequently, hookworm infection is associated with ascariasis. In this case, dithiaza-nine is the treatment of choice.

For treatment of tapeworms, quinacrine hydrochloride is recommended. Dichlorophen and niclosamide have been recently produced abroad and are reported to be effective in the elimination of tapeworms. The antibiotic, paro-momycin (Humatin), has been used with success in treatment of tapeworm cases since 1960.[60]

Infection with pinworms (enterobiasis) is world-wide in distribution. It is estimated that 20 per cent of the general population of the United States harbors this parasite. The reservoir of infection is the infected human. The eggs are transferred by fingers from anus to mouth or by contaminated food, clothing, or other objects. Irritation and itching of the anal region is usually caused. Treatment is with piperazine salts or pyrvinium pamoate (Povan). Probably, the whole family should be treated as a unit to avoid reinfection of individuals.

## Chemoprophylaxis

Any measures that can cut short the period of

illness of a communicable disease and can reduce the time in which the patient is capable of passing on the infection to others are likely to diminish the incidence of that disease. In the preceding pages, specific therapy for a large number of such diseases is outlined. In some infections such therapy, no matter how effective for the patient, will not reduce the spread of the parasite in nature. Histoplasmosis or coccidioidomycosis are such examples. Effective treatment of cases of infectious syphilis, however, stops the threat of transmission of that infection to others within a few hours.

Chemoprophylaxis may be defined as the prevention of the development of an infection, or the progression of an infection to actual manifest disease, through the use of drugs, antibiotics, or other chemical compounds. Such prophylactic measures are usually directed to contacts exposed to certain infections. This control measure is only applicable under limited circumstances: (1) the parasite must be highly susceptible to an available drug of low toxicity, and (2) the prophylactic must be administered at the correct time in relation to the exposure.

For some years, sulfonamides were used widely among populations exposed to meningococcal meningitis. Because of the widespread prevalence of sulfonamide-resistant meningococcal strains throughout the world, sulfonamide prophylaxis should not be undertaken unless the outbreak can be shown to be caused by sulfonamide-sensitive strains. This measure is applicable for the control of outbreaks in institutions and in military populations where supervision of drug administration is possible and where sulfonamide-resistant strains of the organism are infrequent.

In tuberculosis, the use of isoniazid in therapeutic doses for one year has given promising results for household contacts, for those whose tuberculin test has recently changed from negative to positive, and for tuberculin-positive children under three years of age. Trials are now being undertaken to determine whether periods of three or six months on isoniazid will be effective in protecting such persons against the development of active tuberculosis.

The use of antimalarial drugs to protect military personnel and others assigned to live in malarious areas and travelers on short visits to the tropics is well-known. Chloroquine (Aralen)

diphosphate or sulfate, 300 mg. once or twice weekly, is recommended. The drug should be taken for the entire time spent in the malarial zone and for five weeks afterward. Other drugs which may be used are: amodiaquine (Camoquin), 300 mg. once or twice weekly; pyrimethamine (Daraprim), 25 mg. once weekly; or proguanil (Paludrine), 100 mg. daily.[33] For those who have been on suppressive drugs and are leaving an endemic area, primaquine, 15 mg. daily for 14 days, should be taken to prevent relapses.

A well-established procedure to prevent *Ophthalmia neonatorum,* or infection of the newborn baby's eyes with gonococcus, is to instill a few drops of 1 per cent silver nitrate solution in each eye after birth. This is a legal requirement in some states.

The contacts of bubonic or pneumonic plague may be put on adequate doses of broad spectrum antibiotics or of sulfonamides for a period of six days. This applies to medical and nursing personnel as well as to household contacts.

To some extent, prophylaxis is used by travelers to the tropics to prevent amebic dysentery and other intestinal infections. Clioquinol and other halogenated hydroxyquinolines are apparently effective.[59] Caution must be observed in taking these drugs in full dosage for long periods. Occasional instances of eye damage, retinopathy, or optic atrophy have been reported.

Chemoprophylaxis has been strongly recommended for children who have shown evidence of developing rheumatic fever. It is felt that such individuals must be protected as far as possible against subsequent infections with Group A hemolytic streptococci. Oral penicillin in daily doses of 200,000 to 250,000 units or monthly injections of 1.2 million units of benzathine penicillin G are effective. For persons sensitive to penicillin, alternative therapy must be planned.

## CONTROL OF CANCER

Since 1929, cancer has remained the second leading cause of death from all causes in the United States. Approximately 17 per cent of deaths in the United States are caused by cancer. It is estimated that 355,000 will die of cancer in the United States in 1974 and that more than 1 million individuals will be under treatment for cancer. It is obvious that control measures to combat this major health problem are of the highest importance.[61]

To understand the cancer problem, one must recognize that "cancer" is not one disease but a whole group of diseases—skin cancer, lung cancer, and leukemia have some common characteristics, but are quite distinct in their symptoms, their clinical course, and their pathology. All malignant tumors manifest a higher rate of cell growth and multiplication than do the normal tissues from which they arise. Such tumors develop a tendency to invade normal tissues and organs. Late in the disease such cells tend to spread by lymph or blood vessels to distant parts of the body, setting up new growths or metastases that destroy normal tissues and organs.

## Early Detection and Treatment

To a large extent cancer control has been based upon early detection and diagnosis followed quickly by appropriate treatment. Patients whose cancer is diagnosed when it is still localized, or restricted to a limited area, have the best chance for cure. Quite frequently, cancers do not produce symptoms until the disease is moderately advanced. For that reason, regular examinations are recommended, especially for people over 40. In recent years, the examination of cells shed from the stomach, esophagus, lungs, intestines, bladder, and cervix of the uterus has proved to be a valuable method for early cancer detection. The Papanicolaou test, which consists of microscopic examination of stained cells obtained by swab from the uterine cervix, has come into wide use. Many early cases of cancer of the cervix have been detected. Most of these are amenable to cure by surgery and radiation.

X rays provide another important tool for cancer detection, especially for tumors of the lung and digestive tract. The use of X rays to discover breast cancer is gaining wider acceptance. The bronchoscope is a valuable instrument for discovering growths in the bronchial tree, as is the sigmoidoscope for the lower intestine.

Diagnosis of cancer is made by examination of tissues under the microscope by a highly trained pathologist. Cells from some organs are readily obtained, but tissues from inaccessible tumors must be obtained through surgical operation, by aspiration, or by punch biopsies.

Intensive efforts by research workers to discover biochemical tests for the early diagnosis of cancer have been underway for many years. It has been learned that the determination of serum alkaline phosphatase activity aids in the diagnosis of patients with skeletal and liver cancers; acid phosphatase has proved equally useful in patients with cancer of the prostate.

The determination of certain other enzyme blood levels are valuable in following the progress of patients, but not for the diagnosis of the disease.

Another biochemical test has some promise for use in the diagnosis of cancer of the colon and rectum. This test, known as the CEA assay (carcinoembryonic antigen), has been under investigation for some years. There is no general agreement as to its validity.[62]

Attempts to educate the public on the importance of early diagnosis in cancer have been intensive. The public has been instructed endlessly about the early signs and symptoms of cancer. Women have been urged to carry out regular self-examinations of the breast to detect the appearance of lumps. Those who discover any suspicious signs or symptoms are exhorted to visit their physician immediately.

Cancer detection centers where every known means for specific cancer detection are readily available have been established throughout the United States. More than 200 such centers were in operation by 1957. The chief value of these centers has been to evaluate detection procedures and to develop new techniques. In 1973, the first three of 20 planned breast cancer detection centers were announced. Cost of the centers will be shared by the National Cancer Institute and the American Cancer Society. These centers will train physicians and allied health personnel in the techniques of breast examination. The burden of responsibility for finding cancer rests on the practicing physician. Every effort is made by the American Cancer Society and many other agencies to keep physicians abreast of current information and to stimulate their interest in regular physical check-ups to discover cancer as early as possible.

The prospects of early detection are more favorable in cancers of the uterus, mouth, colon and rectum, breast, and skin. It is in the treatment of these cancers that the most satisfactory progress has been made. Meanwhile, medical research is opening up new pathways to diagnosis and therapy. Since World War II, nuclear medicine and radioisotopes have played a vital role in the discovery and treatment of cancer cases. These methods have aided in the detection of cancer of the thyroid, brain, liver, and stomach. Specific radioactive isotopes, such as cobalt 60, have also been used in therapy of cancer of the prostate, thyroid, and bone marrow.[63]

The search for cancer-controlling drugs has already produced several that are promising in the treatment of cancer in laboratory animals. Approximately 100 new drugs have been tested in the treatment of human cancer; a few have had hopeful results. The use of X rays and of surgical techniques has been restudied critically so that the best method of treatment can be selected for individual patients.

## Epidemiological Studies

In recent years, the skill of epidemiologists has been employed in the study of the natural history of cancer with fruitful results. It has been learned that there have been marked changes in the incidence of cancer by site occurrence. The most striking change has been the sharp increase in lung cancer among men. This has been accompanied by smaller increments of lung cancer in women. Since 1930, the mortality rate in men from lung cancer has increased more than 14 times and is going up steadily in women. The incidence of cancer of the pancreas has risen 65 per cent in the past generation.

Mortality for cancer of both the uterine cervix and the body of the uterus has decreased by almost one-half. This is mainly a result of early and successful treatment. Stomach cancer has declined substantially in incidence in the United States for reasons unknown, but remains quite high in Japan (about 7 times the United States rates) and in many other countries. On the other hand, cancers of the breast, ovary, and intestine are five times more common and prostatic cancer four to five times more common in the United States than in some of these countries. Remarkable differences exist between countries as close geographically as France and Germany, or areas such as Puerto Rico and New York. Studies carried out on migrant groups have shown that the migrants tend to assume the cancer pattern closer to that of their new home. It appears, therefore, that the cancer patterns of a population depend upon environmental factors. This provides promising material for studies on the nature of the responsible agents in the environment that produce cancer.[64]

In some types of cancer such carcinogenic agents are already known or are strongly suspected. During the past 25 years, a remarkable association between smoking of cigarettes and lung cancer has been reported by many investigators. The risk of developing lung cancer increases with the duration of smoking and the number of cigarettes smoked per day, and is diminished by discontinuance of smoking.

The sharp rise in deaths from lung cancer began about 1930, some 20 years after cigarettes became widely popularized during World War I. Almost 1 million deaths are attributed to lung cancer since 1930. The scientific community and the health authorities appear to be convinced that the smoking of cigarettes is a causal factor in lung cancer. Still the public is either unconvinced or is not greatly concerned.

Evidence points to an increased incidence of lung cancer in urban, as compared with rural, areas that cannot be explained by smoking habits. Analyses of polluted urban air have demonstrated known carcinogens of the aromatic hydrocarbon group (notably 3, 4-benzpyrene), while other types of carcinogens are believed to be frequently present.

Some occupations are known to be associated with high risks of lung cancer. Among these are the miners of uranium, cobalt, and other products that involve inhalation of radioactive dusts and gases. Other occupational exposures that may lead to development of lung cancer include workers with asbestos, nickel, mustard gas, and chromates. Workers in these industries have risks of developing lung cancer of from five to 30 times higher than the general population (see Table 7.17).

Recently, it has been discovered that fatal liver cancers are occurring among workers exposed to vinyl chloride in their occupation. Some experts believe that the great majority of cancers are attributable to carcinogenetic exposures. In 1971, Miller reported that seven of eight young women who developed adenocarcinoma of the vagina had been born to mothers who had been given stilbestrol during pregnancy because of threatened abortion. This form of cancer is extremely rare in young women.[65]

One of the dangers from widespread usage of chemicals that may cause cancer is through the use of the hormone diethylstilbestrol to increase the weight of cattle in the feeding lots. This use of the hormone has been banned by a number of European nations and by 17 others around the world.

Enforceable federal standards to protect the health of workers exist for only 450 of the estimated 15,000 chemical and physical agents now employed in industry. Experts in occupational health regard most of these standards as inadequate and unenforced.[66,67]

Increased rates of occurrence of cancer of the skin and of the respiratory tract have been reported among workers handling inorganic compounds of arsenic in factories, and extremely high rates of cancer of the scrotum were recently discovered in wax pressmen in oil refineries.

Leukemia is another malignant disease for which mortality rates have been increasing in recent decades. Leukemia accounts for one-half of all deaths from cancer in childhood. Two agents are known to cause leukemia, ionizing radiation and benzol. Persons receiving high doses of radiation have substantially greater risk of developing leukemia. Apparently, however, radiation is not involved in causing one form of leukemia, that is, the chronic lymphatic form.

Evidence is accumulating that the use of diagnostic X rays in the lower abdominal area during pregnancy may increase the risk of children developing leukemia or other forms of cancer during the first 10 years of life.

In regard to benzol, reports of leukemia are limited mostly to rather intensive occupational exposures.

Cancer of the skin is associated with heavy exposure to radium and X rays. Many pioneer investigators of the use of radium and X rays in medicine developed such cancers, especially of the hands. The evidence for the association of sun rays in skin cancer is well known. The incidence of skin cancer is much higher in southern United States than in northern areas of the country. It develops most frequently among farmers and other outdoor workers. Ultraviolet light produces skin cancer in experimental animals.

TABLE 7.17

*Cancer-causing agents often associated with occupations*

| Agent | Sites of Cancer | Areas Where Noted |
| --- | --- | --- |
| Arsenic | Skin, lung | United States, Great Britain, Germany, France, Argentina |
| Coal tar, pitch | Skin, lung | United States, Great Britain |
| Petroleum | Skin, lung | United States, France, Great Britain, Austria |
| Shale oils | Skin | United States, Great Britain |
| Lignite tar and paraffin | Skin | Great Britain, France |
| Creosote oil | Skin | United States, Great Britain |
| Anthracene oil | Skin | Great Britain |
| Soot carbon black | Skin | United States, Great Britain |
| Aromatic amines | Bladder | United States, Germany, Great Britain, Switzerland, and other areas |
| X rays and radium | Skin, lung, leukemia | United States and many other areas |
| Asbestos | Lung | United States, Great Britain, Germany, Canada |
| Chromates | Lung | United States, Great Britain, Germany, Canada |
| Nickel | Lung, nasal cavity, and sinus | Great Britain, Norway |
| Benzol | Leukemia | United States and other areas |
| Isopropyl oil | Lung, larynx, nasal sinus | United States |
| Radioactive chemicals | Bones, nasal sinus | United States |
| Sunlight | Skin | United States, Argentina, Australia, France, and other areas |

Source: *Cancer Questions and Answers about Rates and Risks,* Public Health Service Publication 1514. Washington, D.C.: United States Public Health Service, 1966.

Workers using luminous paint for watch dials have developed cancer of the bone. They swallow significant amounts of radium as a result of pointing up their brushes with the lips.

The use of X rays for prolonged diagnostic or therapeutic purposes appears to lead to increased incidence of cancer in the areas of the body most exposed. For example, cancer of the thyroid occurred with increased frequency among children treated with X rays for enlargement of the thymus gland. An excess cancer incidence has been reported among adults treated by X rays for ankylosing spondylitis, a form of arthritis of the spine.[68]

Some factors relating to cancer of the digestive system are known. Mouth cancer appears to be related to chewing of betel nut and tobacco quids in some areas of the Far East or to tobacco chewing alone in other parts of the world. In India, some cigar smokers keep the lighted end in their mouths. Cancer of the hard palate, rare elsewhere, is not uncommon among these people. There is some evidence that the smoking of pipes and cigars contributes to the development of cancer in the oral cavity. The drinking of hard liquors and the smoking of tobacco both are associated with cancer of the esophagus.

Cancer of the stomach is extremely prevalent in Iceland among men in the northwestern part of the island; it accounts for some 35 to 45 per cent of all malignant tumors. The incidence of these stomach cancers appears to be correlated with the consumption of large amounts of smoked mutton and smoked fish. In the United States, the stomach cancer rates today are only about one-half of what they were in 1930. The reason for this is not clear.

Two conditions that are relatively uncommon appear to have a predisposing relationship to the development of cancer of the colon and rectum. These are a rare inherited form of polyposis of the lower intestinal tract and a more common disease known as ulcerated colitis.

Cancer of the breast shows a marked variation in incidence from one country to another. Rates are generally low in areas where prolonged lactation is common. Single women and women with no children have higher rates of breast cancer than do those who have borne offspring. Women whose ovaries have been removed in early adulthood have only about one-half as many breast cancers as those who have not.

Several factors related to incidence of cancer of the cervix have been established. It appears to be associated with sexual activity. It rarely occurs among nuns. Married women have higher rates than do single women. An earlier age of marriage leads to a higher incidence of cervical cancer.

Women of the lower socioeconomic groups experience higher rates of cervical cancer than do the women in the more favored groups. The explanation for this difference is not clear. Perhaps it is related to standards of personal hygiene.

Jewish women generally have low rates of cancer of the cervix. Puerto Rican women in New York have extremely high rates of cervical cancer, some six times that of non-Jewish white women, and 25 times that of Jewish women.

Cancer of the urinary bladder has been associated with a number of possible causative agents. Chemical workers handling $\beta$-naphthylamine and other products of the aniline dye industry are known to be subject to a higher risk of bladder cancer than is the average. Heavy smokers of cigarettes develop about five times as many cancers of the bladder as non-smokers. No specific chemical agent has yet been discovered to explain these bladder cancers.

In many warm countries where schistosomiasis is prevalent, high rates of cancer of the bladder have been found. The parasitic worms responsible for this disease reside in the veins of the host. Eggs make their way to the walls of the bladder or intestine and cause marked irritation in the tissues before being discharged in the urine or feces. The relationship of schistosomiasis to cancer of the bladder has not yet been adequately investigated, but an association appears probable.

Cancer of the penis occurs in males who have not been circumcised early in life and is probably related with poor personal standards of cleanliness. The incidence of penile cancer is low among western nations, even among the uncircumcised, possibly because of ready access to bathing facilities.[68]

It is difficult to prove that a particular substance or course of action leads to cancer. Recently, it has been demonstrated that certain substances, harmless in themselves, can act with other agents to stimulate cancer development. For example, citrus oils may cause stomach cancer in mice receiving doses of benzpyrene too small to be carcinogenic alone. It may well be that certain potentiators present in the polluted air of urban areas combine with cigarette smoke to produce the carcinogenic effect generally attributed to cigarette smoking. Probably, in most cancers, the etiology involves a number of factors rather than a single causative agent.

## Preventive Measures

Based on current knowledge, a few measures to prevent cancer appear to be practicable:[68]

Excessive and prolonged exposure to the sun and to ultraviolet rays should be avoided. This is especially important for fair skinned individuals who burn rather than tan. For outdoor workers, wide-brimmed hats give protection to the face and neck. To protect the hands, sunscreen ointments are probably the best alternative if gloves are a nuisance.

An intensive and prolonged campaign to inform the public about the dangers of cigarette smoking must be intensified. This campaign should be aimed at youth to prevent the starting of the smoking habit, but should also persuade parents of the influence their own smoking habits in the home have on their children.

Warning labels on each package of cigarettes are already required by law. Perhaps the next step is to prohibit the advertising of cigarettes, especially advertising that is directed to young people.

Successful attempts to remove carcinogenic elements from cigarettes by filters or other methods will probably have to await specific information as to which substances are harmful to man.

In the Far East, public education to discourage betel chewing or the chewing of other harmful mixtures is urgently required to prevent cancers of the oral cavity.

Occupational cancer hazards are widely distributed in many industries. Various protective measures have been successful in reducing and, in some cases, in eliminating these hazards. Technological measures include: (1) replacement of carcinogenic materials by suitable non-carcinogenic products; (2) prevention of dust and adequate cleaning of premises, preferably by an exhaust ventilation system; and (3) a closed or automated system of production.

Employment practices should include the following considerations: (1) Individuals with previous exposure to similar carcinogenic substances should not be employed in a hazardous industry. (2) Because of the prolonged latent periods of occupational cancers, only older persons should be employed. (3) Women in the child-bearing age should not be employed for hazardous occupations.

Excellent methods are available for the protection of workers in industry and in research laboratories from ionizing radiation. Uranium miners are chiefly affected by breathing in radioactive dusts. Industrial hygiene methods are available to reduce this hazard markedly.

Medical and dental examinations with X rays represent an important hazard in all advanced countries. The known genetic effects of such radiations demand that exposure be kept as low as possible. Probably the amount of radiation received by most patients for diagnostic purposes represents only a very slight hazard, and one that may well be outweighed by the expected benefits. The use of X rays over the abdominal area during pregnancy is a dubious procedure.

## Research

As cancer has increasingly become a cause of mortality, the public has become more concerned that something be done to control this fearful malady. Having observed the rapid advances in diminishing the threat of infectious diseases, the demand for effective measures for the prevention or cure of cancer has grown. Congress has responded to the public clamor by providing large amounts of money for research on all aspects of the cancer problem. Funds for the National Cancer Institute have been stepped up from $492 million for fiscal year 1973 to $600 million for fiscal year 1975. During the past 30 years, great advances have been made, some of which have been outlined above. It appears likely that during the coming decade a great deal will be discovered about the basic biological nature of the cancer process. It is most likely that this greater understanding of the natural history of cancer will lead to new methods useful in the prevention of the disease.

From the present position, it may be concluded that the etiology of cancer is almost certainly a complex matter with multiple factors involved. These factors include chemical, hormonal, physical, and viral carcinogens. Genetic characteristics may also be involved.

No doubt new carcinogens will be introduced or at least discovered as the search goes on. This is pointed up by the recent reports that aflatoxins from the mold, *Aspergillus flavus*, and substances from the cycad nut are potent factors in producing liver cancers in animals.[69,70]

Another method of controlling cancer is by chemotherapy. The most active approach to the selection of new drugs is through the use of rodent tumor screening tests. Attempts have been made to select compounds that would interrupt the growth cycle of malignant cells. One group of chemicals acts solely against cells actively synthesizing DNA. A second group also blocks DNA synthesis, but also inhibits RNA and protein synthesis. A third group of compounds form complexes with DNA and can kill cells in all phases of the cell cycle.

Chemotherapy combined with surgery has been successful in the treatment of Wilm's tumor, a malignant tumor of the kidney in young children. When a drug, actinomycin-D, is added to radiation therapy following removal of the kidney, survival rates are almost doubled over the rates for children receiving the same treatment without the drug.

Following the demonstration in 1947 that aminopterin could produce a remission in acute lymphatic leukemia, at least 12 other compounds have been identified as having a therapeutic effect in this disease. These remissions were temporary, but when two or three of these compounds were administered simultaneously, the result was an increase in the percentage of patients achieving complete remission of the disease. Combined chemotherapy and immunotherapy are being studied.

Combination of drugs has also proved helpful in the therapy of lymphomas. In Hodgkin's disease, combinations of four drugs have given far better results than had been previously achieved. Similar therapeutic regimes are now being tried in other malignancies, especially cancer of the breast.

Perhaps the most promising and rapidly moving areas of cancer research is in the investigation of viruses as causative agents of the various forms of neoplasms. As far back as 1908, two Danish scientists transmitted leukemia from one chicken to another by injection of filtered material from the infected fowl. Shortly after, Dr. Peyton Rous succeeded in transmitting a solid tumor by cell-free filtrate

from one chicken to another. Over the years, other animal tumors were transmitted in the laboratory by cell-free materials.[71]

In recent years, the introduction of new instruments, including the electron microscope and improved high speed centrifuges, the development of better tissue culture methods, and the unfolding of knowledge of molecular chemistry have brought new hope to the virologists in investigations. In addition to fowl leukemia virus, more than a dozen leukemia viruses have been discovered that produce leukemia in mice, rats, or guinea pigs. Studies on these viruses indicate that in some instances infection may be passed from a mother to her offspring. Frequently, these viruses remain latent for long periods of time, unless activated by exposure of the animal to radiation or other stimuli.

Attempts to detect viruses in human leukemia patients have yielded several types of particles seen by the electron microscope. Studies on these virus-like particles are now going forward.

During the 1960's came the first evidence of cancer-inducing potential of a known human virus. Adenoviruses, which cause respiratory disease in humans, produce tumors in mice and hamsters. A monkey virus (SV40) was found to induce sarcoma-like solid tumors in newborn hamsters.

Of late, much attention has been focused on the association of Herpesviruses and human cancer. Members of this group are known to be associated with kidney tumors in leopard frogs, with a lymphomatous condition of chickens, and with lymphatic leukemia in marmosets.

A herpesvirus of great interest is the Epstein-Barr virus (EBV) which has been found in association with lymphoma tissues. There is some evidence that this virus may be the causative agent of infectious mononucleosis.

A herpesvirus has also been associated with cancer of the uterine cervix. Evidence suggests that cervical cancer could be considered a venereal disease. Should it be proved that herpesvirus is the cause of cervical cancer, it may be possible to prevent the disease by a vaccine.[71]

An interesting discovery has been the demonstration that two viruses may be combined to form a hybrid strain with enhanced tumor-producing characteristics. This discovery suggests that a relatively harmless virus might activate potentially dangerous ones to induce cancer. Another instance of combined action by two viruses is in the induction of the Rous chicken tumor. The Rous sarcoma virus has been recognized for years, but it now appears that the aid of a "helper" virus, known as Rous associated virus, is necessary to complete the tumor-producing process. A similar situation has also been described in a solid tumor in mice.

Although no cancer-inducing virus has yet been demonstrated for humans, the search goes on intensively. Should viruses prove to have an important role in producing some or all human cancers, it is hoped that new methods to prevent or control such growths can be found. Such measures would probably depend upon the well-known possibilities of immunization or the use of immunological principles in the treatment of established tumors.

In recent years, a great deal of interest has arisen in the possibilities of immunotherapy for cancer. This form of treatment is either (1) specific, or (2) non-specific. In the specific approach, individuals with tumors are treated either by active immunization with material derived from the tumor or by passive immunization whereby sensitized lymphocytes, antibodies, or both are transferred from an appropriately immunized donor to the tumor patient.

In the non-specific approach, agents which cause a generalized increase in immunity are administered to the patient. One of these agents is the BCG (Bacillus Calmette-Guérin) strain of bovine tuberculosis. These approaches to controlling cancer in the human are still in the experimental stage.[72-74]

## EDUCATION OF THE PEOPLE IN DISEASE CONTROL

Education of the public in matters of health has two objectives: (1) to impart information on the nature of disease, its causal factors, and the measures that are effective in the preventing ill health, both for one's self and for one's family; and (2) to motivate people to want good health, even at some financial sacrifice and at the expense of time and energy, or, what is even harder for people to accept, at the cost of changing fixed habit patterns and ways of living. One may assume that almost all people would desire good health rather than bad, if it could be attained without expenditure of money, time, energy, or alteration in living patterns. The function of health education is to persuade people that good health is preferable even at considerable cost to themselves and at the inconvenience of rearranging some of their daily routines.

In the early days of the development of public health, most of the preventive measures were taken at the community level and by fiat of law. Such health-preserving changes as the purification of water supply, the installation of water-borne sewage disposal, and the insurance of clean milk and safe foods were introduced with little disturbance of the equilibrium of most of the population. This was not true of later health measures such as the hygiene of pregnant women and children, the protection of the health of school children, the discovery and treatment of contagious cases of tuberculosis and syphilis, the diagnosis and serum therapy of diphtheria, and the isolation and quarantine of those sick with or exposed to smallpox, meningitis, or scarlet fever. These measures required that the public be kept informed of what was to be done and that people understood the rationale for such actions on the part of their health officials.

In the process of development, public health soon discovered the necessity for highly trained personnel: health physicians, public health nurses, and sanitarians. A great proportion of the time of these health workers had to be devoted to education of individuals, families, and communities about the basis of health protective procedures.

As the 20th century advanced, the rate of new discoveries rose to phenomenal heights; vaccines, sera, vitamins, and new drugs became available at a rapid pace. New screening tests were devised to discover a number of the prevailing chronic diseases. Needless to say, there were real difficulties in keeping the public informed of these complicated technical advances.

At the same time, amazing technological changes were affecting the lives of those living in modern industrial communities. The horse was replaced by the automobile; old-fashioned groceries and meat markets gave way to supermarkets, deep freezers, and frozen foods; telephones, radio, and television gave new dimensions to communication; shorter working weeks brought increased leisure; and labor-saving appliances reduced the drudgery of household chores. The growing urbanization of the population has exposed more people to air pollution, crowding, and dehumanizing conditions. The increase in the use of tranquilizers and other drugs and of alcohol and tobacco has created new health problems. Gradually, the need for sound impartial information and advice on these and other health matters became more apparent.

Some 30 years ago, a number of schools of public health responded to this challenge by setting up courses designed to train new members of the health team to be designated as health educators. Recruits for this new profession were drawn from various sources: schoolteachers, science graduates, psychology majors, nurses, and others. The courses were planned to present the basic curriculum of public health, as well as the special techniques that have been found effective in presenting complex data to the public in an interesting manner.

Graduates of these courses in health education have been eagerly sought by health agencies to direct or assist them with their problems of getting information to people in a manner that will persuade them to seek the health services that are available. Such aid is particularly valuable in reaching low income groups and ethnic minorities. Problems of language barriers and of cultural differences make people-to-people communication with such groups difficult.

Obviously, the optimal period for health education is during the school years, extending from nursery school to university graduate schools. Information presented to children must be adjusted to their particular age groups. Beginning with care of teeth, personal cleanliness, drinking of milk, and other simple practices, teaching proceeds to safety precautions, immunizations, and more sophisticated measures. Junior high schools and high schools discuss health problems of smoking, drinking, and sexual relations. College students are concerned with almost all health problems, especially those related to sexual relations, marriage, pregnancy, and care of young children.[75,76]

To be effective health education must be directed to situations of immediate interest. The woman in the late stages of her first pregnancy or shortly after the birth of her first child is receptive to information on infant care. Young people are not particularly interested in the prospects of chronic degenerative disease

that might come late in life. Probably, the failure of the anti-cigarette smoking campaign is explained by the remoteness of the penalties.

The most successful effort in health education was the immunization campaign against poliomyelitis undertaken in American communities a few years ago. Several factors may explain this success. People fear poliomyelitis, especially for their children. A vaccine became available that could be administered by mouth at a low cost with a minimum of discomfort and little expenditure of time. Another unusual feature of the campaign to promote the Sabin vaccine was that the whole family was called upon to participate, from infants to grandparents. A study of the experiences gained in this campaign will reveal many valuable lessons for health educators.

As research programs unfold new preventive procedures to preserve health, the need for skilled personnel to motivate the public to accept new measures or to alter old patterns of living will become more urgent.

## REFERENCES

1. *A Drop to Drink—a Report on the Quality of Our Drinking Water.* U. S. Environmental Protection Agency, Washington, D. C., June, 1973.
2. *A Strategy for a Livable Environment.* A report to the Secretary of Health, Education, and Welfare by the Task Force on Environmental, Health and Related Problems. Washington, D. C.: Government Printing Office, 1967.
3. *Health Protection: the Target of the Bureau of Disease Prevention and Environmental Control.* Public Health Service Publication 1634. Washington, D. C.: Government Printing Office, 1967.
4. U.S. Bureau of the Census, Statistical Abstract of the United States: 1973. Ed. 94, Washington, D. C., 1973.
5. *Proceedings: the Third National Conference on Air Pollution, December 12-14, 1966.* Public Health Service Publication 1649. Washington, D. C.: Government Printing Office, 1967.
6. Heimann, H. *Air Pollution and Respiratory Disease.* Public Health Service Publication 1257. Washington, D. C.: Government Printing Office, 1964.
7. *Research and Monitoring—Cornerstone for Environmental Action.* U. S. Environmental Protection Agency. Government Printing Office, 1972-0-4700874, October, 1972.
8. Schwabe, C. W. *Veterinary Medicine and Human Health,* Ed. 2. Baltimore: The Williams and Wilkins Co., 1969.
9. Johnson, P. E. Food additives. *Public Health Rep.,* 81: 244, 1966.
10. *Evaluation of Food Additives.* Technical Report

Series No. 488. 15th Report of the Joint FAO/WHO Expert Committee on Food Additives, Geneva, 1972.

11. *Foodborne Outbreaks. Annual Summary, 1972.* Center for Disease Control. DHEW Publication No. (CDC) 74-8185, issued November, 1973.

12. *An Evaluation of the Salmonella Problem.* National Research Council, Committee on Salmonella. Washington, D. C., 1969.

13. *Insect Control Series.* Public Health Service Publication 722, 1961-1963: Part I. Introduction to arthropods of public health importance; Part IV. Sanitation in control of insects and rodents of public health importance. Part V. Flies of public health importance and their control. Part VI. Mosquitoes of public health importance and their control. Part VII. Fleas of public health importance and their control. Part VIII. Lice of public health importance and their control. Part IX. Mites of public health importance and their control. Part X. Ticks of public health importance and their control.

14. WHO Expert Committee on Insecticides. 19th Report. Technical Report Series, No. 475. WHO, Geneva, 1971.

15. *Safe Use of Pesticides,* edited by I. M. West. New York: American Public Health Association, 1967.

16. Soper, F. L., and Wilson, D. B. Species eradication: Practical goals of species reduction in control of mosquito-borne disease. *J. Nat. Malaria Soc., 1:* 5-24, 1942.

17. Logan, G. A., et al. *The Sardinian Project: An Experiment in the Eradication of an Indigenous Malarious Vector.* Amer. J. Hygiene, Monographic Series, No. 20. Baltimore: Johns Hopkins Press, 1953.

18. *Vector Control and the Recrudescence of Vector-borne Diseases.* Washington, D. C.: Pan American Health Organization, 1972.

19. *Vector Control: Briefs.* Atlanta: Public Health Service, National Communicable Disease Center, 1971.

20. *Vector Control in International Health.* Geneva: World Health Organization, 1972.

21. Davis, D. E. Control of rats and other rodents. In *Preventive Medicine and Public Health,* Ed. 10, edited by P. E. Sartwell. New York: Appleton-Century-Crofts, 1973.

22. Scott, H. G., and Borom, M. R. *Rodent-borne Disease Control through Rodent Stoppage.* Atlanta: Public Health Service, National Communicable Disease Center, 1967.

23. *Safe Use of Pesticides.* 20th Report of the WHO Expert Committee on Insecticides. Tech. Rep. Series 513. WHO, 1973, Geneva.

24. American Academy of Pediatrics. *Report of the Committee on the Control of Infectious Diseases,* Ed. 17. Evanston, Illinois: American Academy of Pediatrics, 1974.

25. Foege, W. H. Status of smallpox vaccination in the United States. In *Communicable Disease Control Conference. Houston, Texas, March 13-16, 1972.* DHEW Publication No. (HSM) 73-8172.

26. Hillman, M. R., Buynak, E. B., Weibel, R. E., and

Stokes, J. Jr. Live attenuated mumps-virus vaccine. *N. Engl. J. Med., 278:* 227-232, 1968.

27. *Communicable Disease Control Conference, Houston, Texas, March 13-16, 1972.* Center for Disease Control. Atlanta, Georgia, 1973. DHEW Publication No. (HSM) 73-8172.

28. *WHO Expert Committee on Rabies, 6th Report.* Technical Report Series No. 523. WHO, Geneva, 1973.

29. Linhart, S. B., Crespo, R. F., and Mitchell, G. C. Control of vampire bats by topical application of an anticoagulant, chlorophacinone. Bol. Of. Sanit. Panam. *6:* 31-38, 1972.

30. *Immunization in Tuberculosis. Report of a Conference on Progress to Date, Future Trends and Research Needs.* National Institutes of Health, Bethesda, Md., Oct. 26-28, 1971. DHEW Publication No. (NIH) 72-68.

31. Comstock, G. W., Livesay, V. T., and Woolpert, S. F. Evaluation of BCG vaccination among Puerto Rican children. Amer. J. Public Health, 64: 283-291, March, 1974.

32. Ashcroft, M. T., Singh, B., Nicholson, C. C., *et al.* A seven-year field trial of two typhoid vaccines in Guyana. *Lancet, ii:* 1056-1059, 1967.

33. *Health Hints for the Tropics,* Ed. 6 edited by H. Most. American Society of Tropical Medicine and Hygiene, 1967.

34. *Vaccination Certificate Requirements for International Travel.* Center for Disease Control, Morbidity and Mortality Weekly Report. Supplement to Vol. 22:No. 17. April 18, 1973. DHEW Publication, No. (HSM) 73-8216.

35. Neumann, H. H. *Foreign Travel Immunization Manual.* Springfield: Charles C Thomas, Publisher, 1971.

36. Edsall, G. Passive immunization. *Pediatrics, 32:* 599-609, 1963.

37. Krugman, S., and Ward, R. *Infectious Diseases of Children and Adults,* Ed. 5. St. Louis: C. V. Mosby, 1973.

38. Wilson, G. S. *The Hazards of Immunization.* London: The Athlone Press, 1967.

39. *Tetanus Surveillance, Report 3.* Atlanta: Public Health Service, National Communicable Disease Center, 1970.

40. *Neurotropic Diseases Surveillance: Poliomyelitis.* Annual Poliomyelitis, Summary 1971. Center for Disease Control. DHEW Publication No. (HSM) 73-8214, March, 1973.

41. *Measles Surveillance.* Center for Disease Control, Report No. 9. 1972 Summary. DHEW Publication No. (CDC) 74-8253, August, 1973.

42. *The Work of WHO 1972.* Annual Report of the Director General, Geneva, 1973.

43. Bierenbaum, M. L., Flieschman, A. I., Raichelson, R. I., Hayton, T., and Watson, P. Ten-year experience of modified fat diet on younger men with coronary heart disease. *Lancet, i:* 1404-07, 1973.

44. Mayer, J. Nutritional aspects of preventive medicine. In *Preventive Medicine,* edited by D. W. Clark and B. MacMahon. Boston: Little, Brown, and Company, 1967.

45. Mayer, J. *Human Nutrition: Its Physiological, Medical and Social Aspects.* Springfield, Ill.:

Charles C Thomas, Publisher, 1972.

46. Lowenstein, F. W. Iodized salt in the prevention of endemic goiter: a world-wide survey of present programs. *Amer. J. Public Health, 57:* 1815-1823, 1967.

47. McClure, F. J. *The Search and the Victory.* National Institute of Dental Research. Washington, D. C.: Government Printing Office, 1970.

48. Pratt, W. B. *Fundamentals of Chemotherapy.* New York: Oxford University Press, 1973.

49. Smith, H. *Antibiotics in Clinical Practice.* Baltimore: The Williams and Wilkins Co., 1972.

50. Weinstein, L., and Chang, T. W. The chemotherapy of viral infections. *N. Engl. J. Med., 289:* 725-730. Oct. 4, 1973.

51. Juel-Jensen, B. E., and MacCallum, F. O. *Herpes Simplex, Varicella and Zoster Clinical Manifestations and Treatment.* Philadelphia: J. B. Lippincott Co., 1972.

52. Lehman, J. *para*-Aminosalicylic acid in the treatment of tuberculosis. *Lancet, 1:* 15-16, 1946.

53. Antituberculosis Agents in Drug Evaluations, Ed. 2. Chicago: American Medical Association, 1973.

54. Hazen, E. L., and Brown, R. Two antifungal agents produced by a soil actinomycete. *Science, 112:* 423, 1950.

55. Gold, W., Stout, H. A., Pagano, J. F., and Donovick, R. Amphotericins A and B, antifungal antibiotics produced by a streptomycete. I. *In vitro* studies. *Antibio. Ann.,* 579-586, 1955-1956; *Medical Encyclopedia,* New York, 1956.

56. Grove, J. F. Griseofulvin. *Quart. Rev. (London), 17:* 1-19, 1963.

57. Busch, H., and Lane, M. *Chemotherapy: An Introductory Text.* Chicago: Year Book Medical Publishers, Inc., 1967.

58. Antimalarial Agents in Drug Evaluations. Ed. 2. Chicago: American Medical Association, 1973.

59. Wilcocks, C., and Manson-Bahr, P. E. C. *Manson's Tropical Diseases,* Ed. 17. London: Bailliere, 1972.

60. Ulivelli, A. Paromomycin and taeniasis. *Lancet, 1:* 696, 1968.

61. *1974 Cancer Facts and Figures.* New York: American Cancer Society, 1973.

62. *Biochemical Tests for Cancer.* Interview with Dr. Oscar Bodansky. Ca—A Cancer Journal for Clinicians. American Cancer Society. New York, 23:275-280, Sept.-Oct. 1973.

63. *Progress against Cancer, 1970.* Report by the National Advisory Cancer Council, National Institutes of Health, Public Health Service. Washington, D. C.: Government Printing Office, 1970.

64. Lilienfeld, A. M., Levin, M. L., and Kessler, I. I. *Cancer in the U. S.* Cambridge: Harvard University Press, 1972.

65. *Environment and Cancer.* Published for the University of Texas at Houston, M. D. Anderson Hospital and Tumor Institute, Houston, Texas. Baltimore: The Williams and Wilkins Co., 1972.

66. Welford, H. *The Nader Report—Sowing the Wind.* New York: Grossman Publishers, 1972.

67. Ryser, H. J.-P. Chemical carcinogenesis. *N. Engl. J. Med., 285:* 721-734, 1971.

68. *The Prevention of Cancer,* edited by R. W. Raven and F. J. Roe, London: Butterworths, 1967.

69. Lancaster, M. C., Jenkins, F. P., and Philip, J. McL. Toxicity associated with certain samples of groundnuts. *Nature (London) 192:* 1095-1096, 1961.

70. Laquer, G. T., Nickelsen, O., Whiting, M. G., and Kurland, L. T. Carcinogenic properties of nuts from *Cycas circinalis L.* indigenous to Guam. *Nat. Cancer Inst. J., 31:* 919-951, 1963.

71. Allen, D. W., and Cole, P. Viruses and human cancer. *N. Engl. J. Med., 286:* 70-82, Jan. 13, 1972.

72. *Current Research in Oncology, 1972,* edited by C. B. Aufinsen, M. Potter, and A. N. Schechter. New York: Academic Press, 1973.

73. Hersh, E. M., Gutterman, J. U., and Mauligit, G. Immunotherapy of Cancer in Man. Springfield, Ill.: Charles C Thomas, Publisher, 1973.

74. *Conference in Immunology of Carcinogenesis.* National Cancer Institute Monograph #35. DHEW Publication No. (NIH) 72-334, December, 1972.

75. Conant, R. K., DeLuca, A. J., and Levin, L. S. Health Education—A Bridge to the Community. *Amer. J. Public Health, 62:* 1239-1244, 1972.

76. *New Directions in Health Education,* edited by D. A. Reed. New York: The MacMillan Co., 1971.

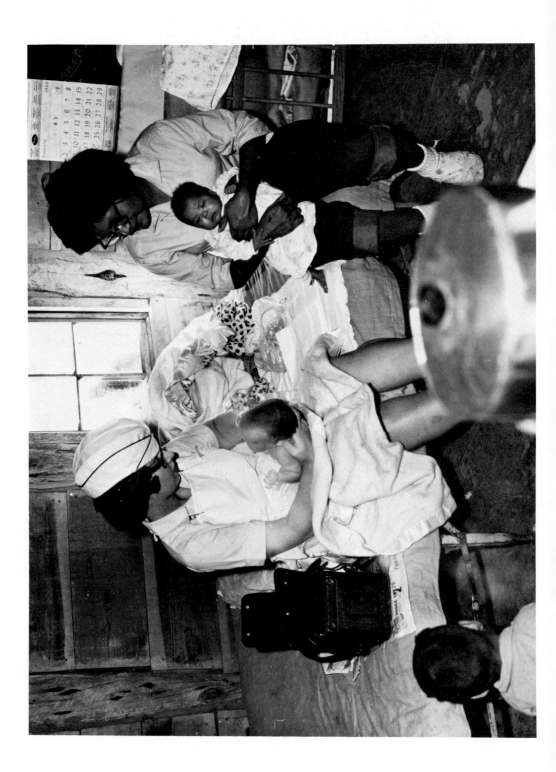

# 8

# Mental health

So neither ought you to attempt to cure the body without the soul; and this is the reason why the cure of many diseases is unknown to the physicians of Hella, because they are ignorant of the whole, which ought to be studied also. For this is the great error of our day in the treatment of the human body, that physicians separate the soul from the body.

PLATO

---

The terms "mental health" and "mental illness" can be confusing sometimes. They may mean different things to different people. Thus, one group may be referring to a national or international movement that concerns research into newer methods to prevent or treat the mentally ill. Another facet of mental health concerns the psychosocial relations to which some mental disorders may be traced, although the terms discussed may also refer to the psychological factors associated with a physical illness. Still another concept involves establishing community clinics, conducting educational campaigns to alter the public's former reservations toward mental illness, reducing the number of institutionalized patients, and establishing halfway houses to help former hospitalized patients return to useful living.

## EXTENT OF MENTAL ILLNESS

Whatever the terms used or the interpretations given, it is increasingly evident that mental illness has become an outstanding health problem in the United States. In February, 1963, President Kennedy sent a message to Congress on mental health in which he made the following statement: " . . . mental illness and mental retardation are among our most critical health problems. They occur more frequently, affect more people, require more prolonged treatment, cause more suffering by the families of the afflicted, waste more of our human resources, and constitute more financial drain upon both the Public Treasury and the

personal finances of the individual families than any other single condition."[1] Throughout the intervening years since this statement was made mental illness still remains one of our most critical health problems. This, in spite of the fact that mental health programs are presently spending more money, employing more people, serving more clients in more varied ways, and providing services of greater scope than ever before.[2]

The problem continues to increase with each passing year. We are informed that at least 10 per cent of the population, an excess of 20 million people, have some form of mental or emotional illness that would benefit from professional help. Twenty-one million families, an average of one in four, are affected by mental illness from someone in their immediate household. However, there are only approximately 23,000 practicing psychiatrists in the United States. The distribution of these specialists is very uneven; five states have more than one-half of all practicing psychiatrists, while two-thirds of all counties in the United States have none at all. In addition, there are approximately 16,000 psychologists, 15,500 psychiatric social workers, and 27,000 psychiatric nurses, resulting in a ratio of 35 mental health workers for every 100,000 people in the United States.[3]

One estimate of the extent of mental illness is related to the number of hospitalized patients. There are more people in hospitals with mental illness, at any one time, than with all other diseases combined, including cancer, heart disease, tuberculosis, and every other killing and crippling disease. Recent figures indicate that approximately 360,000 persons are under psychiatric care in public and private mental hospitals, psychiatric services of general hospitals, and Veterans Administration psychiatric facilities on any one day of the year and that over 1.75 million persons annually receive treatment at these institutions. Readmissions to mental hospitals are also quite common. Of the 972,000 persons admitted to mental hospitals and psychiatric services of general hospitals during the year, nearly 360,000 already had been hospitalized one time or more.[4]

The cost of mental illness is another significant factor. About 3.8 billion dollars are spent annually for the treatment of mental illness in state, county, Federal, and private mental hospitals and psychiatric units of community general hospitals. Tax monies pay approximately two-thirds of this bill, with the other third, 1.3 billion dollars, coming from the private sector. Other expenditures include 64 million dollars for facility development, 93 million dollars for mental · health manpower development, and 110 million dollars for research.[5]

The burden of mental illness on industry is even more impressive. The National Association for Mental Health estimates that people hospitalized for mental illness lose nearly 2 billion dollars per year in purchasing power. In addition, emotional disturbances and mental illness account for at least 50 per cent of all absentees. The annual cost to industry of this absenteeism is 5 billion dollars. Also, emotional disturbances and mental illness are important factors in the cause of 75 per cent of all accidents. Such accidents cost industry 3 billion dollars per year in injury to workers and damage to their machines.

## CARE OF THE MENTALLY ILL

The history of care for the mentally ill in the United States is not a record to be viewed with pride. In the early days, it was believed that persons suffering from mental illness were possessed of demons and that they should be "put away." Affluent families tended to conceal the mentally disturbed persons in their household in attics or cellars. The poor either were left to wander about the countryside or they were placed in jails, poorhouses, kennels, cages, in stocks, or at whipping posts. Some were driven out of town so that the community would not have to provide for their support.[6]

In 1756, Benjamin Franklin was instrumental in opening Pennsylvania Hospital in Philadelphia to the mentally disturbed. It was at this hospital, 40 years later, that Dr. Benjamin Rush raised the study of mental illness to a scientific level for the first time in the United States. In 1773, the first hospital in the United States devoted exclusively to mental patients was opened in Williamsburg, Virginia. Although treatment at that time was of doubtful benefit, these developments revealed a growing concern for the mentally ill.

Perhaps the greatest early reformer in care for the mentally ill in the U. S. was Dorothea Lynde Dix. During the mid-portion of the 19th century this tireless worker crusaded for intelligent and humane treatment. She visited numerous institutions, worked with the press, spoke before many State Legislatures, and made frequent talks to galvanize public opinion. She lobbied bills through Congress and is recognized as the founder of Saint Elizabeth's Hospital in Washington, D. C. In addition, she is largely responsible for awakening the public conscience and stimulating the movement toward the creation of the state mental hospital system.

## Public Supported Mental Hospitals

The concept of a state-supported mental hospital flourished and such hospitals were established in most of the states by the end of the 19th century. The numbers of these institutions have continued to grow until presently there are 327 state and county mental hospitals in the United States.[7] Even though these hospitals provided little more than custodial care, they filled rapidly. Overcrowding and poor treatment became serious problems, leading to the "snake pit" exposes of the 1940's. Newspaper and magazine photographs of dreary rows of hospital beds crowded together and overflowing into corridors, service rooms, and porches prompted some temporary relief in the form of additional hospital construction. The patient load in these mental hospitals increased steadily until the mid-1950's. By that time, the development of psychotherapeutic agents and advanced methods of intensive therapy permitted a much shorter period of confinement for most mental patients. Many of these hospitals have realized a gradual decrease in resident patient load.

The population of the institutions has dropped continually since 1955. In addition to the effectiveness of the psychotherapeutic drugs much of this decrease can be attributed to the development of Community Mental Health Centers. Population growth and increased use of the Community Centers, however, may well reverse the downward trend of the patient curve. Thus, limited though they may be, the state institutions will remain an important factor in the treatment of the mentally ill. The financial burden of these hospitals on the states will not diminish in the foreseeable future, even if the decline in patient population continues, because of the recognized need to improve the quality of services and the continued admissions to these institutions.

Self-help in times of mental stress can be employed only to a limited degree. The very fact of mental illness implies a narrowing of preception and an increase in defensiveness. It is necessary, then, to seek professional assistance. For a great many persons, psychiatric services are unavailable or are prohibitively expensive. The more recent development of Community Mental Health Centers has provided an excellent source of help and service for a large number of these people in need but for many others the state hospitals still serve as a major resource. There has been marked improvement in the conditions in a large proportion of these institutions in recent years, but much remains to be done. For example, at least half of the present mental hospital buildings were constructed before World War I and a few of these have been declared fire hazards. Some of the larger mental hospitals have over 14,000 patients, as large as a medium sized town and much too large to assure adequate treatment and care. Approximately one-third of the patients in state mental hospitals have been institutionalized continuously for 10 years or more. This is due, primarily, to the large number of senile geriatric patients and to the restriction of state funds. The latter seriously limits the administration of intensive therapy, which is needed to restore many hospitalized patients to useful lives. In addition, the physician-to-patient ratio in some public-supported mental hospitals is reported to average less than one per 100 resident patients and the ratio of patients to psychiatrists is even more profound.

The type and quality of care are reflected in the amount of funds spent for each patient. Recent figures indicate that the average daily expenditure for maintenance in public mental hospitals is $20 per patient. By contrast, short-term general hospitals spend approximately $85 per patient per day. It can readily be seen that a welfare institution, wishing to stretch its money, would elect to send patients to a state mental hospital rather than to the psychiatric department of a general hospital.

## Private Psychiatric Hospitals

There are 158 private psychiatric hospitals in the United States. Eighteen states have no private mental hospitals and 11 states have only one.[8] These private hospitals account for approximately 14,300 beds as contrasted with over one-half million beds in public institutions. Because of the more intensive and expensive therapy and care rendered to patients in private psychiatric hospitals, there is a fairly high turnover, with over 92,000 admissions per year. Private psychiatric hospitals offer many obvious advantages to those mental patients who can afford to pay. However, they are unequally distributed throughout the United States. For example, 40 per cent of the hospitals and 25 per cent of the beds are found in two states, New York and California. The opinion is generally held that private institutions will never be a major resource for the treatment of the mentally ill. The reasons given are the relatively high cost of their services, their geographic concentration in a few states, and their frequent isolation from the mainstream of social welfare services.

## Psychiatric Services in General Hospitals

Approximately 785 community general hospitals, or one out of every seven, have separate units for treating psychiatric patients. About twice that number admit psychiatric patients to their regular medical facilities. The number of beds reserved for treating the mentally ill in these institutions is approximately 19,000, but the average stay of patients is only three weeks.[9] Therefore, the psychiatric services in general hospitals account for almost as many admissions as do the state mental institutions. The future of such services is very promising. A number of leading mental health professionals support the concept of a close alliance between mental health and general health services. This alliance is well illustrated in the general hospital. In addition, the growth of insurance coverage for the mentally ill can be expected to be most important in the area of inpatient services in general hospitals. Added to this is the fact that a significant number of Federal mental health programs assign special consideration to those community health centers which are part of or associated with a general hospital.

## Private Psychiatry

Receiving individualized counseling and support from a medical doctor specializing in psychiatry is an optimal form of therapy. The paucity of private psychiatrists, however, limits this personalized professional attention to a privileged few, usually those who can pay for it. Therefore, patients in the upper and upper-middle socio-economic classes are the usual recipients of this type of treatment. Even allowing for some growth in health insurance in this field, it is not likely that private psychiatry will be financially within the reach of a very large portion of the population.

## Community Services

Because the mentally ill historically have been deemed a responsibility of the public and state governments have assumed the obligation of caring for these people for many generations, the development of private and public treatment resources outside the spectrum of the state mental institution has been rather haphazard, piecemeal, and unco-ordinated. A few of the more populous, progressive states, with the aid of active, civic-minded private citizens and aggressive public leaders, have established programs in community health that serve as examples of what can be done. Perhaps the most active of such programs are those associated with outpatient clinics.

There are about 2000 public and private outpatient clinics in the United States serving approximately 900,000 children and adults. Almost one-half of these clinics are in the northeastern states, principally in urban areas. Many are part-time clinics and most of them have long waiting lists. Operating funds have come principally from state, community, and private sources and have been quite limited. This was reflected in the trained manpower that was hired to staff these clinics.

The Community Mental Health Centers program has initiated a pronounced change in outpatient care of the mentally ill. Through

funds provided principally by the Federal government, approximately 400 comprehensive community centers have been established and many additional such centers are in the planning stage. This is the realization of a dream of many dedicated workers in the mental health field who are convinced that the mentally ill should be treated through comprehensive services within their own communities rather than be placed in a distant mental hospital. Historically, local and state sources have spent relatively small amounts on community mental health services but larger sums will be required from these sources as Federal funding decreases.

## CHANGING CONCEPTS AND ATTITUDES

### Introduction

Until approximately 200 years ago, there seemed to be very little hope for the mentally ill. These unfortunate people were confined with criminals and diseased persons, beaten unmercifully, restrained with chains and strait-jackets, and exhibited as curiosities or sources of amusement. Asylums for the insane were established in Europe as early as the 15th century. Regardless of the merciful intent of their founders, the conditions at these institutions became deplorable. Bethlehem Hospital, established in Lambeth parish in London, is reported to have been fairly typical of the very low quality of care and extremely poor treatment given to patients. Its popular name, "Bedlam," was soon incorporated into the English language as a synonym for pandemonium.

Courageous and dedicated people, working against apathy and active opposition, gradually were able to stir the public conscience and promote a more humane treatment for the insane. Outstanding among these humanitarian reformers were William Tuke in England and the team of Jean-Baptiste Pussin and Dr. Phillipe Pinel in France. William Tuke founded the York Retreat in 1766, a Quaker institution where patients were treated as guests in a family environment with religious overtones. In 1792, Dr. Pinel and M. Pussin were credited with changing the worst asylum in Paris from a custodial, repressive institution to a progressive, psychiatrically oriented hospital. By the use of "moral treatment" these men are credited with "striking off the chains' of the insane.[10]

Toward the end of the 19th century, the fields of psychology and psychiatry emerged as important disciplines which demonstrated possible prevention as well as improved methods for treating the mentally ill. As the problem and some of the solutions became more defined, there was established a mental hygiene movement in the United States. The book by C. W Beers, *A Mind That Found Itself.*[11] provided much of the impetus. The first mental health association, the Connecticut Society for Mental Health, was established in 1908 for the purpose of public education regarding mental illnesses and their cause. The National Committee for Mental Hygiene was established in the following year. In 1922, recognition of mental health movements in other countries led to the formation of the International Congress for Mental Hygiene. By 1930, there were mental hygiene societies in 19 states and 15 foreign nations.

In spite of this growing movement, there remained much to be done. Changes in philosophies and public acceptance of mental health objectives and programs came very slowly. Mental disease is not a cause for shame or a sign of moral turpitude, yet victims of this illness were quietly removed from society by their families and placed in mental institutions where they no longer attracted the attention of the public. The mental hospitals were often noisy and the working conditions for the staff were frequently unsatisfactory and unsafe. As a result, it was difficult to attract professionally trained nurses and attendants and the quality of personnel that could be found did not always meet the desired standards. This, in turn, had a deleterious effect upon the mental patient's chances for recovery.

Thus, the victims of mental illness were confined in an impersonal institutional environment and were subjected to restraints and routines that would have seriously threatened even those with sound minds. Barbiturates were used quite extensively; relatively large doses helped to control the hyperactive psychotics, while smaller doses were used to depress those suffering from neuroses. Skilled psychotherapeutic care was available, but the need for it greatly exceeded the facilities and the personnel that could be provided. Other types of treatment were generally limited to frontal lobotomy, insulin shock, and electroconvulsive therapy. The extreme scarcity of progressive therapy and the general conditions in the hospitals often shocked relatives and friends when they visited mental patients. These people frequently came away with their consciences badly shaken.

## Factors Influencing the Changing Concepts

This somewhat discouraging situation has been improved greatly in recent years. As in the case of similar large scale developments, there have been many forces interacting to bring about this change. Some have been stimulated by professional groups, lay groups, communications media, and government agencies. Others seem to have arisen spontaneously in various areas of the country, frequently concurrently. There were some outstanding accomplishments and developments, many overlapping each other, which established the impetus, pointed the way, and provided the means for a substantially improved program in mental health.

### *Public Education*

Through the entire fabric of the enlightened approach to mental health runs the substantial, purposeful, and effective thread of public education. Through medical channels, mental health associations, lay press, radio, and television, the public has been informed about mental illness and the various aspects of mental health. The old ideas of insanity are now being replaced by the concept that patients with mental disease can frequently recover and, regardless, are entitled to as much care, sympathy, and consideration as a patient with any other infirmity. The American people are becoming more sophisticated regarding health problems of all kinds, including mental illness. They are learning to discuss openly mental health and are honestly and sympathetically seeking methods and means to combat this ever growing problem effectively. As a result of increasing attention, there has developed an awareness of the relationship between mental illness and crime, juvenile delinquency, addictions, suicides, and other undesirable social phenomena. The public also has become conscious of the increasing mental stresses of urban and industrialized life. In the light of this growing awareness and concern, it is not surprising that there are significant demands for public health endeavors directed toward the research, care, and prevention of the mentally ill.

### Expanded Definitions of Health

A very significant factor in the comprehensive approach to mental health was the acceptance of a broad definition of the term "health." The negative definition, which was formerly found in most dictionaries, was that "health is the state of someone who is not sick." This limited concept usually referred to the clinical symptoms of illness and did not take into consideration the environmental and social factors which could also serve as etiological agents. Although social workers and health practitioners had long promoted a more positive approach toward maintaining health and preventing illness, it was not until the establishment of the World Health Organization that the expanded definition of health was publicized and gained popular support. According to its constitution, the World Health Organization defined health as " . . . a state of complete physical, mental, and social well-being and not merely the absence of disease or infirmity." This expanded concept presented a challenge to and caught the imagination of health professionals, behavioral scientists, legislative representatives, and the general public. Thus, it was no longer sufficient for surgeons to repair, replace, or remove damaged organs or for physiotherapists to teach the infirm how to use their limbs again. It was reocgnized that the efforts of the best therapists were only partially effective if patients were homeless, lacked elementary sanitation, or were faced with despair.

As a result, the many aspects of mental health assumed much greater importance. The relationship between the mind and the body became better known and psychosomatic medicine was established as a reality rather than a theory. It is now generally accepted that emotional factors are connected with almost all types of illnesses and some doctors have estimated that as high as 70 per cent of their cases are largely psychosomatic. The importance of mental and physiological compatability continues to be stressed. Rabbi Abraham Joshua Heschel, speaking at the AMA Symposium on Medicine and Religion, made the following statement in this regard: "The

doctor must find out the pressure of the blood and the composition of the urine, but the process of recovery also depends on the pressure of the soul and the composition of the mind. Physical vigor alone does not constitute total health. Nor is longevity the only purpose of living. Quality of living is as important as quantity of living. . . . "

Also, another consequence of accepting mental and social well-being as fundamentals of health is the recognition that the line of demarcation between mental health and mental illness does not sharply separate. In mental health, as in physical health, we are now beginning to appreciate that, between normal and severely abnormal states, there extends a continuous spectrum of overlapping characteristics of the mind. This has called for a refinement in diagnosis. What is normal or deviant may vary from culture to culture and even from one authority in the field to another. There are many times when well-trained psychiatrists cannot agree whether a certain patient has a neurosis with depressive manifestations or a manic-depressive psychosis. Thus, a result of this closer scrutiny in matters relating to mental health suggests that arbitrary distinctions in diagnosis and treatment may not always be justified.

The relationship established between mental and physical health has called attention to certain similarities of the two. For example, it is recognized that diseases in either group do not originate from a single cause. There are various stages throughout the development of both types of diseases where it is possible to halt the progress, if certain remedial measures are instituted. Just as environmental sanitation and immunological procedures are stressed in communicable diseases, there is increasing awareness that attention given to psychosocial factors could lower the incidence and severity of mental illness. Communities are responding by marshalling forces which are needed to strengthen mental health programs. It has become apparent that neither physical nor mental health is the exclusive concern of the medical professions and that health problems can be diminished effectively only through co-operative efforts in the community.

### Psychotherapeutic Drugs

It is difficult, if not impossible, to weigh the relative values of the forces and events which brought about such a change in the field of mental health. The development of the psychotherapeutic agents, however, was perhaps one of the most outstanding. Prior to the availability and use of reserpine, the phenothiazines, substituted propanediols, monamine oxidase inhibitors, and similar drugs, there was small chance for rapid recovery. Victims of mental illness were all too frequently condemned to trade the amenities of civilized life for an indeterminate, or even endless, sentence of confinement. Thanks to the psychotherapeutic agents, the periods of hospitalization for most of these patients have been reduced markedly. Psychiatric wards of general hospitals report an average stay of only three weeks. Mental patients are now vastly improved and are more receptive to psychotherapy. The drugs have robbed delusions and hallucinations of their terror and have helped to overcome suicidal depression.

Most mental hospitals have seen marked improvement since the advent of the psychotherapeutic drugs. Patients are happier, more co-operative, and less freightened. The attendants, recognizing that there are hopes for improvement and seeing encouraging signs of progress in their charges, have changed their attitudes considerably. Abuse, agitation, assaults, and filth now have been replaced largely by a clean orderliness. Federal grants from the Hospital Improvement Program and the Hospital Staff Development Program have helped to provide better facilities and to improve the training of personnel.[1][2] In spite of some remaining old buildings and outmoded facilities, the atmosphere of mental hospitals today approaches that of any other medical institution for the treatment of the sick. Friends and relatives are encouraged to visit patients in mental hospitals and most patients now believe that they have been admitted for treatment and not for punishment.

The development of psychotherapeutic medications had other far reaching effects. As attempts were made to determine the site of action of these drugs, there developed the new field of psychopharmacology. Brain neurohormones are being studied, advanced methods in biochemistry and physiology are applied now to the study of the brain, and sources of aberrant discharges of the central nervous system are being detected, probed, and analyzed. The progress which has been made in this field has been most encouraging and has attracted the interest of the public and the government. As a result, considerable funds, public and private, are being spent for research. This concerted drive to disclose the biochemical nature of mental disease promises even more startling developments in the future. The general hunch among investigators is that they are on the verge of a major breakthrough in this field.

Another important effect resulting from the development of psychotherapeutic drugs relates to victims of mental illness who remain in the community. Many of these people have not been confined in an institution because medications have helped to control their conditions. Others, who were hospitalized for comparatively short periods, are now back at their jobs and leading purposeful lives while continuing to take maintenance doses of psychotherapeutic medications. The presence of these persons in the community has had a profound influence upon public acceptance of mental illness and has been of material help in promoting mental health programs. It is readily seen that these people are not greatly different from others in the population who are suffering from physical illnesses and who are taking medications to control symptoms of their diseases. By their examples, these individuals are demonstrating the accomplishments which have been made in the field of mental health. Public minded citizens are, thus, encouraged by these signs of progress and are becoming convinced that the establishment of community mental health programs is well worth the effort and expense involved.

For members of the allied medical professions, there are constant reminders of the necessity to extend their learning and endeavors in the field of mental health as they have in physical health. Victims of mental illness visit their pharmacists each month to obtain prescription refills and they visit doctors' offices and hospitals for routine check-ups. Most of them are constructive members of society and their numbers within the community are growing constantly. It is incumbent upon the members of the health professions to know the problems which face these people, to seek ways to reduce the incidence of the disease, and to help mix sympathetic understanding with community action. Historically, citizens in the community have looked to the medical professions for theoretical understanding, technical knowledge, and representative leadership in

striving toward and maintaining optimal physical health. With the increased emphasis on
mental and social well-being and their relationships to optimal health, the health professions
are again sought for information and leadership.
There is, therefore, an implied obligation to
become informed of the nature, scope, and
possibilities in mental health and to participate
actively in local community programs in this
newest of health endeavors.

*Health Insurance*

Restrictions against mental illness in many
forms of coverage have resulted in a much
lower proportion of the mental health bill being
met through insurance. However, with
improved treatment methods for mental illness
and shorter hospital stays, as well as the
increasing use of the general hospital to treat
psychiatric patients, these restrictions are being
removed, particularly with respect to inpatient
services. Consequently, within the last 10 years,
there has been an increase in the use of
prepayment and other insurance plans to help
pay the cost. Coverage of nervous and mental
conditions is now a basic feature of most
hospital insurance written for groups, but study
data indicate that the current practice of health
insurance agencies is to provide only those
benefits specified by service contracts.[13] For
policies issued to individuals the extent of
coverage is usually quite limited. Medicare and
Medicaid provide some benefits but there are
significant limitations both in duration of
coverage and financial allowance.

For outpatient coverage and partial hospitalization services, the picture is not nearly so
bright. This kind of coverage usually is available
only under an extended benefit or major
medical type of certificate. Even when available, such certificates frequently place special
restrictions which do not apply to other
disorders. In addition, the initial deductible and
co-insurance features have served to discourage
the early referral and treatment that is felt to
be so important. In the majority of these
insurance policies, there is an almost total
absence of coverage for day care and for the
services of psychologists, social workers, and
other professionals who are increasingly important in the treatment of the mentally ill.

With the implementation of the Community
Mental Health Centers program a major portion

of the finances required to initiate newer
services is furnished through Federal grants.
Continued staffing and program expense, however, will increasingly become a local responsibility. While it will be necessary for
communities to provide some subsidies to
operate the centers, it is quite evident that a
significant portion of the financial burden will
fall upon the patients themselves. Their ability
to afford the services rests largely upon the
availability of prepayment and other insurance
programs. The health insurance industry, by
exploring steps to encourage the expansion of
coverage to include mental health, can be an
important factor in providing access to these
new community services. The Task Force on
Insurancy of the National Institute of Mental
Health has developed a number of suggested
concepts for coverage of mental illness. Among
these are the following:

1. Emphasis should be placed on early
referral and short-term, intensive therapy. The
total costs of the first few visits could be
covered completely, with a progressively
decreasing percentage of cost coverage for
subsequent visits, up to a stated limit.

2. In-hospital benefits should be at least as
complete as those for physical illness. Partial
hospitalization, such as in a psychiatric day-
night hospital, should also be included in the
in-hospital benefits.

3. Increased recognition should be given to
all professional skills essential to treatment.
Both the continuing development of the concept of the mental health team and the present
shortage of psychiatrists argue strongly for
covering the services of the clinical psychologist, the psychiatric social worker, the
psychiatric nurse, and rehabilitation specialists.

4. Insurance should not favor a particular
type of treatment. Comparable coverage should
be provided for electroshock, psychotherapy,
and all other forms of treatment so that there
could be free choice in selecting the type best
suited to a patient's need.

5. Prescribed drugs should be covered for
ambulatory as well as for hospitalized patients.
The importance of psychotherapeutic drugs as a
resource for treating mental illness cannot be
overemphasized. This may well be the very
factor which keeps a patient ambulatory
instead of hospitalized.

Experience with a few of the programs that
presently cover mental disorders has shown that
utilization rates are not excessive and costs

incurred are not prohibitive. As the community mental health program develops and more facilities and manpower become available to treat the mentally ill, it is quite likely that periods of treatment will become shorter and the chance for greater insurance coverage will improve. With the improvement of insurance coverage, it is expected that more people will seek psychiatric services earlier, before the need arises for long periods of treatment or hospitalization. This, in turn, could result in even lower insurance premiums with still greater coverage. Thus, there are promising signs that health insurance for mental illness may reach the same levels of acceptance, coverage, and utilization as those attained for physical illness.

## GOVERNMENT PROGRAMS IN MENTAL HEALTH

Mental health, as one of the newer developments in public health, has been the subject of gradual and cautious exploration. A few local and state governmental units such as health departments began introducing various activities relating to mental health, which were admittedly exploratory, experimental, and often combined with some other agency activity. Early direction, support, and suggestions were provided by interested private agencies such as the Mental Health Association, but there was no concerted move to establish a mental health program on a national level. The U.S. Public Health Service had a mental hygiene division, but it was concerned mainly with administering two Public Health Service hospitals for the treatment of narcotic drug addicts and studies of drugs and drug addiction. It was not until 1946, when Congress passed the Mental Health Act, that there was national attention focused upon the scope of the mental health problem and upon the many deficiencies. The Act provided for construction of a mental health facility and for Federal grants-in-aid to states for research, training, and assistance in community health programs. The National Institute of Mental Health was created in 1949 and helped to administer the Mental Health Act. Progress was made as a result of this Federal assistance and interest. One of the notable accomplishments was the additional attention which was directed to the discrepancies and gaps which still existed in the care of the mentally ill.

In 1955, Congress established the Joint Commission of Mental Illness and Health. This Commission, which was made up of leaders of the various health and social science professions, was charged with analyzing the needs relating to mental illness, evaluating the resources of the nation, and making recommendations for appropriate Federal action. The final report of the Commission was issued in 1961 in a volume entitled *Action for Mental Health*.[14] This report pointed out the deficiencies which existed in the public mental hospital system and called for a number of significant changes. Among these were more community clinics for outpatient treatment, increased use of general hospitals for the inpatient treatment of psychiatric illness, and a change in the nature of the public mental hospital. A cabinet level committee was appointed to analyze the report and to provide guidelines. President Kennedy then presented his now historic special message, *Mental Illness and Mental Retardation*, in which he proposed a bold new approach and emphasis to the care of the mentally ill. The new approach was designed, primarily, to use Federal resources to stimulate state, local, and private action to create, at the community level, a significant number and range of mental health services. By such action, it was anticipated that patient loads in state mental hospitals would be markedly reduced.

Federal legislation followed shortly. The Community Mental Health Centers Construction Act of 1963, the Hospital Improvement Program, the Inservice Training Program, the Mental Health Benefits of the Social Security Amendments of 1965, the Mental Health Amendments of 1967, the Community Mental Health Center Amendments of 1970, and the Social Security Amendments of 1973 were but harbingers of numerous mental health bills, acts, and programs which have subsequently been introduced or are in the planning stage. Planning, in its own right, has become a major aspect of the newer Federal mental health programs. Examples of such programs are Comprehensive Community Health Planning, Mental Health Planning, Mental Retardation Planning, Alcoholism Planning, and, the hallmark of repetitive redundancy, Plans for Planning. One government official has stated that "...it seems as if we as a society have finally matured from the so-called age of anxiety to the age of planning."[15]

Governmental involvement in the problems of

mental health and mental retardation is administered primarily through the National Institute of Mental Health. This Institute is dedicated to broadening existing research programs, increasing the supply and variety of mental health manpower, and expanding and improving mental health services. Specially focused effort now is given to such problems as additional development and evaluation of psychoactive drugs, cultural deprivation and mental health, services for the mentally ill offender, behavior of groups, incidences and prevalences of the mental illnesses, and mental health of children and youths.

In addition to the expenses involved with research and service, the extent and costs of mental health facilities also are increasing rapidly. It is estimated that capital outlays for community mental health centers will be 2.93 billion dollars and facilities for the mentally retarded will require 3.34 billion dollars.[16] The present annual Mental Health budget, exclusive of Drug Abuse and Alcoholism programs, is in excess of 400 million dollars. Thus, public health endeavors in the field of mental health are becoming more pronounced in an effort to help the American people acquire and maintain a state of mental and social well-being. These endeavors will involve the allied medical professions to an increasing degree. Similar to the situations pertaining to expanded government activity in the area of physical health, there will be greater utilization of services, more facilities to staff, enlarged needs for health manpower, increased funds to allocate, and additional policies to formulate. Early involvement in program planning and active voluntary participation in program development will assure the allied medical professions a position of leadership in this new venture.

It is well to remember that, even though the majority of health legislation was written and promoted through non-medical channels, it is still administered largely through medically oriented government agencies. These agencies look to the health professions for help and guidance in implementing their programs. Cooperative allied medical groups can influence favorably policies relating to extent of coverage, types of care, and quality of service. If these health professions are recalcitrant or too hesitant, they well may lose their positions of influence through default.

## NEWER APPROACHES TO MENTAL HEALTH—COMMUNITY INVOLVEMENT

The fundamental interests and the ultimate goals of the field of mental health are not necessarily increased facilities and manpower, additional development of psychoactive drugs, and the improvement of psychotherapy and other treatment techniques for the mentally ill. Indeed, these well may be methods to help attain the objectives, but the primary concerns are even more refined. These concerns include earlier and more effective detection of psychiatric and prepsychiatric conditions which cause social maladjustments, the exploration of their sources, and efforts to help eliminate the various factors which precipitate these conditions. Thus, the ultimate goal of mental health is a more satisfying and effective life for the American people, with a reduction in the stresses and strains which may present mental problems. The development of emotionally mature and well-adjusted individuals is the attainment which is sought.

To arrive at this goal, it is first necessary to use existing knowledge to reduce the number of mentally ill and to provide a comprehensive and effective treatment program. The need is so great and the personnel is so scarce that considerable attention is given to possible solutions that would encompass resources other than those of the clinic, the traditional mental hospital, or the private practitioner. It has been found, for example, when alternatives to full-time hospitalization exist and proper screening is employed, that mental patient loads in hospitals are markedly reduced. Up to 50 per cent of all psychiatric patients who are referred for hospitalization can be handled in some other way. It has also been demonstrated that the solutions of complex mental health problems cannot and must not rest in the hands of one group. A community endeavor, therefore, is needed to achieve the progress anticipated in this field and the concept of the community mental health center was thus proposed.

The community health center is not necessarily one physical facility containing all of the program elements relating to the range of services and continuity of care. Rather, it is a number of facilities located in different places throughout the community and fully coordinated to supply the proper combination of services which may be needed for individual cases. Efforts are made to add to existing resources of the community such as the general hospital, rather than to duplicate these resources.

Through community effort and co-operation and with initial financial support from the Federal Government, the comprehensive community mental health centers reflect the modern services and programs that assure a continuity of care. The elements of such a comprehensive plan include the following:

1. Services for early diagnosis and prompt treatment such as case identification and referral, 24-hr. emergency service, and diagnostic and screening services.

2. Inpatient care, usually in the psychiatric divisions of general hospitals, where emphasis is placed on intensive and short-term therapy.

3. Day hospitals for those who can spend their nights at home and night hospitals for those who can work. It has been found that partial hospitalization is less expensive, decreases the tendency toward dependency and regression, and retains the patient's ties with family and community.

4. Outpatient clinics, usually attached to mental hospitals.

5. Availability of psychoactive drugs for maintenance therapy.

6. Halfway houses and clubs to function as self-help, mutual aid supports for former mental patients in the transition from hospitalization to social living.

7. Vocational rehabilitation, using trained counselors and specialists to help restore productive usefulness and purpose to life.

8. Nursing homes, which maintain specially trained personnel to handle senile geriatric patients.

9. Additional community services such as consultation, education, training, and research.

The Community Mental Health Centers Act of 1963 (Public Law 88-164) and the Community Mental Health Center Amendments of 1970 (Public Law 91-211) will probably be considered a major metamorphasis in mental health in the United States. The goal is for the eventual establishment of 2000 community mental health centers throughout the country. The Federal funding for most of these centers is for a period of eight years, on a progressively declining basis. The emphasis on local services required that there be a means of identifying the community to be served. Each center must service a population of from 75,000 to 200,000, known as the center's "catchment area." This terminology is derived from the public health term "catch basin", and is analogous in meaning and concept to the term "service area." The basic concepts embodied in the Act were that each center must provide community oriented programs with accessibility of care, comprehensive services, continuity of care, and an emphasis on prevention as well as treatment.[17] Through the implementation of this legislation, mental patients will be assured of continuous care within their own communities. This large increase in Community Mental Health facilities, however, also requires a concomitant increase in trained personnel. Recent reports indicate that there is a pronounced need to improve the quality of some services, particularly crisis intervention, to a level considerably above the legally required minimum.[18]

The role of the state hospital as the major system for care of the severely mentally ill will diminish as the comprehensive community plan develops. The tide of events is forcing the state mental hospitals to become a more conscious part of a bigger system. During the transitional period, however, they will continue to carry a large share of the load. To prepare for their new role, these institutions have been encouraged, through government support, to undertake demonstration and pilot projects, improve the quality of care, and provide in-service training for staff personnel.

In addition to the preoccupation with efforts to adequately care for the mentally ill, the larger and more diffuse goal of positive mental health remains an ultimate objective. Community activities, attitudes, and co-operation are of vital need in this important endeavor. As a greater percentage of mental patients is treated within the community, the local citizens must adopt an even more open acceptance of mental illness, an acceptance combined with compassion and understanding. There must also be an increased willingness to help former mental patients adapt to normal life in the community.

Leadership in this area continues to be shown by the National Association for Mental Health and the more than 900 local mental health associations. These organizations conduct information services to assist the public in locating appropriate resources for the care and treatment of the mentally ill. They sponsor seminars and workshops promoting better understanding of mental illness and they deal with the employability of former mental patients. Seeking to provide insight into the emotional components of the individual, urging school boards to adopt more liberal attitudes toward teaching mental health in the public schools, and working with mass communication media in their public education campaigns are additional activities which occupy the time and energy of these dedicated people.

Similar to the circumstances surrounding any injury or illness, the prevention of mental illness is far better than any treatment which can be devised. The concerted efforts of all groups and individuals who maintain an active interest in the welfare of the people in their community are needed to promote the positive aspects of mental health. This is particularly true of the various caretaker groups in the population which have contact at key stress points in the life cycle. Thus, the attainment and maintenance of emotional maturity remain as the greatest bulwarks against mental illness. The emotionally mature individual possesses most of the following characteristics.

1. He has developed a sense of identity, self-acceptance, and integrity.

2. He can accept responsibilities.

3. He has developed ability to make decisions.

4. He has learned to love someone or something outside of himself and to show affection.

5. He has developed the ability to carry on when emotionally disturbed and to learn from his emotional mistakes.

6. He has learned to be self-reliant and does not have to depend upon artificial entertainment to occupy his time and thoughts.

7. He can face the past or future without fear and can look at unknown future changes as interesting adventures.

8. He has set suitable goals and has learned to accept limitations that cannot be changed.

This fortunate individual did not attain all of these characteristics completely by his own efforts and determination. As a product of his environment, he had able assistance from family, clergymen, teachers, general conditions and standards of living, and the countless numbers of citizens within the community who touched his daily life. Through continued community support in promoting a positive mental health program, this individual could well be representative of the general population in years to come.

## EMOTIONAL DISTURBANCES

### Introduction

Just as the human body has certain requirements for the maintenance of good physical health in the form of nutrition, activity, rest, and physiological needs, it also has requirements for the maintenance of good mental health in the form of interrelated emotional needs. Some of these needs are security, love and affection, independence, achievement, companionship, self-acceptance, and faith. When these needs are threatened or denied or efforts to obtain them are frustrated, there arise, within the body, emotional disturbances of a marked degree. These disturbances are accompanied by significant physiological responses such as changes in cardiorespiratory rate and depth, perspiration, muscle tension, and gastrointestinal activity. In a highly developed civilization such as ours, emotional reactions may be stimulated by such social situations as public embarrassment, false charges of dishonesty, or denial of earned rewards, yet the emotional response may be physiologically similar to the alarm reaction elicited in a cave man when threatened by a predator. The important difference lies in the increasing number of subtle stimuli which can harrass modern man almost constantly and, thus, lead to an almost perpetual state of defensiveness.

Emotional disturbances may imply either an inner conflict or a conflict against circumstances for which no immediate action is appropriate. Since the conflict cannot be resolved, it is usually prolonged. The victim is uncertain of the outcome, although he is constantly aware of the conflict. One of the more common emotional reactions is anxiety, which is said to be physically and psychologically a fear reaction. Such reactions can occur when the individual is not consciously afraid and they may well be the result of earlier experiences and subtle environmental stimuli. The range of stimuli which will arouse the various emotions is further broadened through learned or conditioned behavior and the reactions to these stimuli are limited by the dictates of our culture. Thus, the permissible amount and manner of expression of emotions are to be confined within the framework of established custom. For example, a man is not expected to cry, he is very limited in the manner to which he can show affection for another man, and he must not display outward signs of inner turmoil. Reservations such as these serve to intensify the physiological reactions which result from emotional stimuli.

Even the well-adjusted, emotionally mature individual presently living in our society cannot expect to be free from anxiety, tension, dissatisfaction, and frustration, nor does he plan to be in a state of constant happiness and contentment. It would be unwise and unhealthy for him to do so. The demands of modern living, the conflicts arising from within oneself and through interpersonal relationships, the squashing of ideas, the thwarting of projected plans, and the frustrations of nonattainment preclude the possibility of living a life completely void of strife. The alternate rise and release of tension, both physical and emotional, are integral parts of normal living and are even more pronounced in the ambitious person who possesses drive and energy.

Indeed, it is well that society does not provide an environment which is free from these emotional forces. A mild degree of discontent and dissatisfaction is beneficial both to the individual and to the society in which he lives. A person who is in a mild state of tension is in a condition of heightened consciousness. He is more aware of circumstances in his environment, he can formulate constructive ideas more effectively, and he possesses more of an incentive, desire, and ability to accomplish tasks. He is the person who moves mountains, who accomplishes the seemingly impossible, who develops into a great leader, and who establishes guidelines and blueprints for further development. A very large portion of the discoveries and progress of mankind throughout history has been a result of the persistence and drive of dissatisfied, unhappy, and restless people who were not content to remain placid and secure in their environment.

In recognition of the alertness and other benefits derived from a mild state of tension in our competitive society, there has been warranted concern over indiscriminate use of the so-called tranquilizers. These psychoactive drugs were developed and marketed to serve the very useful purpose of treating symptoms of neuroses. They help calm the agitated patient, serve to decrease tensions, and are a valuable aid in allaying fears and reducing apprehensions in the excited and frightened individual. Judiciously used, these drugs have helped to shorten periods of hospitalization for mental patients, allow treatment of victims of nervous tension in their own communities without the necessity for hospitalization, and halt the deterioration produced by mental stress. As indicated in an earlier discussion, the development of these and other psychoactive drugs has had a profound influence upon methods of treating the mentally ill and, indeed, upon the entire mental health program. Their high value in this field is well established. It is, however, the misuse and abuse of these drugs which present potential threats.

Rather than face unpleasant situations or endure even relatively minor conflicts or tensions, a distressingly large number of people retreat to the tranquilizing effect of certain psychoactive drugs. As this retreat becomes more established and widespread, there is more than a possibility that a significant portion of these people will no longer be interested in or capable of accepting responsibility. It has been demonstrated that persons under the influence of these drugs are more open to suggestion and there have been reports of inferred reduction of willpower. It even has been postulated that the will of an entire population could be controlled through the tranquilizing effects of drugs, when used by an ambitious and unscrupulous few. The abuse of these psychoactive drugs has been likened to the abuse of alcohol. There are certain similarities between the two. Ultraconservative teetotalers, who would not think of drinking alcohol, may freely take tranquilizing drugs for the same purpose of reducing tensions and seeking relaxation. There are other similarities which may be recognized. These drugs may require more frequent or enlarged doses to produce the same effect; there are dangers associated with overdosage; dependency may develop with prolonged use; and withdrawal symptoms have been produced following cessation of chronically high doses. Attempts to escape the realities of modern life through the abuse of alcohol could cause the same distressing effects. Tranquilizing drugs, therefore, have supplied modern man with another psychological crutch. Crutches are very useful devices when employed during acute periods and for the purposes intended. Too much reliance upon them and continued use beyond the period of need, however, can result in atrophy, degeneration, and contortion. The individual may well lose his native and acquired abilities. He would then find it necessary to depend upon crutches for support and would require additional help to perform his daily activities.

The strength of any nation comes from the strength of its people and the United States has long prided itself on its position of leadership and power among the nations of the world. In order to maintain this position, it is necessary for the citizens of the country to stay alert and concerned. The tendency of larger numbers of the population who take drugs to seek tranquility, avoid conflict, reduce tensions, and avoid facing stark realities poses a potential threat that is worthy of recognition. Complacency and apathy in an individual are sad and unfortunate. These same qualities in a significant portion of the population can be dangerous.

## Adaptive Methods

The ability of individuals to cope with emotional disturbances varies considerably. In a given situation, two people may react differently, depending upon stability, general make-up, and background. Persons with strong characters and a sense of mission often can withstand seemingly overwhelming quantities of tensions, anxieties, and frustrations, although others may have a very low threshold. Apparently, the degree of tolerance is largely dependent upon such factors as environmental conditions to which a person has been subjected, the habits that he has developed for coping with difficult situations, and the basic attitudes of those closest to him. Many people may be able to increase their endurance to these tensions and anxieties, but the range open to them is dependent upon their total environment. Interpersonal relationships during periods of emotional strain are also important. Such relationships may be positive and supporting or they may be negative and cause insecurity,

doubts, and dissatisfaction. Unsuccessful attempts to resolve these emotional conflicts result in mounting tension, generalized ineffectiveness, and still more tension. The farther one moves away from a healthy, productive adjustment, the more his attempts to gain relief from his emotional disturbances are likely to be maladaptive. Only when tensions and conflicts reach high levels and become burdens do they become a threat to the individual and cause adverse effects within the body. When the individual cannot make satisfactory adjustments to his problems, further maladjustments may occur and efficiency and productivity may be impaired. The proper functioning of the nervous system and the capacity for concentration are also affected. In fact, all of the various physical systems react as if the organism were in danger and adverse physiological responses occur so frequently that the maintenance of homeostasis within the body is threatened.

## Defense Mechanisms

Stress for one person is not necessarily stress for another, but, although individuals may vary in the amount of emotional disturbances that they can carry, everyone is subject to breakdown if conditions become too severe. When sustained emotional tensions and conflicts rise above a person's level of tolerance, the individual must find ways to deal with the fear, hostility, and anxiety that he experiences. The characteristic way of coping with these unpleasant realities is to employ various mechanisms to divert or soften the blow. It is important to devise acceptable reasons for unacceptable actions so that the self-concept will not suffer. Collectively, these methods are called defense mechanisms. The following defense mechanisms are among those most frequently used.

1. *Denial* of the existence of pain, displeasure, or sadness, particularly when it poses a threat to the individual or his environment, is one mechanism. Thus, an operation will not hurt, although past experience has proven otherwise; a love affair is really secure, even in the face of mounting evidence to the contrary; and there is no threat of a thermonuclear war, in spite of enlarging stockpiles and increasing world controversies.

2. *Displacement* of emotional reactions onto an innocent person or object is another defense mechanism. The golfer who breaks his golf

clubs, the teacher who displays hostility toward his students as a result of an argument at home, and the irate motorist who is releasing tensions built up in the office are such examples.

3. *Compensation,* which is used to conceal an inadequacy by developing a superiority which overshadows it, is a third device. The successful businessman who has been a failure as a husband and father is representative of this method of coping with unpleasant realities. There are probably many cases of unusual achievement which involved the employment of this mechanism.

4. *Identification,* in which a person seeks to reduce anxiety and tension by assuming the characteristics of a threatening opponent or one in authority, is also used. An example of this is the corporal who takes on the attitude and disposition of his drill instructor and, thus, may show undue strictness and harshness to his platoon.

5. *Projection* of one's own inacceptable impulses and feelings to other people is another mechanism. An individual who harbors ill feelings toward other people may feel that similar feelings are harbored by these people in return. This individual, then, sees his own weaknesses in other people; he may take offense when none is intended and develop a persecution complex. Projection can lead to rather severe distortions of reality.

6. *Provocative behavior* can be an extension of projection. An individual who harbors strong and unacceptable feelings toward other people may set up his defense by actually provoking these people to be hostile toward him. In this way, his original feelings are justified. The person with a constant chip on his shoulder is an example, as well as the one who persists in testing the affection and tolerance of his friends.

7. *Rationalization* is perhaps the most commonly used and most familiar of all of the defense mechanisms. Through this method, an individual can provide an explanation which is acceptable to himself when he has failed or has acted unwisely. All people at one time or another deceive themselves about the real reasons for their actions or inactions. Thus, a person may be late because the traffic was too heavy, fail an examination because the professor was too unreasonable, or do poorly at a given task because he did not have the time.

8. *Reaction formation* is the act of trans-

persecution complex. Projection can lead to lating anxiety-provoking impulses or fears into just the opposite of those which the individual is trying to conceal from himself. Thus, a soldier who fears death may perform extraordinary feats of heroism; a person with repressed cruelty may exhibit an exaggerated concern for others; and the hostile individual may show overpoliteness and deference or he may be extremely humble and submissive.

9. *Regression* is a form of defense mechanism in which the individual reverts to a form of behavior which was satisfactory in an earlier situation. Examples of this may be the person who has completely recovered from an illness but resumes the helplessness of the past week when he was cared for or the older person who may cry helplessly and assume other characteristics of a child when under certain circumstances of stress.

10. *Repression* of thoughts, feelings, and wishes from conscious awareness is perhaps the most fundamental of all of the defense mechanisms. Events sometime occur which are so disturbing to the self-concept that the individual cannot stand to remember them. By driving these memories into the subconscious, the person avoids conscious conflict with the image that he holds of himself, but the repressed material may reappear in dreams or slips of the tongue. Also, repressed material does not always remain in the subconscious. As it is about to emerge into consciousness, the person experiences deep anxiety or guilt without knowing the reasons for these feelings.

11. *Self-depreciation* is an attitude which is sometimes assumed by persons who cannot cope with mixed feelings (ambivalence) toward those whom they love. Many people do not understand that small quantities of irritation, hostility, and negative feelings usually accompany the stronger feelings of love. A mother, for example, feels that she should love her children and cannot tolerate feelings of animosity against them. The same may be true in any family situation between husbands and wives or children and their parents. Failure to cope with this conflict or to repress such irritation and hostility can result in turning such feelings inward upon oneself. The consequence is self-depreciation, often accompanied by depression and apathy.

12. *Sublimation* is the process of translating an unacceptable impulse into a form of

behavior or attitude that is approved by society and is acceptable to the self-concept. Working off anger and frustration through physical exercise and performing community social service work in answer to the need and desire for attention and affection are examples of this type of defense mechanism. The individual who channels his antisocial feelings of hostility and violence into the socially acceptable outlets of military combat, bodyguard, or prizefighter has found a reasonable compromise.

### Escape Mechanisms

Some of the defense mechanisms may require reinforcement and methods which were once suitable may not be effective when used in later life. As the loads of modern living become even more burdensome, the defense mechanisms may not be adequate and the individual may find it necessary to seek still other devices to lessen the strain. Thus, he employs escape mechanisms, frequently in conjunction with his defense methods. An escape mechanism may take the form of sleeping for prolonged periods each day. If the individual is otherwise healthy but sleeps 10 to 14 hrs. without getting "caught up," there is a strong likelihood that this person is attempting to escape from pressures or unresolved conflicts. Another escape mechanism is the constant pursuit of social activity, with bridge games, parties, constantly changing love affairs, and the seeking of new friendships. The person who plays too much tennis or golf and who must be constantly entertained by movies or television is displaying the fact that he cannot be alone with himself and his inner thoughts.

It is significant that all of the defense and escape mechanisms involve some distortion of reality. These unconscious mechanisms, when used in moderation, are within the bounds of normalcy and provide safety valves. While they are often useful in protecting the individual from intolerable anxiety, they do restrict the freedom of the personality. When persons become dependent upon such mechanisms instead of developing more healthy and efficient methods of coping with emotional problems, increasingly serious trouble is indicated.

### Stress

One of the most universal characteristics of living organisms is the tendency to maintain a relatively constant physicochemical equilibrium within the body (homeostasis). In an effort to keep this delicate balance, compensatory changes are initiated in response to any physiological strains or pressures, whether induced by external environmental hazards or inner, psychic conflicts. Biochemical analysis of the stress syndrome demonstrates that homeostasis depends mainly upon two types of reactions, termed syntoxic and catatoxic. The catatoxic response, mainly an alarm reaction, stimulates the production of destructive enzymes which usually accelerates the metabolic degradation of the body. Syntoxic stimuli apparently act as tissue tranquilizers, creating a state of passive tolerance which promotes a type of symbiosis or peaceful coexistence with aggressors.[19] Thus, if emotional disturbances are not too severe, adaptations go on quietly as a part of general life processes and no harmful homeostatic imbalances prevail. Such adaptations may be unconscious defenses and escape mechanisms as well as compensatory physiological changes. When a person cannot adequately cope with his problems, however, either because the conflicts are too great or he is lacking in adequate resources, the damaging effects may be of such intensity or duration that homeostasis is not achieved and both biological and mental harms result.

Stress, then, is defined as a harmful condition resulting from the inability of the organism to maintain an adequate internal equilibrium. When emotional stress becomes too great, symptoms of mental illness may result. Typically, the attention of the individual centers less on what he is doing and more on himself and his unpleasant feelings. He is less able to learn, think, find new solutions to his problems, and see things objectively. He narrows and makes safe the world in which he lives. The important thing to note is that, when stress continues, impaired functioning always results.[20] A person becomes less able to deal realistically and constructively with people, conditions, or tasks.

No organism can maintain itself indefinitely in a state of alarm. If it can survive in the presence of the stressful stimulus, it passes from a state of alarm into a state of adaptation or resistance. Emotional stressors usually provoke a nonspecific pattern of systemic adaptation which increases resistance to damage, as such. The endocrine system is of paramount importance in these adjustments and alterations

separating the various progressive states of mental disorders. In other words, as an individual departs from normalcy there are very few categories of black and white into which he can be placed. Rather, there are varying shades of gray, which represent mixtures of symptoms ranging from normal behavior to those of a severely disturbed patient.

For this reason, it is fallacious to label prematurely a person as neurotic or psychotic or to assign this individual to various sub-classifications within the major groups of mental illness. Indeed, many psychiatrists and psychologists are now classifying their patients according to the patterns exhibited at the time of examination rather than following the classical procedure of grouping patients by the common final clinical picture. The American Public Health Association, in its book on control methods in mental disorders, has strengthened the more definitive classification.[21] In this publication, the emphasis is placed upon the syndromes which are displayed by the patients, and include the following: confusional syndrome, chronic tension state, depressive state, manic syndrome, paranoid syndrome, and severe anxiety syndrome with panic.

## Characteristics of Neurotic Individuals

Whatever the classification, it is recognized that persons with emotional problems and unresolved conflicts may assume certain characteristics which are generally associated with neurotic individuals. For example, these people experience feelings of fear, anxiety, and depression without knowing why. This sometimes makes them fear that they are becoming insane. The worries, tensions, and emotional discomforts are usually exaggerated, continual, and of long duration, or they are not realistic. These emotional disturbances prevent the neurotic individual from reacting to his best interests. They interfere with his work and his ability to get along with people. Personality disturbances such as excessive timidity, shyness, irritability, or melancholia may characterize the individual.

Neurosis, then, is a state of tension or irritability in which the personality remains more or less intact. It is a mental disorder of a functional nature and is generally classified as a less serious mental illness. The person is still "in touch with reality" but cannot function effi-

ciently because too much has been repressed and driven out of the range of his conscious control. These repressed feelings and impulses keep the individual so busy protecting himself that he has not sufficient time or energy left for solving real life problems. He is self-centered, anxious, and pessimistic and may display utter lack of control over his emotions.

## Varieties of Neuroses

A neurotic person may exhibit a variety of symptoms which indicate that he is unable to react normally to life situations. These symptoms vary in degree and in the extent to which they lower efficiency, but they are of such a nature that it is evident that the individual needs help in resolving emotional conflicts upon which such symptoms are based.

### Anxiety Neurosis

Chief among the symptoms of neurosis is anxiety, which occurs when repressed material threatens to reassert itself. The person experiences episodes of anxiety which may vary from mild uneasiness to panic. Sometimes this anxiety is manifested by physical signs such as sweating, dizziness, diarrhea, labored breathing, or angina-type pains. The individual may feel extremely tense and irritable and may awaken during the night in a state of terror. The characteristic feeling is one of anxious apprehension, as if something dreadful is about to happen, but there is no idea what the dreadful thing might be.

### Conversion Hysteria

This is so called because the emotional conflict is converted into a physical symptom. Although there is no actual physical damage like that found with psychosomatic reactions, the symptom which is not real in one sense is certainly real to the patient. The victim suddenly develops a tremor or a paralysis or becomes blind or deaf. A common form of conversion hysteria is loss of sensation in some anatomical portion of the body. The person actually feels nothing when pins are stuck into these areas, even though his nerves are intact. Frequently, the loss of sensation is not even anatomically possible since a section of one nerve might be "dead" while other sections beyond the "dead" area remain sensitive.

Sometimes these symptoms are temporary and disappear as mysteriously as they came, but usually extensive therapy is indicated. Disappearance of the symptom does not necessarily indicate that the problem has been solved and symptoms may appear again unless the underlying emotional conflict is disclosed and resolved.

### Hypochondria

This type of neurosis is of particular interest to allied medical personnel because of the heightened prospect of encountering this condition in daily practice. In hypochondria, the disorders of the mind are expressed through a preoccupation with body functions or organs. The patient is either abnormally afraid of disease or believes that he is suffering from a physical ailment. Body sensations such as vague abdominal discomfort, fatigue, or minor temperature changes assume monumental proportions. Even though the patient may well be in the range of physical normalcy, merely telling him that he has no cause for alarm will not cure the hypochondriacal attitude.

A hypochondriac is sometimes described by physicians as a person who cherishes his ailments and enjoys poor health. Giving up hope that he will be accepted as a worthy individual for his own personal qualities and accomplishments, such a patient seeks to obtain social attention and acceptance by presenting a recital of his symptoms and complaints. Illness becomes a kind of retreat, with a logical explanation for shirking responsibility. The patient can be waited on by friends and family and can get attention from doctors, nurses, pharmacists, and other health professionals. Typically, the hypochondriac can expect very little relief from medications, since he can always imagine new symptoms and other diseases.

With the increase in patient load and the shortage of health manpower, there is a tendency to show little or no sympathy for patients who complain of non-organic symptoms and ailments. The hypochondriac, however, needs special consideration, sympathetic understanding, and psychotherapeutic interviews to help avoid unnecessary surgery and medications. Without this help, such a patient may wander from doctor to doctor until he eventually seeks out an unscrupulous quack who will at least listen to his problems.

### Neurasthenia (Nerve Weakness)

In this condition, a person usually exhibits signs of extreme fatigue. The fatigue is not due to physical exertion and is largely a product of the patient's imagination. The patient honestly may feel too tired or weak to get out of bed or even to express coherent thoughts. This individual can sleep for periods that would be impossible for a normal person or he can simply lie for hours doing nothing. Yet, he is not physically ill and resting does not cure him. Once the emotional problems are resolved, however, this person can resume scheduled activity, sleep his normal 6 or 8 hr., and awake refreshed.

### Neurotic Depression

Other common neurotic responses are chronic depression and grief, sometimes reaching the point of melancholia. Patients suffering from these depressions feel helpless because of a loss that they might have sustained or perhaps even a change in their life's pattern. Their low self-esteem convinces them that they can never cope with such tragedies or radical changes. In the early stages of depression, there may be simply apathy and indifference. Later, other symptoms are experienced such as hopelessness, self-depreciation, embitterment, regret, slowing of mental and emotional processes, and suicidal impulses. These neurotic depressions are so closely aligned with feelings of inadequacy and insecurity that they can be precipitated by events which well-adjusted people accept as every-day living experiences.

Each year in the U S., approximately 125,000 people are hospitalized for depressive symptoms, and another 200,000 are treated as outpatients. These figures probably represent only a small fraction of those who actually suffer from this condition. It is estimated that from 4 to 8 million people in the United States currently may be in need of professional help to relieve their depressive illnesses.[22]

### Obsessive-Compulsive Neurosis

An obsession is an irrational idea that keeps thrusting itself into the consciousness despite attempts to keep it out. Obsessions are generally disguised expressions of repressed impulses. If the obsession is persistent and strong enough, it can serve as an irrational urge or a compulsion for the person to perform some apparently meaningless action without knowing why or without necessarily wanting to do it. Only by performing this action repeatedly can the individual keep his anxiety within bounds.

The most common compulsions are counting or avoiding cracks in the sidewalk, touching wood, and throwing salt over one's shoulder. These actions serve as a type of ritual and an appeal to magical powers. The normal person performs such actions as a joke, because he has been told that they would bring him luck. It is no joke, however, to the victim of such a neurosis. This person performs his rituals because he is extremely insecure.

Other common compulsions include repeated washing of hands, excessive dusting of furniture, arrangement of objects in a room with exaggerated care, and performance of rituals associated with bathing. Most compulsions involve meticulous care in some form or another.

*Phobias*

A phobia is a special form of obsession that involves a persistent, unreasoning fear of objects, situations, or locations which contain no source of fright for the average person. Examples are fear of high places or fear of being confined in restrictive quarters. Some psychologists believe that a phobia is based upon guilt. The victim feels that because he was bad some punishment is inevitable. The essential mechanism in the formation of a phobia is said to be displaced anxiety or repressed impulse. The anxiety or impulse which developed during a particular emotional conflict has been displaced from its original source to an external object or situation that is directly related. Thus, the feared object is apparently in some way symbolic of the repressed impulse or anxiety. Phobias are far more common than is generally realized and can be found even in the most brilliant and creative people.

## Psychoses

The term psychosis was once used to identify any type of mental disorder, regardless of source or intensity. This influence can be seen in medical nomenclature. Thus, a patient exhibiting an emotional disturbance which is characterized by anxiety, restlessness, and depression may be described as possessing an "anxiety psychosis." Confusion of the mind which is caused by infection and exhaustion of the patient is referred to as "febrile psychosis." "Involutional psychosis" is a syndrome involving a mental disturbance which is associated with the menopause or with old age. "Toxic psychosis" is a confusional state caused by poisons, drugs, or autotoxemia and a "situation psychosis" is a transitory emotional disorder in a predisposed person which is caused by a seemingly unbearable situation.

More recently, the use of "psychosis" has been reserved for the more serious mental illnesses; the legal term for these collective conditions is insanity. The individual with a psychosis appears to be out of touch with reality to some degree. In severe cases, this patient may live in his own private world, not seeing or hearing anything that goes on about him. Characteristically, he may possess one or a combination of three typical symptoms commonly identified with psychoses: delusions, hallucinations, and distorted emotions.

Delusions are false beliefs that persist in spite of evidence to the contrary. A person may actually believe that he is Napoleon or one of the famous kings. Representing some of these great names in history, the individual may conduct himself accordingly and expect to be treated as befits his assumed exalted station in life. Other delusions are associated with a belief that the individual is being persecuted or spied upon or that someone is attempting to gain control of his thoughts.

Hallucinations refer to seeing, hearing, or smelling things that have no existence outside the victim's own mind. Smelling smoke and suspecting a fire, having the visual imagery of multicolored and distorted landscapes or portions of the anatomy, and hearing bells, music, or distant voices are typical examples. Although hallucinations are products of the imagination, they are very real to the person experiencing them and the individual reacts accordingly.

Distorted emotions may involve underreaction, overreaction, or an inappropriate reaction. Thus, a person may make no attempt to protect himself when confronted with a life-threatening situation; he may wander around aimlessly instead of trying to escape from a burning building. When presented with news of a tragic loss of a loved one, the individual may smile and remain in a happy frame of mind. A mild stimulus which would evoke little or no response in a normal person could cause a wildly excitable reaction in a psychotic patient.

*Causes of Psychoses*

It is generally recognized that psychogenic factors such as apparently unsolvable conflicts or unconscious threats to the self-concept are causes of a significant portion of mental illnesses. A psychosis, therefore, may represent the culmination and progression of neuroses. There are, however, numerous other conditions to which the causes of mental illness may be attributed.

Infectious diseases such as syphilis, rubella in the first trimester of pregnancy, or various types of encephalitis arising from pertussis, mumps, rubeola, poliomyelitis, pneumonia, diphtheria, scarlet fever, chickenpox, or meningitis may be causative factors. The resultant brain abscesses, lesions, and inflammations commonly precipitate mental illnesses.

Nutritional deficiencies may also be involved. Pellagra, for example, can eventually affect the brain. Avitaminoses and chronically unbalanced diets may play a significant role. In addition, a form of mental deficiency known as cretinism can occur because sufficient quantities of iodine have not been administered to assure proper thyroid function. Other causes may be toxic chemical substances such as lead, large quantities of sodium bromide, bacterial toxins, food infested with ergot, and excessive amounts of alcohol. Brain tumors, persistent anemia, arteriosclerosis, birth trauma, damaging head wounds, and genetic aspects such as the development of galactosemia and phenylketonuria are additional factors which can cause mental illness.

*Functional Psychoses*

Functional psychoses are those which have not been attributed to any physical cause. Since no anatomical lesions or chemical toxins have been disclosed to explain the symptoms, these conditions are said to arise from psychological trauma or biochemical lesions. Representative of the functional psychoses are such diseases as schizophrenia, manic-depressive states, and paranoia.

*Schizophrenia.* The term schizophrenia denotes a split personality or separation of intelligence from emotion. The prevalent notion of a Dr. Jekyll-Mr. Hyde switch in character, however, is not an accurate description of the disorder. Formerly called dementia praecox (early loss of mind), the disorder usually manifests itself during the younger years of life. If an individual has not developed this condition before the age of 33, it is unlikely that he will ever suffer from it. Schizophrenia is by far the most prevalent of all the psychoses. Half of the beds in mental hospitals are now occupied by schizophrenic patients and it is estimated that 2 per cent of the population will have an episode of this disorder some time during their lives.[2][3]

Schizophrenia is a complex disorder and affects all aspects of an individual's personality. It is expressed differently in different people, and within a single individual its characteristics may vary and change. The condition is characterized by unusual realities, hallucinations, fear and loneliness, and disordered thinking. A person does not *have* schizophrenia as he might have a stomach ulcer or a head cold. He *is* schizophrenic; he *is* the disorder and it pervades his entire being. Typically, the condition manifests itself slowly. The patient becomes more and more listless and eccentric and he draws away from reality into a dream world. He reacts to an ordinary situation in a variety of unusual ways; he shows bizarre behavior, deviations from normal emotional response, and evidences of vagueness or incoherence in thought processes. There is usually a lack of attention to personal appearance and hygiene. Some patients may hear voices, develop delusions, demonstrate a violent rage, or exhibit a trance-like withdrawal. In extreme cases, the victims of this disease attempt to retreat from all contact with the world. They assume a hunched-up position, as if they were reverting to the isolation of the womb. They are helpless and completely unresponsive. Since schizophrenia is the leading mental illness for which patients are institutionalized, it is unfortunate that this disease must be treated without knowledge of its fundamental cause. The results of recent investigations, however, have provided considerable promise that the cause of this disease may be detected within the foreseeable future and that methods can eventually be developed to prevent or to treat this affliction effectively. For example, workers have established a positive link between non-paranoid schizophrenia and the presence of a mescaline-like substance known as dimethoxyphenylethylamine, which is a dimethylated derivative of dopamine. This substance was found in the urine of schizophrenic patients, but not in control groups. At present, it is theorized that schizophrenics excrete dimethyoxyphenylethylamine not because their bodies manufacture it, but because some inborn biochemical defect prevents them from breaking it down. Such a substance could be involved in producing some of the characteristic reactions in schizophrenia.[24] Investigators at Tulane University have gathered considerable evidence which indicates that some cases of schizophrenia may involve a disorder of the body's immune system. A substance which was found in the blood of schizophrenics is reported to be an antibody, produced within the body, that attacks nerve cells in the brain. Other investigators contend that there is a familial relationship and state that there is strong evidence to support a genetic hypothesis of schizophrenia's origin.[25]

Schizophrenia is one of the more difficult of the mental disorders to treat successfully, although favorable response frequently has been obtained through the use of psychotherapeutic drugs. Some clinicians support the use of "megavitamin" therapy, employing the use of large doses of various vitamins, particularly nicotinic acid. There is no clear-cut evidence, however, that these drugs are of any particular value in the treatment of acute or chronic schizophrenia.[26] In fact, it is reported that large doses of nicotinamide may cause major hepatic damage.[27] Early diagnosis and treatment of any mental condition are extremely important, but particularly so with schizophrenia. With this disorder, the chances of recovery appear to be closely related to the duration of the condition.

*Paranoia.* Paranoia is a disease associated with undue and extreme suspicion and a progressive tendency to regard the whole world in a framework of delusions. The individual suffering from this affliction takes on a persecution complex and may be convinced that he is surrounded by enemies. Paradoxically, this person may act and sound deceptively normal, although he is very ill. He may demonstrate logical reasoning and adequate memory, while concealing his confusion, false premises, and impaired judgment.

The affliction of paranoia usually develops between the ages of 30 and 50 and is found more commonly among people who have a history of self-centeredness, jealousy, and suspicion. The paranoid becomes increasingly deluded and sees hidden meanings to support his conviction that he is the victim of a plot. He is liable to brood in a state of heightened sensitivity to a point where he misjudges even the most casual remark made by others. Because the paranoid believes that he is being persecuted, he feels quite justified in performing antisocial acts and may strike back at those he believes to be his enemies. This type of an individual is a hazard to society. To neglect medical and psychiatric care for such a patient is to permit the dangerous possibilities of needless damage to property and serious assault on others.

*Manic-Depressive Psychosis.* This disease is sometimes referred to as an alternating insanity because of the extremes of emotional feelings which are experienced. Manic-depressive reactions are principally the results of disturbances of emotion and mood rather than of thought processes. Usually, there is a rhythmical nature of these states of mania and depression, separated by a period of normalcy.

During the manic stage, the person is hyperkinetic. His energy seems boundless and he has an exaggerated feeling of elation and well-being. He may dash about, talking gaily and wildly for many hours without sleep or rest, and is so energetic that he may collapse in exhaustion if allowed to continue without restraints or sedatives. Flights of ideas, usually grandiose and irrational, are often experienced during this period.

The depressive stage is characterized by melancholia and an equally exaggerated and groundless misery. The patient tends to feel worthless and guilty, often over trivial or imagined faults or errors. He is convinced that he and the world are doomed and that all is hopeless. In severe depressions, the patient rarely speaks, has no appetite, shows difficulty in thinking, and may retire from normal modes of living into a state of physical and mental inactivity. Such severely afflicted depressives rarely attempt suicide, as if even that were too much of an effort. Less severe depressives, however, are almost always suicidal threats and are hazards to themselves. In this depressed state, the victims are miserable and wish for death, which they sometimes seek very cleverly. During such periods of depression, the patients require close supervision and should be given the utmost protection.

There is increasing evidence that these depressive states are accompanied by alterations in the sympathetic and endocrine systems of the body. Some studies have shown that the role of both norepinephrine and serotonin are altered in depressive illness. Other workers emphasize the common occurrence of major depressions in certain endocrine abnormalities. Representative of this group are hypothyroidism, hypo- or hyperfunction of the adrenal cortex, and major transitions in female sex hormones as found in premenstrual, postpartum, and menopausal conditions.[28] Certainly, as more work is being done in this field and the information continues to be synthesized from the multiple research projects, there is even greater hope that the efforts to combat these illnesses will become increasingly successful.

## MENTAL RETARDATION

### Introduction

Mental retardation is a condition characterized by subnormal intellectual development. It is an impairment of the mind or intellect and is not classified as a disease or illness. The term mental retardation does not delineate a single entity, but rather comprises a group of varied syndromes resulting from many causes and having many ramifications. The American Association on Mental Deficiency has adopted the following definition for this condition: "Mental Retardation refers to the significantly subaverage general intellectual functioning existing concurrently with deficits in adaptive behavior, and manifested during the developmental period." In less technical terms the mentally retarded person is one who, from childhood, develops consistently at a below average rate and experiences unusual difficulty in learning, social adjustment, and economic productivity.[29]

This definition places emphasis on aberrations that occur before the completion of growth and development, which interfere with learning ability and social adequacy. It, therefore, excludes mental deficiency acquired in adult life and also excludes those conditions in which intelligence may be masked by illness or reactions of emotional, drug-induced, psychiatric, or epileptic natures. For a vast majority of the mental defectives, over 90 per cent, the condition was present either at birth or within the first two years of life and, in over 95 per cent of the cases, it occurred before the fifth year.

The prevalence of mental retardation is about 3 per cent of the population. On this basis, it is estimated that there are well over 6 million mentally retarded individuals in the United States. The condition is four times more common than rheumatic heart disease and nine times more prevalent than cerebral palsy. It affects 15 times as many people as total blindness. One out of every 10 people in the United States has a direct involvement with the problem by virtue of having a mentally retarded person in the family. Slightly more than 100 thousand babies born each year, statistically, are destined to be regarded as mentally retarded. These persons are found among every race, religion, and nationality; every educational, social, and economic background.

The concept which is held about mental retardates at any one time has a profound effect upon the type of treatment and the quality of care which are afforded the individuals so classified. Historically, mental retardation has been viewed, for the most part, as a static, unchanging, and incurable condition. The idea of "once retarded, always retarded" has led, over the years, to the general practice of providing only humane treatment. Until recently, there has been little hope that the afflicted individuals could be improved enough to participate in the competitive world of employment and responsible community activity. It also had been accepted generally that if a person was retarded at all he was retarded in each specific area of human functioning. With this philosophy, it is hardly surprising that little effort was made in attempts to improve the performance of the mentally retarded.

### Classifications of Mental Retardation

Mental retardation is classified by various means, according to the objectives sought.

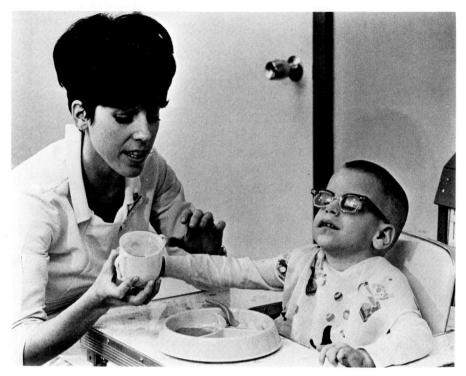

Fig. 8.1. This young boy, a "rubella syndrome" child, was born mentally retarded because his mother had German measles during her first three months of pregnancy. Syndrome children may also be born crippled, with cataracts, heart malformations, small head size and blood disorders. He is being treated at the Child Development Center of the Texas Children's Hospital in Houston, Texas. (Photo Courtesy of Merck Sharp & Dohme, Division of Merck & Co., Inc.)

Thus, mental deficiency can be classified by intelligence quotient (IQ), educational and social prognoses, etiology, clinical criteria, or specific syndromes. It must be recognized that classifications are man-made, however, and cannot accurately fit the natural phenomena of continuous conditions.

*Intelligence Quotient*

This arbitrary method of intelligence evaluation is based upon the results of specially constructed tests that usually have been standardized on the general population. The results of these tests, when properly scored and graded, indicate the individual's level of performance or mental age (MA). In determining a ratio IQ, the MA is compared with the child's actual or chonological age (CA). MA divided by CA and multiplied by 100 gives the IQ, which for a normal, active child, is 100. If a child eight years of age makes an intelligence test grade equal to that of a six-year-old child, the IQ would be MA/CA $\times$ 100, or 6/8 $\times$ 100 = 75. This child would be classified as a borderline mental defective. In determining a deviation IQ, the results of subtests (such as the Weschler Intelligence Scale for Children or the Weschler Adult Intelligence Scale) are used as bases of computation. Based upon such a classification, children with an IQ ranging from 90 to 109 are termed "average." Those with IQ's from 110 to 139 are "superior" and the "genius" category is 140 and above. Children having an IQ of between 80 and 89 are classified as "low normal" and all those registering IQ's of 79 and below are listed as being mentally defective. Those with IQ's ranging from 53 to 79 are listed as "mild" retardates. Within this classification the "borderline" mental defectives have IQ's ranging from 70 to 79, while those who were formerly classed as "morons" have an IQ somewhere between 53 and 69. The "moderate" group possesses IQ's ranging from 36 to 52 while the "severe" defectives, formerly called "imbeciles," are in the 20 to 35 IQ range. The lowest classification, the "profound" group (formerly termed "idiots"), are those with an IQ below 20.

*Educational and Social Prognosis*

The purpose of this classification is to separate children into the special training categories of those who can benefit from the average education facilities and those who may need special training. In addition, this classification also gives some idea of the eventual category in which the child will be able to compete. For these purposes, children with an IQ of 120 or above are termed "superior." Other categories in this classification relate to the previous IQ scale and are divided into sections such as "normal," "educable," "trainable," and "non-trainable." Presumably, all but the normal group need special facilities for education.

The term "exceptional children" now generally refers primarily to those who are mentally below average. With proper educational and vocational training, many of these children may be rehabilitated into normal society and may obtain jobs on farms or as semiskilled laborers. Indeed, for certain types of routine factory or assembly line work, these people are much better suited and will not be as likely to become bored with monotonous work.[30]

There are certain disadvantages to these methods of evaluation. It is well recognized that two individuals having the same IQ may have arrived at this score by several different combinations of strengths and weaknesses on specific items within the test. In addition, the quantitative score tells very little about the nature of the mental deficiency, its prognosis, or the rate of intellectual growth of the child. When psychological measurement is used for classification, there can be a tendency to place too much emphasis on this facet of evaluation and not give full recognition to the equally important factors of cultural and social interaction. Another common error is to maintain the same arbitrary grouping, even though the purpose is no longer the same. The reasons for classification change with age, and categories which were appropriate for children may not be appropriate for adults. Thus, the factors differentiating educable and trainable levels can be quite distinct from the factors determining success in an adult workshop or employment situation. Indeed, for the major portion of the mentally handicapped, the ability to hold jobs after maturity is more likely to depend upon behavior and social graces than intelligence.

The more recent four-level classification (mild, moderate, severe, and profound) was chosen in an endeavor to broaden and increase the flexibility of categories. In combining the criteria of measured intelligence and impairment in ability to comply with the expectations of society, this new classification allows for a better balanced judgment and is a more discriminating tool. Within this framework of categories, it is estimated that only 1.5 per cent of the mentally retarded are in the profound group, 3.5 per cent are in the severe group, 6.0 per cent are in the moderate category, and 89 per cent are in the mild group. The 5.3 million retardates in this latter category are considered educable and can achieve social and vocational skills sufficient for self-support.

*Classification by Etiology*

Classification of mental retardation by etiology gives some insight into the various causes of this deficiency. Actually, there are more than 200 diseases and conditions that can cause mental retardation, yet in over 75 per cent of the cases, the exact cause cannot be determined. If the etiology is known, however, it is logical to surmise the pathology and course of the disease.

Etiological classifications frequently are based upon the time of acquisition such as prenatal, natal, and postnatal. Since it is often difficult to decide whether a given brain involvement was due to prenatal or to natal cases, the two groups frequently are combined to form the "congenital" group. Postnatal causes are usually referred to as the "acquired" group. It is estimated that approximately 90 per cent of all mental deficiencies are due to congenital causes.

Prenatal causes of mental deficiency may be genetic or can be acquired *in utero*. Genetic transmission is reported to be the most common cause of mental deficiency, accounting for approximately 50 per cent of all mental retardates. Conditions acquired *in utero* include maternal infections such as rubella, maternal metabolic diseases such as diabetes and toxemia of pregnancy, and maternal ingestion of such drugs as propylthiouracil and anticoagulants. Additional *in utero* conditions may be anoxia due to maternal carbon monoxide poisoning or severe anemia, autoimmune diseases such as Rh sensitization, and non-inherited genetic changes due to excessive X rays during early pregnancy. Natal factors are primarily traumatic and anoxic, associated with abnormal presentations, accidents of delivery, and oversedation. Postnatal causes are primarily infections or trauma such as encephalitis, skull fractures, and cerebral hemorrhage. Malnutrition, particularly protein and calorie deficiency, is reported to have a detrimental effect due to nutritional deprivation on actual growth of brain cells.[31] Also in this acquired group are the children of neglect. It has been demonstrated that a child can be classified as mentally retarded only because he exists in an environment where physical and emotional needs are ignored, where the child is not stimulated to react, and where parental affection and attention are withheld. A strong case has been made, however, for separating this latter category into a distinctly different group.[32]

The differential diagnosis between true and pseudo-mental deficiency presents a considerable challenge and requires both knowledge and alertness on the part of the evaluator. Actually, there may be a number of conditions which may make a child with normal intelligence appear to be mentally retarded. For example, sensory defects such as poor hearing or poor vision may make a child unresponsive, physical and nutritional deprivation may interfere with normal performance, and children taking psychotherapeutic drugs may react in a dull and confused manner. Some children may have specific perceptual disturbances, so that they can learn by the visual route but not by the auditory route, and *vice versa.* Also, in some forms of epilepsy, a patient may act as if he were retarded but exhibit perfectly normal intelligence between spells.

A particularly difficult problem presents itself when attempting to evaluate the emotionally disturbed. Hyperactivity, emotional instability, or psychiatric difficulty associated with fears and frustrations may interfere with motivation to learn or co-operate. Conversely, the mentally retarded person, because of frustrating experiences, may also develop emotional and social problems which interfere with learning. This creates a vicious circle. It is important, then, to determine whether the emotional problems are primary and responsible for the apparent mental deficiency or whether the mental deficiency is paramount and is responsible for emotional problems.

## Needs and Care of the Mentally Retarded

Why should allied medical professions and society as a whole be interested in the problem of mental deficiency? There are still a vocal few who maintain that the state should take the mentally retarded into custodial care so that our time, money, and effort can be expended more effectively on normal children. Why should we take issue with this position? The reasons are both moral and economic. The more severe mentally deficient patients comprise only a very small percentage of the total number of retardates and the majority of these victims can learn self-care and respond to training on a minimal basis. These people are, after all, our fellow human beings and they need our help and our understanding no less than those who are handicapped in other ways. To write them off as custodial or crib cases is to deny them the dignity and opportunity to develop and improve. This must not be denied any human being, no matter how limited he may be. It is morally incumbent upon society to provide as pleasant and rewarding an existence as possible to all of its handicapped segments.

Disregarding the humanitarian aspects, however, the proper care of the mentally retarded is an economy in disguise. Very few mentally handicapped persons die prematurely; the remainder usually live out a normal span of life. Approximately 200,000 mentally retarded persons in the United States now receive around-the-clock supervision, training, and care in residential institutions. Institutional care costs taxpayers about $40,000 per bed in construction costs and the yearly maintenance of the retarded may range from $2,000 to $10,000. As a result, the aggregate cost of mental retardation in the United States, including such items as support of schools and residential institutions, subsistence payments made to those disabled by mental retardation, funding of demonstration projects, and support for the 12 mental retardation research centers exceeds 3 billion dollars annually. Once institutionalized, it is difficult for a retardate to be released, partly because programs presently offered by most institutions are not strong or varied enough to offer such rehabilitation.

Experience has shown that when properly trained at least 85 per cent of the mentally retarded can support themselves to some degree and the largest classification of mental retardates, the mild cases, usually can learn vocational work quite readily. Many employers have found that the mentally handicapped, when placed in jobs for which they are trained, make capable, reliable, and efficient workers. Therefore, through the expenditure of a fraction of the amount needed for custodial care, the mentally retarded can receive educational and vocational training which would result in the removal of the majority of these patients from institutions and would also permit them to have gainful employment. In this way, such individuals not only cease to be a burden to the taxpayer, but, in turn, become taxpayers themselves. It has been estimated that the average cost to taxpayers of preparing the retarded for employment is approximately the same amount expended for one year of institutional care.

The needs of the mentally handicapped are manifold, but perhaps the greatest need at the present time is for a change in attitude toward those who are mentally deficient. The way in which we treat the individuals considered to be mentally retarded will have a definite effect upon their development. If our concept of mental retardation is static and if we firmly believe that these people are incurable and treat them accordingly, then we can predict, with a high degree of reliability, that they will definitely be limited in their functioning and their ability to deal with problems. If, however, we expect a great deal more of the mentally retarded and take meaningful steps to emphasize their skills and strengthen their weaknesses, then the outlook and potentials are considerably brighter. By providing the training, the opportunities, and the encouragement through which our expectations can be realized, there is a good possibility that these individuals will function at a much higher level than had ever been anticipated in the past.

A basic need of the mentally retarded is recreation. Through this medium, they can experience success, enjoyment, and a sense of accomplishment. Without a recreational outlet to occupy leisure time, retarded people may become social problems. They become shy, withdrawn, and more dependent upon others, particularly their parents. Other essential needs, as discussed previously, are for special educational and training programs and opportunities for employment.

There has been considerable Federal activity in the field of mental retardation in recent years and each succeeding year sees additional legislative proposals in Congress. The Office of the President of the United States has established significant leadership in this endeavor. Starting with the Report of the President's Panel on Mental Retardation in 1962, followed by the President's message to Congress on mental health and mental retardation in 1963 and the establishment of the President's Committee on Mental Retardation in 1966, a framework and blueprint have been established. This has played a major role in the formulation of a comprehensive mental retardation program that shows promising evidence of being responsive to the various needs. For example, special classes for the retarded are reaching 1 million persons, approximately 45,000 mentally retarded people are employed through the Federal-state vocational rehabilitation program, there are approximately 2500 sheltered work shops in the United States which accept mentally retarded clients, several hundred specialized diagnostic clinics have been established, and newer programs providing day care for children of school age and activity centers for severely handicapped adults are being established on an expanded basis. It is recognized, however, that less than one-half of the mentally retarded are having their needs met through these programs. Much remains to be done. Similar to other problems in this category, mental retardation is much more than a medical problem. The fields of education, employment, and social welfare are also areas of cooperative endeavor employed to meet the needs of the retarded. In addition, progress in the prevention of retardation is dependent on advances in programs not directly related to mental retardation. Examples of these programs are adequate general health care for children, adolescent girls, and pregnant women; improvement of education, particularly in early childhood; remedies for poverty through economic progress; and a national scheme of population planning along with genetic counseling.

The bulk of the mental retardation activities of the Federal Government is located in the Department of Health, Education, and Welfare and virtually every service and office of this department have functional programs. Significant activities and contributions are also found in groups outside the Federal Government. Examples of these groups are the Joseph P. Kennedy, Jr. Foundation, the National Association for Retarded Citizens, the Council on Exceptional Children, and the American Association on Mental Deficiency.

## ROLE OF ALLIED MEDICAL PERSONNEL IN MENTAL HEALTH

### Introduction

In the foregoing pages we have discussed the seriousness of the mental health problems and have emphasized the need for more attention and help in this vital area. The mental health program in the United States suffers from many of the ills and obstacles which confront a general medical program.

High on the list of needs are understanding, community acceptance, early screening, referral and information centers, re-evaluation of present techniques, integrated efforts, education, manpower, and facilities. It is true that the Federal Government has become increasingly involved in the fields of mental health and mental retardation and has stimulated considerable interest by encouraging promising programs in various regions of the country. Disregarding political philosophies and loyalties, however, it is fallacious and dangerous to assume that the government is large enough and effective enough to solve all of the problems created within these fields. Regardless of its great size, the capabilities of the Federal Government, even when combined with local and state governments, are actually quite small when compared with all of the resources that are non-governmental in character. Such resources as the allied health professions, voluntary health agencies, religious and educational institutions, hospitals, health programs in organized labor, interested and capable private citizens, business, and industry are all powerful forces that can be applied to reshape and render more effective the mental health and mental retardation programs in this country. Each of these forces, through interest, examination, and application, can make significant contributions toward reducing the frequency and intensity of mental health problems. An example of this is the establishment of Recovery, Inc., originated by a psychiatrist. Recovery, Inc. offers a national program of self-help after-care to former mental patients to prevent relapses.

The allied medical professions, by virtue of their demonstrated concern for others, their experience in working with patients, and their associations with numerous and various segments of the community, are in a position and have the potential for making one of the more meaningful and effective of such contributions. The following suggestions are a few of the many ways in which members of these professions can help to reduce the problems and to promote a more positive mental health attitude.

### Opportunities for Active Involvement

First, become informed. Since there is such a pressing need for understanding and community acceptance, members of the allied medical professions should become informed of the more recent developments in mental health. Once informed, these professional people can serve as sources of information for others, telling the story of mental health and mental retardation and helping to prepare the community for wider acceptance of programs in these fields. It is important to know of the existing problems and methods to handle such problems. A knowledge of Federal, state, and county legislation which affects the mentally ill and an understanding of the concept of the community mental health center is necessary in order to promote positive mental health programs within the community.

Sources of information regarding mental health and mental retardation are numerous. On state and local levels, information can be obtained from health departments, special education divisions of public schools, public welfare agencies, mental health associations, social service agencies, child guidance centers, and associations for retarded children. Information on Federal legislation and programs on a national level can by obtained from sources listed at the end of this chapter. All of these organizations usually welcome inquiries and frequently supply pertinent pamphlets and other materials which explain their programs. These groups are encouraged by the interest and concern shown by those not directly associated with their fields of activity and they will gladly suggest ways in which interested individuals may assist them in their important work.

Materials obtained from these organizations can serve as the nucleus of an information center on mental health affairs. Printed booklets, pamphlets, and leaflets can be placed in pharmacies and waiting rooms of physicians, dentists, hospitals, and medical laboratories. Informed personnel can supplement this printed material by discussing with interested persons the recent developments within their own communities. Other materials such as films and speech outlines furnished by many of these organizations can serve as programs for service clubs and other community groups. In these ways, members of the allied medical professions can help to influence a change in community concepts concerning a very important health problem.

Another way in which allied medical personnel can help is to serve as unofficial primary screeners for those who show evidence of nervous strain and tension. These people are usually less able to resolve their own conflicts and need help. All too frequently, the professionals in the field of psychology are not consulted until the victims have deteriorated to serious levels of disorganization and despair. At this advanced stage, the prognosis for complete recovery is not as promising. There is a great need for early recognition and referral, since timely professional help can often prevent such emotional difficulties from becoming more serious.

Those allied medical personnel such as the pharmacist and the nurse who meet patients directly have an excellent opportunity to render a valuable service in this regard. Because dealing with people is so integrally involved with their daily activities, these professional people soon can learn to recognize signs and symptoms of emotional disturbance. The patient who complains of tension headaches and who frequently asks for something stronger than aspirin, the person who complains of chronic sleeplessness, the husband or wife who complains of marital discord, the parent who talks about delinquent behavior in his child, the patient who visits numerous doctors endeavor-

ing to obtain additional prescriptions for tranquilizing and sedative-type drugs—these are all people who need help.

Through helpful counseling, these people can recognize the fact that a problem exists and usually can be motivated to seek professional guidance. Direct advice giving is of doubtful value and it is equally harmful to become too involved and assume more responsibility than one can handle. Some of these people merely need a sympathetic listener, while others need support so that they will not feel less worthy because they are in trouble or feel that their inability to cope with their problems is a sign of inadequacy. In some instances, it may be fairly obvious that the patient is severely disturbed and needs immediate attention from a trained professional.

Regardless of the need, every community has resources to help, but one of the past difficulties has been the lack of early referrals to these resources. An informed, interested, and concerned body of people in the allied medical professions can do a great deal to lessen the burden which is mounting within this field of mental health. Through the processes of detection, screening, and referrals, these health professionals can be effective and valuable members of the community mental health program.

Still another way in which a significant contribution can be made to the mental health endeavor is to participate actively in the development and implementation of all aspects of mental health planning, both through professional associations and individual involvement. A noteworthy characteristic of recent government programs has been an emphasis upon community participation, citizens' advisory groups, and steering committees made up of interested and informed local citizens. A familiar phrase in planning councils is: "It will be volunteers who will be making the decisions." Here again, allied medical personnel can well be in the forefront of the civic minded people whose daily contacts offer them continuous opportunities to inform themselves and to speak with authority on matters of public importance, particularly as they relate to the public health. These people are needed to encourage and fire the imagination of community health planners and legislators so that mental health programs will be given full consideration.

The various health associations should also be prominent both in the planning and the implementation of mental health programs. The directive from the Federal Government has indicated that all such allied medical associations should be involved, but the chances are quite remote that very many of these associations are represented in community mental health programs. If local allied medical associations do not step forward and participate in matters which so immediately concern them, still another area of responsibility for community affairs will pass from the hands of some of those most qualified to take part in them. This is not a selfish point of view, because the trained professionals are the best qualified to determine how their particular talents can best be utilized in the delivery of health services within the parameters of a community mental health program.

It is important, therefore, for local associations to pass resolutions supporting the concept of community treatment for mental illness, for association presidents to write to the Governor offering consultant services in mental health programs, and for the various associations to work closely with the head of the state mental health division and disseminate information on mental health developments to members through meetings and newsletters. Some of the associations have taken positive steps toward stimulating their members to assume more active participation in mental health programs. For example, the American Pharmaceutical Association House of Delegates has passed a resolution stating that " . . . the Association encourages all pharmacists to participate actively in the development and implementation of all aspects of mental health programs so that the special needs and problems of the mentally ill can be met effectively . . . " These evidences of positive national leadership need to be emphasized at local levels.

However, despite our growing body of knowledge and experience, many of the bases of man's behavior and the mechanisms of his mind remain unknown. We must learn much more about how the brain really works and the roles which certain sections of the brain play in memory, perception, emotions, and personality controls. We must expand our knowledge of the chemistry of the brain, searching out the secrets of its metabolism and the relationship of brain metabolism to mental aberrations and normal mental function. To cope with mental illness and to ensure the mental health which is our goal, we must continually increase our understanding of the whole man. This latter aim demands continuing pursuit of additional knowledge of human behavior and the many physiological, psychological, and sociological factors which determine it.

Information regarding mental health programs on a national level can be obtained from the following sources:

1. The National Association for Mental Health, Inc.
   1800 North Kent Street
   Rosslyn Station
   Arlington, Virginia 22209
2. Department of Health, Education, and Welfare
   330 Independence Avenue, S.W
   Washington, D. C. 20201
3. National Institute of Mental Health
   Barlow Building
   5454 Wisconsin Avenue
   Chevy Chase, Maryland 20015
4. Social Security Administration
   6401 Security Building
   Baltimore, Maryland 21235

The following national offices are sources of information regarding programs in mental retardation:

1. The National Association for Retarded Citizens
   2709 Avenue E., East
   Arlington, Texas 76011
2. Council for Exceptional Children
   National Education Association
   1201 16th Street, N. W
   Washington, D. C. 20005
3. Department of Health, Education, and Welfare
   Washington, D. C. 20045
   a. U S. Office of Education
      Department of Special Education
   b. Children's Bureau
      Welfare Administration
   c. Vocational Rehabilitation Administration
4. Joseph P. Kennedy, Jr. Foundation
   719 13th Street, N W , Suite 510
   Washington, D C. 20005

## REFERENCES

1. Kennedy, J. F. *Mental Illness and Mental Retardation.* Presented at the 88th Congress, 1st Session. House of Representatives Document 58. Washington, D. C., 1963.
2. Feldman, S. *Problems and Prospects: Administration in Mental Health.* DHEW Publication No. (HSM) 73-9050, 1972.
3. *Facts about Mental Illness.* National Association for Mental Health, 1972.
4. *Patient Care Episodes in Psychiatric Services.* Statistical Note 92, Biometry Branch, NIMH, 1973.
5. *Financing Mental Health Care in the United States.* Alcohol Drug Abuse and Mental Health Administration, DHEW Publication No. (HSM) 72-9030, 1971.
6. *Mental Illness and Its Treatment.* DHEW Publication No. (HSM) 72-9030, 1971.
7. *Utilization of Mental Health Facilities.* NIMH, DHEW Pub. No. NIH-74-657, 1973.
8. *Private Mental Hospitals.* NIMH, Series A:10, DHEW Pub. No. (HSM) 72-9089, 1972.
9. *Psychiatric Services in General Hospitals.* NIMH, Series A:11, DHEW Pub. No. (HSM) 72-9139, 1972.
10. Marshall, C. L. *Dynamics of Health and Disease.* New York: Appleton-Century-Crofts, Meredith Corp., 1972.
11. Beers, C. W. *A Mind That Found Itself.* New York: Longmans, Green & Company, Inc., 1908.
12. Windle, C. The impacts of NIMH grants to improve state hospitals. *Health Serv. Rep., 88:* 6, 1973.
13. Gentry, J. T., et al. Provision of mental health services by community hospitals and health departments. *Amer. J. Public Health, 63:* 10, 1973.
14. Joint Commission on Mental Illness and Health. *Action for Mental Health.* New York: Basic Books, Inc., 1961.
15. Brown, B. S. *The Impact of the New Federal Mental Health Legislation on the State Mental Hospital System.* Presented at the Northeast State Governments Conference, Hartford, 1964.
16. Joint Economics Committee of the U. S. Congress. *State and Local Public Facility Needs and Financing,* Vol. 1. 89th Congress, 2nd Session, 1967.
17. Beigel, A., and Levenson, A. *The Community Mental Health Center.* New York: Basic Books, Inc., 1972.
18. Jacobson, G. Emergency services in community mental health. *Amer. J. Public Health, 64:* 2, 1974.
19. Seyle, S. The evolution of the stress concept. *Amer. Scientist, 61:* Nov.-Dec., 1973.
20. Hein, F. V., and Farnsworth, D. L. *Living,* Ed. 4. Chicago: Scott, Foresman and Co., 1965.
21. *Mental Disorders: A Guide to Control Methods.* New York: American Public Health Association, 1962.
22. Medical World News. April 20, 1973.
23. Wienckowski, L. A. *Schizophrenia—Is There An Answer?* DHEW Pub. No. (HSM) 73-9086, 1973.
24. *Research in Schizophrenia.* Mental Health Monograph 4, DHEW Pub. No. (HSM) 72-9016, 1972.
25. Reiss, D. *Competing Hypotheses and Warring Factions: Apply Knowledge of Schizophrenia.* Schizophrenia Bulletin, No. 8, Spring 1974.
26. *The Medical Letter, 15:* 26, 1973.
27. Clin-Alert, No. 24, January 31, 1974.
28. William, T. A., et al. *Psychobiology of the Depressive Illnesses.* DHEW Pub. No. (HSM) 70-9053, 1972.
29. *Facts on Mental Retardation.* National Association for Retarded Citizens, 1973.
30. *America's Needs in Habilitation and Employment of the Mentally Retarded.* The President's Joint Committees on Mental Retardation and Employment of the Handicapped, 1969.
31. Brockman, L. M., and Riccuiti, H. N. Severe protein-calcium malnutrition and cognitive development in infancy and early childhood. *Developmental Psychology, 4:* 3, 1971 (from *Mental Retardation Abstracts, 9:* 4, 1972.
32. Tarjan, G, and Keeran, C. V. Toward accelerated progress in combatting mental retardation. *Pan Amer. Health Org. Bull., 7:* 3, 1973.

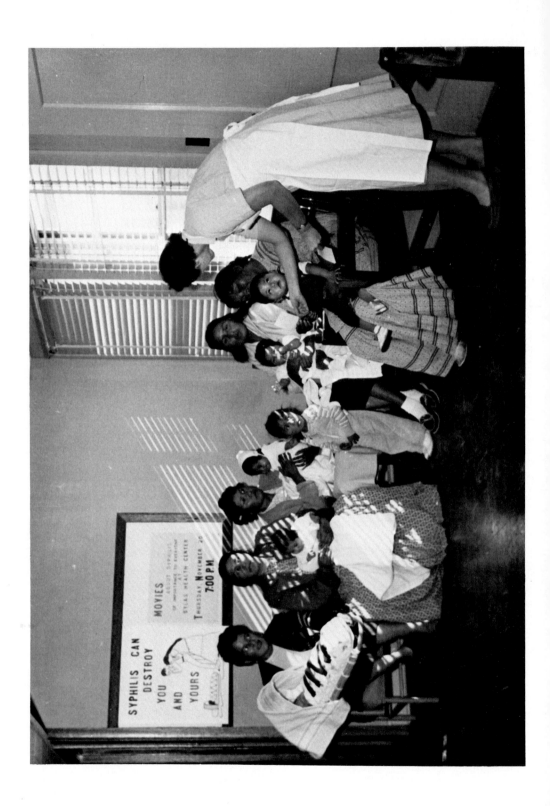

# 9

# Diseases of social origin

We live in a nation where most of the traditional indexes of health are improving, while all around us are the signs of serious illness. The human species is in the midst of an epidemic—a pandemic—of dissatisfaction and maladaptation. And homocide, suicide, accidents, alcoholism, narcotics addiction, and war have moved to the front as causes of death in the productive years of our lives. I do not think we really believe that even such critical mechanisms as prepaid group practice, national health insurance in any form, and training of physician's assistants will bring our nation back to health. I do not think we believe that national health will be restored through air pollution and pesticide control. If we know better than our actions suggest we do, why have we had difficulty putting knowledge into action?

WALTER J. McNERNEY, *Bronfman Lecture*

The citizen of today's industrialized world is confronted with series of paradoxes. He has the opportunity and transportation to live in remote, quiet surroundings and, yet, chooses the noise and confusion and added health problems of the crowded city. He lives in a time when production is at an all-time high, and, yet, the workweek is continually shortening, presenting him with problems regarding proper utilization of leisure time. A significant portion of the serious communicable diseases no longer hold their menacing threat, and, yet, drugs are consumed at a record rate. Modern technology has provided a higher standard of living with material comforts and luxuries never before realized, but people are seeking escape from their modern world along the paths of alcoholism, drug abuse, and suicide at rates which have set new and frightening records.

Modern man not only creates many of his own problems but is the victim of mounting economic and social pressures. As increasing numbers of people congregate in congested cities, as the nerve-wracking pace of competition continues to increase tension and as the social and moral norms continue to decline or remain in a state of flux, the problems resulting from these pressures continue to threaten our social, cultural, and medical equilibrium. Although their causes and origins may be based in the socio-economic aspects of modern living, the results of these turmoils emerge as health problems which affect the entire community.

## SUICIDES

### Introduction

Although all animals can kill and can be killed, only man makes the ultimate decision to kill himself intentionally. The fact of suicide has horrified and fascinated man throughout history. But the tragic and needless loss sustained through this method of taking life has moved the subject of suicide from one of an impersonal, academic discussion to the realm of a public health problem which calls for attention and action among those who have a concern for the welfare of others. There are approximately 22,000 deaths from suicide reported annually in the United States or an average of one such death every 24 minutes.[1] Suicide is the 10th leading cause of death for all age groups and shows evidence of increasing. There are, however, significant variations within this overall average. In the 15- to 19-year-old age group, for example, suicide is the third ranking cause of death whereas in the collegiate age group suicides are exceeded only by accidents in claiming lives. In addition, it must be remembered that these are just the *reported* suicides.

### Legal, Religious, and Moral Aspects

In the United States, suicide is still a crime at common law. Although most states recently have refused to follow this precedent, there are still some states which hold that suicide or attempted suicide is illegal, constituting a misdemeanor or a felony. In all jurisdictions, however, anyone who aids a person in committing suicide is guilty of a punishable offense. Even though the legal implications of suicide have been diminished, the afterglow of the criminal connotation still continues and will be forgotten very slowly.

The religious overtones and sanctions against suicide also influence society's position on this form of death. The Judeo-Christian ethic has instilled in our traditional beliefs that "the Lord giveth and the Lord taketh away," and the judgment of Christianity pronounces that the person who commits suicide is committing a sin. It is quite apparent that, once this sin has been committed, there is no opportunity to ask forgiveness or to seek atonement.

Added to this is the strong feeling held by many in our society that man has a duty to go on living, that he does not have the right to kill himself, and that the act of committing suicide is the act of cowardice. The moral implications are reflected in an Alabama Court of Appeals ruling in 1929 which states that suicide " . . . is a crime involving moral turpitude."[2] Individual reactions toward suicide reflect society's frown of condemnation since the attempt at self-destruction may incite guilt and anger in other persons. This is well illustrated by the report that the attitude of hospital personnel toward a would-be suicide is often overtly hostile and rejecting.[3]

For these reasons, it is known that the actual number of suicides is far greater than those reported. Moral, religious, historical, sentimental, and legal overtones prejudice against suicide to such an extent that there is much concealment regarding the act itself. Thus, it is not uncommon to read that " . . . he died accidentally while cleaning his gun." Other persons, wishing to take their own lives but not wanting to cause friends and relatives additional grief and feelings of guilt, commit suicide in manners that have the true appearance of accidents. These are counted as accidental deaths for statistical purposes. As evidence of this, when the Suicide Prevention Center of Los Angeles and the coroner of that city investigated the psychological histories of persons dying in accidents, it was found that many ostensible accidents turned out to be suicides. Another suggestion of such motives was reported in the findings of a St. Louis County jury which was attempting to learn the cause of rising teenage

traffic deaths. It was found, among other things, that "almost all the subjects had communicated to somebody a desire to end their lives."[4]

Thus, whether the suicide is erroneously reported or is interpreted as an accident, there are considerably more deaths by this method than records indicate. Although men have elected to die at all periods of history, never have so many done so as in the present. Suicide has spread throughout the 20th century. It has been surmised that if a substantial number of suicidal deaths were not otherwise recorded because of religious, social, or moral reasons the annual number of suicides in the United States might actually reach a total of from 50,000 to 60,000.[5]

As suicides increased in number, it was recognized that this was a disease of civilization and was a by-product of pressures and of confusing and rapidly changing times. Most people felt that this disease was a private matter and that "he who wanted to travel should not be detained." Detailed study by a few dedicated men in the fields of medicine and social science, however, revealed that many of these persons did not really wish to travel, that they were using this drastic measure as means of a frantic call for help. It was soon learned that something could be done about suicide, that the potential suicide victim could be recognized, and, through co-ordinated effort, that this cry for help could be answered. It has been only in comparatively recent years that significant attention has been directed toward this problem, that suicide has been recognized as a public health problem, and that government and private health agencies have developed programs in this field.

## Incidence of Suicides

The Vital Statistics Division of the National Center for Health Statistics and the Office of Biometry of the National Institute of Mental Health have gathered information and have analyzed suicide incidence. Although refinements in their programs are planned, they have provided adequate information from which to project a suicide pattern in terms of age, sex, race, marital status, and geographical region. It has been found, for example, that suicides are more frequent in the spring than in any other season, that the rate of suicides in males is approximately three times that of females, and that such deaths are more frequent in the white population than in the non-white. The rates for white males generally increase with successive age groups up through 85 years and over, whereas those for white females reach a peak in the 45- to 54-year age group. Rates for non-white persons are much less and show different and less decided patterns. Geographically, national statistics show that the rate of suicides is highest in the western mountain region and along the Pacific Coast, and, in these regions, the ratio of suicides for males and females is reversed. Nevada has the dubious distinction of maintaining the highest rate. Suicide rates for the Middle Atlantic states are among the lowest in the United States. For those who are concerned with the stress of urban living it is surprising to learn that the rates of suicides in non-metropolitan and rural areas are higher than the national metropolitan rate. As for marital status, the suicide rate is lowest for married persons, slightly higher for single persons, still higher for the widowed, and highest for divorced persons. As a means for committing suicide, firearms are more frequently used, followed by hanging and strangulation. The methods change over the years with an increase noted in the use of automobile exhaust fumes and in overdosages of medications whereas heating and cooking gases are now used less.

Suicidal *attempts,* by comparison, present a different pattern and style. Although there are no national statistics on this topic, it has been reported that eight serious attempts at suicide are made and fail for every one that succeeds. Contrasted to the fact that more males actually commit suicide than females, women are reported to attempt suicide twice as often as men but their rate of completion is considerably lower. The largest number of suicidal attempts are made by people between the ages of 25 and 34, with the next largest number in the 19- to 24-year age group. The incidence drops markedly among people over 35. While older people make fewer suicidal attempts than younger individuals, their attempts more often end fatally.

The popularity of methods used in unsuccessful suicidal attempts also differs. Contrasted to firearms, hanging, and choking, which are the predominant methods used in successful suicides, approximately 70 per cent of the attempted suicides use poisons and drug overdoses. Other methods prominently reported by attempted suicides are body mutilation and gas or auto exhaust.

## Motivation

The results of investigation and of testing hypotheses have provided some basic concepts regarding suicides. For example, leaders in this field of study have stated that the tendency to suicide is a symptom of a hitherto unnamed psychic disease. Rather than genuine mental illness, it is more of a disturbance of mental balance often brought about by unresolved conflicts. It is believed that this disease generally begins in childhood and develops constantly. It is avoidable and its fatal outcome can be prevented. Since there appears to be no conceivable human situation which is unendurable or hopeless enough to drive a healthy person to death, it can be assumed that suicidal patients are ill and are not free in making their decisions to die.

The motivation to attempt suicide is subject to individual variation. As Murphy and Robins state:[6]

The suicidal individual is, after all, primarily an individual. Whatever large sociological trends may predispose him to suicide, there are likely to be some more highly personal factors that are at least necessary, if not sufficient, to bring about the fatal event.

Emotional crises occur from time to time in all lives when people face problems temporarily beyond their ability to solve. If an individual under such stress loses hope and his thinking becomes more distorted and desperate, he is in danger of facing a "suicidal crisis" when suicide is seriously considered. Such a crisis usually passes when the pressures are gone or when the person is somehow able to carry on, but the period is painful and dangerous. Expert help is often desperately needed at this time.

Although the motivations that lead to a suicidal act do not always follow the same pattern, an element of depression is common to the majority of them. By no means do all depressed persons attempt self-destruction but the relationship between depression and suicide is so notorious that professional workers in this field consider it extremely important. Thus, the undermining of confidence and self-esteem may give a susceptible individual the feeling that life is no longer worth living. Men over 40 years of age who are out of work and feel that they are too old to learn a new trade finally have to face the realization that earlier dreams and sought-for goals will never be achieved and, for some of them, life no longer holds any promise or attraction. Women who have reached meno-pause realize that their child-bearing years, their youth, and much of their physical attractive-ness are gone and may feel that they no longer are useful, needed, or wanted. Other people, particularly alcoholics, may attempt suicide because of a lost love or a dead spouse, as an irrational means of being reunited in another world. Others may take their lives as an expiation for past sins and shortcomings, while brooding over illness and prolonged pain is still another precipitating factor.

Young people experience additional prob-lems. Adjustments to the stresses of puberty and of adult living are complex, particularly when one lacks the maturity to find a reasonable solution. Thus, in the heat of anger, disappointment, or frustration, some young people react with impulsive suicidal behavior. Examples of this may be the girl who was not selected by her chosen sorority, the young man disappointed in love, failure in school and the feeling that one is not measuring up to what is expected of him, or the feeling of being pushed beyond endurance by parental pressure. Although these frequently may be only tempo-rary emotional crises, they are recognized as very dangerous situations which could lead to tragedy.

## Recognition of the Potential Suicide Victim

It is now known that, as these severely depressed or desperate people contemplate suicide, the vast majority will signal their preoccupation with self-destruction by words, actions, and symptoms. The old idea that "people who speak of suicide will not commit it" has been refuted. In fact, there is a history of previous, spontaneous, suicidal communica-tions in well over half the suicide deaths.

The thought of suicide is repugnant to most people and when suicidal urges first reach consciousness they may, at first, be disowned and repulsed by the person himself. By the time that the individual gives conscious thought to them and talks of suicide, there is evidence that

he has been harboring these ideas for a long time. It is a mistake, then, to take these statements lightly. Persons who express loneli-ness or a sense of abandonment, who state that their families would be better off without them, or who tell of being tired of living may all be closer to contemplating suicide seriously than most people realize.

Potential suicide patients, particularly victims of depression, frequently display physical symptoms which could serve as signals to the alert observer. The feelings of frustration, inadequacy, guilt, shame, and sadness have an adverse effect on both the autonomic and central nervous systems, as discussed in Chapter 8. Manifestations of this effect may be exhib-ited as insomnia, feelings of self-depreciation, fearfulness, anorexia with weight loss, fatigue, irritability, and loss of interest. In addition, gastrointestinal function may be altered, blad-der function may be speeded up, and blood pressure may fluctuate. Depression takes on a variety of guises in these suicidal risks. Such symptoms as weakness and indecisiveness, diffi-culty with spouse, dizziness, loss of sexual drive, and withdrawal from social contacts are among those commonly listed.

Suicides at any age are sad and a needless loss, but such death among young people present even more of a tragedy. In a study of students who committed suicide in an eastern state, it was found that certain characteristics were prominent. For example, it was determined that suicidal children are often those who do not take part in any of the usual extra-curricular group activities of childhood. Three-fourths of the children who committed suicide were seriously retarded in reading despite average or better intelligence ratings. But the most significant factor was that, in every case of suicide in this study, the child had no close friends.[7] This disclosure is pertinent not only to the suicidal patterns of young people but applies frequently to adults as well. The critical and, literally, life-saving difference between suicide and hope could well be the presence of someone who cared enough to listen, someone with whom to share inner thoughts, and someone to offer help in a time of need. Loneliness is a sickness of our time. It would seem that in the midst of such depersonalizing identities as social security numbers, zip codes, credit card numbers, and computerized state-ments there must be some place for personal relationships, and, yet, there are millions of lonely people throughout our country, particularly in the larger cities and more particularly among the elderly. Man is a social animal and needs the association of other people. Although such association can be supplanted or diverted for short periods, there are times in practically all lives when close companionship is desperately needed. Without this feeling of support in a time of crisis the result could be fatal.

It is true that the majority of people who talk about suicide or even the majority of people who suffer from episodes of depression do not take their own lives, but the incidence of suicides among these groups is far higher than in the normal population. There are additional steps taken by some potential suicide victims which indicate an even stronger purpose and intent. In talking about suicides, for example, these people may discuss the method which they are going to use. Even if done flippantly, these remarks must be taken seriously because they suggest that the potential victim has given considerably more than a passing thought to suicide. The threat becomes even more pronounced if there has been some action toward implementing the stated purpose. For example, the purchase of a gun, the close examination of a tall building, or the collecting of barbiturates gives strong support to a premeditated act. But perhaps the most serious of all is the person who has previously attempted suicide. One suicide attempt greatly increases the likelihood of another. This is usually because the conditions that precipitated the first may still be there to provoke a second. People who have previously attempted to take their own lives are termed "actively suicidal" and it is important that psychological or psychiatric consultation be instituted.

It is equally true that only a portion of potential suicide victims can be positively identified, even by those trained to make such observations. But sufficient progress has been made by investigators and statisticians to show that this is not a hopeless endeavor. By studying trends and specific factors, it can be shown that certain aspects have some frequency in a suicidal population. If these aspects are recognized in advance of the suicide, it is possible that even more effective preventive measures can be employed. By widely disseminating even the present knowledge among members of the allied health professions, therefore, it is very likely that many more suicidal signals would be recognized and many more people would be saved from a tragic and needless death.

## Programs of Suicide Prevention

Based upon the knowledge that the majority of potential suicides actually do not wish to die and will display symptoms or issue a call for help, organizations have been established in several communities to offer service when needed. These organizations have been particularly helpful for the individual who seems to be obsessed with the impulse to die, who wistfully hopes that life can be made livable again, and who realizes that a competent and understanding person can make a life-saving difference at this time of crisis. Seven of the earlier pioneer organizations in this field are located, respectively, in Los Angeles, Salt Lake City, Brooklyn, Worcester, Boston, New York City, and Pinellas County, Florida. Each of these organizations has a history of its own and the resources and methods of operation vary. Religious organizations started some of them whereas others were an extension of emergency psychiatric consultation services. Their common objective, however, is to reduce the toll of suicides. Similar organizations are functioning in Europe. One of the most extensive of such suicide rescue services is the Samaritans, founded in London. It is a highly dedicated volunteer organization and has branches in numerous cities.

Probably the most ambitious of the early programs in the United States was the Los Angeles Suicide Prevention Center. With the aid of a grant from the National Institute of Mental Health, Dr. E. S. Shneidman and Dr. N. L. Faberow established this center and introduced a campaign against suicide in the United States that has had far-reaching results.[8] The members of the professional staff of this center have enriched the medical and psychiatric literature of the world with very valuable books and published papers. Their book, *"The Cry for Help,"*[9] has been one of the most quoted texts in this field. The service which is rendered by this center has set a pattern for similar community services elsewhere. The telephone is a vital instrument. Knowing that a human life may depend upon how a telephone call is handled, the Suicide Prevention Center has developed a philosophy and a procedure for conducting such calls. Patient listening, expert note taking, assessment of the seriousness of the call and of imminent danger, display of sincere interest, and the offering of practical help are all important factors.

Such suicide prevention agencies serve not only as a direct beacon of rescue for potential suicides but offer other community services as well. They are a source of information for other community agencies and for practitioners confronted with special problems. In addition, they serve as a center for therapeutic recommendations and referrals and as a source of research data.

Since suicides have been determined to be a public health matter and since most practitioners agree that the government should help in combatting the disease, the Federal Government has taken definite steps toward organizing programs in this area. Mental Health, for example, has established a center for suicide prevention. The center has five basic functions in support of the development of this nation's capability to prevent suicide. It serves as a focal point to coordinate and direct activities relating to suicide, it compiles and disseminates information and training material, it helps in developing new regional and local programs aimed at reducing suicides, it maintains liaison with suicide programs in other federal agencies such as the Veterans Administration and the Armed Forces, and it serves as a clearinghouse for publicizing results of research conducted by other mental health agencies.

Through the provisions of the Community Mental Health Act there have been established over 200 Suicide Prevention Centers in the United States. Evaluation studies, however, have disclosed no net decrease in numbers of suicides in geographical areas where these Centers are operating.[10] There is a growing feeling among some workers in this field that "... perhaps it is time to redirect the Suicide Prevention Center's functions and goals."[11] Complaints are made that we have disassociated suicide prevention from the bigger arena of society's rejection of the aged, problems associated with retirement, social maladjustment, social isolation, and society's growing disregard for life. Expanded functions of Suicide Prevention Centers are proposed to help combat some of these problems and include programs in active outreach, identification, and follow-up treatment, and intensified community education.

## Assistance by the Allied Medical Professions

In addition to the interest and activities of organized agencies in dealing with the problems of suicide, the contributions which can be made by members of the allied health professions are of inestimable value. Prevention of disease is, assuredly, the new horizon of modern medicine, and this, certainly, should include the disease of suicide. The focus, then, should be placed on recognizing and evaluating potential suicide victims so that they may receive adequate and proper treatment soon enough to abort any drastic actions. It has been reported that approximately 75 per cent of the suicide victims had visited their physicians within six months prior to death. It has not been recorded how many of these victims talked with their pharmacist, their dentist, the doctor's nurse, or others who touched their lives. For those in the allied medical professions who may see these people during the daily routine of practice it is highly important to become more sensitive and reactive to possible presuicidal symptoms. Family, loved ones, and friends are in a position to give emergency assistance but often are too close to the problem to recognize its seriousness or severity. In addition, they may be too emotionally involved in the problem itself to offer much of a solution. Often, a sympathetic listener is all that is required to reduce the tensions and to lessen the chances of attempted suicide. At other times, when cases are recognized as more serious, a frank talk and direct questions are indicated. The answers to these questions plus suspiciously presuicide actions could be the basis for referrals to physicians, psychologists, or suicide prevention centers. Personal interest and a genuine concern are invaluable allies at this time.

It is not enough, then, to recognize that suicides can be prevented through the application of known methods. We must be convinced that suicide rates can be lowered still further by our own personal involvement and by the contributions we make. Without a sensitivity and a concern, we will continue to miss the significant signals of the person contemplating suicide. We will blame our ineptitude on ignorance when, in truth, we know enough to help.

## THE USE AND MISUSE OF ALCOHOL

O God, that men should put an enemy into their mouths to steal away their brains.

SHAKESPEARE *Othello*

### Introduction

Since the time of earliest recorded history, man has used beverages containing alcohol and the consumption of such beverages is still a part of the cultures of both primitive and civilized peoples throughout the world. It is not the author's purpose to take a positive or a negative stand on the discriminate use of alcohol. There are indications that if the use of such beverages had not performed some function this practice would have terminated long ago. Although alcohol affects every organ in the body, it is ingested mainly for its action on the brain. Alcohol is classified as an anesthetic and a depressant, inhibiting the cortical regions first and then the lower areas of the brain. It is to achieve a mild degree of cortical depression, then, that alcohol is used to a large degree. Thus, it serves as a relief from tensions that have built up during the day and, for a significant number of people, secures relaxation before eating a leisurely evening meal. Others, who are far from problem drinkers, feel that a drink before retiring helps to blot out worrisome thoughts so that they need not take their troubles to bed. It is also common practice to serve alcoholic drinks as a gesture of hospitality and to facilitate interpersonal relationships. When used in this fashion, alcoholic beverages present no great health problem.

The indiscriminate use of alcohol, however, is another matter. The accidental deaths and crimes committed while under the influence of alcohol have created social as well as health problems. In addition, the persistent and increased use of alcohol in social situations has made society much more tolerant of the frequent excesses of imbibition. With the lessening of restraints, the borderline between social drinking and problem drinking is not always easy to discern.

When alcohol is taken not as a temporary relief but is used as a substitute for resolving internal and environmental conflicts, the drinker invites further trouble. As this pattern progresses and the individual relies to a continuing degree upon alcohol, there is a distinct danger that such dependency may lead to the beginning stages of alcoholism.

It has been estimated that about six out of every 10 adults in the United States use alcoholic beverages.[1,2] The distribution varies according to age, sex, and geographical location. For example, there are more non-drinkers in the South and, predictably, more drinking in the cities than in rural areas. Persons past middle age do not drink as much as younger people, and men outnumber women drinkers about three to two. Habits of alcohol consumption also vary among religious and ethnic groups.

Drinking among teen-agers appears to be increasing. It is now reported to be a rarity for a young person to graduate from high school without having at least an experimental taste of alcohol. Since most children do not drink and most adults do drink, the majority of young people apparently make the transition in their teen years from abstinence to the drinking patterns characteristic of adulthood. The earliest drinking behavior is reported to occur more likely in the home in the presence and with the approval of adults, usually parents. This drinking under controlled conditions becomes more permissive with the increasing age of the young person. Teen-agers, then, do not invent the idea of drinking. The models and examples have been set for them.

The use of alcohol among young people appears to be quite moderate, and, for the most part, is associated with entertainment, the release of tensions built up from the pressures of school, and the celebration of special events. For a small minority of teen-agers, drinking does appear to get out of hand but for the vast majority alcohol is not the hub around which their lives revolve. Even when they drink frequently and in quantity, young people tend to take reasonable precautions against the consequences of such drinking. Protection is usually provided by peer groups with the result that reports of accidental injury, irresponsible behavior, and antisocial acts are at a relatively low level.

There are evidences, however, that this picture is changing. Currently, significantly more alcohol is being consumed by young people than in the recent past. One reason given for this increase is the lowering of the legal age for drinking in many states. Since the national voting age was lowered to 18, numerous states have reduced the age for legal consumption of alcohol. At the time of this writing, 26 of the 50 states allow the purchase of alcoholic beverages by persons under the age of 21. Also, as young people are turning away from drugs they are reported to be turning towards alcohol, perhaps the most tragically serious and devastating of all drugs.

### Absorption of Alcohol

Once alcohol is ingested it is absorbed directly from the stomach as well as from the small intestine. Ethyl alcohol is a small, water-soluble molecule requiring no digestion and can be absorbed by simple diffusion along the entire gastrointestinal tract, including the rectum. The fastest rate of absorption is when the stomach is empty. Taken in this fashion, the portion of alcohol not absorbed through the gastric mucosa is quickly passed down the intestinal tract. Approximately 80 per cent of it is absorbed from the small intestine as rapidly as it leaves the stomach. Peak blood levels are, thus, acquired approximately 1 hr. after ingestion of alcohol.[13] The rate of absorption of alcohol into the blood stream can be slowed by a variety of factors. When the stomach contains food the rate of passage into the small intestine is decreased and when alcohol is mixed with milk, fat, or meat proteins it is absorbed more slowly. Also, the rate of drinking makes a difference—the slower the rate the lower the blood alcohol level. Dilution is another determining factor. If it is highly concentrated, alcohol exerts a depressant effect on absorption and the irritating nature of the drink stimulates the secretion of mucus which also delays absorption.[13] When alcohol is taken in concentrations of less than 10 per cent the absorption is again slowed due to the dilution. It appears, then, that the most rapid rate of alcohol absorption results from ingestion of beverages containing between 10 and 30 per cent alcohol, as found in wines and highballs. Alcohol can be absorbed through other routes into the body, such as by injections, and although alcohol is not absorbed significantly through the skin, intoxicating blood levels can be achieved through prolonged inhalation of alcohol vapors.

After alcohol is absorbed from the gastrointestinal tract, it passes through the portal vein to the liver and then through the vena cava to the heart, lungs, and arterial blood. The distribution of alcohol throughout the body is in proportion to the water content of the various tissues. The brain receives a larger share because of its high fluid content, with smaller shares distributed to bone tissue and fat deposits. An equilibrium is established between alcohol concentration in the tissues and levels in the blood. A rise in blood level results in an increased concentration in the tissues and vice versa.

### Effects on the Body

To gauge the degree of intoxication by symptoms alone is unsatisfactory since the veteran drinker and the new experimenter may display considerably different symptoms at the same blood level. The determination of the level of alcohol in the blood is one of the most widely used indexes, because it is an objective measurement that aids in estimating the severity of intoxication.

Although the concentration of alcohol in drinks may vary from four to 50 per cent the proportion of alcohol in the blood very rarely exceeds 0.5 per cent. At concentrations as low as 50 mg. per 100 ml. (0.05 per cent), most individuals begin to "feel" their drinks and to exhibit some impairment. When blood levels exceed 100 mg. per 100 ml. (0.1 per cent), even heavy drinkers show undesirable changes and have been shown to exhibit errors in practical driving tests. A blood level of 150 mg. per 100 ml. (0.15 per cent) is generally accepted as the clinical level of intoxication and is not consistent with safe operation of an automobile. Most states have established by law that 0.10 per cent blood alcohol is prima-facie evidence of intoxication. At levels of 0.2 per cent to 0.3 per cent, the individual becomes stuporous and even the most seasoned drinker is definitely intoxicated. When the concentration reaches 0.4 per cent, most persons lose consciousness. Levels as low as 0.35 to 0.45 per cent have caused death whereas those above 0.55 per cent are usually fatal if left untreated.[13]

Because of the many variables involved, such as emptying time of the stomach or rate of drinking, it is difficult to estimate the total amount of alcohol consumed from any given blood level. As a quick approximation, however, it has been estimated that the rapid ingestion of about 2½ ounces of alcohol will yield a blood alcohol level of approximately 0.1 per cent. This is equivalent to five drinks of 100 proof alcohol or about six bottles of beer (see Table 9.1).

The concentration of alcohol in the body is not great enough to irritate tissues directly. The only tissues that may receive such direct damage are the mucous membrane linings of the esophagus and stomach when undiluted distilled liquor is ingested. There are indirect effects of alcohol, however, which are exerted on some biological functions and enzyme systems. For example, one alteration is a decrease in alkali-binding power of the blood. A mild acidosis also results from depressed respiration and there is a build-up of lactic acid within the body.

The chief reason that alcohol is ingested is to depress the brain and to blunt the mind, and the commonly recognized symptoms of intoxication are caused by this depressant action of alcohol on the central nervous system. The areas of the brain affected and the intensity of the reaction are determined by the concentration of alcohol in the blood. Although not completely understood, it is theorized that alcohol interferes with synaptic transmission. The initial action is probably on the reticular activating system, and the effect is to increase the excitability of the cerebral cortex, followed by depression of the cortical centers. These are the areas of the brain which were the latest to be developed in evolutionary man and are the centers which exert the disciplines necessary for civilized people to live together. The properties of restraint, consideration, judgment, and inhibition are but a few of these learned patterns of behavior. With depression of these higher functions, which are capable of reinforcing and inhibiting the action of the lower parts of the brain, the psychological and physical manifestations of drunkenness become apparent. Exhilaration and excitement, loss of restraint, irregularity of behavior, loquacity, slurred speech, incoordination of movement and gait, irritability, and drowsiness are common symptoms and require little elaboration. Research studies also have shown how alcohol acts in less obvious ways. Reflexes are slowed down, reaction time is increased, the ability to understand and to learn is impaired, thinking is dulled, and there is increasing loss of memory. As alcohol concentration increases, progressively more basic areas of the brain become affected, resulting in loss of consciousness. Further increase in alcohol concentration affects the brain stem, or the so-called primitive area of the brain. The medulla oblongata is located at the lower extreme of this brain stem and contains the cardiac, vasomotor and respiratory centers. Depression of this area will seriously affect cardiovascular function and respiration and, if untreated, may result in death.

**Detoxication**

Contrasted to the rapid rate of absorption,

TABLE 9.1

| Quantity | Percent Blood-Alcohol Level | Resulting Behavior |
|---|---|---|
| 3 oz whiskey (2 "shots) | 0.05 | Sedation and Tranquility |
| 6 oz. whiskey | 0.10 | Lack of Coordination |
| 12 oz. Whiskey | 0.20 | Obvious intoxication |
| 15 oz. whiskey | 0.30 | Unconsciousness |
| 30 oz. whiskey | 0.50+ | Death may result |

the rate of detoxication of alcohol in the body is measured and slow. Regardless of the quantity of alcohol ingested, metabolism progresses at a fairly regular, fixed rate. A common estimate is that the body can metabolize about one ounce of whiskey per hr.[14] There is no upper limit to the rate of alcohol absorption, however. One pint of whiskey consumed in a few minutes could be fatal, particularly if the individual should be intoxicated, already. The alcohol would be absorbed into the blood at such a rapid rate that the body could not metabolize it soon enough. Toxic levels in excess of 0.5 per cent could be reached within the hour and would seriously interfere with life functions. The same amount of whiskey taken over a period of 6 to 8 hr., however, could be metabolized, usually, with less difficulty.

Experiments have been conducted with hyperventilation, high protein diets, insulin injections, specific amino acids, pyruvate, and fructose in efforts to hasten the metabolism of alcohol in the human body. This has been a highly controversial area since the number of investigators who have reported an increase in metabolism are balanced by about an equal number who have obtained negative results. It is known, however, that although black coffee, cold showers, exercise, or breathing pure oxygen may alter the symptoms of alcoholic intoxication they have no appreciable effect on the rate of alcohol metabolism. There are reports, however, of research directed towards the development of an acetate tablet that, when combined with acetic acid and a niacin compound (nadide) in the body, will markedly hasten the metabolism of alcohol.

Small amounts of alcohol, ranging from 4 to 10 per cent, are lost into the urine and respiratory air by diffusion and are excreted unchanged. The alcohol in these excretions is in equilibrium with the blood alcohol passing through the kidneys and lungs. It has been shown for example, that 2100 cc. of alveolar air or 1.25 ml. of urine will contain about as many milligrams of alcohol as does 1 ml. of blood. Hence, a determination of the alcohol concentration in respiratory air or urine can be used to estimate blood concentrations for medicolegal purposes.

The bulk of ingested alcohol is detoxified by metabolic degradation. The enzyme that is primarily involved in this process, alcohol dehydrogenase, is located mainly in the liver and the kidney. In cases of ingestion of large quantities of alcohol, another enzyme system is utilized as a supplement. The microsomal ethanol oxidizing system (MEOS) furnishes additional amounts of nadide to assure the maximal operation of the alcohol dehydrogenase system.[15] The liver is the major organ involved in alcohol metabolism whereas the kidney plays a minor role. The overall process by which alcohol is consumed yields carbon dioxide, water, and seven calories for each gram of alcohol oxidized.

The first and slowest stage in the oxidation of alcohol is the conversion of this product to acetaldehyde. A raised level of acetaldehyde probably plays an important role both in the toxicity of the acute phase of alcoholic intoxication and may be involved in the hangover when the individual suffers from headaches and gastritis. In general, it is felt that acetaldehyde acts like a sympathomimetic drug, relaxing the bronchial musculature and stimulating the heart rate. Use is made of this first stage of alcohol metabolism to help former problem drinkers and alcoholics refrain from the use of alcohol. The administration of a drug, disulfiram, will interfere with the removal of acetaldehyde that has accumulated from the oxidation of alcohol. When a patient taking disulfiram also takes even one ounce of whiskey or one glass of beer, the resultant build-up of acetaldehyde produces toxic symptoms which make the individual feel very ill indeed. Characteristically, a reaction occurs consisting of general flushing of the body, rapid pulse and breathing, pain around the heart, and a sense of apprehension. This is followed by a drop in blood pressure, pallor, a feeling of weakness and faintness, nausea and vomiting.

The succeeding stages in the metabolism of alcohol are the oxidation of acetaldehyde to acetyl-CoA, the conversion to acetic acid, then to carbon dioxide and water. These latter oxidative processes can take place in various areas of the body and at a more accelerated rate. The oxidation of alcohol to acetaldehyde is the slowest and, also, is the pacesetting reaction in the chain of metabolic reactions and is largely dependent upon the availability of alcohol dehydrogenase.

Problems associated with drinking become more profound as the drinking increases in quantity and frequency. Alcohol-caused depression of the brain results not only in the dulling of the senses but also affects the brain's normal control over other body functions. In large doses it affects the pituitary and adrenal cortex. Biochemical changes at this level, when repeated over and over as in habitual drunkenness, can cause serious and lasting injury to tissues and organs. The result may be stomach, liver, or kidney ailments as well as various forms of neuritis. Excessive drinking over long periods may result in or be closely associated with serious nervous and mental disorders. Also, it is reported that heavy drinking can affect the heart, depressing ventricular function and producing abnormalities of the myocardium.[16] Added to these conditions, it is known that excessive consumption of alcohol can suppress the formation of red blood cells and blood platelets, with strong suspicions that it can also suppress white blood cell formation.[17]

People who drink regularly but who continue to eat a normal diet are apt to become overweight. A highball or cocktail containing one and a half ounces of whiskey has the same number of calories as six teaspoons of sugar or two pats of butter, and three ounces of whiskey are equivalent to one ounce of fat or oil from a calorie standpoint. Eighty-one calories are found in a bottle of beer or in four ounces of a dry wine. Since wine is fermented from fruit juices and beer is a fermentation product of grain and malt, these alcoholic beverages possess additional nutritional value in the form of some protein as well as a few minerals and vitamins.

Distilled beverages, such as whiskey, rum, gin, and brandy, do not have this extra nutritional value, however, because only the alcohol and flavors are transferred and recondensed in the distilling process. Habitual heavy drinkers of distilled beverages may have their appetites satisfied by the alcohol consumed and frequently fail to eat properly. Calories derived from alcohol in these cases may provide a significant portion of required energy, but they do not support body maintenance, growth, or weight restoration. These people are in danger of developing vitamin deficiencies and diseases that result from inadequate diets. The three deficiency syndromes that are particularly common are polyneuropathy resulting from thiamine deficiency, pellagra resulting from niacin deficiency, and fatty infiltration of the liver and cirrhosis some times resulting from protein and lipotropic amino acid deficiency.

## Alcoholism

The most serious problem resulting from the misuse of alcohol is the development of alcoholism, one of the gravest and most destructive health and social menaces facing our nation. This disease ranks with cancer, mental illness, and cardiovascular disease in its severity, its toll, and its importance to public health. Alcoholism is a progressive illness, epidemic in nature, and affects men and women in all geographical areas without regard to educational, religious, cultural, or financial status. Almost 5 per cent of our citizens over 20 years of age are alcoholic and, statistically, every business and social circle has at least one alcoholic member. Consequently, alcoholism is both a national health problem and a public responsibility.

Of the more than 95 million American adults who drink, about one in 11 develops the disease of alcoholism. In the United States today, there are an estimated 9 million alcoholics, but there are another 36 million family members and associates whose lives are affected and damaged.[18] Less than 10 per cent of the alcoholics fall into those groups described as the chronic drunkeness offender, the skid row type, and the homeless man. Over 90 per cent are trying to lead more or less normal lives at home and at work. Industry estimates conservatively that losses resulting from absenteeism, lowered productivity, and accidents associated with alcoholism exceed 2 billion dollars annually.[13] This, combined with the increased incidence of divorce rates and broken homes, testifies to the fact that many alcoholics are not succeeding in their dual role. In addition, the further loss due to personal and professional deterioration is beyond calculation.

One facet of the public health problem is reflected in reports that alcoholics are subject to distinctly higher than average death rates. According to the National Institute on Alcohol Abuse and Alcoholism, the life expectancy of heavy alcoholic drinkers is estimated to be shorter by 10 to 12 years than that of the general public, the mortality rate is at least two and a half times greater, and a disproportionate number suffer violent deaths. Alcoholism appears as a cause of death on more than 13,000 death certificates yearly.[13] The upward trend in mortality from alcoholic disorders shows considerable variation by sex and race. The rise has been steeper for non-white persons than for white, and also steeper for women than for men. The increase for women was about twice that for men, reflecting the significant increase in alcoholism among women. Deaths from alcoholic disorders were due to cirrhosis of the liver, alcoholism, and alcoholic psychosis. In addition, alcoholic-related deaths from diseases of the digestive system, suicide, motor vehicle accidents, other accidents, and homicides swell the mortality lists to an even more tragic number. Accidental injuries which result in hospitalization and physical impairment present additional problems. It is reported that one-half of all traffic fatalities, highway injuries, and motor vehicle accidents in the United States are directly related to alcohol; 300,000 people are arrested for drunk driving every year; and two-thirds of all alcohol-related traffic deaths each year are caused by heavy, problem drinkers. The report from which these figures were abstracted concludes by stating ". . . and these grisly highway statistics are the end result of 9 million alcoholic people going untreated in a nation with 110 million registered motor vehicles."[19]

Definitions of alcoholics and alcoholism have been evolving for hundreds of years with each definition reflecting the background of the writer. Still, there has been no specific interpretation which is universally accepted. The terms, generally, are used to describe and include a broad range of individual, social, and community problems related to the excessive use or misuse of alcoholic beverages. The term "alcoholism" is defined by the World Health Organization as ". . . a chronic illness that manifests itself as a disorder of behavior. It is characterized by the repeated usage of alcoholic beverages to an extent that exceeds customary dietary use or compliance with social customs of the community and that interferes with the drinker's health or his economic or social functioning."[20] The definition of an alcoholic, according to the National Council on Alcoholism, is "a person who is powerless to stop drinking and whose drinking seriously alters his normal living pattern." Alcoholism, then, is frequently described as a disease within itself, but it is unlike many diseases in some respects. One wife of an alcoholic, for example, stated that this appears to be a disease from which the patient is not anxious to recover. On one hand, there is increasing data obtained from work on alcohol hepatitis, cardiomyopathy, anemias, respiratory diseases, and drug dependency induced by alcohol to argue for a specific disease classification.[21] On the other hand, one of the conclusions of the five-year alcoholism research program at Cornell University is that alcoholism is not a single entity or disease but a symptom associated with several illnesses or syndromes. Whatever the ultimate classification, a separate disease or a symptom, there seems to be various types of this condition and each type responds to a different regimen of treatment. Current studies suggest that one type may be suffering from biochemical deficiencies or malfunctioning enzyme systems. These people may comprise the 10 per cent of victims who become alcoholic from their very first drink, without going through the progressive changes throughout the years.

Wherever man lives he is subject to stresses from his physical and social surroundings. He must adjust to changes within himself, in his living pattern, and to his social environment. When he finds himself confronted with overwhelming difficulty in adjusting, he may take to drinking as a way out of his problems. Alcoholic beverages provide a tension-reducing device. Because alcohol works most strongly against the higher functions of the brain, anxiety is diminished. The immature and frustrated individual seeks more and more frequently the use of alcohol to overcome his intolerance to frustration and finally does so to the exclusion of other more accepted methods to obtain relief.

Of course, not all heavy drinkers become alcoholics but the rate is so dangerously high that there is cause for alarm. As stated earlier, even the specialists in this field have difficulty determining when a patient ceases to be a heavy social drinker and progresses down the road to alcoholism. Personality studies of alcoholics have been conducted to determine what characteristics are common among victims of this disease. It was hoped that the results of such study would help to identify people who are more likely to become alcoholics. Although these studies have not been completely successful, some conclusions can be drawn. Generally speaking, the alcoholic is self-centered, emotionally immature, dependent, insecure, and fearful, possesses feelings of guilt, and has difficulty in coping with the tensions of everyday life. Other characteristics such as heavy cigarette smoking, high standards of perfection, and sensitive, artistic temperament seem to place the victim in greater danger of becoming an alcoholic. For the emotionally immature, alcoholism furnishes the magic carpet back to childhood where there were no decisions or responsibilities and where others furnished the care and protection. Others rationalize their drinking by telling themselves that alcohol makes life more bearable and that it helps them to be less unhappy. This, of course, is one of the serious troubles, because alcohol *does* offer temporary relief in many cases. It is the seeking of this relief over and over again that may lead to dependence on alcohol.

Certainly two of the greatest contributing factors to the prevalence of alcoholism in this country are the psychosocial pressures which stimulate drinking and the permissiveness with which drunken behavior is accepted in our society. Other cultures and civilizations have demonstrated that corrective attention to these two factors has helped to control the incidence of alcoholism. The individual who consistently drinks to cover up or escape from his problems is running the risk of becoming an alcoholic, and an interested and alert community can frequently recognize this problem soon enough to take meaningful action. Through coordinated endeavors of the health professions, social service agencies, rehabilitation specialists, and law enforcement officers, the prealcoholic can be located and helped.

## Steps to Alcoholism

Even though numerous theories have been proposed and supported, there is no conclusive evidence yet available as to the causes of alcoholism. This is a medical-social problem far too complicated for simple answers and no one area of research can be expected to yield complete information. Since alcoholics come from all walks of life with varied family and educational backgrounds and different personalities, they had very little in common prior to being identified as problem drinkers. They become alcoholics for various reasons and cannot be considered as one type of person. Regardless of their varied backgrounds, however, once they become dependent upon alcohol most of them follow a familiar but sad

pattern. They then share a common problem—an inability to control their drinking.

The vast majority of alcoholics reach their condition of development by degrees over a period of years. At any stage in this development, the victim, most probably, can be treated and can recover; however, the individual must seek and earnestly desire help in order for such treatment to be effective. Unfortunately, over 90 per cent of alcoholics and those on the road toward alcoholism do not seek treatment.

The early symptoms of alcoholism, the so-called first stage, usually develop over a period of 5 to 10 years. Characteristic of this stage are those who are using alcohol more and more frequently to help them over the rough spots until such usage becomes a habit. The individual drinks more than is customary among his associates and makes excuses to drink more often. The habit thus develops into a need or a psychological dependence on alcohol to help the drinker escape from unpleasant worries or tensions. These people begin to lie or to feel guilty or sensitive about their drinking. They frequently gulp their drinks and no longer brag about how much they can hold. They take a few drinks before going to a party where alcoholic beverages will be served and feel the compulsion to drink at certain times of the day, after a disappointment or quarrel, or because they feel tired or depressed. As the condition progresses the individual begins to experience blackouts. He does not lose consciousness but, on the morning after a drinking bout, he cannot remember what happened after a certain point in time. If these memory blackouts occur repeatedly or after taking only a moderate amount of alcohol, it is a strong indication of developing alcoholism.[22]

The middle symptoms, sometimes called the crucial or basic phase, are an extension of the early symptoms and, generally, last from two to five years. This stage is characterized by loss of control over drinking. The person finds himself making more promises and telling more lies about his drinking. There are more times when he needs a drink, and when he is sober he regrets what he said or did while drinking. He drinks more often alone, avoiding family and friends, and has weekend drinking bouts with Monday hangovers. After one drink, this unfortunate individual feels a physical demand for alcohol which is so strong that he cannot stop short of intoxication. Suffering from remorse but not wanting to show it, he strikes out unreasonably at others. Family situations become tense and he is in danger of losing his job. As he realizes that he is losing the respect of his associates and hurting his loved ones, the problem drinker tries to get on the "water wagon" but he is rarely successful. He becomes filled with discouragement and self-pity. Because of his continued drinking, his problems become more acute. He loses friends and maybe his job; his family may drift away from him and leave him alone. To get away from these increasing problems he increases his drinking. Memory blackouts and loss of consciousness become more frequent but his drinking has passed beyond the point where he can use it as a way of coping with his problems. At this stage, he may be hospitalized for the first time or attempt geographical escape. Also, drinking in the morning becomes necessary to overcome his depressed feelings. This individual is caught in a vicious circle. His problems lead to uncontrolled drinking which, in turn, leads to more problems and more drinking.

The late symptoms, or the chronic phase, represent the advanced stage of alcoholism which, if permitted to continue, leads to extreme manifestations. The alcoholic has lost concern for his family and for others around him, and he, obviously, is drunk on important occasions such as special dinners or meetings. Drinking bouts last for several days at a time and blackouts and loss of consciousness are quite frequent. The physiological reaction of the person dependent upon alcohol is changed, and a need for alcohol has been created as a result of excessive drinking. There is a marked tendency to develop seizures, often called "rum fits," within 12 to 48 hr. following the cessation of drinking. Also, during this period the patient presents a distinctive clinical picture. He shows a coarse generalized tremor, is alert, startles easily, cannot sleep, and craves alcohol or drugs. Delirium tremens, whether an acute psychosis developed during drinking or an abstinence syndrome, is the most dramatic and serious manifestation. This condition is characterized by profound confusion, delusions, vivid hallucinations, tremor, agitation, sleeplessness, fever, and increased autonomic activity resulting in tachycardia, and profuse perspiration. Not until they reach the point of desperation do most alcoholics seek help, and many never

do. If the habit is not broken somewhere along the line, they ultimately reach the last stage, marked by ethical bankruptcy and admission of defeat. If they can be brought to recognize their illness and accept treatment at an earlier stage, they can save themselves and their families much deprivation and suffering.

Like an iceberg, alcoholism's sinister and devastating effects are not readily apparent and are mostly unheeded, not so much because they are invisible but because they are denied. The vast majority of the millions caught in alcoholism's downward spiral are secret sufferers as are the family members and associates of the alcoholic. Thus, the denial that begins with the alcoholic, as a sign and symptom of his sickness, is endorsed and imitated by the world around him in a conspiracy of silence which usually walls the problem from public view. In the guise of shielding, protecting, and covering up for him, those around him, and society as a whole, perform a disservice. Actually, they join the alcoholic in hiding his illness and, thus, frequently keep him from the treatment he must have in order to recover.

Alcoholics and the effects of their uncontrolled drinking are not always shielded from the public view. Alcoholics are exposed to accidents and injuries while drinking and they are more likely to contract diseases because they frequently neglect good habits of hygiene. Financial waste which accompanies alcoholism can soon be a community problem. A bad environment is created for their bewildered children, and welfare agencies are often called upon for support. The public jails are still the recipients of a large number of alcoholics, and the hospitals must provide care for alcoholics who are unable to pay. Thus, alcoholism is not just a private problem. However, it is the community's denial of alcoholism that hides the early and middle-stage alcoholic who can be most helped by early detection and treatment. This denial, also, permits public attitudes toward the problem to be clouded by myths, misconceptions, and ignorance. When we consider the many costly aspects of this problem, the concern for an adequate public health program becomes more obvious.

### Treatment and Rehabilitation

For many years alcoholics were regarded by the public and health professions as people who could not be helped. Until recently, alcoholics were, generally, considered perverse, weak-willed, and deserving of punishment rather than help. Thus, interest in alcoholism problems grew very slowly. An attempt to control alcoholism by eliminating the use of alcohol was made through passage of the 18th Amendment and the Volstead Act but it is generally agreed that this attempt was unsuccessful. A concerted effort to improve this situation did not begin in the United States until the early thirties, with the establishment of several national organizations and councils to combat the problem.

The first such organization was the Fellowship of Alcoholics Anonymous, founded in Akron, Ohio, in June, 1935. The founders were an ex-stockbroker from New York and a local surgeon, both chronic alcoholics. This organization has grown until there are presently about 12,000 groups in 90 nations. More than 500 such groups are in hospitals of all types and over 700 are in correctional institutions. The groups are largely autonomous, usually democratic, and are served by short-term steering committees of local members. Alcoholics Anonymous (A.A.) is a fellowship of recovered alcoholics who help each other to maintain sobriety and who offer to share their recovery experience freely with other men and women who may have a drinking problem. Their meetings have some of the advantages of group therapy, since they provide opportunity for group discussion of common problems and give members a chance to describe their personal anxieties before a group of understanding and noncritical peers. In addition to emotional support, the social activities of A.A. do a great deal to ease the loneliness which is common to the alcoholic. The A.A. program urges members to appeal to a power greater than themselves for strength in overcoming their difficulties. This approach has the psychological effect of releasing tension and replacing despair with hope.

Alcoholics Anonymous members are men and women from all walks of life, of all age groups beginning with teen-agers, of all races, and with all manner of formal religious affiliations or with none at all. Since the groups are concerned solely with the personal recovery and continued sobriety of individual alcoholics, the movement does not engage in the fields of alcoholism research, medical or psychiatric treatment, or

education. Traditionally, A.A. does not accept or seek financial support from outside sources, and members preserve personal anonymity in all communications at the public level. Anyone who thinks he has a drinking problem is welcome to attend any A.A. meeting. He becomes a member simply by deciding that he is one. Although members recognize that their program is not always effective with everyone who seeks help, an estimated 400,000 alcoholics have achieved sobriety in A.A. Most of these retain their membership in A.A. to help others who are afflicted by this illness.

The national voluntary health agency working for the control and prevention of alcoholism is the National Council on Alcoholism. This agency was founded in 1944 and now has affiliate councils throughout the country. Through education, community services, and research, the National Council is disclosing new facts about alcoholism and publicizing not only the plight of the alcoholic but demonstrating how communities can help to combat the growing menace of alcoholism. An example of this latter endeavor is the popularity of their play "Lady on the Rocks," which serves to increase recognition and understanding of the problems of alcoholism and the alcoholic. The affiliate councils serve as repositories of information concerning alcoholism, act as reference centers for those alcoholics and their families who seek help, distribute educational literature, provide information and suggestions for recognizing prealcoholics and for working with alcoholics, and actively co-operate with other community and government agencies to help reduce the toll taken by this disease. The National Council on Alcoholism is neither "wet" nor "dry". Its sole concern is the disease of alcoholism, not social drinking.

There are numerous other agencies such as Al-Anon Family Groups, Alateen Groups, mayors or governor's councils on alcoholism, state and local health departments, and industrial concerns which have growing programs concentrated on the mutual problem of alcoholism. Also working in this field for several years have been the co-operative Commission on the Study of Alcoholism, the Center of Alcohol Studies at Rutgers, the North American Association of Alcoholism Programs, the National Research Council, the American Public Health Association, the American Medical Association, the World Health Organization, and many, many others.

The Federal Government has taken meaningful and effective steps in setting blueprints for programs on a national basis. The Department of Health, Education, and Welfare, co-ordinating activities through their divisions of education, rehabilitation, social security, welfare, St. Elizabeth's Hospital, and the Public Health Service, has undertaken a major endeavor of research, education, and professional training. The Department's objectives are to make available to alcoholics the best treatment and rehabilitation services, to improve techniques of treatment, and to find effective ways of preventing the disorder. The establishment of the National Institute on Alcohol Abuse and Alcoholism in the Alcohol, Drug Abuse, and Mental Health Administration has helped to coordinate the varied activities associated with a multiple attack on this sickness. In spite of budget cuts in federal alcoholism programs, Congress is still demonstrating active support through passage of additional alcoholism abuse bills.[23] Federal grants from numerous sources have provided the means and the impetus to establish training programs, stimulate pilot demonstrations, and encourage local and state alcoholism programs. Graduate courses and entire Master's Degree programs are devoted to preparing skilled, informed workers to administer alcoholism programs more effectively. Increasing cooperation is also seen at the state level. Presently, 16 states and the District of Columbia have enacted legislation that decriminalizes simple public drunkenness and facilitates voluntary treatment by community-care agencies.

In spite of the excellent work started by selected and dedicated groups and agencies, one of the key factors associated with success or failure of an alcholism program is the attitude of the community. All too often, society as a whole joins in a conspiracy of silence that helps the alcoholic to hide his illness and thereby keeps him from the treatment which he should have. This attitude contributes to the alcoholic's low opinion of himself and fosters his sense of helplessness. Overcoming community denial of alcoholism, therefore, becomes an important first step. Since this condition is an illness, the people within the medical professions and the community as a whole must assume a responsible attitude and gather the resources necessary to combat the problem, effectively, and to reduce both the severity and the incidence. Through a co-operative effort, combined forces can be brought to bear against this illness just as they are against any other disease that poses a threat to the public health.

It is within this area that professionals in the allied medical fields can be extremely useful. With increased understanding of the alcoholic and his plight, it will be possible to teach people more of the facts about alcoholism. All of us can help to overcome many of the superstitions and prejudices that have been linked with alcoholism. We can help to develop intelligent and constructive attitudes about the disease which could pave the way for the community to provide improved treatment and rehabilitation facilities. Even more important, the people in the allied medical professions can learn to recognize, and teach others to recognize, the early signs of alcoholism. Patients in these stages can receive the greatest benefit from therapy and should be encouraged to seek professional help.

The results of working with alcoholics and of research into causes and treatments have changed attitudes and approaches to treatment. It is now recognized that an alcoholic is not just a person who permits his drinking to interfere with his life in one vital area or more but is an individual who is suffering from an illness. Alcoholism is not willful irresponsibility, and there is no gainful purpose to be served in scolding or shaming the victim because he often harbors these same opinions of shame and degradation. The alcoholic uses his feelings, not his mind, when he decides to drink. Once an alcoholic has taken a drink, he is unable to be sure where his drinking will end. He drinks because he feels compelled to, and he keeps on drinking even though he may realize that he is harming his health, endangering his job, and hurting the people closest to him. Alcoholism, therefore, cannot be cured with logic or willpower alone.

It has been demonstrated through new therapeutic approaches that alcoholics can recover. This does not mean that there is a cure for alcoholism, since no method known today can prevent the alcoholic from losing control of his drinking. What it does mean is that, through medical, psychological, rehabilitative, and community support, many alcoholics can be helped to stop drinking and resume normal living; however, they must never use alcohol again. It may be assumed that most alcoholics want help although the desire for help is buried under two fears. First is the fear of losing the increasingly necessary solace of drinking and the second is fear of the stigma in admitting their inability to control their drinking. Therefore, in order to bring about recovery, the victim must accept the fact that he is an alcoholic, that alcoholism is a disease, and that there is no need to be ashamed of his illness as long as he is trying to do something about it. He must seek and accept all of the help that he needs and be confident that he can live without alcohol since thousands before him have succeeded.

The primary goal of treatment, then, is to help the patient remain sober and to handle his problems constructively so that staying sober will not be too difficult. The treatment of the acute phase of alcoholism is primarily medical whereas the treatment of the chronic condition is largely psychological or educational. Medical treatment is becoming more and more important in furthering recovery since new drugs not only help to ease the discomfort of the alcoholic but make it possible for him to be receptive to additional treatment. Psychotherapy is being used increasingly in many clinics throughout the country to help the alcoholic recognize what his problems are, frequently to explore the night-black world of crushing depressions and nameless fears that only liquor seems to wash away, and to enable him to deal with these problems without the use of alcohol. Treatment is usually given by a team of specialists which may include an internist, a psychiatrist, a psychologist, a rehabilitation counselor, and a social worker. The families of alcoholics are also included in these consultations so that understanding support from these members will supply vital help on the road to recovery.

It can be seen, then, that alcoholism takes time to develop and recovery from the condition also takes time. Since this menace is such an important public health problem, it calls for the intelligent and diligent attention and help from all professionals who are interested and concerned about the public health.

## THE MISUSE OF DRUGS

### Introduction

Never before in the history of mankind have drugs been used to the extent that they are today. As a result of scientific research and technology there has been produced an awe-inspiring armentarium of drugs and vaccines for almost every known ailment. These have virtually eliminated many of the previously dreaded diseases and have made significant progress toward limiting the severity of those illnesses that have not been eliminated. Literally millions of lives have been saved because of the judicious use of such medications and mankind owes a debt of gratitude to the drug industry and medical science for their remarkable achievements.

These gifts of life-saving and symptom-reducing medications come to us, however, as a mixed blessing. The taking of drugs has now become an established pattern within the American way of life and more medications are consumed *per capita* in the United States than in any other country in the world. Through the magic of television and other mass media the public is encouraged to visit their local pharmacies and purchase drugs for the common cold, headache, stomach distress, iron-poor blood, allergies, corns, constipation, halitosis, and a myriad of other conditions. Essentially every household has an abundance of proprietary preparations that have been promoted by our modern medicine showmen. Consequently, at the first sign of a cold, headache, or any other physical stress or aberration, the vast majority of the population reaches for one of the so-called panacea which has found such a ready and lucrative market.

It is recognized that over-the-counter drug products serve a useful purpose in reducing symptoms of mild and temporary illnesses. When used with intelligence and restraint they fill an important health need. When taken needlessly, in large quantities, too frequently, or for prolonged periods of time without medical supervision, however, they represent a sickness of our time and their abuse constitutes a hazard.

The medical profession cannot be held entirely blameless in the indiscriminate use of drugs. Most patients feel a little cheated if they walk away from a physician's office without a few prescriptions for medications that will ease their symptoms, whether real or imagined. All too many physicians accommodate their patients in this desire and authorize the use of drugs even when there is no clear-cut therapeutic justification for such prescribing. It has been estimated that up to 70 per cent of patients visiting doctor's offices present symptoms and complaints which have no organic bases, and yet the vast majority of such patients receive prescription medications. Thus, the tired and harried businessman, the gay socialite, the beautiful movie queen, or the frustrated housewife may take stimulants to "get them going" in the morning, tranquilizing-type drugs to "take off the rough edges" appetite suppressants for the weight-conscious, anticholinergics for the nervous stomach, mood elevators for a more positive frame of mind, analgesics and muscle relaxants for vague pains, and sedatives to promote and ensure sleep.

The nature and significance of drug abuse may be considered from two points of view. One of these relates to the interaction between the drug and the individual. The other relates to the interaction between drug abuse and society. The first viewpoint is concerned with drug dependence and emphasizes the pharmacological actions of the drug in relation to the psychological status of the individual. The second viewpoint incorporates the interplay between economic, social, and environmental factors within the community. So, once again, we are confronted with both individual and community health.

In our culture, there is still a degree of religious and public censure associated with the indiscriminate use of alcohol and society almost immediately forces the user of narcotics into his own subculture. People who would be repelled at the thought of using marihuana or who use alcohol with discretion because of its tell-tale odor may have no qualms whatever about abusing sedatives and stimulants. The person feeling the need for an escape from reality has found a new means to do so without stigma or condemnation. Society seems to be particularly lenient on the individual who takes these medications, and those who become dependent upon such drugs can function for a considerable time within the general context of society without being discovered or forced out of their customary environment. Even within the legal channels, then, drug misuse constitutes a major problem.

The most flagrant abuse of drugs, however, is found in the illicit market. Although developed and promoted for alleviation of symptoms of illness, many such medications are being used

for other purposes. Among the most popularly used drugs at the present time are the following: heroin, barbiturates, marijuana, cocaine, diazepam, methaqualone, propoxyphene, doxepin, and certain over-the-counter preparations popularly advertised to induce sleep or prevent motion sickness. These drugs frequently are consumed with alcohol and/or marijuana to gain added effect.[24] With the exception of heroin and marijuana, the medical demand for these drugs requires that they be produced in large quantities by many manufacturers and widely distributed. A system of such complexity and size, therefore, provides many opportunities for illegal traffic.

Dangerous drugs get into the illicit retail trade through various ways. They may be stolen from reputable manufacturers, wholesalers, or pharmacies. Clandestine manufacturers operating illegally in garages, basements, and warehouses produce substantial quantities. Counterfeiters and some registered manufacturers under the cloak of legality make large quantities of dangerous drugs illegally and dispose of them through illicit trade. Reports have been consistent through the past few years that at least 50 per cent of the dangerous drugs seized each year are legally manufactured. In addition, a few registered manufacturers have been reported to ship large quantities of bulk materials to countries beyond the border of the United States. These materials are then encapsulated or made into tablets and are brought back to the United States through the illicit market. For example, the director of the Drug Enforcement Administration told a Senate Subcommittee of the recent seizure of over 26 million barbiturates at the Mexico border and of the diversion of sufficient amphetamine sulphate powder diverted from legitimate international commerce to manufacture 50 million tablets. In a related action, drug enforcement officials have secured a court order asking a U.S. pharmaceutical firm to show cause why its license to export amphetamines should not be revoked.[25]

The people who take drugs, not for medical purposes but as a means of escape or thrill seeking, have created these vast and profitable markets for illegal purveyors. Drug abusers do not conform to any set standard or description. While many have personality disorders which make it difficult for them to face the world unaided by chemical comforts, this is by no means true for all of them. The abuse of dangerous drugs cuts across all social and economic lines. It is as common among high school dropouts as among business executives and is as widespread in the cities as it is in our small towns.

Sometimes the legitimate medical use of narcotics, sedatives, or stimulants is accompanied by the danger of developing drug dependence. The individual who is given narcotics to alleviate extreme, long-lasting pain following severe accidents or extensive surgery may develop both physical and psychic dependence after the medical need for such narcotics is terminated. The compulsive eater who is prescribed amphetamines or other anorexiants for prolonged periods of time may find that he is dependent upon the euphoric effects of the drug long after such medications fail to curb the appetite. Most drug abusers, however, arrive at this condition by other routes.

The National Commission on Marijuana and Drug Abuse has classified non-medical drug use into five categories. First, is the experimental use, motivated mainly by curiosity. Next, is recreational use, occurring in social settings. The sequential, progressive step is termed circumstantial use, motivated by the user's perceived need. Usually this need is to achieve an anticipated effect in order to cope with a specific problem, situation, or condition. The next progressive step is the intensified use, where daily use is needed to relieve a persistent problem. The final category is compulsive use. An individual has reached this stage when drug use dominates the person's existence and preoccupation with drug use precludes other social functioning.[26]

There may be a significant difference between the chronologically mature adult abuser and the teen-age or college age abuser. The adult abuser often feels the need for some type of support to help him through difficult life situations. He may have come to drugs by way of alcohol and finds that drugs offer him a chemical curtain from reality which is socially acceptable. Even though this adult abuser may appear to be successful in his occupation, he has deep feelings of inadequacy and insecurity in a competitive world and dreads to face the decisions, crises, and problems of each day.

Elsewhere in this text, when discussing the subjects of mental health and of alcoholism, reference has been made to the pressures of a competitive society. The urbanization, indus-

trialization, and depersonalization of modern America have imposed enormous burdens on the individual and have presented challenges for him to establish both an identity and a purpose. Unless he makes great efforts to distinguish himself in one field of endeavor or more, he stands in danger of becoming a faceless member in a faceless society. This fear is not restricted to the lower echelons of economic and social functions, nor is it restricted only to the adult.

Although the national voting age has been lowered to 18 there are relatively few other social and cultural recognitions of adulthood at this age. One writer has attributed a significant amount of drug abuse among teenagers to be the result of ". . . an overdose of adolescence in a society whose institutions have generally failed the adolescent."[27] Our society is hesitant to recognize the usefulness or, indeed, even the potential of the younger generation. With the increased emphasis placed upon education the teenager is encouraged to stay in school and the high school dropout soon finds that there is no useful place for him without an education. Those of college age are reminded that they have very few marketable assets until their education is completed, and even then there may be some question. Since these people are students for longer periods of time, they are viewed by many of the older generation as users of resources rather than contributors, and, as such, are not fulfilling a vital need of society. Although former generations were incorporated into society as useful members at an earlier age, the young people of today are not finding such a ready acceptance. There is a heightened frustration because they are not able to compete on an equal basis with those who have established a tentative foothold. The seriousness of our times and the more advanced education of these young people prompt them to reflect upon the meaning of life, the ultimate realities, the purpose of living, the horror of war, the quality of man, and virtues of love. Their quest and the results of their frustrations, however, sometimes take bizarre forms.

The younger juvenile faces even different problems. The progress through adolescence is, even under the best of circumstances, a time of difficulties and stress. The young person does not fully understand himself and often finds little understanding at home. Thus, he seeks refuge among groups of other young people who are going through the same difficulties, and he attempts to satisfy his need to be understood, to identify, and to be accepted. Such groups have their own peculiar code of behavior. Often this code consists of defying legal, social, and parental authority. Results of studies indicate that the more rebellious the adolescent the greater his subsequent use of drugs is likely to be.[28] Environmental factors also have a pronounced influence on adolescent drug use. The most positive correlations are broken families, low income, and sub-standard housing.[29] These insecure and inquisitive young people seek new forms of protest and novel experiences and thrills. Experimentation often begins with sniffing airplane glue, lighter fluid, gasoline, or ether. From there, it may develop into the use of barbiturates or amphetamines. They are then ready for the psychedelic experiences and many seem willing to try almost anything that will "send" them on a "trip."

Since the days of Adam and Eve, a characteristic of young people has been to "test the forbidden." Such attractive temptation is heightened through group action, acceptance, and approval, and the exploring young person finds both the opportunity and the encouragement to try something a little stronger. Added to this are the subcultures which not only use various forms of drugs but, through their publications and the fervent zeal of some of their misdirected converts, actively encourage and promote the use of drugs on a still wider scale.

Aside from the dangers of developing into a confirmed drug abuser, there is yet another tragedy that accompanies this type of action. Some of these drugs are included in Schedule I and II of the Federal Drug law. The penalties for trangressing these laws are very severe and those who are caught using or handling drugs are subject to felony records as drug offenders. Those having such records are restricted as to the types of occupation that they may pursue and are subject to close and continued surveillance by law enforcement officers.

Continued use of dangerous drugs beyond the experimental stage carries with it the eminent possibility of developing into a confirmed drug abuser. As in the stages of alcoholism, these progressive steps are fraught with disaster. The social and legal sanctions associated with illicit use of these drugs forces the drug abuser to associate more and more with other socially maladjusted individuals. It has been confirmed that this association with other drug abusers is an important factor in developing a dependence on drugs. The dependence, in turn, further enslaves the individual to a stereotyped pattern of compulsive drug use.

## Drug Dependence

In the past it has been customary to refer to these persons as "drug addicts" or as "dope fiends." Such terminology is still used to a limited degree, particularly by the lay public, but these descriptions are largely inaccurate and scientifically unsound. In the first place, most drug abusers are not made fiendish by their habit. On the contrary, a great many are deadened and enervated, deprived of personality and will, lose direction in their lives, and frequently are subject to domination and the strong will of others. The term, addict, implies a pronounced physiological and psychological dependence accompanied by severe withdrawal symptoms when the drug is terminated.

The World Health Organization Expert Committee on Addiction-producing Drugs attempted to formulate a definition of addiction that would be applicable to drugs under international control. This was no easy task. With the continuous appearance of new drugs having different pharmacological profiles and containing the abilities to elicit satisfactory and pleasurable responses in at least some of the people taking them, it was obvious that a single definition would have too many exceptions. Definitions of two terms were proposed: "addiction" for the more severe forms and "habituation" to cover other wider and generally less severe forms of drug abuse. These two terms failed in practice to make a clear distinction and they frequently are used interchangeably and inappropriately. It is not uncommon to see or hear the term, addiction, applied to any misuse of drugs outside the medical field. Such broad usage confuses the issue and creates misunderstandings when drugs are discussed from different viewpoints and when constructive programs are proposed to limit drug abuse. Individuals may become dependent upon a wide variety of chemical substances that produce central nervous system effects ranging from stimulation to depression. A characteristic which is common to all of these drugs is that they are capable of creating, in at least some individuals, a particular state of mind that is termed "psychic dependence." In this type of condition the individual develops a feeling of satisfaction, perhaps euphoria, but he also develops a psychic drive to take such drugs continually either to perpetuate the pleasure or to avoid discomfort. Psychic dependence is primarily a manifestation of the individual's reaction to the effects of a specific drug and varies with the individual as well as with the drug. Many authorities in this field are of the opinion that such a mental state is the most powerful of all of the factors involved in chronic intoxication resulting from the use of psychotropic drugs. With certain types of drugs abused, psychic dependence may be the only factor involved.

In addition to psychic dependence, some drugs also induce physical dependence. After taking these drugs for varying periods of time, the body builds up not only a tolerance to the effects of the drugs but so incorporates them into certain bodily functions that there are pronounced physiological disturbances when such drugs are withheld. These disturbances, termed withdrawal or abstinence syndromes, are made up of specific combinations of symptoms and signs of psychic and physical nature that are characteristic for each drug type.

Thus, in order to clarify the problem relating to definitions the WHO Committee devoted much thought and discussion to finding a term that would cover all kinds of drug abuse. They found that the component common to all forms was the development of dependence, whether psychic or physical or both. Hence this Committee subsequently recommended substitution of the term "drug dependence" for both of the terms "drug addiction" and "drug habituation." This recommendation has been supported by leading health and scientific research organizations throughout the world.

The characteristics of drug dependence vary with the agent involved, and these characteristics always must be made clear by designating the particular type of dependence in each specific case. Thus, reference is made to drug dependence of the morphine type, of barbiturate type, of amphetamine type, and so on. The World Health Organization emphasizes that the specification of the type of dependence is essential and should form an integral part of the new terminology, since it is neither possible nor

even desirable to delineate or define the term "drug dependence" independently of the agent involved.[30]

Practically speaking, however, the terms, addiction and habituation, are now written into so many laws in the United States and elsewhere that it seems that all three terms will become a part of drug abuse terminology. Drug dependence will be favored by medically oriented groups and the other two terms will be favored in legislative and law enforcement circles.

## Types of Drug Abused

Although there are many varieties of drugs that are used indiscriminately, the types that are abused to the greatest extent fall into four categories. These are the hard narcotics, depressants, stimulants, and hallucinogens. Each category has its own degree of seriousness and telling effects and many drug abusers do not limit themselves to only one category.

Another classification of drugs recognized by the Drug Enforcement Administration of the U.S. Department of Justice divides drugs into five categories or Schedules according to their abuse potential. Schedule I contains those drugs that have no bona fide medical use but a high abuse potential. Representative drugs of this type are heroin, LSD, and marijuana. Schedule II are those drugs that have a bona fide medical use but also have a high abuse potential. These include the opium derivatives, the short-acting barbiturates, synthetic analgesics such as meperidine, and stronger central nervous system stimulants such as amphetamine. Schedule III contains those medically indicated drugs which have a moderate abuse potential and include most of the intermediate level barbiturates and stimulants. Schedule IV includes those drugs having low abuse potential and a bona fide medical use. In Schedule V are the drugs possessing essentially no abuse potential. Under these Schedules most of the drugs used for non-medical purposes are found in the first two classifications.

### Narcotics

This category of drugs includes opium, the opium derivatives such as morphine, codeine, and heroin, and the synthetic opiates such as meperidine and methadone. Strictly speaking, narcotics are drugs which produce insensibility or stupor due to their depressant effect on the central nervous system. The Federal narcotics laws, however, regulate another drug, cocaine or "snow," which has the opposite effect and produces excitement and stimulation of the central nervous system.

The use of opium dates back at least to the Egyptians in 1500 B C. and it has been important as a medicine ever since. The abuse of this drug apparently was common for many hundreds of years until laws were passed to enable some control. In the United States toward the end of the 19th century, for example, it was estimated that one in 400 had developed psychic and physical dependence on opium or one of its derivatives. Opium is now rarely used in the United States by drug users. Of the hard narcotics the two most commonly abused are morphine and heroin. The problem of the misuse of narcotics continues to exist in this country. The number of chronic abusers of narcotics is unknown. The estimates range from 68,000 to 500,000. Most of these people are located in the large metropolitan centers and the problem remains acute in these areas. For example, it is reported that narcotic abuse has become the leading cause of death between the ages of 15 and 35 in New York City.[31] Other reports, however, are more hopeful and may be indicating more of a wish than fact when stating that narcotic abuse, as a national health problem, seems to be diminishing. Reports from the Drug Enforcement Administration officials state that the heroin population is aging, with a 90 per cent reduction in users under 16 years of age during a recent four-year period. Even among the chronic abusers, their dependence on drugs seems to be decreasing. It is believed that increasing pressure by law enforcement authorities and the severity of narcotic laws have made traffic in heroin more difficult. The so-called "street" supplies are reported to contain progressively lower percentages of the active ingredient and the heroin content of a "bag" is now stated to range between 3 and 10 per cent. Occasionally, the user may unknowingly get a dose containing a much higher percentage of heroin which, if taken undiluted, may cause death. Also, many fatalities in this category have been attributed to hypersensitivity reactions, to impurities, or other substances used to dilute heroin.

The hard narcotics produce a sense of euphoria, reduce both psychological and physical stimuli, and dull the feelings of tension, fear, and anxiety. With chronic use of these drugs, tolerance develops and ever increasing doses are required in order to acquire the desired effect. As the need for the drug increases, the activities of the drug abuser become increasingly centered around the acquiring and using of the narcotic. When supplies are cut off, the user displays the characteristic signs of withdrawal. Such symptoms as nervousness, anxiety, sleeplessness, perspiration, fasciculations, hot and cold flashes, and pupil enlargement occur. Vomiting and diarrhea, severe aches in the back and legs, increased respiratory rate, elevated temperature, and increased blood pressure are still other symptoms. The intensity of withdrawal symptoms, of course, varies with the degree of physical dependence which, in turn, is related to the amount of drug routinely used. The onset of symptoms usually occurs about 8 to 10 hr. after the last dose. These symptoms increase in intensity until they reach a peak in 36 to 72 hr. and then gradually subside over the next five to nine days. Some of the symptoms may persist, however, for several weeks. In extreme cases of drug withdrawal, death may result.

*Depressants*

This category includes varieties of drugs which are used to retard the activity and depress the central nervous system. Included in this group are the sedatives, soporifics and the so-called tranquilizers. Of all the drugs of abuse, the major growth in recent years have been in the use of drugs which tend to quiet people down.[32] The inference from this trend is that significant numbers of people in the United States are seeking, by way of drugs, to become more quiescent. A reduction in stimulation, lowered sensitivity to the social scene, reduced demands for high performance, and less competitiveness appear to accompany this trend. Whether the sought-for quieting affect is simply periodic or whether a significant percentage of the public is seeking chronic tranquility remains to be determined. Certainly, this question is fundamental for our future as individuals and as a society.

The most widely abused among the depressants are the barbiturates and methaqualone, listed under Schedule II of the Controlled Substances Act. The drugs are abused primarily for the alcohol-like euphoria that they give but continued use frequently results in slurring of speech, slower reaction time, loss of balance, quick temper, and a quarrelsome disposition. The abuser is emotionally erratic and may be moved, easily, to tears or laughter. A particularly serious aspect of barbiturate abuse is seen when these drugs are taken in conjunction with alcohol. In these cases, the potentiation of the combined barbiturates and alcohol is greater than the additive effects of each drug taken separately. (In other words, two and two equal five). The results of this combination may well be fatal depression of the respiratory and cardiovascular systems.

Barbiturate abuse is far more dangerous than either narcotic or alcohol abuse. Each year some 3000 persons in the United States die from overdoses of barbiturates, whether by accident or by design. This gives barbiturates the dubious distinction of being the leading cause of death among all poisoning agents.[33] Unintentional overdosage can frequently occur because the drug itself confuses the mind and impairs judgment. Also, since tolerance to the drug develops, even the experienced user sometimes takes dangerously large amounts to achieve the desired effects. Both psychological and physical dependence on barbiturates develop with chronic misuse and excessive doses, and withdrawal symptoms usually are much more extreme than those resulting from narcotics withdrawal. For 8 to 10 hr. following the last dose, the afflicted abuser seems to improve, but pronounced symptoms of withdrawal become apparent shortly after this time. The patient displays signs of increasing nervousness, headache, anxiety, tremor, weakness, nausea, insomnia, and a rapid drop in blood pressure, with postural hypotension. Approximately 24 hr. following the last dose of barbiturate these symptoms intensify and may be accompanied by delirium. Within 36 to 72 hr. convulsions similar to epileptic seizures may be experienced. Unless the withdrawal is accomplished under proper medical supervision, these severe symptoms can result in death.

Methaqualone is the subject of much concern by those who deal with problems of drug abuse. It became a street drug almost as soon as it was marketed and such terms as "sopors" and "luding out" were quickly added to the jargon of drug abusers. It is reported to be the sixth most popular sedative-hypnotic in the United States. Methaqualone is a Schedule II drug since its habitual misuse pattern is reported to be equivalent to that of short-acting barbiturates. There is considerable evidence of psychological dependence with this drug and cases of physical addiction have been documented in reports from the Haight-Ashbury Free Medical Clinic of San Francisco.

A milder, tranquilizer-type drug, diazepam, is the most frequently prescribed drug in the United States. Reports of wide spread abuse of diazepam are increasing, along with severe withdrawal symptoms. The abuse of this drug is particularly serious in the methadone maintenance patient because the central nervous system depressant action of diazepam also potentiates the depressant effect of methadone.[33]

*Stimulants*

This group of drugs acts directly on the central nervous system. They produce a feeling of excitation, alertness, increased initiative and activity, appetite loss, and an ability to go without sleep for protracted periods of time. The two types of stimulants still most commonly abused are amphetamine and methedrine. Methedrine is known as "speed" while amphetamine has acquired many nicknames resulting from both the use of the drug and from the shape and color of the tablets or capsules. The stimulants are usually taken orally but the mainlining of these drugs is also encountered.

Since stimulants tend to make tired people feel alert and depressed people feel rejuvenated and more interested in life, they have a special appeal to some people. They offer optimism, euphoria, and an easy kind of chemical happiness. Many truck drivers have used them to force wakefulness beyond normal physiological limits, and emotionally susceptible teen-agers abuse these drugs as a means to experiment with new sensations, to seek thrills, and to heighten experiences. It has also been reported that stimulants are often relied upon by criminals who use them to reinforce courage during their exploits.

Most medical authorities agree that amphetamines do not produce physical dependence and that there are no characteristic withdrawal symptoms upon abrupt discontinuance of the drug. There is, usually, some mental depression and fatigue but these are not regarded, commonly, as serious effects. But these drugs still produce dependence in the psychological and emotional sense. The dependent user has little impulse to give up the pleasure of his habit. The body develops a tolerance to these drugs, however, and abusers gradually increase their doses, eliciting exaggerated responses. Thus, the abuser may display such signs as restlessness, nervousness, urinary frequency, tremor of the hands, and the usual signs of sympathetic stimulation such as increased heart rate, dilated pupils, dryness of mouth, and increased respiration. He is frequently talkative and excitable, perspires profusely, and suffers from insomnia. Chronic large doses of these stimulants create other problems. As the victim's body uses up its energy reserves there is the danger of complete exhaustion which may cause a blackout. In addition, a drug psychosis resembling schizophrenia develops with delusions and hallucinations, both auditory and visual. These effects are particularly dangerous if the victim is driving an automobile or truck. Other symptoms are paranoid in nature. The victim may think, for example, that he is being followed by enemies or that he hears voices talking about him. In short, the person abusing stimulants may exhibit dangerous, aggressive behavior with antisocial acts. Added to this is the fact that continued abuse can result in high blood pressure, cardiac arrhythmias, low blood sugar, and a higher incidence of cardiovascular accidents.

Another drug listed as a narcotic, cocaine, appears to be increasing in popularity among the street drugs. Because gastric acid hydrolyzes much of the product, cocaine is more commonly introduced into the body either by sniffing or by intravenous injection. Absorption is rapid and the effects last for approximately 30 minutes, depending on dose. Higher doses of cocaine result in a sympathetic discharge with the accompanying increase in blood pressure and body temperature, mydriasis, central nervous system stimulation with euphoria, and increased cord reflexes. Convulsions are not uncommon and medullary response causes rapid, shallow respiration plus nausea and vomiting. Repeated injections or sniffing may lead to sociopathic reactions with a distinct tendency to paranoid behavior. The individual under the influence of this drug with his high body temperature, rapid breathing, dilated pupils, rapid pulse, and frequently demonstrating delirium and paranoia, is the "dope fiend" of literature. Treatment usually consists of

cardiac support, correction of acidosis, and the administration of muscle-relaxants and short-acting barbiturates. There is a certain amount of caution to be observed when treating a patient under the influence of cocaine. When awake, he can be very dangerous; when comatose, he is usually desperately ill.

*Hallucinogens*

A group of drugs which has achieved prominence in recent years is the type which has been shown to affect the mind in rather bizarre fashions. Because they are capable of distorting images and producing hallucinations, these drugs are generally referred to as "hallucinogens." Medical literature more frequently calls them "psychotogens" or "psychotomimetics" whereas a newer term, "psychedelic," has been coined to describe the effects of these drugs. The term psychedelic is defined as "mind-manifesting" and pertains to those drugs whose action seems to expand the consciousness and enlarge the vision.[35]

At present, these drugs do not have general use in clinical medicine, yet, they are being encountered frequently as drugs of abuse. With the exception of very limited and highly controlled research programs, the distribution and use of hallucinogens are illegal. The result, therefore, is manufacturing processes carried out in clandestine laboratories, usually without quality control, or drugs smuggled into this country from foreign sources. In either case, the money used to purchase these types of drugs contributes to the support and profit of those who operate outside the law. As the profits from such activities continue to rise, they attract the interests of organized crime, and there is now substantial evidence that underworld organizations are involved in acquiring and distributing these dangerous and powerful drugs.

Because of their illegal nature, hallucinogens have no standard dosage form or markings that make visual identification possible. They may be encountered as home-made capsules or tablets, or they may be found in nondescript powders or liquids. Herein lies a significant danger. Since there are no quality controls, there is virtually no standard dose or no standard degree of purity of the drugs. Doses of hallucinogens purchased on the illegal market have been analyzed in both public and private laboratories and have been found to contain amounts of active ingredient ranging from 0 to 1000 per cent of purported contents. This may be one of the reasons why little or no reaction is experienced by occasional users although tragic and devastating effects, sometimes, are found.

Another potentially dangerous "rip off" for the buyer of street drugs is the very definite probability that the actual contents are not the same as claimed by the seller of these drugs. Reports from analytical laboratories, including some located in Colleges of Pharmacy, confirm that the buyer is much more likely to get an adulterated product whose alleged chemistry bears little resemblance to that of the actual drug purchased. The collected data suggest that no matter what psychedelic the buyer wishes to purchase, he most often receives lysergic acid diethylamide (LSD).[36] Another common substitute is phencyclidine (PCP), originally produced as a veterinary anesthetic and commonly called "angel dust."[37] One of the dangers associated with this wide-scale deception is in the treatment of acute overdose. It is not unlikely that the indicated treatment for the drug reported to be taken is completely different from the drug actually taken. An example is the substitution of PCP for LSD. Chlorpromazine and related tranquilizers have been used successfully for the treatment of LSD and mescaline intoxication, but the depressant effects of the sedative-tranquilizers are additive with the anesthetic properties of PCP. The combined effect can lead to pronounced depression and possible respiratory arrest.

The wish for instant paradise is older than recorded history and these psychotomimetic drugs seem to offer yet another method to achieve this state of nirvana. Thus, it is small wonder that certain classes of people have sought this route of escape. When the user takes hallucinogens he experiences distortion and intensification of sensory perceptions. There is a lessened ability to discriminate between fact and fantasy and the user may commonly speak of seeing lovely music, hearing beautiful pictures, and tasting exotic colors. Often there is a dilation of the pupils with a hypersensitivity to light, and dark glasses are often worn even at night.

It is difficult, if not impossible, to predict the outcome of a "trip." The user may be restless with an inability to sleep or he may exhibit no noticeable signs of drug intoxication. The mental effects may range from slight deviations to more extreme variations. Thus, illusions, panic, psychotic or antisocial behavior, and tendency toward violence or self-destruction may be experienced. This points up another significant danger. Anatomists, pathologists, physiologists, pharmacologists, clinicians, and biochemists have a rather thorough and sophisticated knowledge of the normal and abnormal aspects of most of the body. When something goes wrong the chances are favorable that accumulated knowledge and technique will dictate a therapeutic regimen that will help restore the body to its normal state of health. This is not necessarily true for the brain. After years of study and research, we probably know less about the brain than any other part of the body. Although medical textbooks confidently refer to the known methods of nerve transmission in the somatic and autonomic nervous systems, there are only theories and general disagreement regarding the exact mechanisms involved in the brain. The neurohormones, their precursors, and degradation products in the brain have been identified but there are still many unanswered questions regarding what they do and how they do it. We do not know whether there is an equivalent in the brain to the two divisions of the autonomic nervous system found in the rest of the body. If there is such an equivalent, we do not know how these two divisions are balanced or how impulses are transmitted or controlled. If, then, we do not know the exact mechanisms involved in a normally operating brain, how can medical science, presently, know what has actually happened or how to restore the functioning of the brain to its normal pattern when something goes wrong? Generally, chlorpromazine or similar medications are administered to those who seek professional help but this treatment is largely symptomatic and there is no guarantee that these same symptoms will not reappear in the patient without warning and without having taken additional psychotomimetic drugs. This is the Russian roulette involved in the use of such drugs since there seems to be no way of knowing in advance whether a trip will be good or bad. Admittedly, there are relatively few bad trips compared to the estimated number of persons who are reported to use these drugs. However, even a few bad trips are too many and unnecessary, particularly when they are measured in wasted lives, ruined plans for the future, and custodial care in mental institutions. The potential users of hallucinogens, especially those students in high school and college who are experimenting, would do well to consider the calculated risk of a bad trip and its possible consequences. There are a significant number of people who have taken such trips from which they have never returned.

Hallucinogenic drugs are derived from numerous sources. Historically, the most common source has been plants. For example, the seeds of some morning glory varieties contain lysergic acid amide, an active principle which is chemically similar to LSD and about one-tenth as potent.[38] Nutmeg, a familiar spice in the kitchen, contains a hallucinogen whose long chemical name has been abbreviated to MMDA. The psilocybe mushroom of southern Mexico was found to contain psilocybin and psilocin, two compounds that have hallucinogenic properties. The peyote cactus which grows in the desert Southwest and in northern Mexico and the lophophora cactus of Mexico both contain mescaline, a trimethoxyphenylethylamine that can produce hallucinations. Dried slices of the peyote cactus are used by certain Indian tribes as a part of their religious ritual and such use is protected by law. The root bark of the Congolese ordeal plant contains ibogaine, a substance having similar properties. Two other hallucinogenic compounds, harmine and harmaline, are found in two additional plants growing in the subtropical regions. One of the newer street drugs in "woodrose" an extract from the seed of a Hawaiian morning glory plant. Other hallucinogenic drugs are more easily semisynthesized; that is, the parent compound is altered through chemical procedures. LSD is such an example. It has been reported that LSD is relatively easy to synthesize when a supply of lysergic acid or one of the ergot alkaloids is available.[39] Lysergic acid, in turn, is either collected from the smut which grows on rye and other grains or is produced by a deep fermentation process with suitable equipment and knowledge. The complete synthesis of LSD is possible but is accomplished only with great difficulty. A number of the hallucinogenic drugs found in nature have since been synthesized in the chemical laboratory. Psilocybin, mescaline, and ibogaine are examples. Another such product is dimethyltryptamine (DMT).

This indole occurs naturally in the seeds of a South American plant, *Piptadenia peregrina*, but it is readily synthesized and, evidently, without too much difficulty. The action of DMT is rather similar to that of LSD but is reported to be more harsh. The onset is more abrupt and the effects last only about 1 hr. Still another synthesized hallucinogen is STP (serenity, tranquility, peace). Its chemical identification, methyldimethoxy - methylphenylethylamine, has been shortened to the letters DOM. This compound, which is chemically related to mescaline and amphetamine, was found to be 100 times as potent as mescaline, and rather severe reactions have been reported following its use. Other compounds have been tested and used as hallucinogens with varying degrees of success and danger. The two hallucinogenic drugs most widely known and used, however, are LSD and marihuana.

## Marihuana

The hemp plant, *Cannabis sativa*, is the source of an intoxicating substance which has been used for centuries in many countries of the world. The drug is known as hashish in the Middle East, charas in Central Asia, ganja or bhang in India, dagga in South Africa, and maconha or djamba in South America. In the United States, marihuana is the term generally used for any preparation of the *Cannabis* plant. The brown resin collected from the tops and leaves of high quality marihuana is called "hashish" and is far more potent than any of the plant parts.[40]

Marihuana is not available legally except by a special license for research purposes, and it currently has no officially recognized medical uses. The traffic in marihuana is very difficult to control, however, since it is not only easily cultivated but can grow wild in various soil conditions in almost any temperate and semi-tropical climates of the world. The use of marihuana was described in the writings of Marco Polo and the countries of Europe and Asia have been plagued with problems of the drug for hundreds of years. Its use in the United States, however, is relatively new. Marihuana was first introduced by Mexican laborers along the southern border in the early 1920's and gained a firm foothold in New Orleans where it was used by jazz musicians.

These artists believed that the drug made them play "hotter." It has been demonstrated, however, through scientific tests and the use of electronic equipment, that musicianship actually declines under the influence of the drug.

It was estimated that thousands of pounds of the dried plant were smuggled into the United States during these early days, and livid stories about the effects of the drug began appearing in newspapers and magazines. The *Cannabis* plant grew in ever greater profusion in various parts of the country. It is reported to have been cultivated, particularly in the midwestern agricultural states, partly for the resinous material in the flowering tops and partly for the hemp fiber. Then, too, one of the large bird seed producers was said to have incorporated some of the plant material into their finished product with the result that birds showed more "life" and sang much more lustily. The bird droppings were credited with a wide scale seeding of this plant throughout large geographic areas.

Sensational reports of the abuse of marihuana and livid accounts of crimes committed under its influence reached a high degree of saturation in the lay press until the drug was brought under the Harrison Narcotic Act in 1937. Marihuana is not a narcotic. Because it was included under the Narcotic Act, however, the penalties provided for the illegal distribution of this drug became quite severe.

Marihuana may be incorporated into spices and sweets and eaten as candy, it may be brewed in the form of tea, or it may be used as snuff. One underground newspaper suggested that marihuana be incorporated into a well-known cookie mix so that the user can "turn on in public with nary a raised eyebrow." Other imaginative ways of using this drug have been explored and publicized, and there are reports of a marihuana cookbook, "Cooking with Pot," which is sold in some bookstores. In the United States, however, marihuana is more generally smoked as a cigarette. The "grass" is frequently mixed with tobacco so that the cigarette will burn cooler and longer. The mixture is rolled in double wheatstraw cigarette paper, both ends folded, and the homemade cigarette is frequently moistened with saliva immediately prior to use. The smoke from the cigarette is inhaled deeply and the user holds his breath as long as practical to allow for maximum absorption. There is no physical tolerance built up to marihuana and the user seems to have a keen sense of knowing how much is needed to get a "high"; there is little tendency to increase the dose thereafter.

*Symptoms*

When marihuana is smoked, the subjective effects usually start promptly and last for about 3 or 4 hr. The user passes into a dreamy, semiconscious state in which ideas and images flow freely and pleasantly and the imagination is untrammeled by its usual restraints. The dreams assume the vividness of visions, are of boundless extravagance, and vary with the character and pursuits of the individual. Accurate judgment seems to be lost, and time sense, spatial relationships, and body images can be markedly distorted. Ideas flash through the mind without apparent continuity, and true hallucinations may appear but are often absent. During this period the consciousness is not entirely lost, for the victim can give a coherent account of his condition when aroused and can answer questions intelligently. There is an intensified perception of auditory and visual stimuli but the sensation of pain is lessened or entirely absent and the sense of touch is frequently less acute. In the company of others, the marihuana user is commonly talkative, laughs easily and to excess, and performs ridiculous movements that he does not seem able to restrain. One reporter at a "pot" party told of a user who was trying to get music out of a guitar by blowing into the end of it while another person was giving a dramatic reading from the *Handbook of Chemistry and Physics.* When alone, the user is more often drowsy and quiet.

The usual mood accompanying the use of this drug is one of euphoria or exaltation. In terms of some effects on behavior, the use of marihuana is, roughly, comparable to modern abuse of alcohol. It tends to loosen inhibitions and increase suggestibility, the user's ability to perform exacting tasks such as automobile driving is seriously impaired, and an individual under the influence of this drug may engage in activities that he would not ordinarily consider.

On the other hand, there may be adverse mood swings and even a predominant depression. Reports of severely deleterious emotional reactions and personality changes are becoming more prominent. In some cases acute mania and convulsive attacks have been developed. Panic, gross confusion, impulsive and aggressive behavior, depersonalization, and paranoid reactions have been reported in the literature, particularly when marihuana is combined with alcohol or amphetamines. In fact, descriptions of both the behavioral and subjective effects of large doses of marihuana are remarkably similar to the effects elicited from LSD, mescaline, and psilocybin. The physiological changes accompanying marihuana use are quite variable. The most consistent and dependable changes are an increase pulse rate, reddening of the eyes, and dryness of the mouth and throat. Other general effects commonly described are headache, dizziness, vertigo, fainting, and perspiration. Other effects frequently associated with marihuana use include urinary frequency, diarrhea, nausea, and vomiting. Contrary to popular belief, hangover effects have been described.[41]

The use of marihuana in the United States continues at a startling high rate. The Internal Security Subcommittee of the U.S. Senate estimated that total consumption of marihuana in 1973 was approximately 17 million pounds and about 500 thousand pounds of hashish. The drug has now been used enough to study some of the longer term effects. Some of these reported effects include tracheobronchitis, damage to white blood cells, reduction in the body's ability to produce DNA, severe personality changes that infer altered cerebral functioning on a biochemical basis,[42] and altered heart functions displayed by electrocardiograms.[43] It is the general conclusion from these later reports that present medical and public approach to education regarding the danger of marihuana use should undergo some reassessment.

Available information indicates that although there is no physical dependence upon marihuana, there is a definite probability of psychic dependence. The combination of the effects of the drug plus psychic dependence may lead to extreme lethargy, indolence, neglect of personal hygiene, and a preoccupation with the drug that precludes constructive activity. In addition, there appears to be a causal relationship developing between the chronic use of hallucinogens and the impairment of both memory and intellectual functioning.

The common names of marihuana are many and varied and reflect the appearance of the prepared plant, the methods of preparation, and the effects. One reference source lists 42 different names and even this does not exhaust the list. The most frequently used names, however, are the following: pot, Texas tea, grass, Mary Jane, Acapulco gold, and Indian hay. A marihuana cigarette is more commonly known as a "joint," "stick," or "reefer," and a butt of such a cigarette is called a "roach." Habitual smokers of marihuana are known, commonly, as "tea heads" or "grasshoppers."

The chief active ingredient of the *Cannabis* plant is Delta 9-tetrahydrocannabinol and it is found in greatest concentrations in the resinous exudate of the flowering tops. Lesser concentrations of this active principle and its congeners, however, are found in other plant parts. The potency of marihuana and its preparations vary with the geographical location where the plant was grown, method of cultivation, time of harvest, how long it was stored, plant parts used, and methods employed in extracting the resin. This variation illustrates a potential threat. There has been considerable discussion in recent years, even among some people prominent in public life, encouraging the legalization of the use of marihuana. There are some cogent arguments for this position. A very large percentage of the marihuana presently used in the United States is reportedly grown in the Mexican state of Sinaloa and some of the other agricultural states of Mexico. Essentially all of the plant except the woody fiber is chopped into fragments and is sold primarily for smoking purposes. As mentioned previously, the "grass" is frequently mixed with tobacco so that the home-made cigarette will not burn so rapidly and so intensely. In addition, some of the sellers of marihuana, in order to increase their profits, are reported to dilute the product with catnip, oregano, or tea. When used in this form, the net result is that relatively small amounts of the intoxicating substance are absorbed into the system and the effects are transient even though disturbing. Mexican marihuana is quite cheap and evidently readily available; when used in moderate amounts there appears to be only a slight chance that it will have a permanent effect on the body; and it produces no abstinence syndrome when the drug is withheld. The suggestions that marihuana be taxed and sold on the open market have found reasonable acceptance among diverse segments of the population because of its widespread use and seemingly impossible task of controlling the drug. When restricted to whole-plant marihuana, these suggestions have some merit, but the proponents of such classification change have not taken into account the recent rapid increase in the reports of serious adverse effects, even among those using this mild form of marihuana. Added to this is the distinct probability that legalization of marihuana would result in the importation of hashish from the Middle East, charas from Central Asia, and other potent forms of the drug found in various parts of the world. The mild euphoria, heightened sensitivities, and vague distortions of time and space accompanying inhalation of the milder marihuana could very easily, and readily, be replaced by the frenzied horror and psychotic behavior which more freqently accompany use of these more potent compounds.

Along this same line, there is another argument that is commonly heard among students. Some of these young people insist that bans against the use of marihuana unduly restrict their freedom and are an unwarranted employment of police power. Yet, it must be remembered that in a communal society the expressions of individual freedom are somewhat limited. These expressions become a matter of public concern and restraint when they abuse and threaten the freedom, safety, and health of innocent members of the same society. Experience has demonstrated that antisocial acts accompanying the distribution and use of marihuana have been frequent enough and severe enough to call for public sanctions. Therefore, the use of police power, or the power to restrict the activities of a few for the benefit of the many, has been found to be both legitimate and justifiable.

## LSD

Few drugs in the last quarter of a century have engendered more publicity and controversy than LSD. Those opposed to the drug cite cases of homicide, suicide, insanity, and perversion to support their views. On the other hand, those who favor unrestrained use of LSD refer to profound, sublime, and emotionally satisfying experiences that the drug is said to give. Literally thousands of articles have appeared in the medical literature regarding LSD and practically every major magazine on the newsstand has contained feature stories and reports concerning this compound. Seldom has so much been claimed for a drug with so little scientifically substantiating evidence.

LSD was first synthesized in 1938 by Stoll and Hoffman in Sandoz Research Laboratories.[44] These investigators used lysergic acid obtained from ergot, a fungus which grows on rye and other grains. Ergot preparations were associated, medically, with their known properties of vasoconstriction and of promoting uterine contractions, as well as beneficial results in cases of migraine headache. At this time LSD was not tested orally in humans. In 1943, five years later, Dr. Hoffman accidentally ingested a micro quantity of the drug and experienced very strange and bizarre reactions. His description of the effects which he wrote in his journal is now classic.[45]

I noted with dismay that my environment was undergoing progressive change. Everything seemed strange and I had the greatest difficulty in expressing myself. My visual fields wavered and everything appeared deformed as in a faulty mirror. I was overcome by a feeling that I was going crazy, the worst part of it being that I was clearly aware of my condition. The mind and power of observation were apparently unimpaired.

In 1953, Sandoz Pharmaceuticals made the drug available in the United States and the Food and Drug Administration agreed to its distribution only to research psychiatrists who were properly qualified to investigate the drug and use it solely on an experimental basis. Subsequently, LSD was used by numerous investigators who reported various degrees of success in treating terminal cancer, different types of mental disorders, rehabilitation of criminals, alcoholism, and character disorders. It was generally agreed, however, that the drug was too dangerous to be administered on a wide basis and its use was discouraged.

During this time period there were increasing reports that the drug was being diverted from legal channels and that it was either being self-administered or was given under less than controlled conditions. In 1959, the abuse of LSD first came to the attention of FDA when it was found that members of certain religious cults in the Pacific Northwest were using it in some of their rites. It was sometime later that a professor in social psychology in a large eastern university experimented with hallucinogenic drugs on undergraduate students. In the early 60's, the use of LSD caught the imagination of certain popular authors, historians, and social psychologists who wrote convincingly of its consciousness-expanding qualities. It was spurred on by sensational publicity and by apostles of the new cult who came to view LSD as a symbol of protest against cultural values held by the establishment. Thrill seekers and non-conformists began to extol the virtues of the drug, and urged others to turn on with LSD. tune in to the message induced by the drug, and drop out of productive society. Adverse effects from uncontrolled usage continued to mount and emergency hospitalizations were becoming commonplace. For example, in 1965, during a four-month period, 27 patients with severe complications resulting from self-administration of LSD were admitted to New York's Bellevue Hospital.[46] The abuse of the drug became so blatant and the results of scientific investigations so involved in controversy that, in 1966, Sandoz Pharmaceuticals withdrew their sponsorship of investigations using LSD and transferred its remaining stock of the drug to the National Institute of Mental Health. Consequently, except for the very limited and highly restricted investigational use through the Federal .Government, all production, distribution, and use of LSD in this country are now illegal. This fact underscores another serious problem.

Previously, when the drug was more widely used by scientists, the chances of a "bad trip" were not nearly so great. The user was assured that he would be taking a known quantity of the drug that was produced by a reputable manufacturer, that he would be in a controlled environment with highly trained personnel observing his reactions, and that he would have adequate protection in case he was moved to perform antisocial acts or self-destruction. Even when the drug was taken outside a controlled environment and the observers were not technically trained, the user was generally assured that the drug itself was of a high quality.

Since the government has restricted LSD and the chemicals from which the drug is made, however, it is reasonable to assume that the illegal drugs now used were made with little or no quality control. LSD is odorless and tasteless and can be placed upon such common items as hard candy, animal crackers, postage stamps, chewing gum, aspirin, and costume jewelry. Indeed, the methods for transporting this drug are limited only by the imagination. The user of illegal LSD, then, is taking a double chance. He is taking a drug not only of untested purity and strength but he has no way of knowing that the aspirin tablet or the chewing gum contains the proper amount of the drug for a "good trip." As was mentioned previously in this discussion, analyzed "buys" of illegal LSD reveal quantities ranging up to 10 times the stated amount and many of these drugs are of poor quality.

Unfortunately, people who are most attracted to the abuse of LSD are those who are most likely to be harmed by it. When these people experiment with illicit drugs of an uncertain quantity and purity, they are making no attempt to direct the drug to specific psychiatric problems. Their only desire is to go on a "trip" without direction, supervision, or knowledge of the psychiatric and physical dangers involved. With untrained peers as the only available assistance, the chances of a bad reaction and the dangers of serious mental damages are multiplied many times over. There is no way of predicting when or why an LSD trip, which is intended to be beautiful and sublime, will become a hellish nightmare.

Among the various hallucinogenic drugs now known, LSD is by far the most potent. Doses as small as 20 to 30 $\mu$g. may produce effects in susceptible individuals although the usual dose taken by a non-tolerant person ranges from 100 to 200 $\mu$g. Tolerance to the drug develops rapidly but usually is lost in two or three days. The physical effects associated with the use of LSD are mainly those which are mediated through the autonomic nervous system. These include an increase in body temperature, heart rate, blood pressure, and blood sugar. Nausea, perspiration, chills, hot flashes, and irregular breathing are additional symptoms. The pupils are usually so widely dilated that the user may wear dark glasses even at night, and sleep becomes virtually impossible until at least 8 hr. after the LSD episode is over.

There is no hindrance to the passage of LSD across the blood-brain barrier, and the most significant effects of the drug are almost entirely upon the central nervous system. Although there is no definite sequence or series of invariable effects from taking LSD, certain typical changes occur. Euphoria may often be the first sign that the drug is beginning to work. Despite the absence of precipitating events, some subjects feel silly and start laughing, some are in a state of contentment, and others are fearful and anxious and feel alone and abandoned. Perception becomes distorted, with visual changes usually the most vivid. Solid objects such as sofas and tables begin to move, and walls seem to close in, expand, or pulsate. A sudden noise may be perceived as a flash of color. Objects which usually evoke little feeling can charge the emotions and seem to be expressionistic works of art. One reporter who served as a peer supervisor at an LSD party told of one user who sat for 2 hr. in a trance-like state admiring his own big toe, while another subject spent an equal amount of time "passionately enthralled with a rather ugly-looking table lamp." Feelings of depersonalization are, also, quite common. One user related how he got out of his body and sat in a corner of the room and watched his body perform. Other users feel that their arms and legs are not really attached to their bodies and additional users feel that they are floating off in space. One subject reported, "I feel as though my body is melting away; I have no boundaries—scoop me up off the floor and tie me up in a sack to give me some limits." Perceptual changes in time are also noted. Subjects may state after several hours that only minutes have gone by or may exaggerate the amount of time elapsed. Time may seem to stand still, reverse itself, become accelerated, or slow down.

LSD also affects thought processes, judgment, and concentration. The subject may show confusion or impaired thinking, and trivial events may assume unusual significance and importance. Limited observations suggest the need to explore the possible impairment of abstract thinking and the ability to reason. Some of these observations have indicated strongly that habitual users of LSD may actually lose their capability to think clearly, to reason lucidly, to create, or otherwise to use their minds productively.

The increasing number of side effects being reported through the use of LSD seems to be proportional to the increased procurement of the drug from illicit sources. Such untoward reactions as self-destruction, impulses toward violence, prolonged psychosis, paranoia with ideas of grandiosity, severe depression, and panic have been reported in the medical literature. Another frightening reaction is the spontaneous reappearance of symptoms and experiences even after relatively long intervals of abstinence from LSD. More recently, however, reports of untoward reactions from LSD appear to be diminishing.

These are the disastrous reactions of "bad trips." However, perhaps even more tragic are the consequences of the many "positive trips." These lead the user to feel that he has finally reached Utopia, that he has found the answer to the frustrations of life, and that his chemically centered religion has introduced him to values that transcend his society and culture. As a result, such users all too often become oblivious to the personal satisfaction resulting from accomplishment and fail to develop skills, discipline, and means of self-expression. They frequently have a tendency toward anti-intellectualism and non-rational thinking, and they disengage themselves from productive activities and drift aimlessly without social achievements to enrich their personal lives.

Whether the illegal use of LSD is a growing menace or a diminishing problem is open to discussion at this time. It may be wishful thinking but there are promising signs that its widespread use has been more of a fad. Although the drug will continue to be prominent in some subcultures, there seems to be a growing conclusion among young thrill seekers that they would rather "turn on" with something a little less potent and dangerous than LSD. Others have seen the effects of LSD on their peers and do not want to take the chance of reacting in such a violent or uncontrolled fashion. The vast majority of young people do not feel the need for such a mind-jarring experience and there is serious question whether such a "trip" is worth the fare that may be exacted.

## Combating the Drug Problem

What is to be done about drug abuse and the drug abuser? Certainly, traditional law enforcement methods alone cannot cope with the situation because they do not take into account the sociological and psychological origin of the drug problems. Education is an obvious answer but here we must be cautious. Intensive educational campaigns do not necessarily educate people although they may do an effective job of imparting vital facts. We are not certain that the public has sufficient background to assimilate these facts adequately, and, even if they can, there is a question whether they alter their behavior toward minimizing abuse. The thin line between educating for prevention or informing for curiosity's sake perplexes us. There is always the sobering possibility that some forms of education may actually make drug abuse more attractive, just as banning a book ensures increased sales. Indeed, considerable evidence has been accumulating the past few years to indicate that traditional drug abuse preventive educational techniques have been somewhat less than successful.[47] Some areas report that drug abuse has actually increased following intensified educational campaigns. Certainly, there is a very little hard data to support the theory that education is a means of reducing drug abuse.[48]

As long as drugs are available to relieve pain, ameliorate moods, and reduce tensions, they will continue to be abused by non-conformists and by those who need a chemical crutch. As new drugs are developed and as naturally occurring products are synthesized, there always will be those who will try them for non-medical purposes.

Endeavors by the Federal Government to limit drug abuse are aimed both at fighting illicit drug traffic and helping to rehabilitate the drug abuser. Theoretically, the ultimate goal of legal control is to help people achieve self-control. To this end, Congress passed the Drug Abuse Prevention And Control Act of 1970. It was this Act that placed drugs into the five Schedules, confining most of the heavily controlled drugs to Schedules I and II. The interests and activities of the Federal government in this field are divided into two large categories. One is the area of law enforcement and the other is the public health activities. Under the Presidential Reorganization Plan No. 2 of 1973, the Drug Enforcement Administration (DEA) was created within the Department of Justice. The DEA resulted from the merger of the Bureau of Narcotics and Dangerous Drugs, the Office for Drug Abuse Law Enforcement, the Office of National Narcotic Intelligence, those elements of the Bureau of Customs which have drug investigative responsibilities, and those drug enforcement-related functions of the Office of Science and Technology. In carrying out its mission, the DEA cooperates with other Federal agencies, foreign as well as state and local governments, private industry, and professional associations.

The public health activities are centered in the newly formed Alcohol, Drug Abuse, and Mental Health Administration. Considerable legislation has been passed in recent years to provide vast improvements in both prevention and care. Under the Narcotic Addiction Rehabilitation Act, habitual narcotic and marihuana users can be civilly committed for treatment and rehabilitation, and receive after-care in their own communities after release from treatment hospitals. The Drug Abuse Office and Treatment Act of 1972 provided for the establishment of the National Drug Abuse Training Center, the National Institute on Drug Abuse, and a formula grant program to assist States in coping with the drug problem. As discussed in Chapter 2, the Alcohol, Drug Abuse, and Mental Health Administration has devoted a significant portion of its resources to the study of drug abuse and is producing answers which promise an even more enlightened method of treatment in the future. This agency has assumed administrative control of the former narcotic treatment hospitals in Lexington and in Fort Worth.

Contemporary treatment approaches to drug abuse tend to be one of two types. These are the peer-oriented therapeutic community such as Day Top Village and Synanon, or a long-term drug replacement therapy such as methadone maintenance. Evaluation reports conclude that neither approach has led to a major reduction in the prevalence of narcotic addiction or other forms of drug abuse.[49] Criticisms leveled at the peer-oriented therapeutic communities suggest that they are essentially extended centers for the drug culture and not truly effective in rehabilitating the drug abuser.[50] The use of ex-addicts in drug abuse treatment programs does not appear to be based on any systematic evaluation of their success in rehabilitating chronic drug abusers. It is questioned whether these people are able to live up to the job demands placed upon them. Although there are many notable exceptions, it is reported that the ex-drug abuser employed as a counselor may continue to exhibit the low frustration tolerance associated with chronic drug misuse and may also feel safe in continued association with the drug world. In many cases, drug dependency is reported to be transformed into an institutional dependency and abstinence from drugs is, in part, a function of a dependency transformation.[51]

Methadone maintenance continues to have both supporters and antagonists. These programs were designed to transfer the heroin user to a semisynthetic narcotic under more controlled conditions. Methadone produces both a psychological and physiological dependence but is considered to be a safer drug than heroin. Those who are enrolled in this program do not have to worry about their continuing supply of narcotics and can usually function more normally in society when this need is fulfilled. In addition, they are usually more amenable to drug treatment programs, reality therapy, and rehabilitation. Those opposed to the methadone program claim that the user is merely transferring from one addicting drug to another. As more work is being done in the treatment and rehabilitation fields it is hoped that the methadone programs will be able to show an improved reduction in the number of chronic abusers and an increase in the number of individuals who are totally rehabilitated and can re-enter a productive society.

Detoxification is not the end product. The subject must be endowed with the capability to cope with stress situations, first, in a protected environment and, then, within his community. Adequate rehabilitation will require concerted community support with simultaneous efforts to provide housing, employment, acceptance, and other aids. Each patient presents a unique therapeutic problem calling for ingenuity on the part of all who endeavor to help.

Prevention, of course, is the preferred approach and here the allied health personnel can help immensely. This is particularly true of the doctors, pharmacists, and nurses who know these drugs and have in many instances observed their effects. It must also be recognized that the non-medical use of drugs is not necessarily a medical problem to be handled only by the medical profession. The general community has all too often been led to believe that drug abuse is a unique behavior which is best left to the drug expert, whose efforts the community must fund. And yet, it is the community that must respond to this challenge. Only an aroused and concerned public can create, mobilize, and implement resources to deal adequately with as serious a problem as drug dependence in all of its forms. Educational endeavors to this end must come from community leaders aware of the needs and from professionals who apply themselves to these needs. In this context, certain searching questions still remain. Why do young people start

using drugs? Why do they continue? In what ways does a community reinforce or inhibit the use and misuse of drugs? What are the viable alternatives to drug abuse? It is generally recognized that the best precaution against drug abuse is a positive purpose in life but how is this purpose instituted in the lives of young people? Certainly, research and treatment efforts must continue but also must be re-assessed and re-evaluated. Additional factors relating to the community appear to be equally important. These include attitudes and values toward drug use, misuse, and the drug user; public policy relating to intervention; the economics of drug use; and enlarged education programming to help both adults and young people understand their own as well as alternate life styles; school programs designed to enhance individual growth, and community programs that increase the involvement and effectiveness of both organizations and individuals who can assist young people; the effect of mass media; and community programs that are sensitive to the different cultures, life styles, and basic needs of young people and ethnic groups. Knowledgeable professionals can help in this meaningful endeavor. To withhold active support is to place additional burdens on the dedicated few who are working so diligently in this field. In the words of Edmund Burke, "All that is necessary for the triumph of evil is that good men do nothing."

Some years ago, Oliver Wendell Holmes, Jr., made this profound statement: "As life is action and passion, it is required of a man that he should share the passion and action of his time, at the peril of being judged not to have lived." At this time in our history the needs and illnesses of mankind must be met and treated not only in our laboratories, our professional offices, and our places of employment, but must be delivered in the main stream of social interaction. The need for allied health professionals to treat these illnesses where they occur has never been greater. Certainly, we must rise to the challenge.

## VENEREAL DISEASE

### Introduction

Venereal diseases are infections acquired chiefly by sexual contact with diseased persons. As such, they may be classified as social diseases. In a larger sense, however, they are representative of another type of social malady and present a commentary on our changing cultural patterns. Because of their mode of transmission, venereal diseases have long been a taboo subject both in public and in private. As a result, the public has shunned any attempts at publicity. Infected persons treated by private physicians are frequently protected from scandal and their cases are not reported. Most schools, until quite recently, avoided the inclusion of sex education in their curricula with the result that half-truths and myths regarding reproduction and diseases have been accepted as fact. Venereal disease constitutes one of the three most important communicable disease problems in the United States and, if it were any other type of disease without social stigma, it would be considered a major epidemic. Unfortunately, lack of public support and understanding as to methods of spread and control as well as lack of knowledge concerning the extent and severity of these diseases have greatly hampered the best efforts of public health workers and others who are concerned with this ominous threat. Public apathy and unwillingness to discuss openly problems associated with sex, therefore, represent a deficiency which mars the effectiveness of adequate control.

Another social effect which is reflected in the seriousness of the venereal disease problem is the current period of rapid culture change. During such a period the lines of demarcation between good and bad, moral and immoral, or right and wrong become blurred. Social scientists are commenting on the increased permissiveness and promiscuity among a significant portion of the population. Patterns of earlier dating, relaxation of parental authority, declining influence of the church, and changes from the home-centered environment have all been included as factors that contribute to this dilemma. The 1973 reported cases of gonorrhea in the United States were 823 thousand, and 25 thousand cases of syphilis (52). These, however, are merely the reported cases and the Center for Disease Control estimates that the actual figures are approximately three times those reported. A true epidemic of gonorrhea is sweeping the country. The Chief of the Venereal Disease Branch of CDC has stated that the alarming increase is characteristic of a classic epidemic completely out of control.[53] Approximately 20 per cent of the total cases of

gonorrhea are in persons under 20 years of age, 60 per cent are younger than 25, and 80 per cent under 29. The incidence of infectious syphilis is greatest in young adults between the ages of 20 and 24, the next largest group are in the 25- to 29-year age span and the third largest number of cases are found in the 15- to 19-year age group.[54] Among the newly reported cases of specified notifiable diseases in the United States, the number of cases of syphilis at all stages and gonorrhea together outnumber the reported number of cases of all other reportable diseases combined.[55] The report for the first 43 weeks of 1974 show 754 thousand cases of gonorrhea and 21 thousand cases of syphilis. If this trend continues, the incidence of gonorrhea will reach even higher levels while the numbers of syphilis cases will show a slight decline.

In former years it was generally felt that prostitution contributed significantly to the high venereal disease rate. Although factual information on this subject is practically nonexistent and, in spite of the fact that up to 17 per cent of the infected individuals had listed prostitutes among their contacts, it does not seem that prostitutes are, generally, a major factor in the current spread of syphilis and gonorrhea in the United States. By the same token, homosexuals are also implicated to a degree since approximately 14 per cent of infected patients have listed contacts of their own sex. Listing of contacts, however, merely indicates that the person named *may* have been the source. By far, the greatest cause of the spread of venereal disease has been attributed to relaxed moral standards and considerably more promiscuity. It is estimated that there are about 800,000 American women who have asymptomatic undetected gonorrhea with a lesser but significant number of asymptomatic males. The asymptomatic infected female patient is reported to be one of the main contributors to the resurgence of the incidence of gonorrhea.[56] Apart from the moral restrictions, there have been, in the past, two deterrents to sexual freedom—fear of disease and fear of pregnancy.

With the advent of penicillin and broad spectrum antibiotics, the fear of contracting venereal disease lost much of its ominous threat. The one-shot treatment was so widely used, however, that there are now appearing resistant strains of organisms. In spite of this, it is recognized that if a case of venereal disease can be treated soon enough there is still a very good chance for complete recovery. The fear of pregnancy has been reduced, at least to a degree, by "the pill." Among those women who lean toward promiscuity, oral contraceptives have been a great relief and have resulted in less restrictions on their activities. Coupled with this, however, is still another threat. Since the male partner no longer has to use a rubber prophylactic or similar protection, the chances for transfer of infection are greatly heightened. With the significant reduction of these two deterrents, then, it seems that our new morality may be not only setting different social norms but provides for an even more widespread dissemination of venereal disease.

Almost too late, we were forced by circumstances to recognize the fact that it would take more than a miracle drug to control venereal disease and to keep it controlled. At least one indicated course of action is to do everything in our power to recognize every outbreak of the disease and to bring it under control with the greatest possible speed and efficiency.

There are no isolated cases of early syphilis. Every case is related immediately to at least one additional case and must be considered with a sense of urgency, whether it be treated in the office of the private practitioner or in the public clinic. The same is, generally, true for the other venereal diseases.

Case finding, then, is an important key. Some cases of venereal disease are disclosed in military induction examinations, premarital blood tests, annual physical examinations, routine hospital admissions, examination of jail inmates, and examination of food handlers. Cases treated by private physicians seem to be increasing but only a small percentage of these are reported to health departments. Apathy and pressure from private patients are mostly responsible for this lack of cooperation.

The most productive work in case finding has been done by health department investigators who interview the infected patients. In addition to the source of his or her infection, the average venereal disease patient may be expected to name three or four other sex contacts, and it is not rare for infected patients to name anywhere from 20 to 70 contacts in a previous three- to six-month period. These contacts are located whenever possible and are examined and interviewed for additional contacts. One such series of a syphilis investigation reported by the Public Health Service started with an infected 24-year-old woman and eventually involved 625 persons, including 220 children and youths under 20 years of age. Although projects such as these are laborious, time-consuming, and expensive, they have yielded excellent results and have helped to limit an even wider spread of the disease. Once again, however, the greatest benefit has come from those treated in public clinics. One five-year study has disclosed that 85 per cent of the patients treated in public clinics and hospitals named sources and contacts who were then located and brought in for treatment by health officers. By contrast, only 17 per cent of those treated by private physicians provided this vital information. Just because one infected person receives treatment does not mean that the reservoir has been eliminated. There is no immunity to the venereal diseases at this time, and the chances for reinfection are equally as great each time the victim dips into the reservoir.

## Types of Venereal Disease

The venereal disease group consists of infectious diseases transmitted chiefly through sexual contact, and, in the United States, there are five such diseases which are of importance to public health. These are syphilis, gonorrhea, granuloma inguinale, lymphogranuloma venereum, and chancroid. Of this group, syphilis and gonorrhea are, by far, the most prevalent and present the greatest public health menace.

### Granuloma Inguinale

This disease is characterized by the development of red, granulating, ulcer-like lesions in the anogenital area that, if unchecked, will spread to the buttocks and lower abdomen. There is a strong, foul odor associated with the exudate from the lesions and deep scarring may accompany healing of sores. In the United States, granuloma inguinale predominates in the Negro race by at least an 8:1 ratio. The disease is caused by Donovan bodies which appear as encapsulated coccobacillary or rod-like forms within large mononuclear cells, and is treated by administration of broad spectrum antibiotics.

### Lymphogranuloma Venereum

This viral disease is found, more commonly, in the tropical regions of the world, and reported incidences in the United States show a 5:1 ratio of Negro to Caucasian cases. It is characterized by a swelling of lymph glands in the inguinal region, frequently accompanied by genital lesions. The virus is reported to be spread chiefly through the lymphatics and causes generalized stiffness and aching throughout the body. Historically, this disease has been associated with sailors and prostitutes but, in addition to sexual intercourse, it can be transmitted by contaminating exudate. Thus, children and others may contract the infection by simple contact with bedfellows, douche nozzles, or infected clothing. The sulfonamides are reported to be the drugs of choice with broad spectrum antibiotics as a second choice. A rather serious complication of this disease is rectal stricture, which may call for surgical management. Lymphogranuloma venereum can be diagnosed by complement fixation or by the Frei test, which is somewhat similar to the tuberculin skin test.

### Chancroid

Chancroid is characterized by the formation of rapidly growing, painful, soft ulcers, usually in the genital regions. It is the least important of the five venereal diseases and may respond to soap and water alone. The disease is caused by the Ducrey bacillus and can be controlled by sulfonamides or antibiotics. Since contaminating exudates can transmit this disease, it may be found among children, doctors, and nurses. Prevention consists of avoiding dangerous sexual contacts and of scrupulous washing after possible exposure.

### Gonorrhea

Gonorrhea is an infection of the mucous membranes caused by the gonococcus, *Neisseria gonorrhoeae*. It is confined chiefly to the membranes of the genitourinary tract, the rectum, and occasionally the eye. A distinct increase is also noted in oropharyngeal gonococcal infection.[57] Eye infections are commonly restricted to the very young. A newborn infant may contract the disease while passing through the birth canal of an infected mother. The resulting infection, ophthalmia neonatorum, may cause blindness. In fact, at one time, it was the cause of about 30 per cent of all blindness. To prevent the possibility of contracting this disease, all physicians are required by law to instill drops of antibiotics or very dilute silver nitrate into the eyes of newborn babies.

Gonorrhea is spread by discharges from infected individuals and, in turn, directly infects the mucous membranes of the victim. It is not necessary for a cut or a scratch to be present for invasion, as in the case of syphilis, and infection by means other than sexual contact is even more unlikely than in the case of syphilis. In the male, symptoms develop within three to seven days after sexual exposure and begin with a painful inflammation of the urethral canal. This is usually noted by a burning sensation on urination and the appearance of a thick, yellow discharge from the penis. Such symptoms usually persist for two or three weeks and the disease is highly communicable during this time. Because of its common localization in the genitourinary tract, gonorrhea is more easily cured in the male.

In the female, the gonococcus first attacks the urethra, producing urethritis. There may be painful urination and vaginal discharge but, frequently, these symptoms are so mild as to go unnoticed. After one or two menstruation periods, the infection progresses through the reproductive system and involves the fallopian tubes and ovaries. Gonococcal salpingitis, inflammation of the fallopian tubes, is not uncommon. This acute infection may present such symptoms as lower abdominal pain and low-grade fever but these frequently are dismissed as being due to other causes. A well-developed case of gonorrhea in the female is more difficult to treat because antibiotics have difficulty in reaching the sites of infection at high enough concentration to eradicate the disease. Untreated, the acute symptoms subside after two or three weeks but the woman retains a chronic infection which may last for years and she remains a source of infection to those who have sexual intercourse with her.

When gonorrhea remains untreated in either sex there is danger of severe complications. Lesions in the reproductive systems of both sexes may cause sterility. In addition, there may be abscesses of the prostate or vulvovaginal glands or a gonorrheal pelvic inflammatory disease. Systemically, the infecting organisms may affect the valves of the heart, may produce a severe arthritis, or may result in gonoccocal meningitis.

The risk of leaving asymptomatic women undiscovered and untreated is fraught with particular danger. Estimates of the frequency of gonococcal salpingitis and pelvic inflammatory disease extend from 5 per cent to 20 per cent.

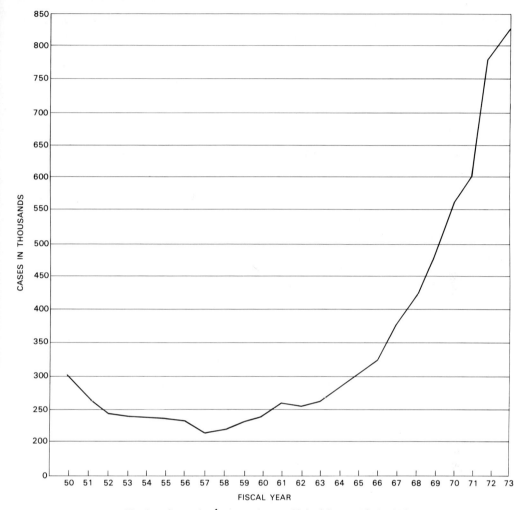

Fig. 9.1. Gonorrhea: reported cases, United States, 1950-1973.

Tragically, salpingitis is the leading cause of female sterility in the United States and a major indication for pelvic surgery. In addition, approximately one of every 200 females with asymptomatic gonorrhea has been estimated to develop a syndrome of gonococcal septicemia and arthritis.[58]

Particular difficulties are encountered when working with the problem of gonorrhea. As mentioned previously, the asymptomatic patient poses a particular problem. Several studies have shown that approximately 80 per cent of women with gonorrhea, confirmed by a positive culture for the gonococcus, are asymptomatic. Conclusions drawn from previous surveys have indicated that among males with gonococcal infection only about 12 per cent were asymptomatic. More recent investigations, however, have revealed a much higher percentage.[59]

Another problem involves lack of proper therapeutic procedures in treating the disease. Studies have shown that approximately 75 per cent of the persons with gonorrhea in the United States are treated by local physicians. A recent survey has disclosed that an excess of 30 per cent are improperly treated by local physicians who are using either inadequate dosages or inappropriate antibiotics.[60] These patients had already sought treatment but the inadequate therapy had failed to remove them from the pool of the infected. Still another problem is the development of resistant strains of gonococcus, both to penicillin and to tetracyclines. Most of this resistance is dose-related, however, and usually can be overcome with massive doses.

Detection of gonorrhea, particularly in females and in asymptomatic males, has been aided by the development of the Thayer-Martin culture media. Samples taken by a bacteriological loop, the cotton swab, or from urine sediment are innoculated on plates containing the selective media and incubated for at least 48 hr. to determine growth of the organism. The search still continues for a rapid, effective screening procedure that can be utilized on a broad scale. At least one pharmaceutical company has marketed a two-minute serological for gonococcal antibody, utilizing *in vitro* latex agglutination, as a screening procedure. Certainly, much remains to be accomplished in this field.

In 1972, the Center for Disease Control of the Public Health Service issued new recommendations for the treatment of gonorrhea. These guidelines call for 4.8 million units of aqueous procaine penicillin injected intramuscularly and divided into at least two doses. Also included in this treatment regimen and preferably administered at least 30 min. prior to the two injections, is 1 gm. of oral probenecid. Penicillin G is still the drug of choice when treating gonorrhea and the other methods suggested by CDC are recommended only as alternatives. In this treatment regimen, probenecid acts by blocking the renal tubular secretion of penicillin and thereby increases serum levels of the antibiotic approximately 50 per cent. In addition, probenecid prolongs the duration of effective serum levels. The recommended oral treatment for uncomplicated gonorrhea is 3.5 gm. of ampicillin with 1 gm. of probenecid, administered simultaneously. Other drugs that are recognized as being effective in the treatment of gonorrhea are spectinomycin, carbenicillin, minocycline, and doxycycline.[61] Unfortunately, in spite of intensified research activities at CDC and other laboratories the chances for producing an effective vaccine within the near future remain rather remote. Researchers have recently demonstrated that both females and males produce specific antibodies within their genital tracts. The appearance of both circulating and secretory antibodies against the gonococcus without evidence of immunity to gonorrhea has raised a question as to the probability of developing a vaccine for the disease. Certainly, the number of gonorrhea repeaters seen in VD clinics has led researchers to believe that little, if any, immunity to the disease does develop.[62] Nevertheless, the pressing need is for prevention of gonorrhea. Since

the current efforts to produce a vaccine seem to be unsuccessful, bolder and more imaginative methods of educating the public about this serious bacterial infection will have to be developed.

*Syphilis*

Syphilis is caused by a spirochete known as *Treponema pallidum.* Outside the body, this organism can ordinarily live but a few seconds. Thus, it is virtually impossible for the disease to be transferred other than by personal contact, usually through sexual intercourse. The disease, then, is not transferred through dirty drinking glasses, eating utensils, toilet seats, towels, unscrubbed bathtubs, or any other similar articles.

The treponeme ordinarily enters vulnerable surfaces of the anogenital, oral, or other mucous or cutaneous surfaces. The disease, unlike gonorrhea which first affects the genitourinary system, is systemic from the onset. The organisms are picked up by the lymphatics, multiply in the regional lymph nodes, and eventually enter the main circulatory system through the thoracic duct. From here they are distributed to virtually every organ and tissue of the body. The infection is rapid and thorough and is accomplished without one outward sign of the disease's course. In fact, during this period there is neither clinical nor serological evidence of syphilis.

Approximately three weeks after infection the first sign appears. This is a lesion, called a chancre, which is found usually in the anogenital region but may occur wherever the treponeme first entered the body, such as the lip, tongue, or tonsil. The chancre is usually a single, eroded, hard papule and is almost always painless. A very common site for a chancre in women is the cervix of the uterus, and such a lesion often is missed in examination of female patients simply because of failure to examine the cervix. The chancre will heal eventually, even without medications or therapy of any kind. To the uninformed, this spontaneous healing may present a sense of false security but, actually, the treponemes are continuing to multiply in the body at a rapid rate. During this primary stage, the serum may be either positive or negative. The best chance of a positive diagnosis at this stage is a darkfield examination of material from a local lesion.

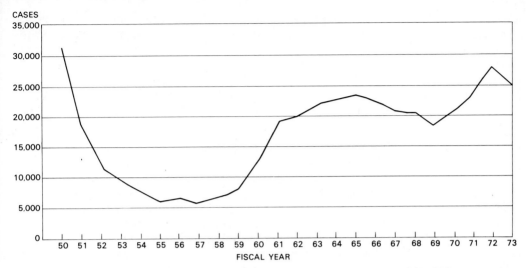

Fig. 9.2. Primary and secondary syphilis: reported cases, United States, 1950-1973.

The secondary stage of syphilis usually appears about six to nine weeks later and is the most contagious stage of the disease. Individual patients exhibit widely varied clinical manifestations at this time. Although constitutional symptoms such as fever, swollen lymph glands, and sore throat are often present, the diagnosis of secondary syphilis is made primarily on the basis of lesions of the skin and mucous membranes. Even at this well-developed stage of infection, the victim can still be cured of the disease through the administration of antibiotics. However, similar to the primary stage, even without treatment, the symptoms of the secondary stage eventually subside and the individual may mistakenly believe that he is cured.

The third stage of the disease is called latent, or hidden, syphilis. This latent period varies widely as to time but averages about six to eight years. The individual remains infectious during the early portion of the latent period, particularly during the first year. A pregnant woman in the latent period is very likely to deliver a baby with congenital syphilis. During most of the latent period, however, the infection appears to lie dormant even though the organisms are still present and viable. The individual will give a positive serological test but there are no clinical manifestations of syphilis at this time.

Following the latent period, the fourth stage of syphilis makes its appearance. In this stage, the infectious microorganisms are likely to be concentrated in circumscribed areas such as the heart, liver, osseous tissue, or the central nervous system. Syphilis has been called the great imitator because the symptoms resulting from infections of these various tissues mimic many other diseases. Thus, there may be attacks on arterial walls causing aneurysms, general increase in connective tissue resulting in hardening of tissues, or sensitivity reactions which produce chronic and destructive ulcers in vital organs. Cardiovascular syphilis is a serious complication, as is neurosyphilis. When the central nervous system is involved, the result may be the development of paresis, locomotor ataxia, blindness, or progressive physical and mental deterioration. Most deaths from syphilis occur in this stage of the disease although the actual cause of death frequently is not attributed to the venereal disease itself.

## Laboratory Identification Methods

For generations, public health investigators have been attempting to improve the reliability and speed with which tests can be used to detect syphilis. The earlier an active case is identified and subjected to treatment, the better will be the response to such treatment. In addition, the sooner the infected individual is located and treated, the less threat there will be to the public health.

About the only effective way of determining early syphilis is by identification of the treponemes in a darkfield examination of blood and sera, or material taken from lesions or regional lymph nodes. Later, about one to three weeks after appearance of the primary chancre, there appears in the serum of the syphilitic individual an antibody complex, called reagin. The serological tests to detect and to measure this reagin employs non-treponemal antigens such as those prepared from beef heart. These tests are, commonly, of two types, the flocculation and the complement fixation procedures. Examples of widely used flocculation tests are the Venereal Disease Research Laboratory slide test, the Kline cardiolipin, and the Kahn standard, while the most commonly used complement fixation procedure is the Kolmer test. The treponemal test currently favored is the fluorescent treponemal antibody absorption (FTA-ABS).[63] A screening test, designed to detect syphilis within 3 to 8 min. without the use of microscopes or centrifuges, is the RPR (rapid plasma reagin) card test. Other tests such as the FPM (filter paper microscopic) and the Chediak blood test are examples of other techniques but they have not, as yet, achieved the popularity and widespread use of the older, established tests. If these later techniques are, indeed, achieving superior results with simplified procedures, they should be adopted at a much more rapid rate than is currently employed.

## Methods of Control

During and after World War II, large amounts of government money were spent to control venereal disease. As a result, the rate declined steadily until about 1955. When the disease was no longer considered a serious public health problem, health department budgets were cut back severely. By 1957, venereal disease again was on the rise. Government funds from the Venereal Disease Program of the Public Health Service were directed to help control this growing problem, again with favorable results. With the passage of the Comprehensive Health Planning and Public Health Service Act, however, there was no longer a specific appropriation for aid to states and localities for venereal disease control. Much of the decisions regarding specific allocations of government funds were determined by the priority assigned to this problem by states and localities. With the resurgence of gonorrhea as a runaway epidemic, national attention is focused on the venereal diseases once again. Physicians are strongly urged to report their contacts and to provide proper dosage of medications. The preferred drug for syphilis is aqueous penicillin G and probenicid, in the same quantities as recommended for treatment of gonorrhea: 1 gm. of probenicid administered orally followed in 30 min. by 4.8 million units of aqueous procaine penicillin G, given in two intramuscular injections of 2.4 million units each. Follow-up treatment is particularly important with syphilis cases. Another method of control is the interviewing of VD cases and tracing of contacts to identify and treat the infectious sources. This is an expensive method since each new case brought to treatment in this manner costs from 6 to 13 dollars.[64]

Since there is no immediate prospect for either vaccines or a marked change in patterns of social behavior, one cannot expect a reversal in the venereal disease epidemic in the near future. The National Commission on Venereal Disease has submitted 19 recommendations to combat this ever growing problem. Among these recommendations are the need for enlarged research programs in all phases of venereal disease, more intensified teaching of venereology in all of the schools of health training, enlarged education programs in the curricula of all public schools, intensified public education through the mass media, and additional support at the local level to control the disease.[65] Intensified education is a very important factor since studies have disclosed large knowledge gaps existing among teenagers and young adults concerning broad symptomology and diagnosis of venereal disease, and available prevention alternatives. Cooperation is needed to encourage these people to report to clinics for diagnosis.[66] The members of the allied medical professions can make significant contributions toward helping reduce this growing spread of venereal disease. Through personal contacts with individual patients, health-related talks to service clubs and PTA groups, the distribution of pertinent literature, and active participation in civic committees, the community can not only be made aware of the severity of the problem but can become convinced that only through community-wide involvement can the programs for eradication be truly effective.

## REFERENCES

1. Statistical Bulletin, Metropolitan Life Insurance Co., Aug. 1973.

2. Penn-Mutual Life Insurance Co. *vs* Cobbs, 1929. 23 Alabama App. 205. *Southern Rep., 123:* 94, 1930.

3. Ansel, E. L., and McGee, R. K. Attitudes toward suicide attempters. Bulletin of Suicidology, DHEW Pub. No. (HSM) 71-9053, 1971.

4. News Briefs. *Rodale's Health Bull., 6:* 8, 1968.

5. Gibson, M. R., and Lott, R. S. Suicide and the role of the pharmacist. *J. Amer. Pharm. Assn., n.s., 12:* 9, 1972.

6. Murphy, G. E., and Robins, Eli. Social factors in suicide. *J.A.M.A., 199:* 5, 1967.

7. Faigel, H. C. Suicide among young persons. *Clin. Pediat.* (Philadelphia) *5:* 187-190, 1966.

8. Schneidman, E. S., and Faberow, N. L. The Los Angeles Suicide-Prevention Center: a demonstration of public health feasibilities. *Amer. J. Public Health, 55:* 21–26, 1965.

9. Faberow, N. L., and Schneidman, E. S. *The Cry For Help.* New York: McGraw-Hill Book Co., Inc., 1961.

10. Lester, D. Effect of suicide Prevention centers on suicide rates in the United States. *Health Service Rep., 89:* 1, 1974.

11. Walu, T. C., and Cam, D. S. Broadening the focus of suicide prevention activities. *Amer. J. Public Health, 62:* 12, 1972.

12. National Institute of Mental Health. *Alcoholism,* P.H.S. Publication 730. Washington, D. C., 1965.

13. *Alcohol and Alcoholism.* DHEW Pub. No. (HSM) 72-9127, 1972.

14. Committee on Alcoholism and Drug Dependence. Alcohol and society. *J.A.M.A., 216:* 6, 1971.

15. Lieber, C. S. Alcohol, nutrition, and the liver. *Amer. J. Clin. Nutrition, 26:* Aug., 1973.

16. Alcohol and Health Notes. National Institute on Alcohol Abuse and Alcoholism, Aug., 1973.

17. Alcohol and Health Notes. National Institute on Alcohol Abuse and Alcoholism, Jan., 1974.

18. Chafetz, M. E. New Federal legislation on alcoholism—Opportunities and Problems. *Amer. J. Public Health, 63:* 3, 1973.

19. Chafetz, M. E. Alcohol and traffic accidents. *PAHO Bull., 7:* 3, 1973.

20. Expert Committee on Mental Health, Alcoholism Subcommittee, Second report. *WHO Techn. Rep. Ser.,* No. 48, 1952.

21. Seixas, F. A. New priorities in diagnosing and treating alcoholism. *Indust. Med. Surg., 42:* 3, 1973.

22. Criteria Committee, National Council In Alcoholism. Criteria for the diagnosis of alcoholism. *Amer. J. Psychiatry, 129:* 2, 1972.

23. Washington Report on Medicine and Health. No. 1387, 1974.

24. Changing face of the contemporary drug scene. *Rutger's Pharmacy Extension News, 24:* 7, 1974.

25. Record high in seizure of illicit Drugs. *PMA Newsletter, 14:* 4, 1972.

26. National Commission on Marihuana and Drug Abuse, Second Report. *Drug Use in America: Problem in Perspective.* Washington, D. C., Gov't Printing Office, stock no. 5266-00003, 1973.

27. DeLone, R. H. The ups and downs of drug-abuse education. *Saturday Rev.,* Nov. 11, 1972.

28. Personality traits predict drug use. *Health Service Rep., 88:* 8, 1973.

29. Johnson, K. G., *et al.* Survey of adolescent drug use. *Amer. J. Public Health,* Feb., 1972.

30. Eddy, Hallbach, Isbell, and Seevers. Drug dependence—its significance and characteristics. *Psychopharmacol. Bull., 3:* 3, 1966.

31. Baden, M. M. Narcotic abuse: A medical examiner's view. *N. Y. State J. Med., 72:* 7, 1972.

32. Blum, R. H. Drugs and America's destiny: Trends and predictions. In *Resource Book for Drug Abuse Education,* Ed. 2. Washington, D. C.; Gov't Printing Office, stock no. 1724-0232, 1972.

33. Saltman, J. *What we can do about drug abuse.* Public Affairs Pamphlet 290, New York.

34. Arieff, A. A. Psychotropic drugs in addiction. (Letters to the editor). *J.A.M.A., 27:* 1, 1974.

35. *Stedman's Medical Dictionary,* Ed. 22. Baltimore: The Williams and Wilkins Co., 1972.

36. Brown, J. K., and Malone, M. H. Some U. S. street drug identification programs. *J. Amer. Pharm. Assn., n.s., 13:* 12, 1973.

37. Rainey, J. M., and Crowder, M. K. Prevalence of phencyclidine in street drug preparations (Letters to the Editor). *N. Engl. J. Med., 290:* 8, 1974.

38. Long, R. E., Penna, R. P. Drugs of abuse. *J. Amer. Pharm. Assn., 8:* 1, 1968.

39. Brown, J. K., and Malone, M. H. *LSD and the Marketplace.* Pacific Information Service on Street Drugs, Bull. No. 2, 1972.

40. *Marihuana and Health.* Report to the Congress from the Secretary, DHEW. Washington, D. C.: U. S. Government Printing Office, 1971.

41. Schwarz, C. J. Toward a medical understanding of marihuana. In Matheson and Davison, *The Behavioral Effects of Drugs.* New York: Holt, Rinehart and Winston, Inc., 1972.

42. Kolansky, H., and Moore, W. T. Toxic effects of chronic marihuana use. *J.A.M.A., 222:* 1, 1972.

43. Kochar, M. S., and Hosko, M. J. Electrocardiographic effects of marihuana. *J.A.M.A., 225:* 1, 1973.

44. Stoll, A., and Hoffman, A. Partialsynthese von alkaloiden vons typus des ergobasius. *Helv. Chim. Acta, 26:* 944, 1943.

45. Smith, J. P. LSD: the false illusion. *FDA Papers,* July-August, 1967.

46. Frosch, W., Robbins, E., and Stern, M. Untoward reactions to lysergic acid diethylamide (LSD) resulting in hospitalization. *N. Engl. J. Med., 273:* 1235-1239, 1965.

47. Einstein, S. Drug abuse training and education. *Amer. J. Public Health, 64:* 2, 1974.

48. Levy, R. M., and Brown, A. R. Untoward effects of drug education. *Amer. J. Public Health, 63:* 12, 1973.

49. Coghlan, A. J., and Zimmerman, R. S. Self-help and methadone maintenance: Are they both failing? *Drug Forum, 1:* 3, 1972.

50. Hart, L. Milieu management in the treatment of drug addiction: Effects on rehabilitation. *Drug Forum, 2:* 1, 1972.

51. Zimmerman, R. S., and Coghlan, A. J. The misuse

of ex-addicts in drug abuse treatment pro-grams. *Drug Forum, 1:* 4, 1972.

52. *Morbidity and Mortality Weekly Report.* Center for Disease Control, PHS, *22:* 52, 1974.

53. Millar, J. D. The national venereal disease problem. In *Proceedings of the 2nd International VD Symposium.* St. Louis: 1972.

54. Brown, W. J. The national VD problem. In *Proceedings of the First International VD Symposium.* St. Louis: 1971.

55. *Venereal Diseases– Recent Morbidity and Mortality.* Statistical Bulletin, Metropolitan Life Insurance Co., Nov., 1973.

56. de Leon, R. Syphilis and gonorrhea. *J. Amer. Pharm. Assn., n.s. 13:* 4, 1973.

57. Wiesner, P. J. *et al.* Clinical spectrum of pharyngeal gonococcal infection. *N. Engl. J. Med., 288:* 4, 1973.

58. Sparling, P. F. Slowing the gonorrhea epidemic. Modern Med., Nov. 12, 1973.

59. Handsfield, H. H. *et al.* Asymptomatic gonorrhea in Men. *N. Engl. J. Med., 290:* 3, 1974.

60. Delf, R. B., and Hofeldt, R. L. Treatment of gonorrhea in Oregon by the reporting private physician. *Health Service Rep., 88:* 7, 1973.

61. Rudolph, A. H. Control of gonorrhea. *J.A.M.A., 220:* 12, 1972.

62. Kellogg, D. S. Current research activities on gonorrhea at the Center for Disease Control. *Health Services Rep., 88:* 1, 1973.

63. Schroeter, A. L. *et al.* Treatment for early syphilis and reactivity of serologic tests. *J.A.M.A., 221:* 5, 1972.

64. Blount, J. H. A new approach for gonorrhea epidemiology. *Amer. J. Public Health, 62:* 5, 1972.

65. Report of the National Commission on Venereal Disease. DHEW Pub. No. (HSM) 72-8125, 1972.

66. Yacenda, J. A. Survey of VD knowledge among young people. *Health Service Rep., 87:* 5, 1972.

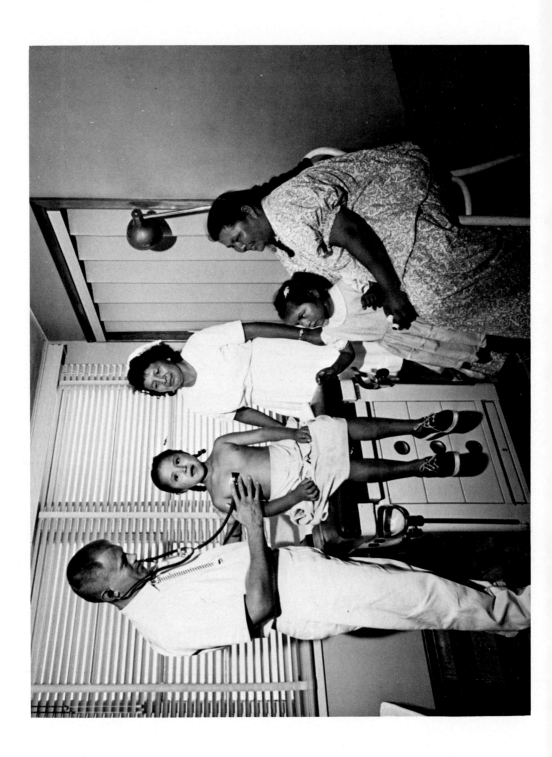

# 10

# Health problems of a modern society

Modern technology has wrought many changes in our society, most of which are highly beneficial. Thus, we live longer and better, have accustomed ourselves to creature comforts and luxuries, and look forward to even more spectacular achievements in the future. Certainly, there has never before been such an advanced civilization in the history of mankind.

There is, however, a shadow side to this bright and golden era. There are public health problems which are created as a result of this same technology and which now appear as dark, brooding clouds on the horizon, posing a serious threat to our advanced society. It sometimes seems that every significant achievement is accompanied by a correspondingly deleterious side action or by-product that poses yet another problem to our social or environmental health. Thus we now have advanced methods of transportation and can cover great distances in a fraction of the time and much more comfortably than did our grandparents. Accompanying this development, however, is the carnage on the highways, the photochemical smog from automobiles, and the smoke trails from jet airplanes landing or taking off. Our increased standard of living has provided us with more material wealth and, correspondingly, with much more trash to discard. The sheer volume of the trash itself as well as methods used to dispose of such waste are posing public health problems of enormous magnitude. In addition, since medical science and advanced technology have combined resources to lower the death rate in the face of continually rising birth rates, our world is now confronted with the very serious problem of overpopulation. The needs created by these increased numbers of people are manifold but food and adequate nutrition are high on the list. Sobering questions are now being asked about the ability to feed these growing multitudes, particularly since the rate of increase in

food production has fallen below the rate of increase of the world's population.

All of these problems have been dismissed as prices which we must pay for progress, and yet the serious student of public health recognizes that such prices are too high. It is not necessary to breathe polluted air, destroy aquatic life in our lakes and streams, bring babies into the world without means to care for them, or threaten to disrupt the delicate balance of nature in our biosphere. The same technology which created these problems can be utilized to solve them. Before such assistance will be forthcoming on a broad scale, however, a concerned public must be willing to co-operate. In problems related to public health the citizens look to the allied health professionals for information, leadership, and guidance. A discussion of the following topics will help to disclose the severity of some of the problems we are facing in our modern society and will provide some suggestions for alleviating these conditions.

## ACCIDENTAL DEATH AND DISABILITY

### Introduction

During a typical year, 55.7 million accidental injuries in the United States killed 117,000 people, temporarily disabled 11.5 million others, and permanently impaired 420,000 additional lives.[1] These figures may be more meaningful if they were equally distributed throughout a 24 hr. period each day of the year. For example, every minute 106 people sustained injuries serious enough to need emergency assistance and 21 of these victims remained in bed for one to three days. Every four minutes, on the average, three people received disabling injuries which were permanent in nature, and one person died from accidents every five minutes. Put still another way, every hour of the day and night an average of 6300 people were injured by accidents and 1300 of these received bed-disabling injuries, 48 people were permanently impaired, and 13 persons died. The economic loss due to accidents including wage loss, medical expense, insurance adjustment and administrative costs, and property loss, amounted to 37 billion dollars. It is small wonder that the human suffering and financial loss from preventable accidents has been compared with the ravages of ancient plagues or world wars.

This neglected epidemic of modern society is the nation's most important environmental health problem and is the leading cause of death in the first half of life's span. It is always sad when older people die. But most of these people have had at least some opportunity to savor the pleasures of life before they fall victims to such terminal conditions as the great killing triad—heart disease, cancer, and stroke. It is not only sad, but is a useless and tragic waste when young people's lives are needlessly and ruthlessly taken, or are permanently disabled due to accidents. The loss is not only to the individuals and their families but to the nation as well. These young people who otherwise could expect to live long and productive lives represent a loss of millions of productive man-years to our society. We have been concerned throughout this textbook with diseases which affect the health of the community and which cause many deaths, and yet, for children aged one to 14 years, accidents claim more lives than the six leading diseases combined. For youths aged 15 to 24 years, accidents take more lives than all others causes combined, and six and a half times more than the next leading cause in this age group. And this carnage continues.

Accidental injuries are responsible for 11 per cent of permanent paralysis and 65 per cent of loss of major extremities. It is estimated that the number of U. S. citizens now physically impaired by injuries is in excess of 12.5 million, including 180,000 persons who have lost a leg, a foot, an arm, or a hand, and 930,000 with varying degrees of impaired vision.[2] The care of accident cases imposes a staggering load on all the allied medical professions and hospitals. Approximately one of every four Americans suffers an accident of some degree each year and about 2 million victims are hospitalized. They occupy an average of 65,000 hospital beds for 22 million bed-days and receive the services of 88,000 hospital personnel. A greater demand for hospital beds and services is created by accident victims than is required to care for the babies born each year or for all the heart patients in the nation, and it is more than four times greater than beds and services required for cancer patients. The campus and its personnel are not immune to this accident toll since it is estimated that one out of nine college students will be the victim of a serious accidental injury during the year. Also, the accidental injury rate for faculty and staff members of colleges is far higher than that for comparable jobs outside the field of education.

But these are only statistics. They do not seem to have the impact and the heart-rendering meaning until they are associated with a member of the family or a very close friend. It is then that the tragedy and the senseless, meaningless loss becomes so overwhelming. Certainly, if an infectious disease was to cause even a fraction of such misery and death there would be such widespread concern that it would border on panic. However, most of our citizens are apathetic. The reports of accidents and deaths have become so commonplace that they are accepted as normal functions of modern society. Otherwise normally intelligent persons reason that since accidents occur unexpectedly and cannot be anticipated they could not have been prevented and no one is really to blame for them. Another fallacy is the general belief that accidents happen only to other people. It is this philosophy that has resulted in the disregard for seatbelts.

A new type of attitude is needed. Each person must become convinced that most accidents result from such causes as poor judgment, alcohol, or thoughtlessness and that these can be either prevented or markedly curtailed. The defeatist, handwringing attitude of impotence in the face of rising accidents and deaths can and should be replaced by a positive approach which convinces each member of our society that safety is everyone's business. An aroused public and a concerted program could result in a decided reduction in this tragic and needless loss to our country and its people.

## Classification of Accidents

Where do these accidents occur, how are they caused, and what can be done to control them? An analysis discloses some interesting facts. For example, the location of the accident, urban or rural, appears to have a significant bearing. Although more injuries occur in urban areas, more deaths occur in rural areas and in towns under 2500 population. Nationally, over 70 per cent of automobile fatalities occur in rural areas. A study of accidental deaths in California disclosed that motor vehicle fatalities were over two and a half times as frequent in flat agricultural counties and five times as frequent in mountainous counties as in the urban areas. Deaths from accidents not involving motor vehicles occurred almost twice as often in the agricultural areas and nearly three times as often in the mountainous areas. It is recognized, of course, that some of the most hazardous occupations, such as farming, lumbering, and mining, occur primarily in rural areas. Also, a portion of the excess fatalities occurring in these areas can be explained by accidents involving urban residents who are traveling or vacationing. But the more apparent reason for increased deaths in the rural areas is the discrepancy in adequate first aid at the accident scene as well as delayed transportation to proper medical facilities. In the above-mentioned California study half of the fatalities were primarily from head injuries and yet, in the rural areas, the majority of head injuries did not involve damage to brain tissue. It is suspected that many of those injured in rural areas died simply because they choked to death from blood, mucous, or vomitus in the mouth and trachea. In addition, of those victims in rural areas who died within 1 hr. after injury, over 90 per cent had not been moved from the accident scene. In another study of highway fatalities in Vermont, generally considered to be a rural state, it was demonstrated that 23 per cent of the victims had died of injuries felt to be either definitely or possibly survivable. Of those who did not die at the crash site but who succumbed either in the ambulance or hospital, about half died of survivable injuries. These latter deaths were attributed to problems and inadequacies throughout the emergency care system.[3]

Classification of accidents usually is made according to location of occurrence, such as highway, home, industry, and public. The latter, public accidents, include the wide assortment of non-vehicular injuries occurring away from home and work. Public accidents account for 2.9 million injuries and 24,300 deaths

annually. A significant portion of these are connected with recreational activities, and three-fourths of those killed are males. The increased national interest in recreation is accompanied by increased accident problems. Hunters, fishermen, and golfers all have an increased potential for accidents. Ski enthusiasts can expect one injury for every 100 participants, and the great increase in pleasure boating has created additional hazards. Approximately one-fourth of the deaths in public accidents was due to drownings and the majority of such drownings took place in rivers, lakes, creeks, and bodies of water not specifically designated for recreation and sports. The number of deaths in this category lend strong support to the American National Red Cross' assertion that half of the people in the United States do not swim well enough to cope with emergencies in the water. Water accidents become particularly acute if the individual has been drinking alcoholic beverages.[4]

The home, usually considered a sanctuary, may not be as safe as formerly imagined. Annual figures total 4.2 million injuries and 27,000 deaths in American homes. Falls are the major cause of death and fires are the next leading killer in home accidents. Every minute of the day, on the average, an American home is destroyed or damaged by fire and approximately 75 per cent of the fatalities in such fires are among children and the aged. The majority of these deaths result from the effects of smoke and lethal gas rather than from flames. In addition to the deaths, The National Fire Protection Association estimates that there are 100 serious injuries for every fatality.

Accidents at work, in one year's time, resulted in 2.4 million disabling injuries and 14,100 deaths. The total cost of such accidents, including loss from business fires, amounted to 11.5 billion dollars. Accidental deaths of workers on the job have decreased markedly, particularly in recent years. This reduction reflects the mutual concern and determination of both labor and management. Most of the larger manufacturing companies have active safety programs to protect both the worker and production schedules of the company. It is interesting to note that member companies of the National Safety Council average 70 per cent lower accident frequency rates and 40 per cent lower rates in severity of accidents. These companies are demonstrating that safety precautions are effective and that a significant number of accidents can be prevented if safety regulations are adequately enforced by both labor and management. Unfortunately, this practice of safety consciousness was not uniform throughout industry and has resulted in needless and tragic accidents that could have been avoided. This, in turn, led to the passage of the Occupational Safety and Health Act which took effect in 1971. This Act provided sweeping coverage for 4 million work places and 60 million workers. Even more pronounced reductions in work accidents are being realized as a result of the enforcement of this legislation.

The leading cause of accidental deaths for all age groups under 75 years, however, is still motor vehicles. In 1972, there were approximately 56,600 deaths, 2.1 million disabling injuries, and costs reaching 19.4 billion dollars. In 1973, however, there were 55,600 motor vehicle fatalities.[5] Lower speed limits and the gasoline shortage which occurred during the last two months of that year contributed to the reduction in the traffic death toll. As fuel economy continues, it is anticipated that the total number of automobile accidents will continue to decline. The National Safety Council states, though, that the severity of accidents is likely to increase due to the larger number of smaller automobiles on the highways.

Drivers between the ages of 15 and 24 were involved in more accidents and suffered more deaths than any other age group. In fact, accidental death rates for this age group have increased steadily and offsets the decline in death rates for most other age groups. The number of drivers under the age of 25 comprise 23 per cent of the driving population and yet account for 37 per cent of the accidents. This is reflected in the increased insurance premiums for younger drivers.

## Causes of Motor Vehicle Accidents

In considering causes of motor vehicle accidents there are three basic elements involved—the vehicle, the environment, and the driver. Characteristics of any of these factors may be altered so as to contribute to the cause or prevention of an accident. In recent years the automobile industry has come under public criticism and congressional scrutiny because

cars were said to be deficient in adequate safety features. It was charged that some models had faulty brakes, improper tires, non-collapsible steering wheels, and protruding fixtures. It was also charged that manufacturers were more concerned with power, speed, and style than with safety of construction and performance. Certainly, the names which manufacturers give to some of their models insinuate that the driver is performing at a famous auto race track or that he has control of a powerful and swift animal. Analyses of automobile fatalities lend support to the need for more safety features and improved design. One such analysis, a four year study in southeastern Michigan, disclosed that collapsing doors caused a significant number of fatalities. Also ranking high as causes of death were impacts with the steering assembly and with protruding instrument knobs. Later model automobiles now possess improvements in design and construction but are still some distance away from the type of safety car envisioned by Cornell and other institutions devoted to safety research. As stated earlier, the increase in sales in compact and subcompact automobiles promises to be a problem for the safety-conscious. One research team has estimated that safety (crashworthiness) decreases 2.5 per cent for each 100 pounds decrease in weight.

Mandatory automobile inspection was promoted to ensure a safe operating condition of the car. However, prior to the passage of the Highway Safety Act, 30 states did not require periodic automobile inspection. It is reported that these states have become dumping grounds for vehicles that fail to pass inspection in the states that do have such laws.

Although automobiles are involved in the greatest number of traffic deaths, motorcycles account for more than their share of mortality. A study in California has revealed that almost 10 per cent of the traffic fatalities are from motorcycles although cycles represent only 3 per cent of the registered vehicles. The past decade has witnessed at 450 per cent increase in the number of registered motorcycles while the number of fatalities to motorcyclists has tripled. The National Safety Council estimates that the mileage death rate for motorcycle riders is approximately four times the overall motor-vehicle death rate. The majority of these deaths are attributed to the absence of adequate protection, where the body is exposed to all of the violent forces without restraint. Because of his low visibility, the motorcyclist must constantly practice defensive driving. The automobile is his worst enemy since collision with other motor vehicles is the predominant type of fatal accidents in which motorcycles are involved.[6]

The roads traveled by motor vehicles also present certain problems. Such items as trees dangerously close to roads, confusing signs, deep ditches next to roads, narrow median strips, poorly built or non-existent guard rails, obstructed vision at intersections, and lack of protection around lamp posts and bridge approaches all contribute to a high accident toll. Rural roads are the greatest threat to modern high speed traffic while the lowest rate of road-related accidents occurs on the interstate highway system.

While it is recognized that automobile construction and poor road design account for many traffic accidents and fatalities, the fact remains that the vast majority, over 80 per cent, of all motor vehicle accidents are caused by the driver. It is this individual who must be studied and analyzed to determine his accident patterns and his fitness to drive. His past is dismal, approaching 2 million deaths since the automobile was introduced. His future is frightening, particularly if the present accidental injury and death rate is allowed to continue. Traffic violations and lawsuits for personal injury have become so numerous that they threaten the American judicial system. Approximately 30 million citations for violations of the traffic laws are issued each year and it now takes an average of 32 months to obtain a civil jury trial in most of the metropolitan areas.

## The Problem Driver

Essentially all drivers at one time or another fail to remain completely alert while driving. Bumped fenders and minor collisions, usually at slow speeds, frequently result from such temporary inattentiveness. Although these cannot be dismissed as inconsequential, the serious threat to traffic safety comes from a smaller and more dangerous percentage of drivers. Actions and attitudes of these drivers lead not only to their demise but also seriously endanger the lives and safety of many innocent victims. Numerous automobile crashes are attributed to personality

disturbances and to uncontrollable, violent behavior. A 3-year study of fatal accidents supports this position. It was found that drivers who cause fatal accidents often are subject to more psychopathological abnormalities, social stress, and acute personality disturbances than other motorists. This study revealed that 20 per cent of the drivers involved in fatal accidents had experienced acute emotional crises, usually violent arguments, within 6 hr. of the accident. Paranoid and suicidal tendencies and depression were significantly more prevalent among drivers in the fatality group. In addition, as noted earlier, young drivers account for a much larger share of accidents than is warranted by their number and by the number of highway miles that they travel. Investigators have attributed much of this increase to inexperience of the driver and to insufficient concern for self-preservation among many young people.

Another serious threat to traffic safety is the problem drinker. It has been reported that an average of 11 per cent of the drivers on the road, at all times of the day and night, have been drinking and have measurable amounts of alcohol in their breath and blood. Investigations have disclosed that drinking is indicated to be a factor in at least half of the fatal motor-vehicle accidents. The main part of this problem is not the social drinker but the person who drinks to excess and is almost constantly under the influence of alcohol.

Despite slogans and campaigns designed to encourage the use of seat belts, shoulder harnesses, and protective helmets, tragic evidence shows that these warnings go unheeded much of the time. Studies at Cornell have shown that in automobiles the risk of serious injury is three and a half times greater in those who do not use seat belts and the risk of death is 5 times greater in those that are thrown from their cars. However, 47 per cent of those killed in auto accidents were thrown from their cars. Another study of 139 automobile accidents in which 177 occupants died revealed that ejection of the occupant from the car was the leading cause of death. The authors of this report postulate that 40 per cent of those killed could have survived had seat belts been worn and an additional 13 per cent would have lived if seat belts and shoulder harnesses had been used. Improvements in recent years have been made with warning buzzers and safety interlocks connected with the use of the seat belt.

There is a discouraging number of motorists, however, who still seek to bypass these reminders and view them as nuisances rather than life-saving devices.

The general health of the driver is another factor which must be considered. Some medically definable conditions of the driver can be expected to cause accidents, although the extent of this factor is unknown. It is known, however, that persons who have alcohol and drug problems, those who suffer from severe uncompensated arthritis, and people who have skeletal and amputation deformities certainly have increased accident potentials. Others who are mentally retarded, who have visual and other sensory defects, who suffer from neuropsychiatric problems, or who have neuromuscular or cardiovascular defects add to this list of high risk drivers.

### Emergency Care

The emergency care following the accident is perhaps of greatest concern to those in the allied medical professions, and it is in this area that much more could and should be done. The Committees on Trauma and Shock, Division of Medical Sciences, of the National Research Council have listed deficiencies at various levels of emergency care which require early solutions. Among those listed are the following:

1. Millions lack instruction in basic first aid.

2. Few are adequately trained in the advanced techniques of cardiopulmonary resuscitation, childbirth, or other life-saving measures.

3. Local political authorities have neglected their responsibility to provide optimal emergency medical services.

4. Fundamental research in shock and trauma is inadequately supported.

5. Potentials of programs in accident prevention and emergency medical services have not been fully exploited.

6. Emergency departments of hospitals are overcrowded, some are archaic, and most are understaffed.

Added to these are other discrepancies which need correction. An Assistant Surgeon General and Coordinator for Public Health Programs has disclosed this rather sobering assessment of emergency medical facilities and lack of ability to meet adequately the emergency needs of our nation.[7] Only 10 per cent of the 5130 community hospitals with emergency facilities are equipped to handle all medical and surgical emergencies and 14 per cent can handle psychiatric emergencies. Fewer than half have blood banks, and 58 per cent are not equipped to handle cardiac emergencies. Only 6 per cent are able to communicate with the ambulances or rescue vehicles that serve them. It is stated that many of the smaller hospitals do not even have the emergency equipment recommended for ambulances. Only 17 per cent of the hospitals have 24-hour physician coverage.

An ambulance should be an extension of a well-staffed and equipped hospital emergency department. And yet, of the 44,000 ambulances in the nation, only about 1300 are operated by hospitals; 4500 are operated by fire or police departments, 4700 by commercial firms, and 11,000 by volunteer groups. In too many towns the ambulance service is conducted by the local mortuary, a situation that gives the victim and his family an uneasy feeling at best. The term "ambulance" is often a misnomer. Almost one-half of the vehicles were not intended as use for ambulances. One-tenth are panel trucks or vans, one-quarter are station wagons, many are actually hearses, and of the 36 per cent that are conventional ambulances, many are too low and too cramped to permit in-transit patient care. Fewer than one-third of the ambulances are reported to carry all of the equipment recommended by the American College of Surgeons. Most ambulances have merely an oxygen tank and a mask, while fewer than one-half have bag-mask resuscitators. Even such basic equipment as splints, backboards, or airways are often missing. Thirty-eight per cent of the ambulances do not have two-way radio communication. Only a relatively small percentage of the ambulance attendents have completed the 80-hour emergency medical technician (EMT) course. In addition, many medical graduates have had no formal training in emergency care and a survey of medical schools showed that less than one-third had courses in the subject.[7]

One of the serious problems today is the broad gap between knowledge of total emergency care and its application. Expert consultants who were in Vietnam or the Middle East War have publicly asserted that, if seriously wounded, their chances of survival would be better in the zone of combat than on the average city street. Lower death rates have been attributed to excellence of initial first aid, efficiency of transportaion, and energetic treatment at emergency centers. Reduction of the time lag from receipt of injury to initiation of medical care is one of the important elements in prevention of death and permanent disability. The director of the Trauma Unit at Cook County Hospital, Chicago, claims that for every 30 minutes elapsing between the time of an accident and the time when the patient receives definitive care, the mortality rate increases three-fold. And yet probably no American community can lay claim to the excellence of emergency service comparable to that of the Armed Services. Certainly, we can learn from these military personnel and adapt their life-saving services to answer the drastic need of our civilian population.

## Constructive Changes

What can be done to combat this overwhelming, acute public health problem of accidental death and disability? Those of us in the allied medical professions should have an uncommon interest in this daily tragedy because it is our professions that are directly responsible for care of the injured. The time is long past for us to scrutinize carefully our educational objectives, to establish systems of positive preventive measures, and to develop focal points of strong leadership.

The most important transformation centers on public apathy regarding the inevitability of accidents. This could be changed into an action program which convinces the public that concerted effort and cooperation can definitely reduce such tragedy and needless loss. Basic to this approach is identification of the individual citizen with a means by which he can satisfy the inherent desire to serve his fellow man. Since the problem of accidents crosses every economic, social, and political boundary, the resources to attack this problem should also be universal. Federal and voluntary agencies have mobilized to prevent and treat birth defects, muscular dystrophy, and palsy, and have launched frontal attacks to conquer heart disease, cancer, and mental disease. There are now some promising signs that the same type of concerted program is being launched against accidents. Conduct of national conferences at the executive level, appropriation of funds by government agencies, pooling of resources through voluntary health agencies, an expanded and intensified research endeavor, and implementation of programs at regional and community levels are now being marshalled to attack accidental death and disability.

The new science of cybernetics, whereby information is translated into constructive performance, has prompted us to take a new look at the effectiveness of our present educational techniques. Such platitudes as "drive safely," "be careful,' and "speed kills" do not really provide the motivations to prevent accidents. Research into the causes of accidents and educational programs aimed at reducing these causes have proven to be far more effective. Such programs must be based on adequate knowledge of the nature of the problem, and motivational techniques, where appropriate, must be much more sophisticated than most of those currently in use. Many accidents, particularly those involving fires, firearms, and misuse of pesticides, have been the result of sheer ignorance rather than poor attitude. Proper educational programs could do a great deal to lessen the toll in these areas of tragedy. The accident situation is usually comprised of a sequential series of events. This stepwise progression starts with the cause of the accident, followed by the crash itself. If the accident involved an automobile, there frequently is the "second collision" of the impact of the victim's body. The additional, important progression in this series is the emergency medical care following the accident. Similar to a disease pattern, focus can be made on each of these sequential steps of an accident situation so that effective control measures can be determined.

The causes of accidents rarely are due to single incidents. It is no more accurate to conclude that an accident is caused by a single action than to state that a disease is caused by a specific microorganism. We have learned long ago that most diseases result from the interaction of the host, the organism, and the environment and that an alteration of any of these factors could affect the course of the disease. By the same token, we must recognize the multiple causes of accidents. Most of us think of an accident as happening very suddenly, and to the victim it does seem sudden. The more that we are able to analyze accidents, however, the more we can observe that accidents and their consequent injuries result from a sequence of events that began a long time before. Attitudes, physical and mental conditions, and the abuse of alcohol and various drugs, inexperience, and failure to observe adequate safety precautions are the basic ingredients which lead to accidents. Concentration on these causes and intensive programs aimed at changing these practices can do a great deal to lower the incidence and severity of accidents.

In spite of these endeavors, however, we know that some accidents will still occur. Our aim here is to lessen the severity of physical injury. Just because a victim is involved in an accident does not necessarily mean that he must sustain a disabling or fatal injury. This is particularly true for motor vehicle accidents. Since it is estimated that at least one-third of the automobiles are destined for collision, we have every right to crusade for adequate regulation of automobile design. With the trend towards smaller automobiles we must be particularly concerned about the protective safety features due to the increased risk of serious injuries.

The emergency medical care following an accident demands our utmost attention, and here the value of a first aid course cannot be overemphasized. Every government and voluntary health organization involved in emergency medical care has recommended strongly that an American Red Cross first aid course or its equivalent should be mandatory for every student and for every licensed driver. The derived value is not only improved effectiveness in rendering emergency care but also the reduction of accidents, since it has been shown that accident rates have been lowered as much as 50 per cent among groups that have received such training. Those in the allied medical professions are expected to have a more thorough knowledge of emergency medical care. They should be encouraged to take the Red Cross Adanced First Aid or the EMT II course, including cardiopulmonary resuscitation. It is further recommended that those community-minded members of the health professions should extend their training so that they may serve as Red Cross first aid instructors. Certainly, few other voluntary services are more greatly needed or could be more personally satisfying.

Medical committees and special task forces of the National Academy of Sciences have recommended new organizational approaches to combat the problems of accidental death and disability. Among other things, they have proposed the conduction of national forums and conferences on emergency medical services, the establishment of a national council on accident prevention, the pooling of efforts of responsible professional and lay organizations to form a voluntary national trauma association, the organization of community councils on emergency medical services, and the creation of a national institute of trauma. The passage of the Occupational Safety and Health Act of 1970 and the Emergency Medical Systems Service Act of 1973 have provided significant opportunities to overcome some of the previous difficulties and to save thousands of additional lives.

Pilot projects in the states of Illinois and Arkansas and in selected counties in Florida, California, and Ohio have demonstrated that effective, meaningful, programs can be placed in operation. Results from these projects have produced criteria, standards, and regulations for an efficient and comprehensive Emergency Medical Services System. This segment is to be regarded as an integral part of the total health care system to assure proper recovery and rehabilitation of emergency patients. These include categorization of emergency facilities, criteria for ambulance design and equipment, model ordinances for the regulation of ambulance services, uniform standards for training, and certification of emergency medical technicians. In communications, a single telephone number for emergency medical services, such as 911, should be instituted throughout the nation. Central dispatch should be provided for all emergency ambulances and radio communications should exist between dispatch centers, mobile emergency equipment, hospitals, law enforcement, and fire units. Greater emphasis should be placed upon rural emergency services. Most rural ambulances are operated on a marginal budget since the cost for maintaining an efficient ambulance service is estimated at $90,000 per year. Provisions in the Emergency Medical Systems Service Act will provide funding for some of these requirements. Certainly, there is a demonstrated need for better equipment and for around-the-clock staffing by allied medical personnel who are trained in all aspects of trauma.

Among the people of our country and particularly among the allied health professionals there is a growing wave of concern about the tragic and needless loss attributed to accidental death and disability. This concern, it is earnestly hoped, prefaces co-ordinated and concentrated action aimed at accident prevention, lessening the severity of accidents, and improving emergency medical care. The hand-wringing attitude is no longer appropriate; something *can* be done about accidents and members of the allied medical professions can demonstrate methods to combat this great public health problem.

## POLLUTION – THE EFFLUENCE OF AF-FLUENCE

We travel together, passengers on a little spaceship. Dependent on its vulnerable reserve of air and soil. All committed for our safety to its security and peace. Preserved from annihilation only by the care, the work, and the love we give our fragile craft.

ADLAI STEVENSON

### Introduction

The problem of pollution is many problems. It has been and continues to be recognized and attacked as a public health problem of ever expanding dimensions. Indeed, much of the present knowledge concerning factors associated with pollution as well as methods to cope with these factors have been derived from public health research and practice. It is also a social problem, an economic problem, a resources problem, and a management problem. The problem of pollution has also found its way into the political arena and almost every community in every state has been confronted with difficulties associated with man's contamination of his environment.

Our main concern regarding pollution is the adverse effect exerted on the health of our people. Whereas the mechanical technology of the 19th century had produced few hazards other than crowding and accidents, the chemical and radiological technology of today has produced new and still ill-defined hazards. Similarly, nuclear industry through its wastes cannot fail to alter the environment.

Thus, the latter half of the 20th century is witnessing a vast process of man-made artificial contamination of the environment. The air that we breathe and the water that we drink contain chemicals resulting from modern technological progress. Just because we do not yet know the true significance of these in their present concentrations cannot obscure the fact that many of these substances are poisonous and that their concentrations are increasing. But on a wider scale, pollution touches the everyday aspects of the majority of our citizens. In a myriad of tangential effects it is deleterious to health and, therefore, is of prime consideration to those in the allied medical professions. The fact is that pollution is everbody's business, and it is necessary to embark on a program of public awareness that extends down to the grass roots level. The problem is of the utmost urgency because many of the effects of pollution on our environment may be irreversible or, at least, may take generations to correct.

### Solid Wastes

Added to the dangers of air and water contamination are the problems of land pollution. Solid wastes will remain in place for long periods of time and until recently, disposal of these materials has had the least scientific consideration of any of the concerns of pollution control. The classical approaches to disposal have become inadequate and we can no longer follow the old procedure of just spreading our refuse around in the hope that it will not be noticed. It has become apparent that elimination of pollution from one area means intensified pollution of another. The former concept of throwing something away must be modified. As the earth becomes more crowded, there is no longer an "away." One person's trash basket may well be another person's living space.

One massively important consideration is that the consumer actually consumes nothing. Our whole economy is based on taking natural resources, converting them into things that are consumer products (sometimes with built-in planned obsolescence), selling them to the consumer, and then forgetting about them. Thus all kinds of materials and food come into the system and are transformed and used. The user employs the product, sometimes changes it in form, but does not consume it. He just discards it. In addition to the millions of automobiles and major appliances manufactured each year, the United States produces about 33 million tons of packaging, including

48 billion cans and 28 billion long-lived bottles and jars.[8] It is estimated that 6.6 million tons of glass and metal containers are produced each year for beer and soft drinks. Only 10 per cent are returned, millions are littered, and the remainder are disposed of in residential and commercial solid waste. Previously, the problem was not as formidable because the tin can eventually would rust away and discarded paper containers would rot. We are faced now, however, with plastic containers and immortal aluminum cans which may outlast the Pyramids.

According to a study published by the National Center for Resource Recovery, the average American generates about 3 pounds of refuse per day.[9] The combined refuse from commercial establishments and households every year amount to approximately 180 million tons.[10] The average composition, by weight, of residential solid wastes has been given as: paper products, 44 per cent; food wastes, 18 per cent; metals, 9 per cent; glass and ceramics, 9 per cent; garden wastes, 8 per cent; plastics, rubber, and leather, 3 per cent; textiles and wood, 5 per cent. Large cities are faced with the greatest problems. Each square mile of Manhattan, for example, produces about 375,000 pounds of waste each working day. In terms of volume, Los Angeles must dispose of 12 million cubic yards of solid waste each year. Thus, the finished products which are used in a city come out as residues in trash trucks, garbage scows, sewers, and the air. Collection and disposal of these wastes costs an average of $30. per ton, resulting in a total national expenditure of well over 4 billion dollars a year. Of course, not all of these wastes are destroyed or buried, as evidenced by junk piles and accumulations of refuse which litter many parts of our country. In addition to aesthetic affrontery, these trash piles are areas of increased fire and accident hazards, they present problems of rodent control, and they serve as breeding places for flies, mosquitoes, cockroaches, and other undesirable insect pests.

But there are still larger considerations. While we have given increasing, although still inadequate, thought to studies of the effects of pollutants on man, we have devoted relatively little effort to the effects of this great and growing family of pollutants on our land, air, and water. Man is fouling his nest and if allowed to continue unabated may push nature

beyond its limits. The earth is a closed system and the various factors which nurture mankind are in a delicate balance. The sheer volume of gaseous, liquid, and solid residues produced each year is enormous and continues to grow, and yet the capacity of the resources into which these materials are now injected is essentially constant. It should be obvious to those who seriously consider this problem that the atmosphere, the water, and the land cannot continue to be places in which to empty the trash basket.

What, then, can be done to reduce the volume and to improve the quality of our discarded wastes? Some answers have been provided and workable suggestions have been made. Man has been ingenious in learning to mine, process, and distribute resources for his benefit and well-being. Until recently he has given relatively little systematic thought and attention to the problem of wastes. But the same technology that has resulted in the pollution of our environment can also be used to reverse the procedure.

Instead of a long, straight line from raw materials to finished product, to the user, and then to the trash pile, considerably more thought and action should be devoted to cycling many of these products back for modification so that they may be used again. We must seriously consider whether we really want to discard all of the materials that we have expensively mined, transported, and processed. Efficient techniques have been developed for salvaging lead and copper and using them again but known methods for extracting other metals have not been employed to their full potential. Automobiles, with but slight sacrifice to model change, could be cycled back to modification plants for replacement of worn parts and installation of new innovations. Presently, an average community of 10,000 people discards about 1000 tons of paper and 172 tons of metal per year from packaging materials alone. The packaging industry could render a profound service to our society by switching to materials that rot on an accelerated schedule, or adapt containers that can be consumed or dissolved. Actually, the ideal container is the ice cream cone.

Much of our waste could be reconstituted and used again but at the present time and in the confines of our present economic system it has not proven to be a profitable enterprise.

Research and development on selected and limited amounts of certain organic fractions of industrial wastes have developed such products as bone meal, industrial alcohol, molasses, acetic acid, vegetable oils, building tile, and wallboard. For the most part, however, economic factors such as rising labor costs and difficulty in marketing have limited the practical application of these methods, and such salvaging operations have actually decreased. Local governments and operating agencies have generally been so preoccupied with the false economy of keeping refuse disposal costs to a minimum that they have lost the overview. It is difficult to obtain risk capital to build plants of unproven design which may operate at a loss and it is equally difficult to attract private research and development groups to enter this field without financial incentives. But the serious alternative to these choices of recycling waste products may be far more expensive than we can possibly imagine. We have the technology to reduce this ominous threat to the health and well-being of our people; how much are we willing to pay to avert a possible disaster?

The Federal and state governments until recently, have essentially ignored solid waste disposal because this function traditionally has been a local government obligation. As a result, there is a lack of coordinated jurisdiction and there have been no national standards or specifications established in this field. With the encouragement of the National Center for Resource Recovery and financial assistance through both local sources and the Environmental Protection Agency, resource recovery systems have been shown to be effective and economically feasible. Demonstration projects and full scale operations have been established in Franklin, Ohio; Chicago; St Louis; Menlo Park; LaVerne, California; New York; and Lowell, Massachusetts. From these projects an ideal system of handling solid waste has been proposed. Through the use of radically new collection methods, the mass of garbage is delivered to a hammermill where it is shredded into small pieces. A magnetic separator then removes the majority of the steel. If there is a need for recycled paper the shredded refuse can pass through a series of air classifiers where paper, wood, and plastic are first extracted, then the non-ferrous metals are recovered and sold. The glass is further separated by paramagnetic devices into clear and colored glass

and sold as cullet. The organics are destructively distilled by pyrolysis with the resulting methane gas being used for fuel. If there is no need to recycle paper, the refuse could be either incinerated in water-walled incinerators with the resulting steam sold to users or to generate electricity, or the refuse could be pyrolyzed with recovery and sale of methane gas and activated carbon. The resulting ash consisting of metals and glass which are burned or pyrolyzed could further be processed by a system of screens, magnets, and other mineral processing methods and separated into aluminum, clear glass, colored glass, and steel, all of which could be sold for profit. This system is not a figment of the imagination. There is not a single element in the proposed plant which does not exist at the present time.

To the extent that man is directly or indirectly contaminating his environment and introducing factors that render it harmful, the citizens' best interests are served by the adoption and enforcement of regulatory measures to prevent, minimize, or remove undesirable contamination. Since all types of pollution are interstate problems to one degree or another, the Federal Government has rightfully adopted equitable measures of control. State governments also have a vital interest in the problems of pollution and waste disposal since state expenditures in this field are exceeded only by tax monies spent on schools and roads. But the problems of pollution cannot be solved completely without the wholehearted co-operation of communities and the citizens within those communities.

Although it is true that the health dangers associated with pollution do not readily align themselves with a cause-effect relationship such as found in communicable disease or trauma, it is equally true that ignoring the consequences of unabated pollution may have far more disastrous results. Most of us in the allied medical fields were attracted to our professions, at least partially, because of our concern for our fellow human beings and for society as a whole. The problems and the implied threats to society resulting from the pollution of our environment are large enough and serious enough to challenge us to action. We should be willing to exert our energies and influence on both an individual and a collective basis to reduce this hazard to the health of people and to the welfare of our country. Through personal contact, community action boards, service clubs, state organizations, regional committees, and political affiliations the impact of dedicated health professionals can be effective in instituting and implementing methods for adequate control. Convinced of the need for positive action, we can demonstrate our concern for the public health and can convince others that a constructive use can be made of the effluent from an affluent society. Above all, we should strive to live in harmony with nature, not to conquer it.

## AIR POLLUTION

### Introduction

Unless gas masks are to become an accepted part of our dress, we must recognize the dangers and adopt adequate measures to reduce air pollution in our country effectively. Approximately 90 per cent of our urban population lives in localities which have air pollution problems. Many of these localities are large urban complexes which spread across state boundaries. It is estimated that all of the 212 standard metropolitan areas with populations greater than 50,000 and approximately 40 per cent of all other communities in the United States have problems caused by air pollution. Rural areas are affected also since air pollution has such a deleterious effect on vegetation. Current national estimates of economic damage, including injury to livestock and vegetation, corrosion and erosion of masonry and metal, and reduction of property values exceed 11 billion dollars annually.

What is air pollution? If a substance is present in the atmosphere in concentrations great enough to interfere directly or indirectly with a person's comfort, with his safety and health, or with the full use or enjoyment of his property, then that substance is considered an air pollutant. A collection of these substances varying in composition and intensity in different regions of the country constitutes air pollution. The Air Conservation Commission states that the air is termed "polluted" when wastes are produced so rapidly or when they accumulate in such concentrations that the normal, self-cleansing or dispersive propensities of the atmosphere cannot cope with them.

### Types of Contaminants

Pollutants in the air surrounding the earth did not originate with the industrial revolution. Tornado winds, dust storms, forest fires, and volcanic eruptions have long made their contributions. The terpenes which are emitted from large fir forests produce nature's equivalent of photochemical smog, as seen in the Blue Smokies of North Carolina. Gases from decaying animal and vegetable matter and pollens from flowering plants further promote air pollution.

Added to the natural contaminants are the by-products of an urban and industrialized civilization. Once man learned to master fire he was superbly equipped to surpass nature in polluting the air, since the pollutants which threaten the health of our citizens are the products of combustion. This combustion furnishes power for most of the transportation, and it generates electric power, heats homes and buildings, plays a vital role in manufacturing, and consumes much of the refuse.

Until the 1930's concern with air pollution was limited to smoke or other pollutants that could be seen or smelled. These pollutants were often tolerated because smoke in a community meant busy factories, more business, and more jobs. Gradually the public began to demand curbs against excessive smoke and a number of American cities, led by St. Louis and Pittsburgh, enacted control legislation. Advances in technology have furnished industry with methods to control much of the particulate matter which was sent indiscriminately into the air. Other technological advancements, however, have furnished scores of new contaminants. It is estimated that the present level of combustion in the United States annually produces 240 million tons of potential pollutants.[11] Thanks to the Air Quality Act and the Clean Air Amendments of 1970, a significant portion of these pollutants are trapped or rendered inactive before they escape into the atmosphere. A dangerously large quantity, however, still pollute our air. As contrasted to the 1930's, the vast majority of these contaminants, approximately 90 per cent, are invisible gases. They do much more harm but they cannot be seen.

The gaseous air pollutants with which we primarily are concerned include carbon monoxide, sulfur oxides, hydrocarbons, and the photochemical oxidants such as ozone, peroxy-

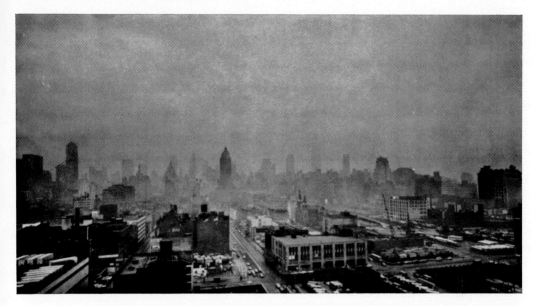

Fig. 10.1. Polluted air in a large U. S. metropolis. Source: Robert A. Taft Sanitary Engineering Center, Cincinnati.

acyl nitrates (PAN), and nitrogen dioxide. Carbon monoxide is the most common pollutant in urban air and its major source is the burning of gasoline in automobiles. In concentrations of 100 p.p.m., a level which has been found in heavy traffic or major cities, carbon monoxide produces symptoms such as dizziness, headache, and lassitude. Levels beyond this concentration can be severely hazardous. Experimental evidence suggests that carbon monoxide may inhibit proper response in a complex situation, such as driving in traffic. The effects have been compared to those of alcohol or fatigue. In fact, carbon monoxide may be doubly dangerous when a driver is tired, has had an alcoholic beverage, or has been taking tranquilizing-type drugs.[12]

Since the less expensive fuels used for heating and power generation contain elemental sulfur as an impurity, the burning of these fuels discharges large quantities of sulfur dioxide and, to a lesser extent, sulfur trioxide into the air. Inhalation of sulfur dioxide can irritate the upper respiratory tract and when the gas is adsorbed on particulate matter and carried deeper into the lung it can cause more serious damage. Recent studies have shown that increased mortality rates are associated with the use of these cheaper forms of heating fuel.[13] Sulfur trioxide combines with water vapor to form sulfuric acid and, as such, not only injures body tissue but causes considerable damage to crops, stone statues, and building materials. For example, Cleopatra's Needle, a stone statuary brought to New York in 1881, has deteriorated more since its arrival in New York than it did during the 3000 years that it spent in Egypt. These consequences are particularly important since the recent fuel economy has placed added importance on the increased use of coal. The American Public Health Association has stated that the conversion of power plants from the use of natural gas and oil to the burning of coal, without adding more pollution control devices, could cause 91,000 additional attacks of chronic respiratory disease and approximately 3800 excess deaths over the course of one year.[14]

The hydrocarbons which are discharged from dry cleaning establishments, refineries, and gasoline engines are usually considered to be directly harmful only in high concentrations. It has been found, however, that some of these products are carcinogenic and are identifiable with similar substances extracted from cigarette smoke. Further studies have linked lung cancer not only with cigarette smoking but also with inhaling heavily polluted city air. The death rate from lung cancer in urban areas is considerably higher than in rural areas and this difference is not explained completely by the differences in smoking habits.

The most noticeable effect of hydrocarbon pollution, however, is the production of photochemical smog. This mixture of gases and particles result from the intermixture of pollutants, catalyzed by the sun's energy, to form additional products commonly known as oxidants. An oxidant level in the air of one part per 10 million is sufficient to cause eye irritation and some respiratory distress and almost every urban area experiences at least a few days of this unpleasantness each year.

One of the oxidants in photochemical smog, ozone, can severely irritate mucous membranes. At levels comparable to those found in severe smog, ozone produces coughing, choking, severe fatigue, and reduces visual acuity. Another of the more recently studied oxidants, peroxyacyl nitrates, also causes eye irritation and impairs lung function. The nitrogen oxides are responsible for the whiskey-brown haze seen over most cities. Nitric oxide is a common and relatively harmless by-product of combustion but the same conditions which lead to the formation of photochemical smog greatly accelerate the conversion of nitric oxide to the more dangerous nitrogen dioxide. Experiments with animals have shown that exposures of 10 to 20 p.p.m. of nitrogen dioxide produce persistent pathological changes in the lungs and increase the susceptibility to infection. These tests with laboratory animals have profound implications in considering what levels of air pollution should be tolerated. If the person who is suffering from disease is to be protected we must set much more rigorous standards than if we were to consider only the robust individual.

It has long been known that industrial exposure to air-borne asbestos dust is causally associated with a specific form of pulmonary fibrosis, along with the possibility of developing cancer of the lung. However, it was found that asbestos contamination was not limited only to the industrial environments but was found in the lungs of a representative population. This air-borne noxious substance comes to us not only from mines and processing plants but from building materials, floor tiles, insulation, and the wearing away of automobile brake linings.

Environmental health workers are particularly concerned about the hazards of lead intoxication. Lead is a cumulative poison; it is taken into the body through food, water, and inhaled air, and is excreted very slowly. There are adequate studies to show that lead concentration in a significant number of people in the larger urban communities is now at a threatening, subtoxic level and is particularly dangerous to young children and pregnant women. Blood dyscrasias, cardiovascular and renal injury, and damage to the central nervous system can result from lead poisoning. The major contributor of atmospheric lead in the past has been the combustion of gasoline containing organic lead. During combustion the organic compound is broken down and the lead appears in engine exhaust as a complex inorganic halogen salt. Reports of studies in various cities have shown that these emitted lead-containing particles are the proper size to be inhaled and, quite likely, absorbed from the lung. It is anticipated that the decrease of leaded fuels will result in a marked reduction of this problem.

## Sources of Air Pollution

What are the major sources of air pollution? As formerly indicated, the pollution of the air we breathe is an indirect result of our pursuit toward more material goods, faster transportation, warmer and more comfortable homes and offices, and man's penchant to live in close proximity to his fellow man. The combination of advanced technology and the abundant resources of this country have created the most powerful and the most prosperous nation in the history of mankind. We have been so intent upon reaping the benefits of our accomplishments, however, that we have failed to give enough attention to the attendant problems which these successes have created. Air pollution, then, is the shadow side of prosperity and progress. The very industries that provide us with the materials of the good life also contribute a major share of the pollutants that contaminate the air that we breathe.

The major industrial contributors to air pollution in the United States are pulp and paper mills, iron and steel mills, petroleum refineries, and smelters. Added to this list are the chemical manufacturers who produce such diverse items as fertilizer and synthetic rubber.

Most of the electricity consumed in the United States is generated by burning coal and oil. With the emphasis on fuel economy, additional plants that have been using natural gas are being encouraged to switch to coal, which is found in greater abundance in this country. The sulfur that is contained in these fuels as an impurity provides the sulfur oxides, which represent one of the most serious and prevalent forms of air pollution in the United States today. Governmental restrictions enforced through the Environmental Protection Agency have helped to reduce some of these pollutants but with the emphasis on conserving scarce fuels it is feared that there will be a relaxation in the enforcement of Federal standards. There are relatively few restrictions placed upon residential heating, however. It is estimated that the fuel burned to heat homes and offices each year discharges approximately 3 million tons of sulfur dioxide, 2 million tons of carbon monoxide, and 1 million tons each of nitrogen oxides, hydrocarbons, and particulate matter.

The aforementioned sources of air pollution have all been stationery. They can be located geographically and are under the jurisdiction of local political subdivisions. A major source of air pollution, however, is not stationary. This group consists of cars, trucks, trains, and planes which must generate power for propulsion. The diesel engines in trucks and railroad engines contribute their share of visual pollutants as well as invisible gases. Also, it has been reported that a four-engine jet plane releases an average of 88 pounds of pollutants into the air with each take off. When this figure is multiplied by the number of planes in the United States, times the number of take offs per plane, the contribution of airplane traffic to air pollution is rather significant.

The greatest offender of all, however, is the automobile. There are in excess of 114 million motor vehicles in the United States. In spite of the use of catalytic converters and other pollution control equipment, motor vehicles still discharge into the atmosphere millions of tons of carbon monoxide, hydrocarbons, nitrogen oxides, sulfur oxides, and particulate matter. In addition to being the major source of carbon monoxide, they also supply the main ingredients for photochemical haze. The automobile owes its supremacy as a source of air pollution to the inefficiency with which it burns its fuel. Hydrocarbons escape through the exhaust, from the fuel tank, and from carburetor vents, and slow driving in heavy traffic greatly increases the rate of emission. A further contribution of the automobile to air pollution is in the form of highly pulverized rubber and asphalt, generated by abrasion of tires upon streets. With the rise in gasoline prices, the increased number of smaller automobiles, and the added emphasis on mass transit there are hopes and expectations that some of these problems will be reduced. At the time of this writing, though, that expectation is still in the future. Department of Public Safety officials report that the attitude of the average motorist seems to be that fuel economy is for someone else and that there should be a reduction of other automobiles on the highways so that the "average" motorist will have more room to drive. We hear and read much about coordination and control but there are relatively few who are willing to be coordinated or controlled.

Chemical analysis divides the polluted atmospheres of the world's cities into two major types. One is classified as the London type, composed principally of sulfur compounds from the burning of low-grade fuel, and the other is the Los Angeles type which is composed principally of hydrocarbons from petroleum products. Most cities have various mixtures of both. Since the use of automobiles is so widespread, all cities suffer to some degree from air pollution by hydrocarbons, and in those geographical areas where low-grade fuels are burned for power and domestic space heating, the air may also be polluted with sulfur compounds.

Both the nature and the seriousness of the problem of air pollution can vary according to geographical location, the season of the year, and even the hour of the day. The major variables include the types and quantity of pollutants, wind speed and direction, topography, sunlight, precipitation, vertical air movements, and the susceptibility of individuals to particular combinations of pollutants. Most of the major cities of the world are located in natural basins at the confluence of rivers, around bays, or in flat areas backed up by mountains. In many cities these basins are natural traps for any kind of wastes that can hang suspended in the atmosphere. Within their envelopes of haze the city skylines are sometimes more easily imagined than seen.

The strong breezes that attend the movement of great air masses over the continent generally disperse these pollutants, and in the absence of breezes the air may be cleaned by updrafts that dilute and carry away the particulate matter and gases. These natural ventilation processes sometimes fail, however, and there may be no movement of air over a particular area for various periods of time. One of the more troublesome mechanisms interfering with vertical air movements is the phenomenon of temperature inversion. Here, a blanket of warm air forms at higher altitude and traps a layer of cooler air next to the ground. The pollutants which are discharged into stagnant air from heavily populated regions are not diluted or dispersed and they continue to build in concentration until favorable meteorological factors restore normal air flow. Although temperature inversions occur more frequently in some areas than in others they are not restricted to geographical sections. Indeed, these phenomena occur a considerable number of days each years in virtually every region of the country.

### Effects of Air Pollution

Serious students of the problems associated with air pollution have predicted that if and when air contamination increases beyond the capacity of the atmosphere to cleanse itself then the life of mankind will be threatened with gradual suffocation by its own effluents. This situation, fortunately, has not occurred on such a cataclysmic scale but there have been hints and warnings that the skies can be poisoned by man beyond their endurance. One such warning occurred in the industrialized town of Donora, Pennsylvania, in October, 1948. A heavy fog held down by a thermal inversion blanketed the town for four days while zinc fumes, coal smoke, and waste gases from steel mills, slag-processing plants, and sulfuric acid mills continued to be poured into the thickened atmosphere. Grime began to fall out of the smog and within 48 hr. visibility had become so limited that residents had difficulty finding their way home. By the third day of constant smog, 5910 of the town's 14,000 residents became ill. Particularly affected were people 65 years of age or older and those persons who had a history of bronchopulmonary disease. Twenty persons died, with 17 deaths occurring on the last day. Then, a heavy rain fell, the smog disappeared, and the epidemic stopped immediately.

Another such episode presented itself in London, on December 5, 1952. On that day a thick fog rolled into London and was held down by a temperature inversion. The pinned down air was steadily thickened by the soot and smoke of the coal-burning city and within three days the atmosphere was so heavily polluted that vision was severely limited. Policemen wore respiratory masks, and the sun was described as having no more brilliance than an unlit Chinese lantern. Thousands of people became acutely ill from respiratory diseases and the hospitals were soon filled to overflowing. During the five days that the smog smothered London there were 4000 more deaths in that city than would have occurred under normal circumstances.

Similar episodes, but with less tragic results, have since occurred in many of the great cities of the world including Tokyo, Rome, Paris, the Ruhr Valley, and the heavily congested New York-New Jersey coast. Air pollution has become such a world-wide preoccupation that the belching smokestacks which long symbolized prosperity in the industrialized countries are now viewed as a source of irritation and the foul air that had been accepted as an inevitable part of busy cities is becoming intolerable.

The most obvious effect of air pollution is the limit that it puts on visibility, creating hazards for land, water, and air transportation. Air pollutants also crack rubber, corrode metals, and cause further extensive damage to materials of all varieties. One of the most widespread effects of polluted air is damage and destruction to vegetation, including "salad" crops, citrus, and ornamental plants, and the damage to livestock has been calculated in the millions of dollars. The most serious effect of air pollution, the problem which concerns those in the allied medical professions, is the contribution to disease and premature death.

Although oxygen requirements are the most critical of man's daily physical needs, he does less to control the purity of the air than he does to ensure the wholesomeness of his food and water. It is rather likely to assume that pollutants which injure plants and erode stone also exert damaging effects on humans. Indeed, this assumption has been shown to be correct. Reference previously has been made to the association between air pollution and such physical ailments as heart disease, cancer, dermatitis, and systemic poisoning. Oxidant air pollution also has been shown to reduce the level of athletic performance. The most common afflictions either caused or worsened by contaminants in the air, however, are the bronchopulmonary diseases. These may range from the common cold to lung cancer.

In the London and Donora tragedies there were no unusual pollutants which were foreign to the area and no single smog component was present in a higher relative concentration than usual. The disquieting conclusion is that the same smog breathed by all elements of the population during one or two days of heavy air contamination, without immediate ill effects, may be highly injurious to a significant portion of the people when it is breathed continuously for just a few days more. It will be recalled that 17 of the 20 deaths in Donora occurred on the last day of the smog. It can be only conjectured what the number of deaths would have been if the heavily polluted conditions had remained for another 48 hr.

Another serious consequence of these disasters was the subsequent health history of many of the inhabitants. Prior to the tragedy the citizens of Donora displayed a normal health history comparable to those in the rest of the country. For nine years after the episode, however, those people who had become ill from the smog showed a higher mortality and illness rate than did those people who were present and did not become ill. In London, an excess of 8000 people died during the two months following their heavy smog episode. The majority of these excess deaths were due to respiratory diseases and medical experts strongly suspect that they were a direct result of the period of acute air pollution.

It is true that the majority of the people who are most seriously affected by air pollution are those who suffer from some type of respiratory distress. More recent studies, however, have identified air pollution as the cause of an increased number of cardiovascular deaths.[15] But apart from the conditions caused by air pollution it is also true that an increasing number of our population is suffering from bronchopulmonary illnesses. Since the advent of sulfonamides and broad spectrum antibiotics our people are recovering from many respiratory illnesses which formerly would have taken their lives. The majority of these people usually are left with a residue of lung or bronchial damage. Also, Asian, London, and Hong Kong flu epidemics and other virus-caused diseases have caused their share of respiratory cripples.

What is not generally known is that more people die as a result of influenza *after* the epidemic than during it. In large measure these excess deaths occur in people with damaged pulmonary structures or chronic heart disease. Generally, these are the same type of victims who are in danger of serious illness from continued exposure to heavily contaminated air. The toll is taken in respiratory diseases that usually involve microbial agents at some stage of their course. But in many cases these agents would not be able to multiply in the body if some other factor had not intervened to decrease the body's general resistance.[16]

But the irritation and debility associated with air pollution is not necessarily restricted to those afflicted with previous disease conditions. The so-called Tokyo-Yokohama (T-Y) asthma is an example. This affliction first appeared among American troops and their families living in Yokohama and was noted later among troops living in Tokyo. The asthma-like symptoms did not respond to medications but when patients were promptly removed from the immediate area they usually recovered. It is interesting that most of those stricken had never shown asthmatic symptoms before. Studies showed that the incidence and severity of the disease were best correlated with the levels of air pollution originating from the Kanto Plain, a heavily industrialized section extending between Yokohama and Tokyo. There have been similarly caused epidemic outbreaks of asthma attacks in Okinawa, Memphis, Pasadena, and New Orleans, which lead health experts to predict that this type of illness may well become more widespread if there are no adequate checks placed on the pollutants that contaminate our atmosphere.

The most important air pollution health effects, then, occur from irritant materials which reach air-exposed membranous surfaces. The response elicited in the individual may vary according to the major type of pollutant involved. For example, sulfur dioxide is rapidly dissolve in the aqueous wall coatings of the upper airway while nitrogen dioxide and ozone reach deeper into the lungs. Irritation of the upper airways causes such symptoms as sneezing, coughing, slowing of ciliary movement, increased production of thickened mucus, and narrowing of the airway. A greater irritation may induce an inflammatory response with tissue congestion, loss of cilia, and cellular metaphasia. Irritation in the lower airways may cause all of the above symptoms as well as pulmonary edema. It can readily be seen that inhalation of these gases in any measurable quantity could result in damage to the tissues involved in respiration.

Whether caused by or aggravated by air pollution, respiratory diseases continue to plague man at an ever increasing rate. Medical conditions which are related directly to air pollution are chronic bronchitis, acute non-specific upper respiratory disease, chronic obstructive ventilatory disease, pulmonary emphysema, bronchial asthma, and lung cancer. Emphysema is the fastest growing cause of death in the United States, and both the incidence and death rate are much higher in congested cities.

Apart from the health aspect lies an even more ominous threat, because man has tended to ignore the fact that he is utterly dependent upon the biosphere. Technological man, the builder of bigger and bigger industrial societies, is so aware of his strength that he is unaware of his weakness—the danger that his distortion of the iron laws of nature may provoke disaster on a vast scale.

The earth is basically a closed system and the winds which ventilate the earth are only six miles high. Air and the valuable oxygen in the air are not a limitless resource. Through the process of photosynthesis growing plants supply oxygen in a delicate balance of nature; approximately 30 per cent of this oxygen is obtained from vegetation on earth and 70 per cent comes from phytoplankton floating passively on the earth's oceans. Through the excess burning of fossil fuels, however, considerably more carbon dioxide is being produced than can be used by the plants in photosynthesis. The result is a reduction in available oxygen and an excess of carbon dioxide. It has been estimated that atmospheric carbon dioxide has increased 10 per cent since the turn of the century. Some scientists contend that the gas creates a "greenhouse" effect in the atmosphere which prevents the heat of the earth from escaping back into space. The result is a warming trend that, in a matter of decades, could start to melt the polar ice caps and threaten major cities on the coastline. Another major effect of air pollution is the fact that it effectively prevents a significant portion of the sun's radiant energy from reaching the earth. This, in turn, could alter weather conditions

and cause a serious reduction in the world's food supply.

**Corrective Measures**

There is no question that the problem of air pollution has become acute and that adequate steps must be taken, and soon, if we are to preserve our environment and assure the health of our people. But what are these corrective measures and why have they not been adopted earlier? To be truly effective, controls on air pollution need the compulsion of law, and even with this compulsion the processes for reducing contaminants at their source is very expensive. It is not surprising, then, that the accused industries take a defensive position, first against general legislation, then against specific provisions, then against law enforcement. Their arguments are familiar and realistic: "It will drive jobs out of town, or price our product out of the market." "There may be offensive odor, but you have no conclusive proof that it is a menace to health." "Our plant has been here for 50 years. Why are we suddenly accused of performing a dis-service to our community?" Today's contamination is not the work of evil men or even slovenly neighbors. As mentioned previously, these air pollutants are the impersonal consequence of a highly industrialized society and corrective measures must involve all of the varied interests of society. Public health officials alone cannot be expected to secure the agreements and cooperation of all the private and public interests and the countless numbers of businesses, transportation officials, legislators, and taxpayers. What is needed is a more concerted citizen's movement to help control environmental pollution.

Definite steps have been taken. The leadership, almost by necessity, has been assumed by California. In that state, drastic restrictions have been placed upon all potential sources of air pollution, from backyard incineration to cars and oil refineries. In fact, Los Angeles has been called the world's most smog-controlled city. Indeed, if such drastic control was not enforced in that heavily congested basin which is plagued with thermal inversions, Los Angeles would most probably be suffering from series of disaster days reminiscent of Donora and London. By contrast, if most of the cities in the United States observed the restrictions on air contamination now practiced in Los Angeles, these cities would have little or no air pollution problems.

Spurred by aroused citizens, local newspapers, and concerned public officials, considerable State and Federal legislation has been passed in attempts to control air pollution. Essentially all levels of government have air pollution control programs with sanctions against those who do not voluntarily comply with published restrictions. Since polluted air is no respector of political boundaries, the problem is being approached through multistate cooperation. Through the provision of section 303 of the 1970 Federal Clean Air Act, if states and local governments cannot or will not move against major polluters of air, particularly in emergency situations, the Federal government is empowered to bring suit on behalf of the United States. The purpose of this suit is to immediately restrain persons causing the air pollution and to stop the emission of air pollutants. This power was granted in order to avert another Donora tragedy. The first use of the Federal air pollution injunctive authority was exercised in Birmingham in November, 1971.[17] Under Federal legislation the Environmental Protection Agency designated air quality control regions in the United States, published air quality criteria and reports on available control techniques. The individual states, in turn, were required to set air quality standards and establish comprehensive plans for implementing such standards. These were then submitted to the Federal government for review. It is the responsibility of the states to control air pollution in accordance with the standards and implementation plans submitted.

But much remains to be done. The polar ice caps need not melt, and citizens with respiratory diseases do not have to live in fear of an ominous threat from the skies. Technological man who has produced our affluent society not only can but *has* developed methods and procedures to prevent potential air pollutants from reaching the atmosphere. The real question is whether enough people want action enough to see that adequate controls are instituted.

In regard to pollution from stationary sources, most of the contaminants can be captured before they reach the air. Industrial gases can be washed out by scrubbers, adsorbed on charcoal filters, or burned to form harmless products. Particulate matter can be removed by filters, ultrasonic vibrators, cyclonic separators, or electrostatic precipitators, and the open burning of a city's trash can be replaced by sanitary landfill or by efficient incineration. Pollution by sulfur oxides can be reduced drastically or eliminated through removal of sulfur from fuel oils prior to use or by restricting fuels only to those of low sulfur content.

Pollution from mobile sources, such as automobiles, may be reduced by even more efficient smog control devices but it appears that some other type of motor will have to be developed. Electric cars, gas turbine engines, and greater use of deisel power and nuclear energy will help a great deal to reduce the pollutants now discharged by automobiles.

There are three very important sequential needs in order to control the problem of air pollution. The first is the need for recognition of the dangers which are present and which will be multiplied if air pollution is allowed to continue unabated. These dangers must be recognized by the citizens and their governments. The second need is for the enforcement of sound standards that are attainable and can be maintained, and the third need is for the continuation of impartial rules to govern the producers of pollution.

All of us, particularly those in the allied medical professions, have a real interest in the health aspects of air pollution. We have seen the tortured efforts of those who are fighting for each breath and we are concerned about improving the health of the public. It is important, therefore, to use our influence, privately and professionally, to refute the fallacy that nature exists only to serve man. We must convince those within our sphere of influence that air pollution is a threat to health and that it can be controlled through organized community action. Participation in town meetings, citizen's councils, governor's committees, and regional conferences will furnish opportunities for speaking to interested civic leaders and others who can influence public opinion. Convinced of the inherent dangers of continued air pollution, we must do what we can to help guarantee to all mankind the right to breathe.

## WATER POLLUTION

### Introduction

Water has multiple meanings for most people. To the scientist the chemical combination of hydrogen ions and hydroxyl groups is of prime consideration. To a drowning man water may mean death, while to a man dying of thirst it may mean life. Water is an essential substance in many industries and still remains a source of recreation to the fisherman and to those who participate in aquatic sports, and who can forget the moonlight shimmering across a lake or river on a beautiful evening? Water is such an integral part of our lives that we tend to take it for granted and seldom recognize that clean water, like clean air, is not a limitless resource.

The extent of a nation's water supply is determined largely by the total precipitation and is supplemented frequently by underground storage deposits. The total annual rainfall in the United States averages about 30 inches, unevenly distributed by geography and seasons. The rain forests of Washington state receive more than 100 inches and large sections of numerous states in the southeastern United States receive over 50 inches annually, while Death Valley in California gets less than two inches. Most of the rainfall and thus the greater availability of water is in the eastern portion of the nation and yet there is a steady migration of people toward the West, the more arid region. Of the average 30 inches of annual precipitation for the United States as a whole, about 22 inches are returned to the atmosphere by evaporation. Only about half of the remaining eight inches can be tapped and the rest flows into the seas. Of what remains, only about two inches presently are available to man on a dependable year-round basis.

Our need for water is outstripping our supplies, and the situation will worsen in coming years unless we place a higher priority on curbing water pollution. In order to assess the magnitude of the pollution problem the quantities of wastewater must be considered in relation to the total available supply of fresh water. The annual average stream flow that discharges into the oceans from the continental United States is representative of our available supply of fresh water; this stream flow amounts to approximately 1100 billion gallons daily.[18]

Modern living demands vast quantities of clean water. Uses of water around the household, including bathing, laundering, and watering of plants, amount to approximately 50 gallons per day for each person in the home, representing a daily national total of 10 billion gallons. To irrigate one acre of farmland takes approximately 750,000 gallons of water and total irrigation in the United States requires about 141 billion gallons daily. Most of this water cannot be recovered for additional use and that which is recovered is contaminated with dissolved minerals plus pesticides and fertilizers that have been used on crops. The major users of water, however, are industries. Approximately 200 gallons of water are needed to manufacture $1 worth of paper, 500 gallons for one yard of woolen cloth, 65,000 gallons used in the manufacture of an automobile, 320,000 gallons required to produce one ton of aluminum, and 600,000 gallons to make one ton of synthetic rubber. The total use of water by industry in the United States amounts to approximately 200 billion gallons each day. The daily use of water throughout the country, including such other uses as mining and steam-generating plants, adds up to an excess of 400 billion gallons. With increased population and increased demand for goods and services, the use of water will continue to be accelerated. The projected need for water in 1980 is 597 billion gallons a day, including 394 billion gallons for industry alone. By the year 2000 it is anticipated that the daily need for water in the United States will be 969 billion gallons. At that time, the Public Health Service estimates that 95 per cent of the population of 280 million people will reside in urban areas and waste which is discharged through municipal sewer systems will average some 132 gallons per day per person.

In discussing the need and the application of water, it may be noted that the term "water consumption" was not employed. Although about one-third of the water is not reclaimed, largely because of evaporation and transpiration, the remainder of the water used in the United States is returned, for water, like air, can be cleaned and used again. It is obvious that we do not have enough "new" water to meet the growing needs of the nation and that greater emphasis must be placed upon recycling processes so that more efficient use can be made of the water that is available. This re-use of water is already a common practice in certain sections of the country. Along the Ohio River during particular times of the year water is used approximately four times as it passes from Pittsburgh to Cairo, and the author recalls a jocular sign in Easton, Pennsylvania, which implored the user to "flush the toilet twice— Philadelphia needs the drinking water."

Since water must be used over and over again

it must be kept clean enough to meet the standards for municipal water supplies, industry, and agriculture. Prior to World War II there was relatively little difficulty with polluted streams and waterways. Most of the pollutants were biodegradable and the oxygen content of the water supported microorganisms which fed on these contaminants. At least two factors have changed this situation, however. One is the rapid increase in population with its attendant increased use of water and the other is the development of chemicals such as man-made fibers, insecticides, and synthetic detergents that are not biodegradable. These new chemicals reach the lakes and streams from manufacturing processes and from consumers' use of products and little is known of their pollutional characteristics or their long-range toxic effects on man. As pollution continues to grow and as more complex contaminants find their way into our water supplies the processes for treating water become increasingly expensive and difficult and the resulting product becomes poorer in quality.

## Classification of Pollutants

Pollutants entering watercourses have been broadly classified into eight categories:

*1. Domestic Sewage and Other Oxygen-Demanding Wastes.* As mentioned previously, these wastes are ordinarily reduced to stable compounds through the action of aerobic bacteria that require and obtain oxygen from the water. At excessive residue levels, however, the resultant oxygen reduction can have serious impact on the life in the water. According to the Naitonal Academy of Sciences, the oxygen-demanding fraction of domestic and industrial waste is growing much more rapidly than the efficiency of waste treatment. The first massive warning was seen in Lake Erie where most of the lake's center was robbed of its oxygen content and aquatic life was catastrophically diminished.

*2. Infectious Agents.* Modern disinfection techniques have greatly reduced the dangers from disease-causing organisms. All of the threats have not been removed, however. For instance, the filtering mechanisms are quite effective in removing bacteria but not viruses. Health authorities are constantly wary of diseases such as infectious hepatitis, the virus of which is suspected of being water-borne. An-

other threat from infectious agents arises when heavy runoff overloads the treatment facilities of those cities that maintain combination storm drains and sewers, so that raw sewage enters the watercourses.

*3. Plant Nutrients.* In small, moderate amounts these pose no problem but the nitrates and phosphates which are present in domestic, industrial, and agricultural wastes are now so concentrated that they encourage excess proliferation of algae and plant growth. This in turn causes changes in the color and taste of water, alters aquatic life, and interferes with proper utilization of waterways.

*4. Organic Chemicals such as Insecticides, Pesticides, and Detergents.* These substances are usually very toxic at low concentrations and have been responsible for spectacular kills of fish and wildlife. Adequate information is lacking regarding long-term exposure to these products and efforts to treat or remove them from water supplies have been largely unsuccessful.

*5. Other Minerals and Chemicals.* This group of industrial wastes includes chemical residues, petrochemicals, salts, acids, and sludges. In combination with other pollutants they form still other chemical entities. Many of this group are known to be toxic or carcinogenic and methods of removal are poorly developed.

*6. Sediments from Land Erosion.* This additional loss of natural resource necessitates expensive treatment of water supplies, reduces a stream's ability to assimilate oxygen-demanding wastes, and covers fish nests and food organisms.

*7. Radioactive Substances.* Although contamination from this source is minimal at present, the anticipated large increase in nuclear power reactors poses threatening additional challenge.

*8. Heat from Power and Industrial Plants.* The amount of dissolved oxygen that water can contain decreases as the water temperature increases. Introducing heat into a stream, then, has an effect equivalent to that of introducing oxygen-consuming waste. This lowers the ability of water to purify itself and presents a serious threat for fish and other aquatic life.

## Sewage Disposal

The majority of cities in the United States now have some type of sewage treatment plants although a small per cent of municipal wastes are still dumped into our rivers and streams as raw sewage. Another small per cent are given only primary treatment, which removes just the settleable solids. But even this cursory treatment represents a considerable advance.

Historically, the growth of cities as a result of the industrial revolution led to problems not previously encountered. Ditches had been dug in most towns for drainage purposes and some of the larger cities constructed elaborate storm drains. Wastes, however, were not allowed to be placed in these drains because it was believed that toxic fumes from such matter would cause the spread of disease. It was not until 1815 that London admitted sewage into its storm sewers, followed by Boston in 1833, and Paris in 1880.

The development of sanitary procedures was quite slow. Although water closets were invented in 1778, they were adopted very slowly and, of course, were not highly efficient unless connected with a sewer system. Hamburg, Germany, built the first comprehensive sanitary sewer system in 1843. This system discharged its sewage into a river and provisions were made for a weekly flushing. A similar system was started in Chicago in 1855, and Brooklyn began discharging its sewage into the tidewater in 1857. No one weighed the possible consequences of emptying large amounts of putrescent matter into the watercourses of the land. In fact, no one then could have conceived the tremendous amount of wastes generated by supercities and by industries. As the streams became steadily more noxious some cities took remedial action, but continued progress in sanitation was rather hesitant until forced by untoward events. The cholera epidemics in London and Paris and typhoid in Chicago, for example, were the compelling forces which prompted these cities to improve their sewage facilities. The waste treatment plants which were built, however, also included storm drainage. In fact, most of the systems built to serve large population centers before 1940 were combined storm drains and sewers. A recent Public Health Service inventory of municipal sewage facilities lists over 1300 communities with combined sewers and another 650 communities with both combined and separate systems. This represents the sewage from approximately one-half the total urban population.

The veiled threat associated with these combined storm drain sewer systems is the inability to handle all the runoff of an intensive storm. The overflow, including raw sewage, is dumped into the rivers and contaminates the water supply of communities downstream. The public health problems of such contamination is evident, but there is also the problem of economics. It has been estimated that the complete separation of sewage systems throughout the country, an ideal situation, would cost on the order of 20 to 30 billion dollars.

Approximately 99.9 per cent of sewage entering a treatment plant is water. Although the remaining 0.1 per cent may seem small, in 1 million gallons of sewage this amounts to over four tons of solid matter. The purpose of the treatment plant is to remove the solids and contaminants and to purify the water so that it can be used again. The most efficient systems utilize two processes, a physical separation and screening of the waste water followed by bacterial treatment of this water. The processes are known as primary and secondary treatment.

The sewage entering a modern treatment plant first passes through a bar screen which catches such large objects as sticks and rags. Then the water flows slowly through a grit chamber which allows sand, gravel, and other objects to settle. From there it flows to primary sedimentation tanks where the solids settle to the bottom and are pumped to the sludge thickeners. These combined processes comprise the primary treatment of sewage and remove approximately 35 per cent of the contaminants.

In secondary treatment, the remaining water, called effluent, is treated by bacterial action. One method is the flow of effluent through trickling filters. In this process the effluent is trickled through a large, circular bed of crushed rock three to eight feet deep and up to 200 feet in diameter. Complex colonies of bacterial slime, algae, and microscopic organisms are attached to the rocks and consume organic wastes as the water trickles by. In recent years, however, the use of trickling filters has been discouraged. Another process of secondary treatment is known as the activated sludge method. Here, the effluent from the primary settling tanks flows to aerated tanks and is mixed with sludge, a jelly-like mass consisting of colonies of bacteria and other microorganisms which digest the remaining sewage. The water from either of these processes of secondary treatment then flows to secondary sedimentation tanks where the remaining suspended solids settle out. The final effluent is then chlorinated and released. This process, though, still fails to remove adequate amounts of detergent, viruses, and dissolved impurities which have adverse effects on both color and taste. To remove these impurities the use of a more expensive tertiary method is employed on a limited scale. These methods use alum or lime for coagulation-sedimentation processes and activated charcoal filters to remove the dissolved refractory organics. Other methods of tertiary treatment include electrodialysis and a unique process called reverse osmosis.[19] Technology is presently available for the removal of most of the harmful constituents of municipal and industrial waste waters. The limitations on existing capabilities are restricted primarily by available funds.

## Control Programs

But the gap between possible technological achievement and existing conditions is all too evident. Water pollution is jeopardizing our water supplies, menacing the public health, destroying aquatic life, threatening our economic growth, and disgracing our environment. In many cities drinking water is becoming less palatable because of chemical additives, and bathing beaches, picnic areas, and boating marinas are less safe for people to use. Miles of streams in most states are being lost to fishing and useful aquatic life, and in suburbs all over the country detergent foam is a familiar sight on the surfaces of rivers and streams. The pollution load in our rivers is approximately six times as much as it was 60 years ago. Unfortunately, a common description given to the Potomac River which flows through our nation's capital is that "... the water is too thick to swim in and too thin to plow."

Constructive efforts are being expended to combat this serious problem. Since the basin of a great river encompasses many thousands of square miles and crosses numerous political boundaries, it soon became evident that all those who were in the watershed area were directly involved in problems of pollution and control, but there was no organizational structure to promote co-operation. Existing local governments were interested primarily in conditions within their immediate environment, the various states in the basin did not have standardized laws, and many pollution hazards had their origin or exerted some of their potentially most serious effects in communities too small to be able to provide effective control. In answer to the need for a uniform, co-operative approach to the problem of pollution, various interstate stream commissions were established. One such agreement was the Ohio River Valley Water Sanitation Compact, whereby each of eight states pledged to the others faithful co-operation in the control of future pollution in the rivers, streams, and waters in the Ohio River basin. Another similar compact was the Interstate Commission of the Potomac River which enabled four states and the District of Columbia to develop and carry out joint programs for controlling water pollution on this river. Other agreements were the Delaware River Commission and the Missouri River Basin Engineer's Health Council.

In addition several comprehensive basin studies were done which formed the foundation for further compacts between various states and included Federal participation. One such plan was the Arkansas-Red River Basin which involves 180,000 square miles in Kansas, Oklahoma and Texas. Somewhat similar studies were conducted in the Colorado River Basin, the Great Lakes-Illinois Waterway area, the Delaware Estuary, the Columbia River Basin, and Chesapeake Bay.

The Federal Government, through the strengthened Federal Water Pollution Control Act, is becoming more involved in attempts to solve the problem. Money is furnished to pay 30 to 50 per cent of construction costs for new and enlarged treatment plants and Federal agencies are conducting research into new ways to prevent or reduce water pollution. River basin planning is also a project of the Federal Government as well as enforcement of pollution laws on interstate streams. The Water Quality Improvement Act of 1970 added emphasis to research in controlling oil pollution, acid mine drainage, vessel pollution, and pollution problems in the Great Lakes.[20] A particular problem is found in recreation boating. Approximately 6 million registered boats are afloat in the United States, excluding most sail boats.[21] Federal regulations require an acceptable sewage disposal system for each boat but it is anticipated that difficulties will be encountered in preventing continued discharge of raw sewage from these boats into the waterways. Many officials and environmentalists are rightfully concerned about the future of lakes, rivers, and seashores favored by boating enthusiasts. Therefore, even more Federal and State regulations are being formulated.

But none of this is enough. Our population is

growing and becoming more concentrated, thereby creating acute and special problems of waste disposal. No longer can the use of our waterways as receptacles of uncontrolled wastes be accepted as a legitimate use of water. Whatever may have been acceptable or unavoidable in years past, our goal now and in years ahead must be to prevent as much water pollution as possible. All users of waters have a responsibility for returning those waters to the stream as clean as is technically possible.

For water pollution control programs to succeed, we must have an informed and aware public which understands the problem and supports the necessary programs of action. To gain this, it is necessary to show the public the dimensions of the problem and demonstrate ways of solving it. No real progress in solving any health or social problem can ever come about without the support of an informed and determined public. People in each community must become aware of what is happening to their own waterways and realize that the same thing is happening in other areas. Those in the allied medical professions are particularly concerned about the quality of water and the potential dangers of constantly being exposed to trace elements that are deleterious to health. Encouragement of abatement programs and participation in community and state pollution control endeavors will demonstrate our determination to combat this threat. A water quality index has been proposed and we should give this proposition our full cooperation.[22] Other methods for obtaining water quality objectives are to establish effluent standards based upon water quality standards and then impose pro-rated fines on the amount of waste discharged in excess of these standards.[23] By joining in this struggle for clean water, the allied health professions can play an important role in maintaining the health of our people and in assuring the future prosperity of this country. An adequate supply of clean water will help immensely in making it possible to achieve these goals.

## POPULATION INCREASES

Within human reason, conception is good only if it can be expected, through the essential help of parents and society to result in a healthy, constructive, adult component of family and group. It follows that conception is bad if parents and society cannot protect, sustain, and train the infant through childhood and adolescence. Exploding populations make this quite impossible today over large parts of the globe. Obviously, to man's God-given reason, man is not intended to beget young merely to have them die of starvation or violent death after a bare, beastly existence. Reason manifests that man's intellect was provided, among other objectives, to prevent this, but without violating his sexual nature or his marriage, through which this is fulfilled. Toward this end, his intellect, I submit, has evolved "the pill."

JOHN ROCK, M.D.[24]

## Introduction

A great deal has been written in recent years of the time bomb which has erupted in the form of the population explosion. Since most of this increase in population has occurred in Asia, Africa, and Latin America, the people of North America and Europe have viewed the reports as a distant problem. We have tended to believe that much of such reporting has been work of sensationalists and that emotions have distorted reason.

We must realize, however, that uncontrolled growth of the world's population is perhaps, other than the threat of nuclear war, the most urgent problem of our age. The almost indiscriminate multiplication of human lives is out of proportion to present and prospective increases in world economic development and, as a result, the standards of living which are already below the minimum in almost two-thirds of the world will sink to even lower levels. The necessity to supply adequate public health services to this burgeoning population is already acute and the demands of the future pose problems of enormous proportion.

The safety, health, and welfare of humanity have been threatened from many sources throughout history. Man has been remarkably successful in reducing these threats and has supplied the means to live not only better but longer. Within the past few decades medical science has concentrated on the disease problems which threaten human life and has developed techniques and medications to combat most of these problems effectively. This knowledge has been shared with the underdeveloped countries of the world and has helped to reduce mortality rates drastically in all nations of the globe. But, although death rates have been lowered markedly, there has not been an attendant decrease in birth rates. A brief review of population development will demonstrate the magnitude of the problem with which our world is now confronted.

## Growth of the World's Population

At the time of Christ the world population was approximately ¼ billion. It was not until the middle of the 17th century that this number had been doubled to ½ billion. By 1830, approximately 200 years later, the population had doubled again to 1 billion. It took less than 100 years to add the next billion and about 37 years for another billion in population. With man's control of famines and mass killer diseases and no drastic reduction in birth rates presently in sight, the next billion increase in total population will take only 15 years. It must be remembered that this is an *increase* in world population and such an increase is equal to the total present population of North America, all nations of Europe, and all other areas of the world except Asia, Africa, and Latin America. The world population, approaching 4 billion persons at the time of this writing, is growing at a rate of about 2 per cent per year. This may not appear to be an extraordinary increase but it is the fastest rate in recent history. Population growth, like compound interest, is self-accelerating and a few simple calculations will show that if this rate is unchecked it will take only 35 years to add another 3½ billion and less than 35 years after that to produce an increase of an additional 7 billion. By the end of this century then, if present rates of growth continue, we can expect almost 7 billion population and, carried to its ridiculous extremes, within two centuries there could be 150 billion people on this earth.[25] Of course, it is anticipated that there will be instituted some drastic changes long before that time but, barring major disasters, it appears that substantial growth in every region of the world will continue at least throughout the remainder of the 20th century.

The rates of population growth are not the same, of course, in all parts of the world. The less developed areas of the world, including Asia, the southwestern Pacific Islands, Africa, the Caribbean islands, and Latin America, will double their population in 20 to 30 years. In such countries as Mexico, Venezuela, Iran, Madagascar, and Tunisia, birth rates still exceed 35 per 1000 population.[26] Between now and the year 2000, if present rates continue, Latin America is expected to add nearly 350 million to its present population of 250 million, North America is projected to add approximately 80 million, and the population in Asia alone is expected to almost equal the current total world population. Estimates of India's current rate, about 39 per 1000, suggest 20 million births there each year and the United Nations' estimate of the annual number of births in China approach 25 million. Japan and most of the countries of Europe, on the other hand, are growing relatively slowly and may take 70 to 100 years to double their populations (see Fig 10.3).

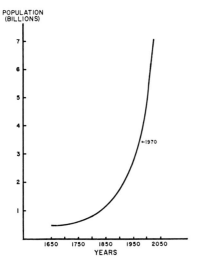

Fig. 10.2. Growth and projected increase of the world population

## World Problems of Uncontrolled Growth

The implications and attendant problems of such a phenomenal increase in population, particularly for the poorer and less-advanced countries, border on the disastrous. Already over half of the world's population lives on a bare subsistence, with an annual *per capita* income of around $100. The increasing numbers of people are placing demands upon nations that cannot meet the needs of their citizens even now. It is reported that the underdeveloped countries have no schools for some 300 million of their children, even though their school enrollment has increased by 80 per cent in the last decade.[27] The former President of the World Bank has stated that population growth threatens to nullify all of our efforts to raise living standards in many of the poorer countries and that it is optimistic to think that even present living standards can be maintained. Underscoring the seriousness of the problem in his country, the former President of Pakistan has said that if his people continue to increase at the present rate it will ultimately lead to a standard of living little better than that of animals.

The reasons for these statements can readily be seen. Increasing population creates increasing needs. One of the immediate needs is food, both quantity and quality. Even with improved methods of high density agriculture there is a grave question regarding the world's food-producing capacity in the face of continued population growth. It is estimated that the world wheat production must increase by 15 million tons per year just to meet world population growth. Within the next 15 years, for example, India will be trying to feed an

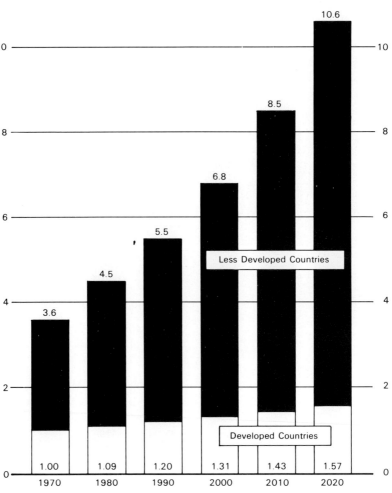

POPULATION EXPLOSION
In The Less Developed Countries

Fig. 10.3. World population: less developed countries' growth projected at the current annual rate of 2.5 per cent, developed countries' at 0.9 per cent. Source: Agency for International Development, FY 1974 presentation to the Congress.

TABLE 10.1

*World population growth*

| If Annual Per Cent Rate of Population Increase Is | No. of Years Required to Double the Population Is |
|---|---|
| 0.5 | 139 |
| 1.0 | 70 |
| 1.5 | 47 |
| 2.0 | 35 |
| 2.5 | 28 |
| 3.0 | 23 |
| 3.5 | 20 |
| 4.0 | 18 |

increase in population about equivalent to the present population of the United States. The nutritional adequacy presents another sobering problem since studies indicate that millions of people in many countries not only receive inadequate calories but that there is an even more serious shortage of specific nutrients such as proteins, minerals, and vitamins. These shortages are particularly evident in children. Such undernutrition and malnutrition not only lower resistance to disease but produce permanent physical and mental retardation. This results in massive losses of human capital and places an even greater burden on developing countries.

In addition to the need for quantity and quality of food, the burgeoning population must be provided with at least minimal shelter. Already, overcrowding and inadequate housing have led to social problems and the spread of disease. Then, too, the spectacular decline in death rates in the less developed countries has primarily affected infant and child mortality with the result that children under 15 years of age now constitute at least 35 per cent of the population of these countries. Such a large percentage of dependent population adds enormously to the burden of education and prevents families from saving any of their meager income, or from buying materials and equipment that would enable them to increase productivity or income. Illiteracy remains high in these countries and in spite of attempts at progress a large percentage of the children are still not enrolled in school. Until this sad situation is improved there is little hope of obtaining the skilled manpower needed to raise the standard of living. Despite United States expenditures of well over 100 billion dollars in foreign aid since World War II, population

growth continues to outrun economic growth and increases the human, economic, and political problems.

Although death rates have declined, almost all of the developing countries have a high incidence of disease. Of the 150 countries in the world, approximately 100 of them are in the less developed category and the need for health services is greater here than in the more advanced countries. Significantly, these are the regions where health and medical facilities are very limited and where health personnel are relatively rare. The physician-population ratio in the United States is 1:630. In Africa it is 1:4,000 and in rural India it is 1:23,000. But the lack of other supporting health personnel is perhaps an even more acute problem. Even with the scarcity of physicians, some developing countries have more doctors than nurses. The other allied medical personnel who figure so prominently in our medical team are just beginning to be developed in many countries.

## Population Increases in the United States

In the United States the situation is somewhat different. There is no acute shortage of food and classic cases of severe malnutrition are quite rare. It is true that agricultural land is decreasing rapidly because of construction of highways, factories, homes, and airports, and that agricultural research in the future will not necessarily increase efficiency of food production, but the capabilities to supply food still exceed the projected demands for local consumption.

The problems associated with education present many formidable obstacles but education through high school is at least theoretically available to all applicants. There are presently around 3 million new first graders each year. High school enrollments have been climbing steadily due to the greater numbers remaining in school. Present enrollment figures in high school are slightly less than 15 million students. College enrollments to 1980 have been projected by the Bureau of the Census and indicate that between 1960 and 1980 such enrollments will treble in size. Since this advanced training requires more elaborate and expensive facilities, the cost of educating such increased numbers is extremely high. Also, with the emphasis on educating large masses at the college level there is the distinct danger of reducing the quality of instruction and lowering the performance standards of students.

The growth of population in the United States has been somewhat erratic. The first census, taken in 1970 showed a count of 3.9 million persons in the original 13 states. Only 5 per cent of these people lived in cities. High birth rates and large immigration numbers contributed to rapid increases and the population doubled about every 25 years until the Civil War. Rates fluctuated and slowed after this period but growth continued. In 1900 the population was 76 million. It reached 93 million in 1910 and by 1962 this number was doubled in 186 million. At precisely 11:00 a.m. on November 20, 1967, the U.S. Census Bureau's population clock, which recorded an additional citizen every 14½ sec. registered 200 million population in the United States. The present population in the United States is somewhat in excess of 210 million persons.

The present rate of growth in the United States is the lowest in the nation's history. The death rate in the United States has remained almost stationary at 9.5 per 1000 for a number of years while the birth rate of 15 during calendar year 1973 produced a net gain of 1.16 million persons for the year. Even at this reduced rate the annual increase in population is sufficient to form additional cities that do not presently exist.

### Growth Problems in Industrialized Societies

The problems associated with population growth in the United States and other industrialized nations differ considerably from the problems in the underdeveloped countries. In the poorer nations most of the increased growth is more evenly distributed throughout the rural, agrarian sections of the country. In the United States such factors as modern transportation, the growth of industry, and the economic forces and mechanical methods affecting agricultural production have combined to accelerate the movement of people from the farms to the cities. This migration from the rural to the urban community will continue, and it is estimated that 90 per cent of the United States population will be living in cities in the not-too-distant future. Although every part of the country has experienced some measure of population growth and urbanization, there is not an equal distribution. Instead of the additional millions of citizens going into

the countryside to form new towns, this increasing population is being absorbed into already crowded cities. People are gregarious and tend to group in large population centers. In the United States this has caused phenomenal growth in some sections of the country, particularly the eastern seaboard, the west coast, the Washington, D.C. complex, and the Great Lakes region. Substantial gains in population are also noted in the desert southwest and in Florida, while the least apparent growth appears to be the plains area of the midwest.

The heavy congregation of people into congested cities has created problems of enormous magnitude. The serious threats of air and water pollution, sewage disposal, and accumulations of solid waste, trash, and rubble are discussed elsewhere in this chapter. The by-products of living result in concentrated filth unless these discarded residues are disposed of by the city. Also, the high population density of many cities makes it necessary to employ numerous firemen and policemen. The low income groups that live in central cities frequently are the most fertile, necessitating expensive school-building programs, and the overcrowding of old housing units leads to costly expenditures for urban renewal. Thus, the central cities face rapidly rising costs and a diminishing tax base since the higher income groups are moving out into the suburban sprawl.

On a more defined basis, the lower socio-economic groups tend to congregate into low rent areas that frequently are the backwash regions of an expanding city. Such regions usually are located in a rather drab buffer zone between the inner city and the more affluent residential areas. Many of the older housing units in these districts have subminimal plumbing and ventilation, are infested with insects and rodents, and have become virtual fire traps. However, units such as these are housing increasing numbers of people. It is not uncommon to find 10 or 12 people packed into living spaces built to accommodate three or four. In these crowded districts in virtually every city there are marked increases in communicable disease, maternal and child mortality, venereal disease, borderline malnutrition, and enteric diseases. The health problems are greatly accentuated but the people are less able to pay for adequate health care, thus increasing the load on existing public health facilities and personnel.

## TABLE 10.2

*Provisional vital statistics for the United States[1]*

| Item | Number | | Rate | | | |
|---|---|---|---|---|---|---|
| | 1974 | 1973 | 1974 | 1973 | 1972 | 1971 |
| Live births | 3,142,000 | 3,237,000 | 15.0 | 15.5 | 17.1 | 18.2 |
| Deaths | 1,969,000 | 1,955,000 | 9.4 | 9.4 | 9.4 | 9.3 |
| Natural increase | 1,173,000 | 1,282,000 | 5.6 | 6.1 | 7.7 | 8.9 |
| Marriages | 2,276,000 | 2,259,000 | 10.8 | 10.8 | 10.7 | 10.6 |
| Divorces | 917,000 | 849,000 | 4.4 | 4.1 | 3.7 | 3.5 |
| Infant deaths | 55,200 | 59,700 | 17.6 | 18.4 | 19.0 | 19.8 |
| Pupulation base (in millions) | | | 210.0 | 208.4 | 206.4 | 204.5 |

[1] Twelve months ending with January. Issued March 27, 1974, the National Center for Health Statistics.

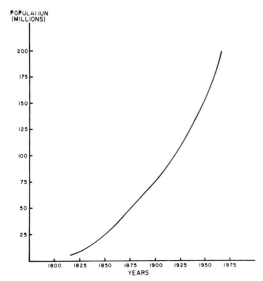

Fig. 10.4. Population growth in the United States since 1815

## Unwanted Children

Significant numbers of the increasing population were neither planned for nor wanted. Using the familiar accident slogan as a reference, one wag has stated that "90 per cent of the people are caused by accidents." Regardless of religious beliefs or social pressures, when unwanted children are brought into the world the results can be tragic for both the child and the parents. Certain groups and categories within our society are more seriously affected than others. One such group is teenagers.

The choices available to pregnant young girls are both limited and dismal. They can either face the censure of society and place their babies for adoption; keep their babies to be raised by grandparents, babysitters, or in a fatherless home; have an abortion; or prematurely enter into marriage. Studies have shown that the younger a girl is at the time of her marriage the greater are the chances that she is pregnant on her wedding day. The younger a woman is at marriage, the greater the chance that her marriage will end in divorce.

Another group which adds to the double tragedy of an expanding population are the married couples, who, for one reason or another, definitely do not want children. These may be young people attempting to complete their education, professional people dedicated to business careers, itinerant couples whose free movements would be hampered by children, the more mature couple who have already raised children, and those self-centered couples who are jealous of the time and trouble demanded by newborn babies. The unfortunate children of such couples soon learn that they are unwanted. Through no fault of their own they frequently are deprived of love, adequate care, supervision, and a harmonious home which form the foundations for emotional stability. Instead, they are faced with a life of rejection, loneliness, and despair. A tragic reminder of this is the "battered child" syndrome which has become increasingly familiar to U. S. physicians.[28]

Perhaps the greatest increases in unplanned population in the country, however, are among the impoverished. In these groups the multiplication of people has posed many problems to a nation which is committed to caring for the health and welfare of its citizens. Large families are still commonplace among the poor. According to government statistics, 57 per cent of all families with five children or more live below the poverty line and they account for almost half of America's deprived youngsters. The children in families of very limited means often do not have adequate food, shelter, or clothing and frequently do not possess the intelligence levels or education for skilled jobs. In an attempt to get away from a poor home environment many of them marry early and start producing children of their own, continuing the vicious cycle of poverty and more population.

Departments of Public Assistance report that second and third generations of children are on welfare roles and that up to 40 per cent of their cases come from sons and daughters of former welfare families. By conservative estimates there are approximately 6.2 million indigent women of child-bearing age in the United States. According to a Planned Parenthood Center's study approximately 50 per cent have been served by family planning services.[29] The others, it may be assumed, are continuing to experience unplanned pregnancies. Of course, not all of the indigent women are married and there is a steadily increasing number of children born out of wedlock. In some agencies approximately 14 per cent of all welfare cases involve unwed mothers and their children. In fact, one interesting local report told of a single woman who listed a different father for each of her 12 children. With the advent of legalized abortions these figures are showing a decline.

## Control Methods

What is to be done to limit the almost uncontrolled expansion of our human population? One scientific group came to the conclusion that "either the birth rate must go down or the death rate must go up." Since our civilized world is dedicated to the principle of conserving life and relieving suffering we certainly cannot consider famines, natural disasters, or thermonuclear warfare as acceptable alternatives. The widespread use of abortions has served to reduce the number of births but this

method is still opposed by certain religious groups and some conservative members of society. The most obvious answer lies in some method of birth control. Since advances in medical technology have made significant contributions toward death control, this must be balanced by adequate birth control.

Efforts to limit the number of births are as old as recorded history but, until recently, few have been notably successful. Telling a married couple to refrain from sexual intercourse is nothing short of ridiculous. The practice of periodic continence, the so-called rhythm method, is little more than a pious hope, particularly among peoples of low culture and literacy. Even if the method were perfected, periods of abstinence are difficult to attain, especially among societies where sexual gratification is one of the few pleasures available to the masses. The Kinsey Report stated that the average person experiences approximately 5500 intercourses throughout his lifetime. Certainly without some method to prevent conception a significant number of pregnancies can be expected to result from such activity.

Several methods are presently available to limit conception. These include voluntary sterilization through such surgical procedures as salpingectomy or vasectomy, the introduction of foams and jellies, and the use of mechanical obstructions such as diaphragms and condoms.[30] Other newer methods emerging from the laboratories are the use of silicone plugs for the fallopian tubes, anti-pregnancy vaccine, and the use of prostaglandins.[31] Another method, a variation of an old technique, is the insertion by a physician of an intrauterine device (IUD). The device is usually a coil or twinlooped plastic material which is inserted through the cervix. The presence of this foreign substance in the uterus is highly effective in preventing conception, although authorities are still not in agreement as to the reason why this is so. As mentioned earlier, the use of the IUD stems from a much older practice. Many generations ago Arab camel drivers were said to have inserted rocks into their female animals to prevent conception while on long caravan trails.

The most effective method of birth control at the present time is the routine administration of an oral contraceptive tablet containing estrogen and progestin, and known universally as "the pill." Since these tablets inhibit ovulation, the fear of pregnancy has been virtually eliminated in those women who take them regularly and on schedule. Although no one person can be credited with the development of oral contraceptives, the two men most commonly associated with the pioneering work are Dr. Gregory Pincus, a physiologist at the Worcester Foundation for Experimental Biology, and gynecologist Dr. John Rock of Harvard University. Working on methods to regulate the cycle of subfertile women, these men decided to use a synthetic progestin. Subsequent work determined the effectiveness of this medication to prevent conception.

The use of oral contraceptive drugs has been approached cautiously by some medical and lay people and there have been a few reports which provide statistically significant evidence linking the drugs with an increased thromboembolic disease. Despite this, however, their use has not been discouraged by the majority of the leaders in the field. Authoritative medical consultants believe that the serious psychological consequences of fear of pregnancy, unwanted pregnancy, potential physical risks of pregnancy, and abortion justify the use of oral contraceptives by many women.[32]

## Programs in Family Planning

Today, birth control is a subject of medical inquiry, scientific research, and social philosophy. This was not always so. Fifty years ago there was a restrictive atmosphere regarding birth control and many states had laws prohibiting the distribution of contraceptive information and devices. A great deal of the credit for changing the laws restricting birth control and much of the enlightened discussion and current literature concerning methods and purposes of contraception are due to the determined efforts of one woman, Margaret Sanger. Through her experiences as a nurse, Mrs. Sanger was deeply moved by the tragedies of unwanted children, induced abortions, and the almost complete lack of knowledge regarding methods to prevent conception. She determined to devote her life to "freeing motherhood throughout the world from the shackles of unwanted pregnancy."[33] After obtaining needed information on the subject in Europe, Mrs. Sanger returned to the United States where she wrote prolifically, appeared in numerous court battles, coined the term "birth control," and emerged as the central figure in this dynamic movement. The first birth control clinic was opened in 1916 by Mrs. Sanger in Brooklyn. It was raided by the police almost immediately and closed as a public nuisance. In 1921, Mrs. Sanger founded the American Birth Control League, which later became the Planned Parenthood Federation of America. In 1960, the Federation merged with the World Population Emergency Campaign to form a single organization, the Planned Parenthood-World Population. This organization now has over 100 affiliates in the United States alone and continues as one of the outstanding leaders in the struggle to make effective family planning available to everyone.

Programs of family planning and birth control have now been instituted in many clinics and hospitals, both public and private. In addition, colleges of medicine, pharmacy, nursing, and schools of other allied medical professions are teaching pertinent information regarding methods, techniques, and philosophies of birth control. The Ford Foundation, Rockefeller University, and other philanthropic organizations are supplying needed help for research activities such as the University of Michigan's Center for Population Planning. Federal, state, and local governments have incorporated family planning programs into essentially all levels of health service. Also, since the Supreme Court established a woman's right to obtain an abortion during her first three months of pregnancy, legalized abortions are being performed on an ever increasing scale. The risk involved with these legal abortions is very small. A study in New York state, involving 400,000 abortions, disclosed the mortality ratio to be 5:100,000.

On the international scene, the United Nations and the Pan American Health Organization have endorsed reduction of the rate of population increases through family planning and are now at work in this field. The Soviet Union, other Iron Curtain countries, and mainland China have launched programs to reduce birth rates. The British, Swedish, and Japanese Governments are also active in foreign assistance for this type of need. The United States Government not only has included family planning in much of its recent legislation here at home but through its Agency for International Development some 39 foreign countries have been given substantial help.

Thus, the world is awakening to the population threat. But, despite these still rather limited beginnings there is a great deal left to be done and there is still a very wide gap between services and needs. At the present time, over 70 million people are added to our world population each year. We are confronted, then, not only with the filling of the health manpower needs to provide wider, more extensive services for the present population but also to supply the basic health needs of these additional millions. In the coming years allied health manpower will be required to an extent never before witnessed. In foreign countries as well as the United States it is possible that much of the future shortage of physicians may be remedied by better ways of using other allied health professionals to serve much larger numbers of people effectively but the need remains acute.

In confronting the problems of over-population the health professionals in the more advanced countries can ill afford a do-nothing attitude. The welfare of the world, our country, and ourselves is involved in the solutions developed for these problems. Current knowledge indicates that the leadership and participation furnished by the allied medical professions will be vital in developing such solutions. Perhaps never before in history have the health professions occupied such a crucial role in determining future history.

## REFERENCES

1. *Accident Facts.* National Safety Council, 1973.
2. *Impairments Due To Injury.* Vital and Health Statistics, 10: 87, DHEW Pub. No. (HRA) 74-1514, 1973.
3. Walker, J A. Rural emergency care: Problems and prospects. *Amer. J. Public Health, 63:* 7, 1973.
4. Dietz, P. E., and Baker, S. P. Drowning, epidemiology, and prevention. *Amer. J. Public Health, 64:* 4, 1974.
5. *Accidental Death Toll in 1973.* Metropolitan Life Insurance Co., Statistical Bulletin, *55:* 1, 1974.
6. *Motorcycle Accident Fatalities.* Metropolitan Life Insurance Co., Statistical Bulletin, Aug., 1973.
7. Hanlon, J. J. Emergency medical care as a comprehensive system. *Health Services Rep., 88:* 7, 1973.
8. The age of effluence. *Time,* May 10, 1968.
9. The treasure in trash. *Environmental News Digest, 39:* 5, 1973.
10. Kupchik, G J. Recycling and reclamation. *Amer. J. Public Health, 62:* 8, 1972.
11. *The Sources of Pollutants.* Air Pollution Primer, American Lung Association, 1971.
12. Lehr, E. L. Carbon monoxide poisoning: A preventable environmental hazard. *Amer. J. Public Health, 60:* 2, 1970.
13. Love, L. B, and Seskin, E. P. Air pollution, climate, and home heating: Their effects on U. S. mortality rates. *Amer. J. Public Health, 62:* 7, 1972.
14. Statement warns excess deaths to result from conversion to coal. *The Nation's Health,* Jan., 1974.
15. Jacobs, C. F., and Langdoc, B. A. Cardiovascular deaths and air pollution in Charleston, S. C. *Health Service Rep., 87:* 7, 1972.
16. Dubos, R. Health and Environment. *Amer. Lung Assn. Bull.,* Sept., 1973.
17. Hardy, G E. *et al.* FIrst use of the Federal Clean Air Act's emergency authority. *Amer. J. Public Health, 64:* 1, 1974.
18. *Clean Water, It's Up to You.* Izaak Walton League of America, 1970.
19. *A Primer on Waste Water Treatment.* Federal Water Pollution Control Administration, 1969.
20. Dominick, D D. Crusade for clean water. *Forensic Quart., 44:* 3, 1970.
21. Massachusetts Dept. of Health. Boating and Health. *N. Engl. J. Med., 289:* 19, 1973.
22. Brown, R M *et al.* A water quality index—Do we dare? *Water and Sewage Works,* Oct., 1970.
23. Hunter, J. S. Shortcomings and remedies for the water quality improvement programs of the U. S. *Amer. J. Public Health, 63:* 4, 1973.
24. Rock, J. Population growth (editorial). *J.A.M.A., 177:* 58-60, 1961.
25. Merrill, M. H. An expanding populace in a contracting world. *J.A.M.A., 197:* 8, 1966.
26. *Current International Birth Rates.* Metropolitan Life Insurance Co., Statistical Bulletin, June, 1972.
27. *Population Planning and Health.* Agency for International Development, FY 1974, Presentation to the Congress, 1973.
28. *The Ecology of Birth Control.* Chicago: G. D Searle & Co, 1971.
29. Family Planning Programs Reaching 50 Percent of Neediest, *Emko Newsletter,* Aug., 1973.
30. Huff, J. E., and Hernandez, L. O-T-C Contraceptives. *J. Amer. Pharm. Assn., 14:* 3, 1974.
31. *Protaglandins.* George Washington University Medical Center, Population Report, G:2, 1973.
32. Oral contraceptives and thromboembolism. *Med. Letter, 14:* 17, 1972.
33. Sanger, M *My Fight For Birth Control.* New York: Farrar and Rinehart, 1931.

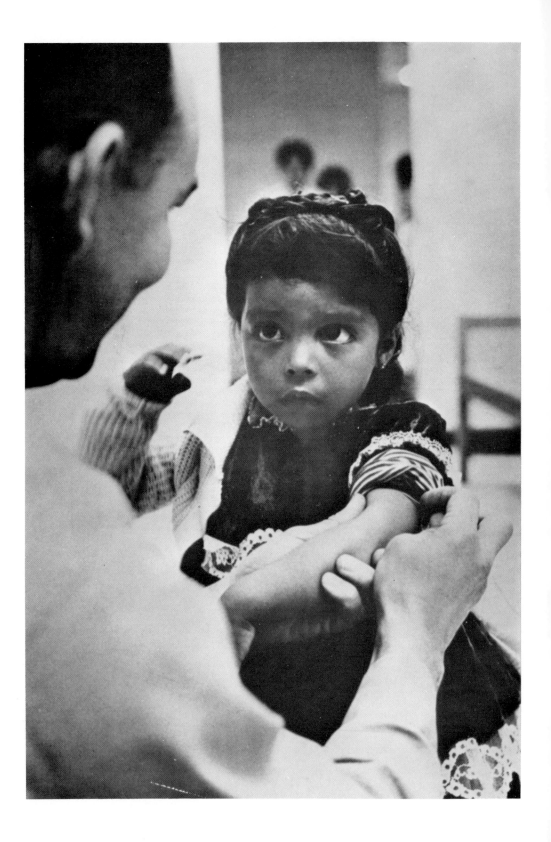

bradycardia, decreased metabolic rate, and the development of edema and anemia.

The major source of calories in diets throughout the world is furnished by carbohydrates. These may be found in foods such as cereal grains, potatoes, beans, peas and fresh fruit. Most of these foods are produced in large quantities, are relatively cheap, and can be stored quite easily. Other carbohydrates are ingested in refined form and are lacking in minerals and vitamins which are lost during processing. Representative of such foods are white flour, polished rice, refined sugar, and syrups.

The most potent source of calories is found in fats, primarily in the form of triglycerides. When taken in excess of dietary needs much of this material can be converted to storage fat to be mobilized and metabolized when additional energy is required. Weight-conscious individuals and those on crash diets avoid fats as much as possible but fats serve useful purposes. In addition to making food more palatable and supplying essential unsaturated fatty acids, they are also carriers of the fat-soluble vitamins A, D, E, and K. Those people who avoid fats or who use mineral oil in excess are subject to significant deficiencies of these vitamins. Further, it has been reported that dietary fat offers some protection against tuberculosis and other diseases.

Proteins, although available for production of energy, are particularly important to the body as sources for building, replacing, and maintaining tissues. They also help to regulate the acid-base balance of the body, help to form body hormones and enzymes, and help to build resistance to disease. Through proteolytic enzymes, proteins are reduced to the basic amino acids which, in turn, are used as building blocks in the body. Twenty-two different α-amino acids have been identified in dietary food and all are utilized in the body. A greater number and assortment are found in meat proteins whereas plant proteins are lacking both in variety and quantity. Some of the amino acids can be synthesized within the body from other nitrogenous compounds but certain important ones cannot be so synthesized and must be provided in the diet for proper nutrition. These are referred to as essential amino acids and include the following: leucine, isoleucine, lysine, methionine, phenylalanine, threonine, tryptophan, and valine.

A complete protein food contains all of the essential amino acids plus a good representation of the non-essential ones, while incomplete proteins are lacking in one or more of the essential amino acids. The absence from the diet of one or more of the essential amino acids can result in serious dysfunction of the body. Representative of this group are: hyperprolinemia, characterized by fever, vomiting, diarrhea, drowsiness, frequent convulsions, and hearing loss; cystathioninuria, a condition found in certain mental defective patients; histidinemia, associated with mental and speech retardation; alkaptonuria, recognized and diagnosed by the darkening of urine, the deposition of ochre-yellow pigments in various parts of the body cartilages, and the development of arthritis. Another related disease in which there is an abnormality in metabolism of some of the branched chain amino acids is known as maple syrup urine disease. This disease occurs in infants and is early recognized by the maple sugar odor of the urine. Symptoms include irregular respiration, reflexes absent or abnormal, intermittent stiffening of muscles, head retractions, and, if not treated, rapid deterioration resulting in death.

Body requirements for protein are greatest, naturally, in periods of rapid growth. Thus, a child may require as much as 3 or 4 gm. of protein per kg. of body weight in the daily diet. This should be in the form of complete proteins instead of the incomplete forms found in substandard diets. As we are becoming more and more concerned with health problems throughout the world we recognize that nutritional deficiency diseases are both serious and widespread. Such a disease is kwashiorkor, a term thought by some to mean "red boy," and by others, "displaced child." This disease occurs primarily in infants and young children on diets grossly deficient in protein and water-soluble vitamins and was first noted on a large scale among African natives. The patient has edema, a pot belly, depigmented skin, enlarged liver, loss or change in hair color, and reversed albumin-globulin ratio of the plasma, and passes bulky stools containing undigested food. The disease is endemic and has a high rate of mortality among children in Africa, India, and Central and South America. Generally, without reference to a specific disease, extreme cases of protein deficiency may result in poor muscle tone and posture, lowered resistance to

### Table 11.1

Food and Nutrition Board, National Academy of Sciences–National Research Council recommended daily dietary allowances, revised 1973

Designed for the maintenance of good nutrition of practically all healthy people in the U.S.A.

| | From Up to years | Weight kg. | Weight lb. | Height cm. | Height in. | Energy kcal. | Protein gn. | Vitamin A Activity r.e. | Vitamin A Activity i.u. | Vitamin D i.u. | Vitamin E Activity i.u. | Ascorbic Acid mg. | Folacin μg. | Niacin mg. | Riboflavin mg. | Thiamin mg. | Vitamin B$_6$ mg. | Vitamin B$_{12}$ μg. | Calcium mg. | Phosphorus mg. | Iodine μg. | Iron mg. | Magnesium mg. | Zinc mg. |
|---|---|---|---|---|---|---|---|---|---|---|---|---|---|---|---|---|---|---|---|---|---|---|---|---|
| Infants | 0.0–0.5 | 6 | 14 | 60 | 24 | kg. × 117 | kg. × 2.2 | 420[4] | 1400 | 400 | 4 | 35 | 50 | 5 | 0.4 | 0.3 | 0.3 | 0.3 | 360 | 240 | 35 | 10 | 60 | 3 |
| | 0.5–1.0 | 9 | 20 | 71 | 28 | kg. × 108 | kg. × 2.0 | 400 | 2000 | 400 | 5 | 35 | 50 | 8 | 0.6 | 0.5 | 0.4 | 0.3 | 540 | 400 | 45 | 15 | 70 | 5 |
| Children | 1–3 | 13 | 28 | 86 | 34 | 1300 | 23 | 400 | 2000 | 400 | 7 | 40 | 100 | 9 | 0.8 | 0.7 | 0.6 | 1.0 | 800 | 800 | 60 | 15 | 150 | 10 |
| | 4–6 | 20 | 44 | 110 | 44 | 1800 | 30 | 500 | 2500 | 400 | 9 | 40 | 200 | 12 | 1.1 | 0.9 | 0.9 | 1.5 | 800 | 800 | 80 | 10 | 200 | 10 |
| | 7–10 | 30 | 66 | 135 | 54 | 2400 | 36 | 700 | 3300 | 400 | 10 | 40 | 300 | 16 | 1.2 | 1.2 | 1.2 | 2.0 | 800 | 800 | 110 | 10 | 250 | 10 |
| Males | 11–14 | 44 | 97 | 158 | 63 | 2800 | 44 | 1000 | 5000 | 400 | 12 | 45 | 400 | 18 | 1.5 | 1.4 | 1.6 | 3.0 | 1200 | 1200 | 130 | 18 | 350 | 15 |
| | 15–18 | 61 | 134 | 172 | 69 | 3000 | 54 | 1000 | 5000 | 400 | 15 | 45 | 400 | 20 | 1.8 | 1.5 | 1.8 | 3.0 | 1200 | 1200 | 150 | 18 | 400 | 15 |
| | 19–22 | 67 | 147 | 172 | 69 | 3000 | 52 | 1000 | 5000 | 400 | 15 | 45 | 400 | 20 | 1.8 | 1.5 | 2.0 | 3.0 | 800 | 800 | 140 | 10 | 350 | 15 |
| | 23–50 | 70 | 154 | 172 | 69 | 2700 | 56 | 1000 | 5000 | | 15 | 45 | 400 | 18 | 1.6 | 1.4 | 2.0 | 3.0 | 800 | 800 | 130 | 10 | 350 | 15 |
| | 51+ | 70 | 154 | 172 | 69 | 2400 | 56 | 1000 | 5000 | | 15 | 45 | 400 | 16 | 1.5 | 1.2 | 2.0 | 3.0 | 800 | 800 | 110 | 10 | 350 | 15 |
| Females | 11–14 | 44 | 97 | 155 | 62 | 2400 | 44 | 800 | 4000 | 400 | 10 | 45 | 400 | 16 | 1.3 | 1.2 | 1.6 | 3.0 | 1200 | 1200 | 115 | 18 | 300 | 15 |
| | 15–18 | 54 | 119 | 162 | 65 | 2100 | 48 | 800 | 4000 | 400 | 11 | 45 | 400 | 14 | 1.4 | 1.1 | 2.0 | 3.0 | 1200 | 1200 | 115 | 18 | 300 | 15 |
| | 19–22 | 58 | 128 | 162 | 65 | 2100 | 46 | 800 | 4000 | 400 | 14 | 45 | 400 | 14 | 1.4 | 1.1 | 2.0 | 3.0 | 800 | 800 | 100 | 18 | 300 | 15 |
| | 23–50 | 58 | 128 | 162 | 65 | 2000 | 46 | 800 | 4000 | | 12 | 45 | 400 | 13 | 1.2 | 1.0 | 2.0 | 3.0 | 800 | 800 | 100 | 18 | 300 | 15 |
| | 51+ | 58 | 128 | 162 | 65 | 1800 | 46 | 800 | 4000 | | 12 | 45 | 400 | 12 | 1.1 | 1.0 | 2.0 | 3.0 | 800 | 800 | 80 | 10 | 300 | 15 |
| Pregnant | | | | | | +300 | +30 | 1000 | 5000 | 400 | 15 | 60 | 800 | +2 | +0.3 | +0.3 | 2.5 | 4.0 | 1200 | 1200 | 125 | 18+ | 450 | 20 |
| Lactating | | | | | | +500 | +20 | 1200 | 6000 | 400 | 15 | 60 | 600 | +4 | +0.5 | +0.3 | 2.5 | 4.0 | 1200 | 1200 | 150 | 18 | 450 | 25 |

466

disease, premature aging, anemia, stunted growth in children, tissue degeneration, and slow recovery from illness or surgery.

Early in the present century it was demonstrated that normal foods contain minute traces of substances which are essential to health. These were first termed "accessory factors." Because of the vital nature of these compounds and because they were first thought to be amines, it was proposed that the group name be changed to vital amines or vitamines. Classification by solubility was then suggested. Thus, the fat-soluble antixerophthalmic factor which cured nutritional eye disease was differentiated from the water-soluble compound which prevented beriberi in pigeons. It was later found, however, that fat-soluble antixeropthalmic factor did not contain an amine group and exacting scientists hesitated to label a compound with a misnomer. A compromise terminology was then proposed, dropping the final e in vitamine and assigning the word "vitamin" as representative of the entire group. The antixerophthalmic factor was called Vitamin A, the compound used to prevent beriberi was called Vitamin B, and the antiscorbutic principle was called Vitamin C. As additional vitamins were identified they were assigned succeeding letters of the alphabet. Exceptions to this rule are Vitamin K, representative of the Danish word koagulation, and Vitamin H which is the older designation for biotin and refers to the German word for skin (haut).

Confusion regarding nomenclature was further compounded when it was recognized that the crude preparations which relieved beriberi also contained many factors which were essential nutrients. Thus, the compounds which were isolated from yeast, liver, and other sources of water-soluble B were given subscripts of either numbers or letters. It is not uncommon for nutrition articles in scientific journals to refer to Vitamin $B_{15}$ or Vitamin B$x$. The recent trend, fortunately, has been promotion of chemically related names: thiamine for Vitamin $B_1$, riboflavin for Vitamin $B_2$, and ascorbic acid for Vitamin C. Vitamin nomenclature is not settled yet and there are strong indications that it will undergo additional modifications before we finally arrive at a consistent and rational system.

Although numerous compounds have been studied and the designations of Vitamins W, X, and Y have already been assigned, the vitamins which ave been found to be essential in human nutrition are relatively few in number. The fat-soluble group includes Vitamins A, D, E, and K. The water-soluble vitamins are thiamine, riboflavin, pyridoxine, Vitamin $B_{12}$, ascorbic acid, niacin, pantothenic acid, folacin, and biotin. A brief description of the functions of selected vitamins and their attendant deficiency diseases underscores the importance of these essential nutrients.

Vitamin A is required to maintain normal body growth and to ensure the health and integrity of certain specialized epithelial tissues. It helps in the adaptation of vision to dim light, aids in keeping skin smooth and soft, and helps to maintain healthy mucous membranes.[8] Severe deficiency of this vitamin may result in night blindness, dry eyelids and reddened eyes, increased susceptibility to infection, and defective tooth formation. As mentioned earlier, the use of mineral oil as a substitute in salad dressings is to be discouraged since one ounce of mineral oil will dissolve 140,000 international units of Vitamin A. It also interferes with the absorption of Vitamin D, calcium, phosphorus, and Vitamin K.

Vitamin D is actually a group of vitamins. There are seven known compounds in this group, most of them formed by irradiation of ergosterol or of 7-dehydrocholesterol. Vitamin $D_3$ occurs solely in the higher animals and is formed through a photochemical process.[9] New metabolites of Vitamin $D_3$ have been discovered which are many times more potent than the parent compound.[10] Vitamin D, in moderate amounts, promotes retention of calcium and phosphorus and maintains concentrations of these elements in the blood that help in the formation of bone tissue. It is also thought to aid in converting organic phosphorus when needed. Excessive doses of Vitamin D may be toxic and even fatal as a result of the mobilization of calcium and phosphorus from bony tissues and redeposition in tissues such as blood vessel walls, kidney tubules, bronchi, and the heart. The deficiency disease associated with avitaminosis D is rickets. The first signs of this disease are deformities of the skeleton such as severely bowed legs, followed by the development of soft spots in the skull, deformities of the ribs, bending of the pelvis, and delayed tooth formation. If treatment is delayed the deformities may persist through life.

Vitamin E has suffered from early enthusiasm

that attributed rather remarkable benefits to be derived from the use of this compound. The precise biochemical function of Vitamin E, or α-tocopherol, in man has not been conclusively established. This vitamin has been recognized as an essential nutrient and there is general agreement that the body needs for Vitamin E are related to the amount of polyunsaturated fatty acids in the diet and in tissue. The vitamin appears to participate as a biological antioxidant that limits lipid peroxidation reactions and protects cells from membrane damage.[11]

The group of nutrients known as the B vitamins, or B complex, often are found together in foodstuffs. For convenience, they may be divided into two groups—those involved in the release of energy from foods and those active in the formation of red blood cells. The energy-releasing vitamins are thiamine, nicotinamide, riboflavin, pantothenic acid, and biotin, whereas folic acid and $B_{12}$ belong to the hematopoietic group.

Thiamine not only helps convert carbohydrate to energy but, also, aids in digestion and assimilation of food and helps in the proper functioning of the heart, nerves, and muscles. Gross deficiency of this vitamin may result in poor appetite, retarded growth, nervousness and irritability, poor digestion, and abnormal fatigue. The nutritional disease associated with lack of thiamine is beriberi. This disease affects the heart, central nervous system, and gastrointestinal tract. The symptoms that characterize this disease may include weakness, emotional disturbances, tachycardia, irregular pulse, shortness of breath, cardiac enlargement, anorexia, nausea, vomiting, and constipation.

Riboflavin helps to maintain good vision and clear eyes, builds healthy skin and mouth tissues, and promotes well-being and vitality. Extreme deficiencies of this vitamin involve the eyes, lips, and skin. The eyes are reddened and oversensitive to light, there is vascularization of the cornea, and cataract-like symptoms develop. Cracks and maceration occur at the angles of the mouth, the tongue may be inflamed and painful, and premature aging of the skin occurs.

Nicotinamide is an essential part of the enzyme system concerned with hydrogen transport in the living cell. As such, it functions to build and maintain healthy skin and tongue, aid digestion, and reinforce the nervous system. Deficiencies of this vitamin result in rough and inflamed skin, mental depression and nervousness, and digestive disorders. The disease associated with niacin deficiency is pellagra, a name derived from *pelle* (skin) and *agra* (rough). Early symptoms include glossitis, stomatitis, insomnia, anorexia, abdominal pain, numbness, forgetfulness, morbid fears, vertigo, and changes of bowel functions. Lesions first appear on the mucous membranes of the tongue, mouth, and vagina. Dermal lesions then appear first on the normally exposed portions of the body such as the face, arms, and feet, and then in such protected areas as the elbows, knees, the perineum, and under the breasts of women. Factors which either precipitate or intensify the lesions are sunlight, heat, and friction. The lesions, in early stages, closely resemble segments of sunburn and then develop into raised patches of intense erythema with itching, pain, and blister formation which more closely parallel the lesions in erysipelas. Tremor, rigidity, paralysis, and insanity frequently occur in untreated cases. In the advanced stage pellagra is recognized by the classic three d's—dermatitis, diarrhea, and dementia.

Ascorbic acid is utilized in collagen formation, is involved with the metabolism of certain aromatic amino acids, and is reported to function as a hydrogen carrier. As such, this vitamin helps to maintain firm gums, helps to build and maintain bones, tissues and blood, aids in the proper utilization of iron, builds resistance to infection, and helps in the healing of wounds and fractures. Gross deficiency of ascorbic acid may result in possible bleeding in any part of the body, weakened bones which may become deformed, a tendency to bruise easily, and swollen, painful joints. Scurvy is the deficiency disease and is characterized by various hemorrhagic manifestations, delayed healing of injured soft tissues and fractured bones, edema, gingivitis, loosening of the teeth, secondary anemia, general weakness, and emaciation. Most of the deficiency symptoms are probably due to adverse effects on collagen formation, but the anemia reflects the value of ascorbic acid in enhancing the absorption of iron in food and, thus, is indirectly effective in preventing iron deficiency anemia.

It must be emphasized that although the above vitamins and their deficiency disease were discussed separately it is quite rare to find only one vitamin which is lacking. More commonly, when an individual suffers from decreased vitamin intake enough to exhibit clinical symptoms there is strong probability that he is deficient in other vitamins as well. Studies with vitamin-dependent genetic disease have shed considerable light on the biochemical role normally played by vitamins. Most of these compounds serve as coenzymes to facilitate a variety of metabolic processes.[12] It follows that a reduction or lack of these coenzymes will markedly alter body metabolism. Vitamin deficiency diseases often accompany poverty, chronic alcoholism, dietary peculiarities, fever, hyperthyroidism, pregnancy, and stress of injury or surgical procedures.

Mineral requirements of the body range from the so-called trace elements to those of greater concentration and wider utilization. Included in the trace elements are cobalt, copper, iron, iodine, fluorine, manganese, selenium, and zinc. The minerals used in greater quantity are calcium, chlorine, sulfur, potassium, phosphorus, sodium, and magnesium. All of these minerals are important in regulation of body functions, maintaining an optimal acid-base balance and electrolyte levels, and controlling or catalyzing essential metabolic processes. A diet that is low in essential metals may make a person more vulnerable to heart attack. Conversely, manipulation of certain metals in an individual's diet may offer a way to control dangerous levels of blood lipids.[13]

Calcium, for example, helps to develop and maintain bones and teeth, helps in the proper clotting of blood, promotes normal action of muscles, and aids in proper functioning of nerves. Deficiency of this mineral may result in poorly formed bones and teeth, precipitation of tetany, and onset of rickets. Iron helps to form hemoglobin and transports oxygen to body tissues. Inadequate quantities of this element may cause hypochromic microcytic anemia, characterized by listlessness and weakness, gastric disturbances, pale and dry skin, shortness of breath and dizziness. The role of zinc in the processes of growth, synthesis of nucleic acids and proteins, body maturation, and improvement of sensory impairments is now being reported and promises to be a source of further interesting study.[14] Simple goiter, or hypertrophy of the thyroid gland, occurs as a result of inadequate amounts of iodine in the diet. This condition is now quite rare in the United States since the practice was adopted of adding iodine to table salt. Currently 100 mg.

of potassium iodide are in 1 kg. of purified salt, giving a concentration of 1 part in 10 thousand.

In addition to the primary causes of undernutrition and the development of nutritional deficiency diseases, there are problems of secondary undernutrition which are not due to a poor diet. These problems arise from the individual himself and may be due to a number of factors. One such factor may be reflex or functional disorders of the stomach caused by nervous tension, hyperchlorhydria, achlorhydria, rapid eating, or poor mastication. The indigestion complaints accompanying this disorder are well known and include nausea, abdominal pain, regurgitation, heartburn, distention, and flatulence. Microbial contamination of the intestines with its accompanying diarrhea is an additional cause.[15] Other factors include such organic diseases as peptic ulcer, gastroenteritis, hiatus hernia, stomach cancer, and diseases producing visceral pain. Such gastrointestinal diseases are not only numerous but may be quite serious. Data from the National Health survey indicated that 17 million people suffer from the 10 leading chronic digestive conditions.[16] An excess of 120,000 deaths from gastrointestinal diseases has been reported in the United States in a single year. Absorption of food from the gastrointestinal tract may be limited by diseases of the liver or pancreas, by biliary obstruction, or by hypermotility of the intestine. Sometimes the nutrients which are absorbed cannot be utilized because of improper functioning of diseased organs such as cirrhosis of the liver and diabetes. Certain pathological conditions in the body such as hyperthyroidism, cardiac decompensation, convulsions, and increased temperature heighten the need for essential nutrients. For example, for each centigrade degree of increase in body temperature the basal metabolic rate is increased 13 per cent. Regardless of the cause, when the body requires nutrients of which it is deprived the result may be clinical manifestations of malnutrition. The wealthy industrialist suffering from a series of digestive complaints may exhibit the same symptoms of malnutrition as the lower class natives in India, Africa, or South America.

In the United States, and most of the other technically advanced nations of the world, malnutrition is also a problem but of a different nature. A significant portion of the people in these nations suffer either from the effects of overindulgence or from the results of deliberately choosing an improper diet. The consequences of these nutritional patterns are not without serious complications and invite potential danger.

## Obesity

The consumption of excessive quantities of food results in the development of obesity, in which body weight is grossly abnormal due to an overabundance of adipose tissue. Associated with obesity are significant compromises of health and increased risks to life. For example, obesity has a causal relationship with an increased incidence of diabetes mellitus, gallbladder disease, degenerative arthritis, hernia, postoperative thromboembolism, and diseases of the cardiovascular-renal system including advanced atherosclerosis. It has been estimated that between the ages of 45 and 55 an excess weight of 25 pounds increases the chances of death within the next year by 25 per cent and a 50-pound excess increases the chance to 50 per cent. Obesity, therefore, must be considered as important a problem of malnutrition as is undernutrition or deficiency disease.

The estimated number of persons in the United States that are sufficiently overweight to be classified as clinically obese is approximately 20 million.[17] Most of these people are past middle age but the number of adolescents who are overweight is larger than is generally realized. The results of a study in Boston led the investigators to conclude that 12.0 per cent of the girls and 9 per cent of all boys between the ages of 12 and 19 are obese. Since there are approximately 29 million young people in this age group in the United States, the total number of obese adolescents is significant. Concern for overweight in children appears to be well founded. Two 20-year retrospective studies have shown that overweight children tend to remain overweight as adults. In one of the studies involving 100 subjects, 87 were still obese 20 years later. The remaining 13 had to watch their diets continually.

The causes of obesity are manifold; some are not completely understood. Certainly, psychic factors are of great importance in the development of obesity. The pleasure of eating greatly influences the desire for food and may be used to replace other satisfactions of living. An occasional adolescent will engorge himself with food as a substitution for fulfillment of his more basic and social needs. Adults may utilize the pleasures of food to take the place of emotional outlets which are otherwise denied through unhappy marriages, personal losses, or maladjustments. As research into the causes of obesity continues to develop, it becomes increasingly clear that continued consumption of food in excess of bodily need is motivated by personal insecurity and emotional instability.

It is a mistake, however, to assume that all cases of obesity arise from emotional or psychic problems. Many women are overweight simply because of their position in the home and their ready access to the refrigerator. The lower income groups may have a higher rate of obesity because they must eat low-cost carbohydrate food instead of the more expensive proteins. Then, too, the fact that obese children tend to remain fat in adult life has led researchers to investigate the biochemical differences between normal and obese persons. In years past, the claims of fat people that they were the naturally heavy type or were the victims of glandular trouble were met with derision and denial.

A symposium on the endocrine aspects of obesity, however, has focused attention on newer work in the field of nutritional biochemistry.[18] Investigations have been conducted relating insulin to obesity, the utilization of carbohydrates and the efficiency of energy metabolism in the obese, glucocorticoid-induced obesity, and the cause-effect of obesity and diabetes. Throughout the symposium was the underlying current that there are indeed significant biochemical differences in the obese. Some of these may have been acquired whereas others probably were inherited. If these aberrations can be identified, positively, and substantiated, perhaps additional hope can be offered to those who are hopelessly obese.

For the majority of obese people who have an intense desire to lose weight there are available various types of dietary aids. These range from proprietary soaps, salts, and salves to dietary candy, which seems to be a contradiction of aims. Most of these products do not live up to their advertising claims and usually are not worth the money spent on them. Low-calorie liquid diets are a popular form of weight reduction but it is recommended, usually, to replace only one meal a day with such substitutes. One of the problems with liquid diets is the low residual bulk. If used to excess, constipation may result unless high-residue foods are also ingested. This can be a particular problem with older people. Other over-the-counter agents which may be used in attempts to lose weight include hydrophylic bulk producers such as methylcellulose, wafers or gum containing benzocaine, the low-calorie foods, and artificial sweeteners. For the dangerously obese, a complete program of weight reduction under the direction of a physician is recommended.

Although the practice is generally discouraged among medical groups and associations, there are still some physicians that prescribe various central nervous system stimulants to suppress the appetite. The anorexigenic effect of these drugs is well known but their widespread misuse, even abuse, has created major problems and has caused much adverse criticism and discouragement. Unfortunately, these drugs are used, often erroneously, as the major or even sole treatment for obesity, a procedure which dooms such treatment to immediate or eventual failure. Appetite suppression by means of drugs is only a minor but integral part of a total individualized therapy for obesity. These drugs are of practical value only to eliminate or reduce the discomfort which initially accompanies a sharp reduction in calorie intake and are most effective during the period when education, indoctrination, and mental adjustment are taking place. To extend their use beyond this stage is an unwise procedure since they not only lose their effectiveness as anorexigenic agents but the patient may establish a psychological dependence on such drugs.

## Nutritional Practices in the United States

The dietary habits and food practices of the people in the United States have caused uncommon concern in recent years because of the occurrence of borderline malnutrition in this land where food abounds. Department of Agriculture figures tell us that the average American consumes approximately 145 gm. of fat and 110 gm. of sugar per day. In one year's time this same American consumes an average of 174 pounds of beef, veal, pork, and lamb which amounts to a total of more than 36.5 billion pounds of meat for the country as a whole. All of this seems to tell us that food is in

abundance and that problems of malnutrition are more imagined than real. Indeed, officials of the U. S. Food and Drug Administration have publicly stated that most Americans eat foods which provide all the vitamins and minerals normally required for good health.

Contrasted to this position, however, is the report of the U. S. Department of Agriculture (USDA) in which a total of 15,000 households throughout the United States were surveyed to ascertain food practices. The findings of the survey show that only 50 per cent of American families eat a nutritionally good combination of food and that 20 per cent eat poor diets when rated by the USDA's standard. The remaining 30 per cent ranged somewhere between good and poor. When compared to a similar survey conducted 10 years prior, it was found that the number of families on good diets had decreased by 10 per cent and the number on poor diets had increased by 5 per cent. It is interesting that families from both the upper and lower income groups were represented in the nutritionally poor category. The reason for this downward trend has been attributed to decreased use of fruits, vegetables, milk, and milk products plus an increased use of ready-made baked goods and soft drinks. The nutrients which were consistently short in the diets were calcium, thiamine, riboflavin, Vitamin A, and ascorbic acid.

Some of the reasons for such poor nutrition in a land of plenty relate to improper eating habits. Although breakfast is recognized as the most important meal of the day there are pattern changes which contradict this recognition. The results of a nationwide, technically organized, market research disclosed that three-fourths of all American families do not eat breakfast together, that breakfast is largely a do-it-yourself project, and less than 20 per cent of all family members eat a breakfast that the housewife considers nutritionally complete. A study of 3500 high school students in Massachusetts disclosed that 11 per cent of the boys and 19 per cent of the girls had no breakfast while an additional 40 per cent of the boys and 50 per cent of the girls ate a nutritionally poor breakfast.

Of the various age groups, it is found that teen-agers generally have the poorest food habits. This cannot be attributed to their lack of knowledge concerning nutrition. In a four-year study of 1000 high school students in

Berkeley, California, there was disclosed a refreshing knowledge of proper foods and eating habits. There seemed to be little relationship, however, between the students' views on eating and their actual practices. In another study in North Carolina, 13 per cent of the students in the ninth grade missed a meal. This increased to 18 per cent in the 10th grade and to 25 per cent in the 12th grade. Snacks made up some of the deficit. A survey in Iowa revealed that about one-fourth of a teenager's calories comes from snacks. When these are made up of fat, sugar, and starch the diet will be nutritionally incomplete. Still another problem involves the youthful food revisionists who are proponents of organically grown, or health foods. Many of these people reject the findings of both the United States Department of Agriculture and the Food and Drug Administration that some of these foods are either adulterated or toxic. Instead, they consult with health food store proprietors for both medical and dietary advice. In at least some cases it has been observed that when the retailer assumes the role of the physician, professional medical care is often delayed.[19]

Other reasons for borderline malnutrition are attributed to custom, fad, ignorance, stress, shortage of time, overindulgence of favorite foods at the expense of balanced diets, the conviction that certain foods do not agree, and preoccupation with pleasing the palate instead of ensuring an adequate and balanced meal. Thus, the harried college student, the two-martinis-for-lunch businessman, and the fashion-conscious matron are all subject to the dangers resulting from malnutrition. Education and motivation can change some of these patterns of behavior but experience tells us that the prognosis is not too favorable.

Nutritionists tell us that an optimal diet consists of the basic seven foods. Daily servings of these foods include: (1) one ration or more of leafy, green, and yellow vegetables; (2) one serving or more of foods having a high Vitamin C content such as citrus fruit, tomatoes, and raw cabbage; (3) two servings or more of potatoes or other starchy foods; (4) milk—one pint for adults and one quart for children and pregnant women; (5) one serving of meat, nuts, dried beans or peas, and at least four eggs per week; (6) one ration of whole grain or enriched bread and cereals; (7) butter or fortified oleomargarine. For those who fall short of this balanced diet it would seem that supplemental vitamins are indicated.

Notions about food and digestive processes are frequently based upon both fact and fallacy and can sometimes be the source of distorted nutritional practices. The vegetarian, for example, is in danger of depriving himself of essential amino acids which are found in meat proteins. Comparisons are made by these people to the apparent good health of grazing animals but it must be remembered that herbivores can synthesize vital food factors which man cannot. Another distorted notion is the belief that the extent of hunger is an index of the quantity of food to be eaten. Actually, hunger and appetite, although related, are two separate entities. Hunger is the combined result of reduced blood sugar and rather vigorous muscular contractions passing over the wall of the stomach, and it acts as a stimulus to seek food. Appetite, on the other hand, is usually a pleasant sensation based on previous experiences with the taste, smell, texture, and appearance of food. It promotes the desire to eat but is not an accurate indication of either the amount or nutritional value of the food to be ingested.

Through the medium of television, radio, and the printed page, advertisers try to persuade the public to buy their products to treat bodily ills, whether real or imagined. One such example is advertisers of alkalizers who try to create an acid condition of the body, a condition which is far less common than we are led to believe. Their success is reflected in the report that antacids account for annual sales of over 82.5 million dollars. This includes 43 million dollars spent on 300 different kinds of tablets, gums, lozenges, and wafers, about 33 million dollars for the 175 various liquids, and 6.5 million dollars for the 100 varieties of powders.[20] Some of the most tragic victims of this advertising are those who suffer from peptic ulcer disease.[21]

One of the most exploited of all notions is that dealing with regularity or one-a-day habit. Advertisers of laxative products find a fertile field for their promotional claims because, historically, excrement has been associated with filth and evil and the elimination of these waste materials from the body has been identified with expiation of guilt. There are now more than 700 proprietary laxatives on the market in almost every dosage form and their annual sales amount to an excess of 200 million dollars. It generally is not known that bowel movements may vary from two or three per day to one every four or five days and still remain within the normal limits of health. A person may become constipated because of faulty eating habits; faulty stool habits, mental and nervous strain, or prolonged use of certain drugs. Some people ingest an excess of low-residue foods such as meat, eggs, cheese, or liquid diets and there is not enough bulk remaining for properly formed stools. Many cases of constipation can be relieved by the intake of adequate quantities of fluid and the increased consumption of fresh vegetables, fruits, and grains. Laxatives and cathartics frequently do more harm than good. They propel the intestinal contents too rapidly along their course and the individual loses the full nutritional value of his food. Their use over prolonged periods of time is to be discouraged.

It is abundantly clear that if the nutritional level of the general public is to be brought up to USDA standards there will have to be considerable change in established eating patterns. One method of bringing about this change is through nutrition education. Those in the allied health professions recognize the value of good nutrition and are in a position to offer sound advice regarding the practice of good health habits. Valuable assistance in this endeavor is offered not only through government agencies such as the Department of Agriculture, Food and Drug Administration, and the Public Health Service, but through professional associations as well. Organizations furnishing information and assistance in nutrition education include the American Heart Association, the American Home Economics Association, the American Dietetics Association, and the American Medical Association.

The companies which produce the nation's food have also assumed an outstanding and laudable responsibility for nutrition education. One notable example was the establishment of the Nutrition Foundation by a group of food industry leaders. This foundation has taken the lead in support of research and education in the science of nutrition. Trade groups within the food industry spend millions of dollars annually in obtaining and disseminating nutrition information about a particular type of food product without regard to brand name. Associations such as the National Dairy Council, the National Live Stock and Meat Board, Wheat Flour Institute, Evaporated Milk Association, Poultry and Egg National Board, Sugar Research Foundation, and the United Fresh Fruit and Vegetable Association promote better health by acquainting the public with the nutritional value of their products and how they fit into a well-balanced diet.

One can only surmise what the eating habits of our citizens would be without these educational endeavors and we may inquire as to the effectiveness of these endeavors in actually changing established eating practices. Perhaps nutritional knowledge has poured forth more rapidly and in greater abundance than can be accepted and practiced on a personal basis. Then, too, more intensive investigation should be directed in the area of motivational research. We do know that we are far from our established goals, and that until these goals are nearer realization, borderline malnutrition will continue to be a public health problem of considerable significance.

## GERIATRICS

All who work in the allied medical professions can point with understandable pride to the accomplishments which have characterized the progress of medicine in the past 75 years. Advanced knowledge of the basic and applied sciences, development of a drug armentarium unequaled in history, the application of newer procedures and techniques in therapeutics, and public health endeavors in the areas of environmental sanitation and preventive medicine have markedly reduced both the threat of disease and the tragedy of premature death. A concerned and dedicated profession has presented mankind with its most dramatic success story. Along with this success, however, have come attendant complications and the creation of new areas requiring public health attention.

In Chapter 10, in the discussion of population increases, it was pointed out that a decrease in death rate was not accompanied by a decrease in birth rate. The result has been a constantly increasing population in the world. Another effect of reducing the death rate during the most productive years of life has been the lengthening of life expectancy, and the presence of many more aged people in our society. In 1900 the life expectancy was 47 years; today it is somewhat greater than 72 years. In 1900 there were approximately 3 million persons in the United States who were

65 years of age and over. Today there are more than 21 million. Approximately 40 per cent of these people are over 75 years of age. It has been estimated that approximately 4000 people in the United States reach the age of 65 each day and about 3000 of the over-65 age group die each day, resulting in a net increase of 1000 people. If present low birth rates continue, it is projected that by the year 2000 there will be almost 29 milion in the aged population in the United States, or one out of every nine citizens.[22] Worldwide, according to United Nations estimates, those people over 65 years of age now number about 200 million. By 1985, the number is projected to 275 million and by the year 2000, approximately 400 million.[23]

Along with these advancing years have come numerous changes—some insidious and some profound. For many industries this is the mandatory retirement limit and those without active hobbies or outside interests have too much time on their hands to worry, to reflect, and to become lonely. Prolonged survival frequently brings physical handicaps and problems which, in many cases, originated from illnesses incurred in earlier life. The aging of tissues, the appearance of wrinkles, and other numerous evidences of increasing years serve as constant reminders that the individual's life is drawing to a close. Compounded with these problems are the new hazards of a changing society that no longer reveres the aged, does not benefit from their past experiences, views the aged as liabilities instead of assets, and generally is unprepared for the flood of the elderly. The need is apparent for renewed and enlarged efforts in the field of gerontology, the scientific study of all of the phenomena of aging. Also, advancing age is usually accompanied by health problems of greater frequency and magnitude. Particular emphasis should be placed upon the study of geriatrics, which is a branch of medicine dealing with the physiological and pathological problems of older persons.

The distribution of the aged throughout the country is not uniform. Proportionally, more people 65 years of age and over are found in New England, in the West North Central region, the States of West Virginia, Florida, Arkansas, and Oklahoma. In terms of actual numbers, the majority are found in the four most populous states: New York, California, Pennsylvania, and Illinois.[24] With a more mobile society and greater ease of transportation, increasing numbers of the elderly are moving to Florida and the Desert Southwest to escape much of the harsh winter weather. Migration of younger people to these states, also, has been heavy so that the percentage of composition of the populations has not changed markedly. The predominant number of aged are women who outnumber men by a ratio of about 1.4 to 1. More than one-half of the women are widows whereas more than two-thirds of the men are married. This reflects the fact that 40 per cent of older married men have wives who are under 65 years of age. All of these factors are important in assessing the needs and in planning programs of preventive medicine and rehabilitation for the elderly.

Increased longevity without health is much more than an individual tragedy; it is a dangerous family and social economic liability. The types of disability associated with the aging process fall into three main groupings. One of these is the disability due to the aging process itself. Actually, there are conflicting reasons for the changes in tissues which develop with advancing years. Some authorities believe that this is an involutionary process which is inevitable in the modification of cells, tissues, and fluids. Others feel that degenerative changes and impairments are the result of infections, trauma, cumulated toxins, and nutritional disturbances which have exacted their toll through the passing years. It is thought by some that the diminution or cessation or meaningful work results in the atrophy and structural involution which are characteristic of old age. Other authorities subscribe to the theory that the aging process is a gradual depletion of tissue reserves which were inherited or built up in earlier stages of life. As a result of such depletion the aging individual becomes less able to withstand the rigors and unusual stresses which are handled capably by younger persons. With such a mixture of ideas and theories, it is evident that considerably more investigative work is needed in this field to supply the specific information required to overcome or prevent some of the problems associated with aging.

Other types of disability related to the aging process are those associated with long-term illnesses. In the discussion of degenerative diseases in Chapters 5 and 6, reference was made to the kinds of illnesses which are more common in the elderly. Among these are chronic conditions associated with circulatory impairments, metabolic malfunctions, the various types of arthritis, and both benign and malignant neoplasms. Such diseases increase the burden, lessen the enjoyment of retirement years, serve as psychological depressants, and may be the ultimate cause of death. Approximately 80 per cent of those persons 65 years of age and older have some chronic illness which actually or potentially requires medical care or is disabling.[25] The leading causes of death in this advanced-age group have been listed as heart disease, cerebral vascular lesions, cancer, general arteriosclerosis, pneumonia, and influenza. These are among the leading causes of death for the nation as a whole and contrast markedly with the major killers of 50 years ago when the communicable diseases, diarrhea, and enteritis were high on the list. It appears that medical science has now succeeded in keeping a large percentage of the people alive long enough to die of cancer and degenerative diseases.

The third type of disability is associated with psychological problems, mental deterioration, and socio-economic disturbances that frequently accompany old age.[26] Much of this difficulty is caused by wasting away of body tissues and mental faculties as a result of enforced idleness. Other sources are the result of worry over economic and social insecurity. It is no secret that the older age groups generally do not fare well financially compared with younger age groups. Only about one-third are in the labor force and earning capacity frequently is diminished even for these few. An increasing number of the elderly are receiving some type of retirement benefits from former employment, but for a large portion of the aged their only source of income is a combination of Social Security and government old age assistance programs.

A deplorably large percentage of the elderly are lonely people. They feel abandoned by their families, believe themselves neglected, and become apathetic and withdrawn. Realizing that they are becoming a burden on others they feel useless and believe that their lives are pointless and hopeless. With large quantities of time on their hands, they reflect increasingly upon their own infirmities, develop psychosomatic disorders, and think excessively about their approaching death. One study estimates that over 50 per cent of persons residing in homes for the aged display depressive symptoms severe enough to justify psychiatric attention.[27] These patients are problems in hospitals and nursing homes because they demand constant attention, are uncooperative in the treatment program, and are restless, agitated, hostile, noisy, and belligerent. Other problems arise from the elderly patients who act childishly, require constant supervision, are confused and disoriented, have poor eating habits, are personally untidy, and seek to avoid taking medication.

The largest portion of the aged who are not institutionalized live in their own households, but the poor economic status of older people all too often forces them into substandard housing found in low-rent areas. Approximately 25 per cent of the elderly live with children and relatives but the increasing trend toward urbanization of the population with apartment-house living makes it more difficult for children to take care of their older parents. When the aged become so physically and emotionally fragile that they create abnormal problems in the home there is a tendency for families to place them in institutions. More often the family circle is then closed to the patient, his room is turned over to someone else, those who look after him make other plans, and there is no intention of returning him to his family. Long-term care facilities are needed for the aged but in their absence mental hospitals often must provide this service.

With the increasing number of older people in our present population, it is imperative that the variables associated with the care of geriatric patients be minimized. Successful attempts are now being made to transfer most of these people into nursing homes and with the help of Title 18 and the Older Americans Act, this transition can now be made with less difficulty. The Veterans Administration, concerned with the increasing number of geriatric patients in their hospitals, has made a study to determine whether patients placed in nursing homes can adjust physically and behaviorally. The results of the study showed that the majority of the patients preferred to live in nursing homes rather than hospitals because of the freedom and home-like atmosphere prevalent at these institutions. Other approaches to the care of the aged include the placement in foster homes. This procedure has been adopted in Louisiana and has been found to be highly satisfactory.

Still another method of care is the state geriatric hospital such as the facility in operation in Minnesota. This facility was specifically designed to remove from the mental hospitals non-psychotic patients who are 65 years and older. Patients admitted to the geriatric hospital have been reported to improve considerably in their attitudes and outlook on life because there is more concentration on enjoyment of what life has to offer.

The aged do not necessarily have to face a terminal period of loneliness, despair, and chronic illness. Although much remains to be done in the field of gerontology and additional research is needed in geriatrics, great progress has been made in helping the elderly adjust to the vagaries of old age and in helping society adjust to the increasing numbers of older people. Of course, the elderly must retain certain responsibilities for their own well-being. The privilege of longevity bears with it an obligation of personal effort and concern for one's own health protection and maintenance.

This is particularly true in the area of nutrition. Researchers have provided foods with built-in safeguards, and modern methods of storage and rapid transportation have given us a variety of fresh fruits and vegetables for year-round use, yet the majority of the aged suffer from some form of malnutrition. The first obstacle is usually overweight.[28] By age 60 the average person in the United States has accumulated about 15 extra pounds. From here, there are two deviations from a sensible dietary regime. For some, eating excessively is their main surviving pleasure, a sedative which brings drowsiness, immobility, and obesity with its attendant problems. For a significant number of the elderly, the loss of teeth and resultant loss of masticatory function markedly reduces digestive efficiency.[29] Other lonely people do not take the trouble to prepare balanced diets and eat skimpy, irregular meals. This is the chief cause of progressive malnutrition among the elderly.[30] Actually, with the exception of decreased carbohydrate intake because of reduction in physical activity and the need for about 10 per cent increase in proteins, there is no separate and distinct retirement diet. Older people should be encouraged to eat three equally balanced meals each day and follow the general patterns of good nutrition which were outlined in the first section of this chapter.

In addition to proper nutrition, the elderly should be encouraged to learn new hobbies, to involve themselves in social activities which are being provided in ever increasing numbers, and to volunteer their services to the Red Cross or to other charitable and health organizations who need help. Loneliness and apathy seldom mix with these types of activities and those people who continue to be needed in some way are less prone to become ill. Much of the deterioration usually attributed to the aging process can be traced to mental and physical unfitness, and programs which will keep older people active, alert, and involved in projects and objectives beyond themselves can greatly diminish medical care problems.

The community also has an obligation. We cannot ignore our responsibility to these senior citizens. Those people who reach age 70 still have a statistical prospect of 11 to 12 more years and the community should assure the opportunity for these remaining years to be spent as pleasantly as possible. Through the combined efforts of individuals and agencies, additional arrangements for recreational and educational facilities can be made. Assistance in self-employment, better housing to accommodate the aged, and improved economic status from retirement and government programs are further goals which a concerned community can attain. In the practice of geriatric medicine, greater attention should be directed toward the preventive aspects. Periodic health examinations to detect early signs of chronic disease, screening examinations for large-scale detection, and geriatric clinics provide the elderly with an opportunity to help restrict and control the diseases which are associated with old age. It is also the firm belief among those who work with geriatric patients that long-term care should be provided in the community, and not in state mental hospitals or public state facilities removed from the community. Conferences in comprehensive community mental health centers and regular health centers provide more adequate planning for the aged at the local level. The family, the physician, and the providers of health care can work together for the greater benefit of the patient.

All of us have a personal interest in gerontology and geriatrics, not only because we are in the allied medical professions and an increasing number of our patients are among the elderly, but because we see ourselves in this category in the years to come. The preparations which we as individuals, as a profession, and as a society make for the aged may well be the foundation upon which such services are administered when we are among the senior citizens. Our concern with older age groups, then, is not only because of the public health problems of today, but because the subject becomes more personal with advancing years.

## DENTAL CARE

The human mouth needs more daily care and probably receives less than any other part of the anatomy. The practice of not brushing teeth after eating, the ignoring of dental caries, the preponderance of sweets in the diet, and general inattention to oral hygiene have resulted in a high incidence of dental defects. It appears that the more affluent society becomes, the more numerous are the incidences of oral disease. The most common defect is tooth decay which is exceeded only by the common cold as the most prevalent disease of man. It is estimated that 98 per cent of the people will experience tooth decay sometime in their lives and that six out of 10 persons in the United States have untreated cavities in their teeth.[31]

We are all familiar with the admonition to visit your dentist at least once each year and, yet, the Public Health Service estimates that only 36 per cent of the population visits a dentist yearly. Thirty-three percent of the children between the ages of five and 14 have never visited a dentist; of those who do visit a dentist only 23 per cent of the carious lesions have been treated.[32] The cause-effect relationship is noted in the results of a survey which showed that people who stayed away from the dentist for three years lost twice as many teeth as those who had dental treatment every year and 16.7 per cent of the people in this group had to have complete dentures. Another report indicates that, by the age of 35, approximately 70 per cent of the population need bridges or dentures to replace lost teeth. An additional government survey led to the estimate that 20 million men and women in the United States are edentulous or completely lacking in natural teeth. In addition, there were approximately 91 million others who had on the average 18 decayed, missing, and filled teeth.[33] It is currently estimated that 36.5 million adult people in the United States need dental care.[34]

Contrasted to this is the fact that the civilian population of the United States already spends in excess of 2 billion dollars per year on the care of its teeth. The vast majority of these expenditures, unfortunately, are for secondary treatment rather than primary prevention. The 100,000 dentists in this country are kept busy with their present patient load and if all of the people who need dental treatment actually tried to receive such care at any one time the appointment books would be clogged for months. The American Dental Association estimates that between five and 10 times the annual productive capacity of all of the dental personnel in the United States would be required to meet the existing dental needs of the population at any given time.

The dental profession, along with the nursing profession, has taken the lead in the utilization of auxiliary personnel in helping to perform routine functions and thus release the professional for more exacting tasks. Thus, the dental hygienist, the dental assistant, and the dental technician are becoming more prominent in sharing the patient load in the dentist's office. The numbers of these trained personnel and their proper utilization must increase markedly, however, before we can seriously expect that all people who need dental care can receive it within any reasonable time. For example, the dental hygienist has repeatedly proven her worth in the cleaning of teeth, instructing patients in proper care of teeth and prosthetics, prophylaxis, and similar methods of improving the dentist's productive capacity, and, yet the Survey of Dental Practice reports that still a minority of the dental practices in this country utilize the services of a hygienist. Another method to reduce unmet dental treatment needs, particularly in indigent rural populations, is the increased use of dental student manpower.[35]

As noted earlier, tooth decay is almost universal and is the most distinctive dental disease of the child and young adult. (Generally, people past 40 incur fewer new dental caries.) As most of us know from past experience, tooth decay is the chief cause of toothache, it is the major source of pulp and root abscesses, and it is a very common reason for the removal of teeth. It is a disease, a localized infection which destroys tooth structure and produces cavitation, and is not a vague and mysterious rotting of the teeth which must be accepted fatalistically. In spite of its prevalence, dental caries is far from a natural or unavoidable condition. We have enough knowledge to prevent most cases of tooth decay but experience has shown that all too few people follow the necessary procedures.

Dental caries always start on the outside of the tooth, attacking the hardest and most dense tissue in the body, the enamel. This substance is slightly porous material composed of hydroxy-apatite, a crystalline form of calcium phosphate .and calcium carbonate. As such, in spite of its hardness, it has low resistance to acids. In the progress of tooth decay a film or plaque of bacteria on the surface of the tooth converts sugars to acids which, in turn, dissolve the enamel and expose the dentin, the underlying structure also composed of apatite but containing more organic material. Here the rate of decay is much more rapid, the cavitation becomes larger and eventually reaches the pulp. If not treated by drilling out the offending material and filling the cavity, the infection penetrates the tooth and develops abscesses in the root canals.

By reason of the high correlation between the number of *Lactobacillus acidophilus* in the saliva and the incidence of carious lesions in man, it has been assumed by numerous writers throughout the years that this organism was primarily responsible for the acid production that precedes dental decay. Other writers in the field believed that dental decay can be caused by any acid-forming microorganism acting on any carbohydrate substrate. Reports from dental research, however, state that these ideas no longer are accurate. Dental caries is recognized today as an infection caused by a disease; the hole in the tooth is a very uncomfortable symptom. The cariogenic bacteria thrive upon specific carbohydrates, particularly sucrose, and react to produce dextran and acids. Evidently, an index of their cariogenicity is the ability to produce dextrans from their carbohydrate substrates. Some types of sugars, such as fructose, lactose, glucose, and sorbitol, do not provide a suitable substrate and produce very little or no decay in experimental animals and man.

In the prevention of dental caries the most effective method is to eliminate the cariogenic organisms from oral flora. This can be done by specialists who practice preventive dentistry and is not an easy task. Another method highly recommended is the elimination of concentrated sweets from the diet. Most dentists believe that the number of cavities could be reduced by at least 50 per cent if children and teen-agers would substitute such non-cariogenic foods as popcorn, vegetables, cold cuts, cheeses, and fruits to replace cookies and candy as between-meal snacks. It also has been suggested that a high protein diet may increase the salivary urea level which may neutralize acids produced from the bacteria fermentation of the sucrose.[36] Still another effective and positive way to reduce the number of caries attacks is to eliminate all infected enamel and dentin by filling the cavities as early as possible. However, leaving even one small cavity untreated leaves a colony which is a source for the growth of new cariogenic streptococci and, in turn, invites new cavities. Since colonies of bacteria adhere to the teeth in plaques, an additional preventive measure is to keep all tooth surfaces clean by brushing and by eating coarse, fibrous foods such as apples, oranges, celery, and carrots.

A definite relationship has been established between the amount of fluoride ingested and the incidence of dental caries. This was first noted in parts of Oklahoma, Texas, and the Desert Southwest. The fluoride content in the natural water supply in some of these areas was great enough to cause a mottling of the enamel, yet the incidence of dental caries was remarkably low. It has since been established that 60 to 70 per cent reductions in dental caries can be expected in those populations which consume 1.2 p.p.m. of fluoride in their water supplies during tooth development. The first controlled test on a broad scale was performed in the State of Michigan in 1945, when the fluoride content of the water in Grand Rapids was increased. Muskegon, which had a natural fluoride content of 0.2 p.p.m. in the water supply, was used as a control. After 10 years, the caries rate in the permanent teeth of children born in Grand Rapids after fluoridation was 60 per cent less than the comparable rate in Muskegon. Another dental care study compared Newburgh, New York (a fluoridated community) with its non-fluoridated neighbor, Kingston. Dental costs per child in Newburgh were half of those in Kingston.[37] Practically every major medical and dental group in Canada and the United States unequivocally endorses the fluoridation of public drinking water as a means of reducing tooth decay among children. Prenatal fluorides taken by the pregnant mother pass in thresh-old-safe amounts through the placenta to the fetus. Here they are incorporated into the apatite crystals of enamel and dentin to make these structures highly resistant to the action of acids produced by the cariogenic microorganisms. Similar processes take place when the infant and child ingest fluorides through the communal water supply. Once the crown of the tooth is completed and erupts into the oral cavity, however, it is no longer possible to incorporate the fluoride ion into the apatite structure by way of the systemic circulation. Topical application of fluoride solutions and dentrifice, however, will incorporate the ion into the surface layer of the enamel. An even more effective method of reducing the solubility of tooth enamel has been achieved by mixing two fluoride compounds, stannous fluoride and acidulated phosphofluoride.[38]

Other types of dental abnormalities include those due to developmental deformities of the teeth and jaws. The enamel surface of the tooth, for example, gives evidence that teeth are extremely sensitive to various nutritional and other metabolic influences during the period of formation and calcification. Abnormal pits and grooves caused by faulty formation of the enamel, a condition known as hypoplasia, as well as hypocalcification of the teeth can result from nutritional disorders such as rickets. Diseases occurring in early childhood such as congenital syphilis, measles, and scarlet fever may also be reflected in faulty tooth development. Discoloration of the teeth may result from excessive intake of fluorides or from intensive and prolonged use of tetracyclines.

A more common condition, affecting about 30 per cent of all children, is malocclusion. This is an all-inclusive, descriptive term which merely describes the end result. Included in this general category are teeth which are poorly aligned, irregular, overlapping, or protruding at abnormal angles. One of the causes for this condition is heredity. The child who inherits small bone structure from one parent and large teeth from the other is in trouble. Secondary oral influences can also contribute to this condition. Premature loss of deciduous and permanent teeth, prolonged thumb-sucking and lip-biting, and failure of the teeth to erupt at the proper time can all serve as causative factors. Malocclusion interferes with mastication and digestion, promotes food deposits and irritated gums, eventually causes damage to the teeth that must sustain the entire force of the

bite, and leads to facial deformities. Preventive dental measures may include preservation of some teeth, the extraction of deciduous teeth interfering with emergence of permanent ones, and the reserving of adequate space for teeth which erupt later. Corrective measures usually require the services of an orthodontist.

The diseases affecting the supporting tissues of the teeth are referred to as periodontal diseases. The periodontal tissues consist of the gum tissue, or gingiva, the periodontal membrane, and the adjacent alveolar bone that lines the tooth socket. The most prevalent periodontal disease is gingivitis, or inflammation of the gums, and is promoted by the packing of food between the teeth, the accumulation of calculus or tartar around the necks of teeth, mechanical injury as a result of poor tooth brushing, or the improper use of toothpicks and dental floss. In this condition there is bacterial invasion of gum tissues resulting in swelling and redness. If untreated, the gums recede from the teeth, form pockets, and bleed easily. A similar disease which is much more acute and destructive is an ulcerating gingivitis known as Vincent's disease, or trench mouth. This disease causes ulceration and necrosis of gum tissue and is accompanied by bleeding, increased flow of saliva, a slight fever, and a foul odor. The organisms usually involved in Vincent's disease are *Bacillus fusiformis* and a spirochete, *Borrelia vincentii.* There are conflicting opinions regarding the communicability of this disease but it probably is not transmitted effectively to a normally healthy person.

Perhaps the most serious of the periodontal diseases, accounting for more lost teeth in adults than any other cause, is a condition incorrectly but generally known as pyorrhea. The most common form of this disease, periodontitis, originates as gingivitis but progresses beyond the superficial lesions of the gum and extends to the alveolar bone and periodontal membrane. The gums withdraw from the surface of the teeth and form pockets of pus. The periodontal fibers shrink; the support of the teeth becomes seriously damaged because of bone resorption; the teeth become loose, can be moved easily and, if unresponsive to treatment, are lost. The less common type of pyorrhea is periodontosis in which the patient develops a rather extensive breakdown of supporting bone tissue without the more obvious signs of gingivitis. Loss of teeth is common in this condition inasmuch as early diagnosis is more difficult and treatment is less effective.

In this enlightened age when much more knowledge has accumulated regarding dietary deficiencies, effective preventive measures, and advanced restorative techniques, it would seem that tooth decay, periodontal diseases, and general neglect of the teeth would be diminishing. Instead, the problem appears to be increasing, not only among the economic and culturally disadvantaged but also among the large middle class. As the resources of trained personnel for the administration of secondary dental treatment are extremely limited when compared to the need, renewed efforts must be directed toward the preventive aspects of oral disease. Allied medical personnel can perform a distinct service in this area. This is particularly true of the pharmacist who sees far more people with dental problems than the average dentist. In addition, more than 17 million prescription orders, written by dentists, are dispensed yearly by the nation's pharmacists.[39] In this day of multiple drug use and increased emphasis on drug interactions it is of paramount importance that the pharmacist and the dentist work together for the betterment of the patient.[40] However, knowledge among the general population of the most characteristic dental structures is still incomplete and many persons are not convinced of the real value of practicing good oral hygiene or the importance of individual initiative in seeking dental care. It is obvious that further implementation is needed for more widespread dissemination of knowledge about preventive dentistry, for further study into motivational factors, and better utilization of auxiliary dental personnel in order to reduce this widespread and costly national health problem.

## VISUAL DISORDERS

Of the various senses which man exercises to adapt and live in his environment, vision is the most useful. During most of the waking hours the eyes are constantly being moved through the combined and co-ordinated action of the six external eye muscles. In addition, the ciliary and sphincter muscles, through nervous control, are almost equally busy adjusting to the proper focus and allowing the correct exposure to light. The eyes, however, exist not in isolation, but in relation to the entire mind and body. It is estimated that more than three-fourths of all impressions come through the eye. The optic nerve is the largest afferent nerve in the body and conducts visually activated sensations to the brain through approximately 1 million fibers. This very important system cannot be regenerated and the gift of sight is recognized as one of our most valuable possessions. However, most of today's citizens take their sight for granted and far too many do not follow recommended procedures for preservation of good vision. This is emphasized by the sobering fact that approximately one-half of all cases of blindness could have been prevented if proper precaution had been taken or if early warning signs had been heeded.

A very brief review of the process of vision will serve as a reference when describing functional defects. The object that we perceive as a visual image is the source of reflected light waves, unless the object itself is a primary light source such as a lamp or fire. These light waves travel in parallel columns and it is necessary to bring them to a focus on the retina of the eye in order to see properly. The first refraction occurs when the light waves pass through the curved cornea of the eyeball. These slightly bent rays then travel through the aqueous humor and pass through the colored iris, whose circular and radial muscles control the quantity of admitted light. The reflected light waves then pass through the lens, which is a semi-fluid or jelly-like body encased in an elastic capsule. Attached to the capsule are the suspensory ligaments which in turn are attached to the ciliary muscle. Through autonomic control, the action of the ciliary muscle determines the shape of the lens and, thus, the extent to which the light waves are focused on the retina. If accommodation for near vision is required, the ciliary muscles contract and advance which release tension on the suspensory ligaments and allow the lens to assume a more oval shape for greater refraction. If distant vision is required, the ciliary muscle relaxes which increases tension on the ligaments and, thus, flattens the lens. The image is then focused on the retina that has many rods and cones which convert light waves to nervous impulses. The impulses, in turn, are transmitted to the optic chiasma by the optic nerve and from there, to the occipital region of the brain for interpretation.

Certain visual disorders are associated with one or more of the functional processes of sight. One of these conditions is myopia, or nearsightedness. In myopia, the lens of the eye is thicker and more convex and the eyeball is longer than normal. The result of this combination focuses the entering light rays before they reach the retina. The wearing of concave lenses shifts the focus point back to its proper position. This condition is found in approximately 5 per cent of the population.

Another visual defect is hyperopia, or farsightedness. Because the eyeball is too short and the lens is thinner than usual, visual images close at hand cannot be brought to a proper focus, even with maximum accommodation of the lens. The result is blurred vision for objects nearby and clear sight for distant objects. Many mild cases of hyperopia are tolerated without treatment but the more pronounced cases are corrected by glasses with convex lenses which reduce the divergence of the entering light rays and shorten the focal length.

An eye condition rather similar to hyperopia is found in older people and is called presbyopia, a Greek derivative meaning old eyes. In presbyopia the lenses have lost much of their elasticity and will not alter their configuration sufficiently to accommodate for near vision, although distant vision usually remains clear. This condition necessitates the use of convex lens glasses for reading, sewing, and similar close work.

Still another error of refraction is astigmatism, caused by the irregular curvature of the cornea or lens. Astigmatism means without a point, and parts of the image formed on the retina are blurred or distorted because light rays focus on different points instead of converging at one locus. In attempts to secure a proper focus on the retina the individual frequently develops eyestrain, resulting in nervous tension and headaches. Astigmatism is usually congenital although it may result from an injury or inflammation. The only method of relieving this condition is through the use of properly fitted eyeglasses. It must be remembered, however, that glasses do not cure any of the errors of refraction. They merely compensate or counterbalance existing errors.

A serious result of functional eye defects may be the development of lazy eye blindness or amblyopia ex anopsia. In this condition an eye that appears healthy actually has low or poor vision because that portion of the eye which is used for careful vision has not been developed to its full potential. It is usually due to muscular imbalance, refractive error, or other defect that was not corrected during the early years, below the age of six. For example, a child with eye trouble that causes him to see a double image may suppress the weaker eye and use only the stronger one. When this becomes a habit the vision in the weaker eye is gradually lost. This is one of the important reasons why the eyes of all children should be checked at least by the age of three or four.

Most, if not all, visual defects in children can be detected if parents are alert to symptoms displayed. If the child attempts to brush away blurs, blinks more than usual, rubs his eyes frequently, squints when looking at distant objects, or frowns excessively he is most probably suffering from visual disturbances. Additional symptoms include the child who stumbles over small objects, is unduly sensitive to light, or has swollen or encrusted eyelids, recurring sties, or inflamed and watery eyes.

In addition to focal defects the eye is subject to various infections which impair vision and, if left untreated, may result in blindness. The most common is conjunctivitis, an inflammation of the membrane lining the eyelids and the front portion of the eye. Mild forms of this condition frequently accompany colds and more pronounced inflammation is seen in other systemic diseases such as measles. More frequently causes of conjunctivitis are exposure to dust, wind, pollens, salt or chlorinated water while swimming, chemical irritants and fumes, or excessively bright lights. A contagious form of conjunctivitis is pink-eye, caused by infection of various bacteria. Symptoms of this condition are irritation, lacrimation, swelling of the lids, sensitivity to light, and the discharge of pus.

Blepharitis is another inflammatory condition of the eyelids in which the edges are covered with small grey scales consisting of dried, hardened secretions. This condition usually occurs in children who are malnourished and is more pronounced if eyestrain already exists. Ophthalmic antibiotic ointments are usually the drug of choice.

Trachoma was at one time a common cause of blindness in the United States, particularly among the American Indians. Proper diagnosis and treatment have virtually eliminated this disease in the more advanced countries of the world but it is still a serious problem in some of the underdeveloped nations. The disease, known as granular conjunctivitis, is caused by a virus and is spread by such means as flies, contaminated hands, towels, and clothing. The infection causes granulations on the conjunctiva with severe scarring of the lids and cornea and eventual blindness. Trachoma responds to treatment with penicillin and some of the broad spectrum antibiotics but prevention relies upon the elimination of poverty and the application of hygienic practices among affected populations. The disease remains prevalent in areas of the world where poor nutrition and crowded living conditions prevail and where the climate is hot, dry, and dusty.

Ophthalmia neonatorum is an acute infection of the conjunctiva in the newborn infants caused by a variety of infectious agents. The two main types are acquired by contact with the mother's birth canal during delivery. The disease in the past has been due largely to the gonococcus. The most prevalent type of infection at the present is inclusion blennorrhea. Staphylococcus, pneumococcus, and other pyogenic organisms sometimes give rise to mild conjunctivitis. With the development of Crede's method for installation of silver nitrate in the eyes of newborn infants, ophthalmia neonatorum has almost disappeared.

Other eye diseases which are not infectious in nature develop usually with advancing age. Periodic examinations and screening clinics, frequently, will disclose the onset of these insidious diseases in time to exercise corrective measures or to initiate operative procedures. One of these diseases, glaucoma, is the second leading cause of blindness among adults in the United States. This disease, characterized by intraocular tension and its resultant effects upon the retina and vascular bed, may be either acute or chronic. The acute form develops suddenly with severe pain, congestion, and reduced vision. The chronic type, which is much more common, works slowly and painlessly. The victim is only vaguely aware of the symptoms which are transient but recur with greater frequency and intensity. Consultation with a physician is frequently postponed until the patient is in grave danger of losing his eyesight. During the first stages of glaucoma the quantities of aqueous humor build up faster than they are drained away. The result is an increase in fluid pressure throughout the interior of the eyeball. The most pronounced effect of this increased pressure is on the retina which gradually deteriorates. At first the damage is only to those retinal fibers concerned with side vision. In the final stages of the disease the pressure destroys the nerves which permit central vision and all sight is lost. The use of drugs such as pilocarpine or surgical intervention may be indicated to halt the progress of this condition. Symptoms of glaucoma include loss of side vision, blurred or foggy vision, rainbow-colored rings around lights, inability to adjust the eyes to darkened rooms, and frequent change in glasses, with no improvement in vision. As the onset of this condition occurs far more frequently in people over 40 years of age, the best defense is a medical eye examination at least every two years after reaching middle age. The instrument used for detection of intraocular tension is the tonometer. Although the Schiotz tonometer has been most widely used in the past, another instrument, the Mackay-Marg tonometer, is finding wide acceptance. One of the new instruments rapidly growing in popularity is an applanation tonometer which measures intraocular pressure by means of an airpulse instead of direct mechanical contact with the eye.[41] Whatever the method used, prompt diagnosis results in early and carefully supervised treatment which can prevent visual field loss.

The most important single cause of blindness among adults today is cataract, the loss of transparency of the lens. If the cloudiness within the lens remains slight and does not markedly interfere with vision, the patient learns to adapt to the impairment. On the other hand, if it becomes extensive enough and thick enough to cause an opacity of the lens, preventing light from entering the eye, the result is blindness. The exact cause of cataract is never identified in the majority of cases. There have been some relationships established with nutritional deficiencies, injury, iatrogenic diseases, senility, and heredity, but, for the most part, the evidence is far from conclusive.[42] Generally, it is known that cataracts cannot spread from one eye to the other, are not contagious, and cannot be cured by ointments, eyedrops, or any other type of drug. Sight is restored to the eye by the surgical removal of the opaque lens. Experimentation and testing are currently being conducted to determine the feasibility of substituting an artificial lens in the vacant capsule. Until this procedure is further perfected and more widely adopted, most persons operated on for cataracts must wear corrective glasses to compensate for the missing lens.

In addition to the visual disorders and infections already described, the eye is subject to damage from other sources. Both acuity and degree of eye muscle imbalance are known to be affected by the individual's physical condition, in particular, body fatigue.[43] Chronic diseases such as diabetes, anemia, and cancer take their toll. Hemorrhage in the eye, injury to the corneal surface, retinal detachment, hypoxia, excessive heat, radiation, and the ingestion of methyl alcohol can all be factors which restrict or impair vision and can introduce their victims to the night-black world of the blind.

In the United States, approximately 470,000 people are blind,[44] and, despite continuous progress in efforts to prevent blindness, an estimated 30,000 more lose their sight each year. The number of blind persons in the world has been estimated at 10 to 15 million.[45] In addition, there are other millions of persons whose sight is so limited as to be a severe handicap for employment. Unless the trend and statistics are reversed, another 750,000 people now living in this country will become blind before they die. The cost of caring for the blind has been largely assumed by voluntary and government agencies in the fields of health and welfare and amounts to approximately 150 million dollars annually. This includes expenditures for braille and talking books, education, seeing-eye dogs, pensions, and related services. In contrast, all too little funds are expended for research, screening clinics, and education for prevention.

One of the bright hopes for the blind is the opportunity which is presented through vocational rehabilitation. Through a step-by-step process of counseling, physical examination, vocational diagnosis, medical services, personal adjustment, vocational training, and job placement the blind are returned to a useful purpose and positive direction. All of these services are furnished at no cost to the patient and, in addition, assistance is given in the form of tools, equipment, initial stock, and licenses to help the blind person establish a small, independent business. This program serves a two-fold purpose. It not only helps the blind person to become self-supporting but also converts a welfare recipient into a taxpayer.

Various employment opportunities are open to the blind and co-operative efforts between vocational rehabilitation programs and industry are establishing additional fields of work. As the blind must rely upon their other senses and memory to a much greater degree, they have proven to be a valuable asset in jobs where vision is not a prerequisite. One of the more challenging fields is the use of the blind as computer programmers.

The health professionals primarily concerned with problems of vision include the ophthalmologist or oculist, the optometrist, and the optician. The ophthalmologist is a medical doctor who has specialized in the medical and surgical care of the eyes. This specialist can prescribe glasses and drugs and is qualified to recognize signs in the eye of diseases elsewhere in the body.

The optometrist specializes in vision analysis through tests and eye examinations. Although he is restricted in the prescribing and use of drugs, he can administer such forms of treatment as visual training and orthoptics and can prescribe lenses and other aids to vision. Through his training and background he can recognize potential visual difficulties before irreparable damage has occurred.

Opticians fit and adjust eyeglasses according to prescriptions written by ophthamologists and optometrists. They do not examine eyes or prescribe treatment. Frequently, the optician is aided by an optical technician who performs the actual grinding and polishing of the lenses and assembles them in a frame.

The public health aspects of visual problems are becoming more apparent. Advanced nations throughout the world are recognizing their obligation to ensure adequate health and safety for all of their citizens, and the diagnosis and treatment of eye disorders are certainly included as an essential service.

The importance of community-based planning and development programs in the area of eye care cannot be overemphasized. Many cases of blindness can be prevented if the eye disorders are detected soon enough, but public education regarding eye care and the advantages of early diagnosis and proper treatment need to be stressed to a much greater degree if such programs are to succeed. Two of the national voluntary health agencies that help in programs of education and motivational research are the National Society for the Prevention of Blindness and the American Foundation for the Blind. The Lions Clubs have also been outstanding in their community service endeavors for the blind. In many cities they have sponsored eye banks for corneal transplants, a service which is also performed by the Eye Bank for Sight Restoration, Incorporated. Certainly, the co-ordinated, co-operative efforts of all interested agencies, public and private, are needed to reduce the incidence of visual disorders and blindness among the people of our country and around the world.     ·

### Hearing Loss

Next to sight, the sense of hearing is the most important aid in helping in the learning process, adapting to environment, and adjusting to social situations. Approximately one-eighth of all impressions are transmitted through the ear and the loss of this function robs the individual of a great gift. It places him in a special category of loneliness because his powers of communication are weakened. However, approximately one out of every ten people in the United States has some hearing impairment and about 250,000 cannot hear human speech. The frequency of hearing loss increases with advancing age. Testing of school children with audiometers has disclosed that from 3 to 5 per cent of these students suffer from some important hearing loss. The incidence becomes much higher in middle age, usually because an ear infection in childhood did not receive proper attention. In old age, hearing loss is quite common, affecting the majority of persons in this category.

The process of hearing involves the air conduction of sound waves in the outer ear, mechanical conduction in the middle ear, fluid conduction in the inner ear; and nerve transmission to the brain. The auricle and the external auditory meatus direct sound toward the tympanic membrane which separates the outer ear from the middle ear. The lining of the external auditory meatus secretes cerumen, a dark brown wax, which protects and preserves the eardrum and external tissue.

The middle ear is primarily an air space in the temporal bone containing the three auditory ossicles, the malleus, incus, and stapes. The malleus is connected to the tympanic membrane limiting the outer ear and the stapes is sealed against the oval membrane of the inner ear. Vibrations of the tympanic membrane or ear drum, initiated by external sound waves, are incredibly minute. During ordinary conversation, for example, displacement of the drum is only the diameter of a molecule of hydrogen.[46] These vibrations are converted into intensified movements of the three auditory ossicles and, through lever-like action, transmit these movements onto the surface of the oval membrane. The outer and middle ear, then, are conducting mechanisms and hearing loss associated with malfunction of these structures is referred to as conduction deafness. The middle ear is connected to the superior-posterior portion of the pharynx by means of the eustachian tube which serves to equalize pressures in the middle ear when changing altitudes. Nasopharyngeal infections accompanying numerous diseases are spread to the middle ear through the eustachian tube and result in otitis media. This process is facilitated if the patient blows his nose too vigorously, particularly if the nortrils are partially clogged.

The inner ear is set deep in the temporal bone. In addition to the labyrinth, associated with balance, the inner ear contains an endolymph-filled, spiral-shaped cochlea with its hair cells of the organ of Corti. Pressure waves created by the vibrations of the oval window pass through the endolymph and stimulate the appropriate hair-like sensory cells. In this manner, motion is converted to nervous impulses which, in turn, are conducted through the auditory nerve to the brain for interpretation.

Progressive loss of hearing may be caused by conduction deafness, by damage to the sound-perceiving apparatus in the inner ear, or by disease of the auditory nerve which results in nerve deafness. Conductive hearing loss may be caused by a blockage in the external auditory meatus, pressure against the tympanic membrane, perforation of the membrane, or restriction in movement of the ossicles. Impacted wax is the most common form of blockage, and rarely produces permanent loss of hearing. When excess cerumen is secreted it frequently hardens and impedes the sound waves. The patient may complain of a ringing or buzzing in the ear or of mild vertigo. It is best, usually, for a physician to remove the build-up of impacted wax. Otitis media is the most common cause of conductive hearing loss. The infection of the middle ear not only accumulates pus which impairs the proper functioning of the ossicles but, if unchecked by antibiotics, can spread to the air cells of the mastoid bone, resulting in mastoiditis. Over 50 per cent of all cases of deafness can be traced to otitis media.

Otosclerosis is another cause of deafness. In this condition there is an ossification between the base of the stapes and the oval window of the inner ear which fixes the stapes against the window and prevents vibrations from being effectively transmitted to the fluid of the inner ear. Otosclerosis is usually restricted to young adults and nearly always the hearing loss is evident before the age of 30. It can be corrected by an operation called fenestration in which a new opening is made in the hardened bone overlying the inner ear.

Meniere's disease can also cause loss of hearing. As a result of increased pressure in the endolymph of the inner ear abnormal stresses are placed on the sensitive cells of the organ of Corti. The disease is characterized by intermittent attacks of dizziness and nausea with some difficulty in hearing and ringing in the ears. Other causes of sensory-neural hearing loss are heredity, congenital defects, and prolonged exposure to high intensity sound. Also, loss of hearing is a side effect associated with the administration of several drugs. Patients are more likely to develop this ototoxicity if given aspirin, kanamycin, neomycin, gentimycin, paromycin, ethacrynic acid, or quinidine. Patients receiving such medications for prolonged periods should have regular hearing examinations in order to protect against this insidious side effect.[47]

Deafness has been defined as the invisible disability. Perhaps because it has been concealed as much as possible, the public has been unaware of its prevalence and indifferent to its problems. Deafness is one of our most common physical disabilities, and, yet, it is one of the last physical handicaps to enlist public sympathy and support. The deaf person carries the stigma of social rejection because he cannot communicate with his fellow men. People with normal hearing find it difficult to converse with a deaf person and soon stop trying. In spite of public apathy, nevertheless, more progress in research, treatment, and rehabilitation has been made in the last 30 years than in all of the previous centuries of history.

The congenitally deaf person, slow to learn and often speaking with a strange voice, is set apart and doomed to a life of loneliness. Since he is isolated from the hearing world and unable to communicate with others, he develops unique psychological and emotional problems and is often met with frustration when attempting to become a part of the normal society. Therefore, he frequently becomes passive and prefers only the company of the deaf.

The adult who gradually becomes hard of hearing faces a different set of circumstances. At first he is unaware of his hearing loss and, although he cannot understand too well, it is only after substantial impairment has developed that he realizes his difficulty. This unfortunate individual, all too often, follows a characteristic behavior pattern. He grows insecure, suspicious, and socially withdrawn and, as his personality changes, he further avoids his friends, who finally reject him. Inasmuch as his disability is invisible and because he, himself, believes that it is a social stigma and additional evidence of advancing age, he tries to conceal his deficiency and refuses to wear a hearing aid or seek medical help. He does not understand that his deafness is more apparent to others than he realizes, and he willfully places himself at a great disadvantage in the hearing world. Often such a person refuses to admit the oncoming disability until he suffers serious personal and vocational maladjustment.

The tragedy of deafness is that, so often, it can be helped if assistance is sought in time. Even congenitally deaf children can be trained to take their places in the normal world and live a useful, purposeful life, but the disability must be recognized early enough to take remedial action. Certain well-defined symptoms are usually present in the deaf baby. For example, the child fails to develop speech at the proper age, he does not exhibit a startle reflex at a sudden or loud noise, he will not be pacified by his mother's voice, and he tends to play silently by himself without the usual childhood imitation of motors, airplanes, or the blast-off of space rockets.

The early symptoms of approaching deafness in the adult may be more difficult to detect. The victim may complain that people no longer speak clearly and that he can hear sounds but not understand speech. He may begin to speak too softly or too loudly, depending upon the type of hearing loss, and his own voice may sound intensely loud to him. His own chewing sounds may drown out his ability to hear his dinner companions. He cannot follow jokes or rapid repartee. His employer may notice that he no longer carries out verbal instructions. As the disorder progresses the victim may hesitate to go out from the security of his own home and he loses interest in movies and television. Any one of these symptoms is sufficient reason for seeking competent medical advice.

It is obvious that a person who is deaf or hard of hearing needs expert help to improve or restore hearing and to enable him to learn how to communicate with others. The family physician may refer the patient to an otologist, a specialist in diseases of the ear. From here the patient may be sent to a hearing and speech clinic with the necessary electronic measuring equipment or to a clinical audiologist, a person specially trained in the science of hearing.

Treatment depends upon the type of deafness as determined by the audiological examination and diagnosis and may involve one or a combination of surgical, medical, or audiological procedures. Surgical treatment may consist of the fenestration technique described previously or of repair or reconstruction of the hearing mechanism in the middle ear. Medical treatment is most effective for persons suffering from Meniere's disease.For those whose hearing cannot be returned through surgical or medical procedures, audiological rehabilitation, generally, is indicated. Most of these people can be helped by a properly selected and adjusted hearing aid. Sometimes speech correction is necessary if the hearing loss has produced changes in the patient's voice or speech. Most of the modern methods involved in the optimum rehabilitation of the patient include a combination of auditory training, speech reading, and hearing conversation.

Inasmuch as workers in the allied medical professions are becoming increasingly concerned about the total health of all of our people, the problems associated with hearing loss cannot be overlooked. As more and more is learned about auditory functions, newer surgical techniques, and improved audiological methods, the necessity for an individual to go through life in total silence is markedly decreased. A significant percentage of all deafness can be prevented by prompt attention to beginning symptoms and the remainder can

be helped immeasurably if we address ourselves more fully to this public health problem.

## MATERNAL AND CHILD HEALTH

The vast majority of public health endeavors are concerned with the population as a whole. There are, however, certain categories of people who merit particular consideration because they are subject to special health risks. Some of these, such as the aged, blind, and deaf have been discussed previously. Traditionally, two groups that have warranted exceptional attention throughout the years have been pregnant women and infants. There are sound reasons for this special consideration. The health of the pregnant woman is important in protecting this adult member of society at a time when she is undergoing a period of unusual stress. It is also recognized that undesirable influences during the prenatal period affect the subsequent health of the infant and may even jeopardize his life.[48] The risks to life are greatest during the early stages of most rapid change and the most pronounced changes in the body occur during the period from conception to maturity. A high risk is present at this time because aberrations may not only distort the path of growth but may become compounded because growth continues in its fundamental pattern. The drastic changes associated with childbirth and the immediate neonatal period present additional threats to the infant and carry considerable risks to the mother as well. The entire population is involved in promotion of maternal and child health because preventive measures taken during the formative years will eventually affect everyone. Thus, programs undertaken for the mother and the infant must be evaluated both in respect to immediate benefits and to the long-range view of establishing a firm foundation to assure a healthy beginning of life for all people in the nation.

The child in his full ecological setting, from conception through adolescence, is the orientation of maternal and child health. The maternal component of maternal and child health centers on the promotion of the general physical and emotional health of the mother surrounding her reproductive experiences. In this connotation, maternal health encompasses the preparation for parenthood, counseling in child rearing and child care, as well as family planning and genetic counseling. Because of such great breadth, maternal and child health programs rely upon both the science and art of medicine. Programs in pediatrics, obstetrics, psychiatry, nursing, social work, hearing and speech, nutrition, dentistry, and neurology are representative of the disciplines utilized. The general categories of concern in this large and important area include maternal health, fetal development, delivery, newborn and infant health, the handicapped child, child growth and development, and the child in society.[49]

In planning parenthood, the young couple is well advised to take advantage of both family planning services and genetic counseling services. The latter is particularly important if there has been a history of abnormalities in the families of either the man or woman. Some of these abnormalities may be cleft palate, Down's syndrome, cardiac anomalies, or X-linked recessive disorders such as hemophylia and muscular dystrophy. Through chromosome analysis, adult carriers of hereditary diseases can be advised of risks to future children. Also, using amniocentesis, withdrawing amniotic fluid from the uterus through a hypodermic needle, study of the fluid and fetal cells early in pregnancy can tell whether the fetus has certain inherited conditions.[50]

Another determination to be made by the expectant mother is whether, indeed, she wishes to carry the baby to full term. Since the Supreme Court ruling, guaranteeing this right to terminate pregnancy during the first trimester, the opportunity has been presented to make a thoughtful determination. It is generally well known that babies born to teen-age girls and to women in their terminal years of childbearing activity have a much greater chance of stillbirth, neonatal or infant death, or birth abnormalities.[51] The health of the prospective mother is another item for serious consideration particularly among teenagers. Historically, the teen-age population generally has been regarded as robust and healthy but increasing reports are questioning this assumption. For example, a study of apparently healthy adolescent girls attending a contraceptive clinic in New York disclosed that two-thirds of the group had undiagnosed medical conditions requiring treatment and over 50 per cent reported psychosocial problems.[52] These and other considerations such as the socio-economic status of the prospective mother, have been shown to exert an unfavorable influence on maternal mortality in the past. Liberalized abortion laws have permitted terminations of pregnancy when conditions were less than favorable and have been credited with much of the reason for the marked reduction in maternal mortality in recent years.[53]

The safest and least difficult time to perform an abortion is during the first trimester of pregnancy. The most common method currently used is vacuum aspiration, in which a thin tube attached to a vacuum line is inserted through the dilated cervix into the uterus to remove the embryonic material. Another method is dilation and curettage (D & C) in which a curette is passed into the uterus through the dilated cervix and the newly conceived embryo is scraped away. In more advanced stages of pregnancy, up to the 24th week, abortions are performed by the saline induction method. In this process a long needle is inserted through the abdominal wall into the uterus and amniotic fluid is removed. This fluid is replaced by a salt solution which kills the fetus. This process is followed by a period of active labor during which the fetus is expelled.[54]

If the expectant mother decides to carry the developing embryo to term it is highly important to seek medical care so that health status can be determined. Women who are a particularly high risk during pregnancy are those with medical complications such as heart disease or diabetes, those with a history of difficult pregnancies, and those who have had abortions or stillbirths. Nutrition plays an extremely important role during this period. Recent studies have confirmed that caloric intake is a determinant in the birth weight of a baby; and increased dietary protein increases the retention of nitrogen and potassium.[55] Malnutrition during the period of pregnancy is a determining factor in the low birth weight of the infant. And there is considerable evidence concerning the overwhelming influence of birth weight as a factor in determining infant mortality. Approximately 90 per cent of babies born at less than 1000 grams die shortly after birth.[56] Diseases associated with pregnancy, the neonatal, and congenital abnormalities are discussed in Chapter 4 of this textbook.

Remarkable progress has been made in the saving of lives of expectant mothers and their infants in the past half-century. Specific figures on infant mortality in the United States were lacking during the beginning years of the present century. In 1913 the nation did not know accurately how many babies were born each year, how many died, or why they died. It was estimated that about 2.5 million children were born each year and that about 300,000 babies died before they were one year old—a rate of about 124 per 1000 live births.

The Children's Bureau, which was in its own infancy, attempted to determine the reasons for such a high death rate by conducting investigations in nine representative cities. These studies were the first of their kind ever undertaken by any nation and showed that the greatest proportion of infant deaths resulted from conditions which existed before birth and which could have been remedied. It was found, for example, that death rates of babies decreased as the fathers' earnings increased, that sanitary conditions were very important, that breast-fed babies had a better chance to survive the dangerous first year than bottle-fed babies, and that a baby with his mother in the home during the first year of life had a better chance than a baby deprived of his mother's care. These findings, although basic and common-place to us, were revolutionary at that time. With the progress in medical information and techniques, public health education, preventive measures, and improved prenatal care, infant mortality fell substantially during the subsequent years. The present infant mortality rate is somewhat below 20 infant deaths per 1000 live births. The major causes of infant deaths have been attributed to postnatal asphyxia and atelectasis, immaturity, congenital malformations, birth injuries, hyaline membrane disease, and ill-defined diseases peculiar to early infancy, including nutritional maladjustments.[57]

Obviously, the decline in mortality rates cannot continue indefinitely. At some point the irreducible minimum must be reached. How-ever, there is abundant evidence that the United States has not reached this optimum level. The infant mortality rate in the United States is currently higher than the rates for the various Scandinavian countries, the Netherlands, Switzerland, England and Wales, Australia and New Zealand, and is slightly higher than some additional European countries, Israel, and Japan. Added to this is the fact that in a few of these countries of low mortality, particularly Denmark and the Netherlands, the rates continued to decline more rapidly than in the United States. Because of the change in the mortality trend, the present situation in the United States is less favorable relative to other countries than was the case 30 years ago.

Similar but less complete studies and programs were conducted on behalf of the mother because it was realized, fortunately, that infancy could not be protected without the protection of maternity. In the 1915 to 1919 period, maternal mortality was 728 per 100,000 live births and the rates changed only slightly until the middle of the 1930 decade. After more concentrated instruction of the mother, improved prenatal care, more stringent observance of hygiene during confinement, and similar measures to make childbearing safer, the rates began to drop rapidly. As mentioned previously, now that a legal choice can be made regarding pregnancy and childbirth, maternal mortality in some sections of the country has been reported to decrease by as much as 50 per cent. Causes of maternal mortality can be considered according to whether the condition arises during pregnancy, delivery, or puerperium. There has been great improvement in rates of mortality from those complications which arise during pregnancy. Other causes are toxemia, hemorrhage, infection, and ectopic pregnancy.[56] Even with the persistence of the downward trend in maternal mortality it is too

Table 11.2

*Infant mortality rates by age and color, 1969*

| Color | Under 1 year | Under 28 days | 28 days — 11 months |
|---|---|---|---|
| Total | 20.9 | 15.6 | 5.3 |
| White | 18.4 | 14.2 | 4.2 |
| All other | 32.9 | 22.5 | 10.4 |

Source: *Monthly Vital Statistics Report, 22:* 10, 1974.

early to contratulate ourselves and rest on our laurels. As long as there are needless deaths there is still room for improvement.

The United States has long prided itself upon being the world's leader in power, industry, wealth, and standard of living. However, this nation is found relatively far down the list when comparing standards of maternal and child health, and mortality rates of mothers and infants. There is increasing cause for concern when other nations are demonstrating that death rates can be lower and, indeed, are widening the gap, further, between their constantly lowering death rates and the rates in the United States. We must realize, however, that international comparisons of vital statistics must be kept in perspective. For comparative purposes, it is preferable to use countries of roughly the same size, comparable economic level, similar population composition, and similar levels of medical care, but the available alternatives are limited.[58] It is recognized that in some international comparisons the data are not comparable, but it is also recognized there are still significant differences that cannot be explained away.

Numerous inquiries have been conducted to determine why this discrepancy exists and why greater progress has not been made. The answers are many and varied and involve social, economic, cultural, religious, ethnic, legal, and moral factors. Some answers are more obvious than others.

Reasons for higher mortality rates may be attributed to cultural patterns and availability of health services. It is accepted, generally, that socio-economic class is a very important discriminating factor. In a survey conducted by the Health Information Foundation and the National Opinion Research Center, University of Chicago, it was found that family income and the educational level of the mother were correlated with the proportions of women who visited a physician early in their pregnancy, the actual number of prenatal visits, the length of hospital stay, and the total expenditure for services. Unfavorable economic conditions of families in the United States are intensified by the fact that medical care is not as freely available to them as it is in some of the European countries. In addition, no maternity allowances are given to cover the extra financial burden of a delivery, and no maternity benefits are given to working pregnant women. In the

majority of countries whose maternal and child mortality rates are below those of the United States, additional steps are taken to protect the infant and his mother. In the Netherlands, in addition to the complete care afforded during all stages of pregnancy and childbirth, a special organization provides maternity care and help in the household for the family and temporarily manages the household duties. In Denmark all women are allowed nine free consultations during pregnancy, and special public health nurses have been employed to supervise infants under one year in private homes. For the infants, 12 visits are made during the year, and the nurse advises the mother on nursing and feeding, recommends free prophylactic medical examinations, and routinely conducts phenylketonuria tests. In addition, each child less than seven years old may be examined nine times free of charge by a physician, three of which are during the first year of life. Although these preventive and remedial measures were developed under a program of national health insurance, the results of these endeavors have paid off in lower mortality rates. As the various health agencies and medical disciplines, under the financial encouragement of Federal legislation, further explore questions and possible answers regarding maternal and child health in the United States, perhaps the examples set by some European countries may serve as guidelines.

Certainly, the problems in the United States are far from being solved. This is particularly true within cities of a population of over 500,000. As there has been an influx of lower income and higher mortality risk groups to the large cities, there has been a corresponding increase in the number of people who are dependent upon tax-supported medical services. Compounding the problem is the fact that this same group seeks prenatal care late in pregnancy or not at all, and, at the same time, this is the group with an excessive rate of low birth-weight babies.

Together with these worsening social factors is the increasing cost of hospital care with a decrease in the ability of voluntary institutions to provide free prenatal and hospital delivery care. The result has been an increase in the number of deliveries in tax-supported hospitals without an increase in bed capacity.

The many hazards which accompany pregnancy, childbirth, and infancy call for truly multidisciplinary concern and responsibility. All divisions of the allied medical professions are involved to various degrees, and the goals of ensuring safe pregnancies and deliveries as well as healthy infants can be approached only through a broad, co-operative public health program in maternal and child welfare. In order to formulate and act upon an organized program, however, we must ponder some of the problems. Why is it that during a period of economic advancement and allocation of economic resources to medical care, the infant mortality rate has undergone only minor reductions? We are faced with a series of paradoxes. Although there is widespread use of certain diagnostic tests, such as PKU for phenylketonuria, other tests for the evaluation of women with various suspected metabolic or endocrinological disorders require highly sophisticated techniques utilizing expensive equipment and can be conducted only in the great medical centers; thus, these services are limited to a very few. Changes in patterns of living and transportation have enabled the establishment of regional clinics to service a community of small towns in rural areas, and the development of hospitals large enough to provide more complex services for broad geographical areas. Contrasted to this, many of the underprivileged groups, particularly in large cities, cannot or will not take advantage of medical services that are not in the immediate vicinity of their homes. Perhaps a new evaluation and a reorientation are in order. There is a growing philosophy among allied medical workers concerned with public health that is not enough to establish these services in a given place and then sit back and expect all needy people to come for aid. Economic, educational, and cultural backgrounds of significant population groups dictate otherwise.

The level of the community's general health program is the foundation upon which specialized maternal and child health services must be built and directly affects the health of mothers and children. In the area of general health services the community characteristically provides environmental health services, community nursing services, nutrition programs, and health programs for migrant worker families. Activities in the environmental health field have concentrated on the provision of safe milk and water supplies and adequate sewage disposal, resulting in marked reduction of diarrhea, tuberculosis, and typhoid. Another environmental health interest is the use of diagnostic X-ray and fluoroscopic examinations. There is no longer any disagreement on the harmful nature of the biological effects of ionizing radiation and young, growing tissues are more susceptible than are mature tissues. For this reason, a minimum use of X-ray on pregnant women and children is encouraged and fluoroscopic examinations are practically contraindicated.

The public health responsibility of community nursing services has traditionally been divided between voluntary visiting nurse associations and the official nursing services of health departments. There has been a trend toward consolidation of the two types of services but the progress has been slow and spotty. The public health nurse is the vital link in reaching the high-risk groups early in pregnancy and in maintaining and ensuring care for women who have had an unfavorable outcome of a previous pregnancy. The need to concentrate the limited nursing manpower on those health problems which are most acute has resulted in decreased attention on home visiting for routine prenatal and newborn care. In addition, the rising demands for bedside nursing has depleted supplies of available nurses so that even the high-risk groups do not receive adequate attention.

The value of optimum nutrition for the expectant mother cannot be overemphasized, and, yet, nutrition programs directed mainly toward pregnant women may be relatively ineffective because they may not reach the most vulnerable groups. Women who have late or no prenatal care remain outside the scope of the programs. Also, the early age at which first pregnancies frequently occur suggests that any nutritional deficiencies during adolescence carry over into pregnancy. As previously noted in the discussion of nutrition in this chapter, unbalanced diets and food fads are frequent among adolescent girls at all social levels in the United States. An indication of the consequences of poor nutrition in the expectant mother can be seen in reported animal studies. It was found that when the mothers were underfed by as little as 25 per cent during pregnancy and lactation their offspring exhibited stunted growth, reduced capacity for antibody production, lowered resistance to hypothermal stress, required more food per unit of body weight, and lost more nitrogen through urinary excretion. These conditions did not improve when the offspring were freely fed adequate diets. A more recent study of nine- and ten-year-old children in Taiwan evidences support of the findings in animals.

The migrant farm worker and his family suffer the general disadvantage of being on one of the lowest rungs of the economic ladder. Also, their constant transiency interferes with their ability to make use of local health services. For these reasons grants of Federal funds have been made available to the states for special health programs for migrants and their families. In spite of the progress which has been achieved in this area, it is still very difficult to maintain a continuity of health care as the migrant laborer and his family follow the crops. This raises a particular difficulty in maternal and child health.

More specialized health programs for mothers and infants are, usually, the result of the combined interests and support of the community, state, and Federal agencies. Usually, the specific activity is administered by a local or state agency with the funding shared by all three levels of government. Maternal health programs of the past, often using itinerant clinics, concentrated on promoting regular prenatal care through health education and the provision of demonstration prenatal care services. The great majority of women with babies delivered by private obstetricians today, however, have had regular prental care from the first trimester of pregnancy. The prenatal visits, which are spaced more closely together as term approaches, include routine medical examinations and laboratory tests. This highly personalized type of routine care has probably been the major factor in reduction of incidences involving toxemia and other serious complications of pregnancy.

As pointed out earlier in this discussion, the problem today seems to be focused among the indigent groups in major metropolitan centers. Prenatal and postpartum care for these groups is provided in Neighborhood Health Centers or through outpatient clinics housed in either municipal or voluntary hospitals. The same population shifts that have increased the pressure on inpatient facilities have affected outpatient clinics as well. In some areas the pressure has become so great that clinic patients may have to spend an entire day for a single prenatal visit. Inasmuch as there are many factors which interfere with the provision of adequate prenatal care to women in the lower socio-economic groups, gross inadequacy in the volume of clinic services is, undoubtedly, an important element. This serves to further discourage prenatal care among groups which may not be motivated to seek care in the first place, and it well may be an important reason why some major municipal hospitals report a relatively high percentage of women who had no prenatal care at all and first came to the hospital after labor had started.

Diversity, complexity, and change are the outstanding characteristics in the patterns of maternal and child health care in the United States today. Ranging from individually financed care by general practitioners and specialists through complete services supplied by voluntary or tax-supported agencies, there is so much confusion, duplication of services, and gaps in service that it is difficult to match the need with available help. Each agency and foundation has its own policies. Some limit their activities to health education, others support research, and still other groups promote and support special clinical facilities and services or finance individual patient care. Coordination of these services is needed if continuity of care is to be attained in the best interest of the patient.

Of the many agencies which have made major contributions to maternal and child health throughout the years, the Children's Bureau is the most prominent. Prior to the establishment of the Children's Bureau there were organized efforts to contend with the problems of pregnant women and infants that gradually focused attention upon the need for special consideration for these groups. The American Medical Association organized a section of obstetrics and diseases of women and children in 1873. Three years later the Society for the Prevention of Cruelty to Children was formed, followed by the establishment, in 1888, of the American Pediatric Society. Milk stations were developed in New York City in 1893 and served as the forerunner of the present-day well-baby clinics. The first Bureau of Child Hygiene was started in New York in 1908 and the series of White House Conferences on Children began in 1909.

The impetus for the creation of the Children's Bureau was due largely to the efforts of two women, Lillian Wald and Florence Kelley. The thrust of their approach was—"if the government can have a department to look after the nation's farm crop, why can't it have a bureau to look after the nation's child crop." The first bills proposing a Federal Children's Bureau were introduced in both houses of Congress in 1906, and failed. Similar bills were introduced during each of the following six years and gathered growing support due to activities of parents' organizations, labor unions, health workers, and women in general, and Presidents Roosevelt and Taft. Finally, in 1912, the bill passed both houses of Congress and was signed into law. The Constitutional base for the law was the general welfare clause. The Children's Bureau was first assigned to the Department of Commerce and Labor, and, then, in 1913, to the newly formed Department of Labor. In 1946 the Bureau was transferred to the Federal Security Agency which, in turn, was incorporated into the Department of Health, Education, and Welfare in 1953.

The mandate assigned to the Bureau was to find the facts that can lead to better health and welfare for mothers and children, and to report those facts to the nation so that they can be of maximum use to parents and to professional groups, both public and voluntary. A very large portion of all Federal legislation involving maternal and child health is administered through the Children's Bureau. Acts of Congress such as the Sheppard-Towner Act of 1921, the Social Security Act of 1935, the Emergency Maternity and Infant Care Program of 1943, the Vocational Rehabilitation Act of 1954, research and demonstration projects in 1960, health-planning legislation, and sweeping changes and additions to the Social Security Act in 1963, 1965, and 1972 are representative of the support and broad based activities of the Bureau. In spite of Federal legislation and government involvement there still remains much to be done, particularly in the field of child care. The White House Conference on Children has addressed itself to this problem and has issued a plea for the creation of a child advocate system to protect the interests and, indeed, the lives of children.[59] The preamble to the Conference Report issues the following warning:

Our children and our families are in deep trouble. A society that neglects its children and fears its youth cannot care about its future. Surely this is the way to a National disaster.

The chairman of the Senate Subcommittee on Children and Youth has listed some of the findings related to health. Some of these findings are the following: 12 million children with eye conditions, 3 million with speech impediments, and 2 million with orthopedic handicaps are not getting the special care they require; less than half the children who need mental health services ever receive them; and 35 per cent of the children under the age 15 have never seen a dentist.[60] In efforts to counteract these and other conditions, additional programs have been introduced at the Federal level. Among these are Headstart, Children and Youth Projects under Title V, and Maternal and Infant Care Projects. Most of these newer programs emphasize a multidisciplinary approach to health and welfare problems.[61] Programs administered through the Federal Government include maternal and child health services, crippled children's services, child welfare services, juvenile delinquency services, and grants for research or demonstration projects, for training professionals for care of crippled children, and special project grants for maternity and infant care, and for health of school and preschool children. Other organized programs to promote maternal and child health have been developed in state and local health departments and through the endeavors of societies and agencies such as the American Public Health Association, the American Academy of Pediatrics, the National Congress of Parents and Teachers, and the National Foundation.

Nevertheless, with all the available programs and interested help, the actual delivery of maternal and child health services is performed in the community on a local level. There is no other special category of public health which requires more co-operative endeavors of all the allied medical professions. Particular emphasis is placed upon the economically and culturally deprived not only because the need is greater here but because the disadvantaged must have preferential treatment if they are to catch up. The efforts of all those in the health fields are needed to promote adequate levels of family planning, organization and availability of high quality medical care, and personal health practices of the population.

## ACCIDENTAL POISONING IN CHILDREN

A child drinks an unknown quantity of

hair-curling solution, another ingests cream deodorant, and still another drinks some perfume. Additional calls which come into the Poison Control Center reports the child who drank bleach from a cup that his mother had placed near the washing machine, who drank kerosene from a soda pop bottle in his father's workshop, or who swallowed 18 to 20 children's aspirin tablets because they looked and tasted like candy. These children were not trying to commit suicide. Their energetic spirit and restless curiosity prompts them to explore the world about them, to experience new sensations, and to use their bodily senses to acquaint themselves with their environment. It is characteristic of infants to place any and all objects in their mouths, and young children will glibly eat items that would nauseate a more mature person. They have their own frame of reference in regard to what tastes good and what tastes bad, and the toxicity of the products does not restrict their choice.

The products which are ingested usually are not considered in terms of their toxicity. They do not have a skull and crossbones on them nor do they have the word, poison, emblazoned in red letters across the label. Nonetheless, when taken in adequate quantities they can make the child very ill indeed, and may be life-threatening. These items and similar products are found, literally by the thousands, lining the shelves of supermarkets, pharmacies, auto supply stores, nurseries, feed stores, and a myriad of other outlets. Compounding this problem is the fact that a significant number of products capable of causing toxic reactions in humans may not have the contents listed on the label. When ingested, valuable time is lost in attempting to secure this information before specific antidotal treatment can be initiated. With the passage of the Child Protection Act and the Federal Hazardous Substances Act the danger to the consumer has been reduced but it is still the responsibility of the individual household to eliminate the hazards.

The actual number of accidental poisoning cases per year in children is not known although estimates range from 500,000 to 2,000,000. The National Clearinghouse for Poison Control Centers tabulates annually the poison report forms voluntarily submitted by 505 poison control centers in 47 states. It is recognized that these statistics do not represent the total national incidence of ingestions because many of the poisoning cases are treated by private physicians and hospitals not directly associated with the Poison Control Center network. Although the number of reports received are greater each year, this does not necessarily reflect an increasing number of accidents. Instead, it may indicate a higher percentage of reporting. The mortality data are more complete inasmuch as they are received from the National Vital Statistics Division of the U. S. Public Health Service and are derived from death certificates submitted by the states. In 1971 the National Clearinghouse received reports of 84,370 ingestions among children under five years of age, and deaths from accidental poisoning in this age group number 245. That this latter figure is not substantially higher is a testimony to the dedicated work of pediatricians as well as to combined efforts of all of the health professionals involved in poisoning control.

An analysis of the various reports submitted reveals some interesting facts concerning accidental poisoning in children. Ninety per cent of the reports involve children under the age of five. Almost one-fourth of the total occurred in children between the ages of 18 and 24 months. Approximately three-fourths involved children between the ages of 12 and 36 months. Almost all of the cases of poisoning involved either household products or medications. Of the medications, aspirin accounts for 10 per cent of the cases. The household products most commonly ingested by children are cleaning and polishing agents, pesticides, turpentine and paints, pertroleum products, and cosmetics.[62] The danger hours for children seem to be during the early morning just before the parents arise and between the hours of four and six in the evening. About one-third of all poisoning accidents occur in the kitchen. In almost two-thirds of kitchen accidents the substances were not in their customary storage places, and in over one-fourth of all kitchen accidents the materials were not in their original containers at the time of ingestion. Ninety-three per cent of the time, an adult member of the family was at home when poisoning accidents took place, and public health officials declare that 95 per cent of all poisonings are definitely classified as preventable.

The Committee on Toxicology of The American Medical Association has estimated that as many as 250,000 trade name products contain substances that are capable of causing toxicity when ingested in sufficient quantity. A requirement of the Occupational Safety and Health Act of 1970 is the publication of a Toxic Substances List. This publication, available from the National Institute for Occupational Safety and Health, currently contains 25,000 chemical substances. The publication also attempts to identify all known toxic substances which may exist in the human environment and provide pertinent data on their effects.[63] The physician, although well informed concerning toxic effects of most medical agents, cannot be expected to know or remember· the ingredients or to realize the potential harmfulness of even a small percentage of commercial products found in the home. Poisoning is the number one pediatric emergency, and time is an important factor that will determine whether or not the child survives a poisoning incident. Reliable, up-to-the-minute information regarding the contents of these products, their possible toxicity, and the proper means of combating accidental poisoning by them can make a vital difference in the outcome of treatment.

To meet this need, a repository of readily available information, emergency equipment and antidotes, and specially trained personnel are essential. The first Poison Control Center was organized in Chicago in 1953 by the American Academy of Pediatrics, the Chicago Board of Health, the Illinois State Toxicology Laboratory, the University of Illinois, and six major teaching hospitals. Other pioneers in this development were New York City and the states of Florida and Arizona. There are now approximately 590 poison control centers listed in the United States[64] and about 85 per cent of them are associated with the National Clearinghouse network. These centers may range from limited quarters in a portion of a hospital emergency room to large, complex treatment centers with full supporting facilities. Some are operated independently of any other service but most are co-operative endeavors and are a part of statewide systems. The centers, of course, are not restricted to childrens' poisoning and, although there are significant differences between facilities, each center has several features common to all. A 24-hr. telephone service is maintained to furnish immediate information, and references are on file to supply additional data. Appropriate therapeutic agents are kept handy for emergency use, and a pharmacist is usually immediately available for consultation regarding overdoses of medicinal agents. A physician, serving as poison control officer, usually supervises treatment given by residents, interns, and nurses. Pertinent facts concerning the circumstances and nature of each poisoning, the

Table 11.3

*Accidental ingestions among children under 5 years of age*

| Types of Substance | 1971 | |
|---|---|---|
| | No. | Per cent |
| Medicines | 39,917 | 47.3 |
| Internal | 33,610 | 39.8 |
| Aspirin | 8,529 | 10.1 |
| Other | 25,081 | 29.7 |
| External | 6,307 | 7.5 |
| Cleaning & polishing agents | 13,199 | 15.7 |
| Petroleum products | 3,663 | 4.4 |
| Plants | 4,636 | 5.5 |
| Cosmetics | 6,200 | 7.4 |
| Pesticides | 4,513 | 5.4 |
| Gases & vapors | 95 | 0.1 |
| Turpentine, paints, etc. | 5,051 | 6.0 |
| Miscellaneous | 6,195 | 7.4 |
| Unknown | 701 | 0.8 |
| Total | 84,370 | 100.0 |

Source: Adapted from National Safety Council, Accident Facts, 1973 Edition.

treatment administered, and the outcome are recorded to determine trends and patterns.

Statewide poison control networks have proven to be an effective system and are found in an increasing number of states. The State of Arizona is representative of this type of organization. In this state, the Poison Control Committee of the state medical association directs the program. The Poison Control Information Center is located in the College of Pharmacy and treatment centers are located in the emergency rooms of hospitals strategically located throughout the state. The director of the Information Center is a professor of pharmacology who also directs toxiciological research, courses in toxicology, and continuing education in the various aspects· of poisoning prevention and treatment for physicians and lay personnel. It was in the laboratories of the College of Pharmacy at the University at the University of Arizona that research was conducted which led to the affirmation that large dilution of stomach contents before attempted emesis is contraindicated, and that the administration of activated charcoal is more efficacious as an antidote than use of the so-called universal antidote. Another highly effective state-wide program with even more comprehensive technical and professional assistance is Poison Central in the State of Kentucky. The focal point of this program is the Institute of Environmental Toxicology and Occupational Hygiene located in the College of Pharmacy at the University of Kentucky.[65]

With the rapid growth of poison control centers throughout the United States, the need was soon seen for a central coordinating agency to receive reports and to disseminate information on a national basis. In 1957 the Surgeon General, at the request of the American Public Health Association, established the National Clearinghouse for Poison Control Centers. This Clearinghouse, referred to previously in this discussion, regularly supplies the poison control centers with information on toxicity of trade name products for their card file index systems and a periodical bulletin on current poisoning topics. The information which is voluntarily supplied to the Clearinghouse from the various centers serves as the basis for much of our current knowledge regarding poisonings.

With the renewed interest in the incidence of poisoning and concerted activity among health professionals who are working on this problem, a number of beneficial results have accrued. A new assessment of traditional ideas and practices has been called for and fresh concepts have been introduced. For example, some widely used drugs such as boric acid, oil of wintergreen, camphorated oil, and ammoniated mercury ointment have now been indicted not only as comparatively useless but actually dangerous. In reference to warning signs on labels, the Michigan State Pharmaceutical Association conceived a label featuring a striking snake over the words "Warning—Keep Out of the Reach of Children." Their departure from the time-honored skull and crossbones symbol of danger was prompted by the observation that television and motion pictures have made the skull and crossbones a too familiar symbol in other fields. Following publicity in a national news magazine, a flood of request for labels was received from government officials, the military, industry, civic leaders, physicians, and pharmacists. Another renewed practice which is receiving wider acceptance, at this time, is the use of safety caps on certain types of medicine containers. It is recognized that such closures are not satisfactory for all purposes. Parents may be lulled into a sense of false security with these containers and relax their safety precautions by not reckoning with the agility, mobility, and ingenuity of youngsters. The locking device never has been recommended as a substitute for educational and information programs, however. Comprehensive implementation of the Poison Prevention Packaging Act of 1970, administered by the Consumer Products Safety Commission, calls for even more stringent regulations.[66] Not only are pharmacists responsible for providing safety caps on prescription medications but child-protection packaging standards are required for all non-prescription drugs which are subject to the Act.

Although emesis is contraindicated in cases of poisoning by acids, alkalies, and petroleum distillates, and usually is to be discouraged if the child can be brought promptly to a poison control treatment center, there are significant numbers and seriousness of cases where prompt and effective emesis is highly important. Recognizing that stimulation of the gag reflex is not always dependable, the American Academy of Pediatrics has recommended the use of syrup of ipecac. This procedure has been approved by medical groups and government agencies,[67] and syrup of ipecac, which was formerly restricted to prescription use, can now be purchased in pharmacies in limited quantities for emergency use in the home. This medication is generally considered to act both centrally and in the gastrointestinal tract to cause vomiting. The average time required for this emetic action is between 15 and 30 minutes.

It is not enough to establish poison control centers and to devise better ways to treat poison cases. If these cases could be prevented there would be little need for extensive remedial measures. In recognition of this fact Congress, through Public Law 87-319, authorized the President to proclaim the third week in March of each year as National Poison Prevention Week. This time of the year was chosen because of spring housecleaning when cleaning chemicals are often lying about the house in easy reach of small children. Twenty-one agencies comprise the National Planning Council for National Poison Prevention Week and each organization cooperates in publicity regarding this important occasion. One week of emphasis is hardly enough, however, to control this public health problem. The threat of accidental poisoning is present whenever active, inquistive children are in the presence of potentially toxic products. We, as health guardians of our community, can contribute materially to educating the public toward reducing accidental poisonings in children through our everyday contacts with patients, by directing the attention of Parent-Teacher Associations and other civic-minded groups to the gravity of the problem,by outlining the steps needed to solve it, and by direct involvement in prevention programs.[68]

## REFERENCES

1. Berg, A. *The Nutrition Factor: Its Role in National Development.* Washington, D. C.: Brookings Institution, 1973.
2. Shank, R. F. Ever-widening horizons. *Amer. J. Clin. Nutr., 21:* 10, *1968.*
3. Latham, M. C., and Cobos, F. *The effects of malnutrition on intellectual development and learning. Amer. J. Public Health, 61:* 7, 1971.
4. Johnston, P. V. Nutrition and neural development. *Food Nutr. News, 45:* 3, 1974.
5. AMA Council on Foods and Nutrition. Malnutrition and hunger in the United States. *J.A.M.A., 213:* 1970.
6. Henderson, L. M. Nutritional problems growing out of new patterns of food consumption. *Amer. J. Public Health, 62:* 9, 1972.
7. Nutrition survey shows dietary deficiencies. *Health Resources News, 1:* 6, 1974.
8. Roels, O. A. Vitamin A physiology. *J.A.M.A., 214:* 6, *1970.*
9. *Vitamins. Documenta Geigy.* Basle, Switzerland: Ciba-Geigy Limited, 1970.
10. DeLuca, H. F. New forms of Vitamin $D_3$ and their potential applications. *Nutri. News, 36:* 4, 1973.
11. Vitamin E as a biological antioxidant. *Dairy Council Digest, 42:* 4, 1971.
12. Rosenberg, L. E. Vitamin-dependent genetic disease. *Hospital Practice, 5:* 7, 1970.
13. Essential dietary metals may control blood fats. *Health Services Rep., 88:* 2, 1973.
14. Sandstead, H. H. Zinc nutrition in the United States. *Amer. J. Clin. Nutr., 26:* 1251, 1973.
15. Gracey, M. Microbial contamination of the gut: Another feature of malnutrition. *Amer. J. Clin. Nutri., 26:* 1170, 1973.
16. Prevalence of selected chronic digestive conditions. *Vital and Health Statistics, 10:* 83, DHEW Pub. No. (HRA) 74-1510, 1973.
17. What you should know about obesity. *Amer. Druggist, 169:* 4, 1974.
18. Albrink, M. J. Endocrine aspects of obesity. *Amer. J. Clin. Nutr., 21:* 12, 1968.
19. Frankle, R. T. and Heussenstamm, F. K. Food zealotry and youth. *Amer. J. Public Health, 64:* 1, 1974.
20. Penna, R. P. *O-T-C Antacids. Handbook of Non-Prescription Drugs.* American Pharmaceutical Association, 1967.
21. Hirschman, J. L., and Herfindal, E. T. Peptic ulcer disease. *J. Amer. Pharm. Assn., 11:* 8, 1971.
22. Brotman, H. B. The fastest growing minority: the aging. *Amer. J. Public Health, 64:* 3, 1974.
23. Shanas, E. Health Status of Older People. *Amer. J. Public Health, 64:* 3, 1974.
24. *Number of Elders Growing Nationwide.* Metropolitan Life Insurance Co., Statistical Bulletin, 54: 1, 1973.
25. Elwood, T. W. Old age and the quality of life. *Health Services Rep., 87:* 10, 1972.
26. *Human Aging II—An Eleven Year Followup Biomedical and Behavioral Study.* NIMH, DHEW Pub. No. (HSM) 71-9037, 1971.
27. *NIMH Research on the Mental Health of the Aging.* National Institute of Mental Health. DHEW Pub. No. (HSM) 72-9133, 1972.
28. Severinghaus, E. L. Nutritional problems after fifty. *Food Nutr. News, 43:* 6, 1972.
29. Gordon, R. H. Meeting dental health needs of the aged. *Amer. J. Public Health, 62:* 3, 1972.
30. Selected aspects of geriatric nutrition. *Dairy Council Digest, 43:* 2, 1972.
31. Harris, R. S. Phosphates: A promising agent for use in the control of dental caries. *Nutr. News, 34:* 1, 1971.
32. Mello, A. F. *Dental Public Health—What Is It:* Paper presented at the 42nd Annual Meeting of the Arizona Public Health Association, 1972.
33. Need for dental care among adults. *Vital and Health Statistics, 11:* 36, 1970.
34. National health survey measures the national health. *Health Resources News, 1:* 5, 1974.
35. Heise, A. L. *et al.* Meeting the dental treatment needs of indigent rural children. *Health Services Rep., 88:* 7, 1973.

36. The impact of food and nutrition on oral Health. *Dairy Council Digest, 44:* 3, 1973.

37. *Fluoridation–No Better Health Investment.* Division of Dental Health, NKH, 1970.

38. Shannon, I. L. and Feller, R. P. Enamel solubility reduction by mixtures of stannous fluoride and acidulated phosphofluoride. *J. Dent. Assoc. S. Afr., 27:* 9, 1972.

39. *The Dentist and the Pharmacist.* American Dental Association, 1970.

40. Hussar, D. A. Interactions Involving drugs used in dental practice. *J. Amer. Pharm. Assn., 13:* 5, 1973.

41. Forbes, M., P. Guillermo, Jr., and Grolman, B. A noncontact applanation tonometer. *Sight-Saving Rev., 43:* 3, 1973.

42. *Cataract: Fact and Fancy.* National Society for the Prevention of Blindness, Inc., Pub. G-4, 1974.

43. Roberts, J. Vision test validation study. *Vital and Health Statistics, 2:* 59, 1973.

44. *Profile of Blind Persons.* Metropolitan Life Insurance Co., Statistical Bulletin, July, 1973.

45. Prevention of blindness. Pan-American Health Organization. *PAHO Bull.,, 7:* 3, 1973.

46. Myers, D. *et al.* Otologic diagnosis and the treatment of deafness. Ciba Pharmaceutical Co. *Clin. Symp., 22:* 2, 1970.

47. Deafness. St. Louis College of Pharmacy. *Pharmaceutical Trends, 9:* 6, 1973.

48. Smiley, J. *et al.* Maternal and infant health and their associated factors. *Amer. J. Public Health, 62:* 4, 1972.

49. Cornely, D. A. and Broussard, E. R. Maternal and Child Health and Mental Health, in Mental Health Considerations in Public Health. Washington, D. C., PHS Pub. No. 1898, 1969.

50. Clinical genetics gain notice. Medical News Section, *J.A.M.A., 213:* 13, 1970.

51. Bender, D. E. *et al.* Factors affecting postneonatal mortality. *HSMA Health Rep., 86:* 5, 1971.

52. Fiedler, D. E., Lang, D. M. and Carlson, J. M. Pathology of the "healthy" female teenager. *Amer. J. Public Health, 63:* 11, 1973.

53. Liberal state abortion laws affect maternal mortality. *Health Service Rep., 87:* 5, 1972.

54. Marshall, C. L. *Dynamics of Health and Disease.* New York: Appleton-Century-Crofts, 1972.

55. Munro, H. M. Report of a conference on protein and amino acid needs for growth and development. *Amer. J. Clin. Nutr., 27:* 1, 1974.

56. Erhardt, C. L., and Chase, H. C. Ethnic Group, education of mother and birth weight. In *A Study of Risks, Medical Care, and Infant Mortality.* Amer. J. Public Health, 63: Supplement, 1973.

57. Final Infant, Fetal, and Maternal Mortality, 1969. *Vital Statistics Rep., 22:* 10, Supplement, 1974.

58. Chase, H. C. The position of the United States in international comparisons of health status. *Amer. J. Public Health, 62: 4, 1972.*

59. White House Conference on Children. Newsletter, Nov. 1970.

60. Remarks of Senator Walter F. Mondale. *Amer. J. Public Health, 62:* 7, 1972.

61. Stoeffler, V. R., Meyer, R., and Smith, D. C. Lessons to be learned from new child health programs. *Amer. J. Public Health, 62:* 11, 1972.

62. National Safety Council. *Accident Facts,* 1973 edition.

63. *25,000 Chemicals Included in NIDSH Toxic Substances List.* The Nation's Health, Jan. 1974.

64. Directory, Poison Control Centers (FDA), *72:* 7001, 1971.

65. Luckens, M. M. Developing total service capabilities in poison information centers. *Amer. J. Public Health, 62:* 3, 1972.

66. *Weekly Pharmacy Reports, 23:* 7, 1974.

67. Initial management of acute poisoning. *Med. Letter, 13:* 9, 1971.

68. Norwood, J. G., and Rotello, N. D. An accidental poisoning prevention program. *J. Amer. Pharm. Assn., 13:* 3, 1973.

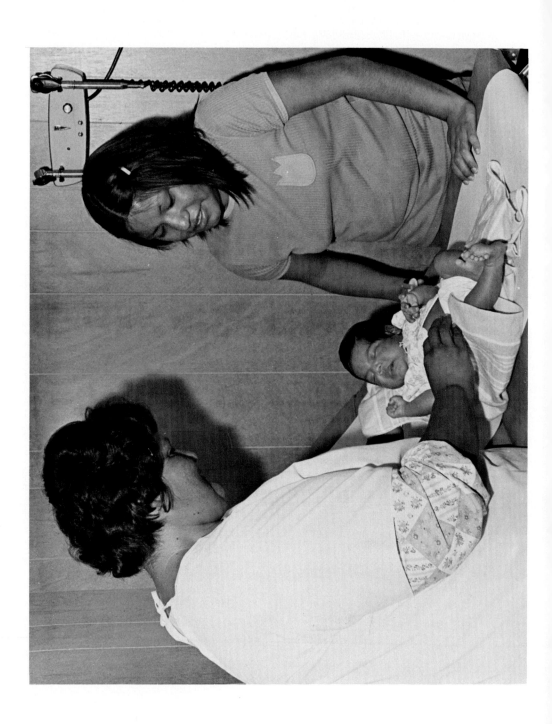

# 12

# The health professions

It is arguable that if disease is defined so that it would be treatable by a complex of medical, welfare, religious, mental health, and educational services, the conceptual effort to synthesize these services will be negated by the practical need to have the services delivered by a doctor, welfare worker, minister, mental health worker, or teacher.

HAROLD RASHKIS[1]

With the advent of newer health programs, with vast increases in the numbers of people seeking medical care, and with new health facilities developing in virtually all segments of the nation there are now demands for health services which greatly exceed present capabilities to deliver such services. Because of its current failure to meet demands, contemporary health care is being challenged, and it must be assumed that all those professions participating in health services will have to make changes in their contributions to the total program.

One of the answers to this great demand for high quality services is to produce large numbers of trained medical personnel to continue performing their historic functions within the discipline of their individual professions. Obviously, however, the training of such personnel takes considerable time, and there is every indication that medical needs will continue to mount so that even an increased supply will not meet the growing demand.

Adjunctive to the preparation of additional health workers is the need for each profession to re-examine its role and duties, some of which are protected by law, and others which professional prerogatives have reserved for a limited segment of medical practitioners. Most health professions have lived in an era of professional isolation and have been concerned primarily with improving health care within the parameters and limitations of their own disciplines. In rethinking their roles the health professions must ultimately address themselves to the fundamental and crucial issue of how best to deliver total health services. They must determine who can best perform certain functions with the greatest effectiveness and efficiency regardless of previously imposed limitations. Every professional involved in health care performs duties which are standard, routine and which others could do equally well, if not better. An answer to the health manpower shortage, then, may be to reassign such duties to responsible persons with lesser training, and to reserve for the professional those decision-making, highly skilled procedures which utilize his background and intensive preparation. It is recognized that professional qualifications, political concern, and prestige will be challenged in the reassignment of duties. Medical personnel are historically conservative and adopt change rather slowly. But such a procedure will help, objectively and constructively, to build the matrix of a new and vigorous health care system.

One of the problems that had plagued the medical care field was the lack of appreciation of the health team concept, and the failure to broaden the horizon of interprofessional rapport and understanding. Indeed, the health team has been referred to as a paper team,[2] and "team care" is a concept to which many people give lip service but which still has far from optional implementation.[3] For example, an assessment of a team effort during a seminar on interprofessional education concluded that each member of the team maintained his own professional role and identity. The team members appeared preoccupied with changes occurring in their own professions, seeing themselves as resource persons rather than as team members. Another example of still widespread professional isolationism was the report of aborted efforts to change State laws regulating health manpower in Minnesota. A committee was convened, composed of representatives from nine of the leading health professions plus professional licensing boards. The report states: "The intensive and at times heated deliberations of this committee did not result in achieving a concensus because of irreconcilable professional differences."[4] In our efforts to protect our own profession we may be in danger of losing sight of our main objective, the care of the patient. Certainly, the old, settled way by which the members of the health professions have related with one another no longer seems functional.[5] It has only been within recent years that the valuable contributions of each of the allied medical professions have been recognized as complementary to the total program of preventive and clinical medicine. The technology of therapy has become so complex that all of the requisite skills cannot be developed in a single person or a single profession.[6] In recognition of this fact a new philosophy has emerged regarding the concept of the health team. The physician is viewed no longer as a sergeant commanding a platoon of subordinates. In contrast, the physician now may be likened more to a quarterback on a football team. It is necessary for someone to co-ordinate the efforts and to assume responsibility for the total regimen but the co-operation of each member of the team is needed to assure the success of the entire program. At one time the education of the physician was clearly superior to that of the other health professions and he dominated the field without any challenge. As the education of various health professions moved to university settings, however, a substantial upgrading in the training has served to close the gap. This is particularly true for the allied health practitioners who return for graduate level training. Also, newer methods of health care delivery, such as HMO's encourage the effective utilization of a true health care team. Each discipline represents one portion of the skills needed to carry patients through the period of diagnosis, treatment, and rehabilitation.

Subsequent paragraphs in this chapter describe various allied medical professions as separate entities. It is recognized, however, that each is a member of a team of dedicated health professionals who achieve their most significant objectives when they work together. Most of these professions have increased requirements for training and standards of performance within recent years, and practitioners within the professions must pass comprehensive examinations and meet other criteria for certification, registration, or licensure. Certainly, in order to meet the growing need for more comprehensive health services each of the health professions must enlarge its sphere of activity, and must utilize each member of the medical team to his most appropriate and utmost capacity.

## ACTIVITIES AND FUNCTIONS OF SPECIFIC HEALTH DISCIPLINES

### The Medical Doctor

The medical doctor must know and understand as fully as possible the functions of the human body and mind. He must also understand the disease itself and the treatments and drugs available in order to master the disease. Academically speaking, he must have a thorough comprehension of anatomy, physiology, histology, and pathology as well as all the remedies, mechanical and medicinal. The physician must diagnose, treat, and cure disease or relieve the unpleasant symptoms as much as possible. He also must be prepared to relieve pain from injuries and to restore damage which has occurred.

The work of the physician is difficult and detailed. Certainly there is glamour and drama, but much more of it is prosaic and frankly unpleasant. The reward is in the satisfaction of relieving suffering and saving life itself. The financial rewards and prestige, however, are not to be disregarded.

Becoming a physician demands intellectual, physical, and emotional stamina. The medical doctor must be able to master all of the biological, physical, and chemical sciences in a minimum of 7 years after high school, although most doctors today continue their studies for 10 to 15 years. He must be capable of alertness at all hours and must often be able to move accurately from one disease to another with little rest. He must not fall prey to disease despite constant exposure. Most of all, he must have the ability to face human tragedy so as to be an effective as well as a sympathetic helper. His work depends on his intellectual background, his keen observation and acute analysis, his sound judgment, and his sense of duty.

Medical schools in the United States award a degree of Doctor of Medicine (M.D.) after successful completion of three or four years of work. Until recently a premedical course in a liberal arts college was advised as preparation, but, because of the higher degree of intensity and specialty now encountered, a major in a particular scientific field is more favorably looked upon for entrance. There is a greater tendency to specialize in the undergraduate curriculum, with the courses more abstract, deeper and narrower, and less relevant to real life. This trend is resulting in the entering medical student's being deficient in some of the basic sciences and the biology of organs.

Not only has the academic background of the medical student changed, but also his socio-economic background. No longer is a medical education a privilege reserved for the upper class. With the greater availability of scholarships and a more enlightened approach to education in general, capable students from poorer families now have a much greater opportunity. The Association of American Medical Colleges reports the cost of educating a medical student to be between $16,300 and $26,400 a year. Of that amount, a student pays an average of $4600 annually.[7] Private sources and medical associations help to pay for some of the remaining costs but the bulk of the educational expense is paid through tax funds. Officials in HEW are predicting, however, that much of this Federal money may soon diminish, as reflected in the following statement: "We are now questioning very seriously whether it is appropriate for the Federal Government to bear so substantial a share of the cost of preparing individuals for careers that offer about the highest earning power in our society. We simply have to question whether taxpayers should continue to be expected to subsidize tuition costs for medical students, but not for students in other fields whose income expectations fall far below that of the physicians."[8]

The number of medical schools has not risen in proportion to preparatory colleges, and the numbers of students applying for admission. This means that the standards are rising even higher with the increase in competition. The student now accepted into medical school is generally better prepared than in former years; he must be qualified to handle material which has increased not only in volume but also in complexity. This all but eliminates the possibility of working one's way through either college or medical school. As the problems of financing an education become more acute to the student, he takes his education more seriously. Even in his extracurricular activities he has become more professional. This is generally true not only of the medical student but of all students in the allied medical professions. The

excellent work being done by the Student Health Organization is but one example. Today's serious students, particularly those in the health professions, are much more committed to academics.

Specialization in medical school is also encouraged. No longer is it necessary for one physician to know essentially all of the broad spectrum of medical information. With modern communications, storage and retrieval of information, and medical teams working together, a thorough knowledge in one field has become customary. The core curriculum has been pruned to allow more electives in the student's desired specialty, and more courses are offered in specific disciplines that are subdivisions of broader fields. In addition, the student is encouraged to spend any remaining free time in clinical studies and research. The first years of medical school are no longer cloisters solely devoted to classroom and laboratory work, with clinical experience completely reserved for the last years. From practically the beginning of his educative endeavors the present medical student has patient contact colaterally with his scientific studies. The methods of study themselves have been updated with the most modern of audio-visual teaching aids.

Upon completion of his three or four years of medical school, the medical doctor must be licensed by the state board of examiners in order to practice. Some states require one year of internship prior to examination. Not all states will accept licensure from other states. Most, however, accept the certificate of the National Board of Medical Examiners. The first part of this examination is taken after two years of medical school, the second part after completion, and the th d part after one year of internship. Should he want to specialize, the physician must spend at least two more years as a resident doctor in a hospital service in his field. Once he becomes a physician he may join the American Medical association and/or the National Medical Association as a full member.

The emerging physician is primarily a scientist. Psychological knowledge seems to be more important to him than the psychology of social patient contact or his traditional role as a clinician. Technology and automation are now incorporated into his routine and the physician is finding himself working with the engineer to develop more sophisticated ways of helping the patient. Recognizing that dependable, high quality ancillary assistance is readily available in hospitals, greater numbers of physicians are allying themselves and spending more of their time in these institutions, despite the growing ideaological concept that the real need lies within the disadvantaged areas of the community, and that the people living in these areas must have at least equal quality of service and mechanical assistance. Newer medical schools and those revising their curricula are acknowledging their responsibility in this field by including courses in community medicine and in social concepts of medical practice. Departments of Family and Community Medicine appear to be exerting a more positive influence in helping to remove some of the criticism regarding emerging medical students. Two of the common criticisms are that the new physician has very little understanding of the impact of the various health systems on his medical practice, and that very little has been done to train him in the delegation of tasks and responsibilities or in how best to utilize the services of others.

Many physicians, recognizing the advantages of a "one-stop medical shopping center" are opening their private offices in hospitals, and many more are establishing practice in affiliated medical centers. Approximately 22 percent of non-Federal physicians have a hospital-based practice.[9]

Because modern medicine has made life expectancy longer, which increases, ironically, the number of diseases possible over a prolonged lifetime, many of the patients in hospitals have chronic or at best interrupted diseases. In these cases they come to the hospital physician only after social and emotional factors of causation, prolongation, and treatment have set in. Acute pain and urgent medical need is the focus for them. But because the object of the hospital is not to establish long term care but a rapid turnover of improved patients, the physician needs the assistance of others in the health team to extend chronic treatment. Liaison with community agencies, nurses, pharmacists, social workers, physical therapists, and rehabilitation counselors is essential. Hospital-type treatment must be brought into the home to rehabilitate the patient. Family-centered patient care is the new objective.

The old concept of the family doctor is sadly disappearing. Not only is there too much for him to do and to know, but also he can provide for his patients much better by working with other specialists. Less than two-thirds of the physicians are in private practice and the rate has been declining. There are approximately 335,000 doctors registered in the United States; the numerical ratio is 159 per 100,000 population. This ratio is impractical, though, because many doctors are inactive or not involved in patient care. Approximately 279,000 are involved in patient care, giving a more realistic ratio of 133 per 100,000 population. Nearly one-half of the physicians have a specialty to which their work is primarily or entirely limited. In the past the doctor went to the patient, but today the patient not only goes to the doctor, but in many cases he also diagnoses his disease in order to choose which specialist to see.

Four major categories constitute the specialties of medicine. These are: (1) medical specialties, which include otolaryngology, endocrinology, dermatology, internal medicine, pediatrics, orthopedics, cardiology, and anesthesiology; (2) surgical specialties, including general surgery, cardiac surgery, obstetrics, gynecology, ophthalmology, and urology; (3) psychiatry and neurology; and (4) miscellaneous specialties such as administrative medicine, pathology, radiology, rehabilitation, preventive medicine, and public health medicine. Returning to the emphasis on the family doctor, a new specialist rating has been created, a Specialist in Family Medicine. This certification and membership in the American Academy of General Practice requires an additional three years in training beyond the M.D. degree.[10]

Since public health medicine is relatively new and promises to be such an important field in the future, it would be well to note that a physician specializing in this field has not only an M.D. but may have a graduate degree in public health. Under his jurisdiction is the control of communicable diseases, chronic diseases, maternal and child health, environmental health, and all public health aspects of mental health. His services are desperately needed on the local, state, and Federal levels, and sometimes with voluntary health agencies.

The future of medical practice is bright, but calls for the visionary physician who can change with the changing patterns of delivering medical care, and who is not hesitant to share with others in the allied medical fields the responsibility for the welfare of the patient.

## The Osteopathic Physician

That the osteopathic physicians receive a different degree (Doctor of Osteopathy, D.O.) from the physician of medicine (Doctor of Medicine, M.D.) indicates less an unequal training and range of services than a basic divergence in their interpretation of the science of cures for sickness and injury. The distinction was first made acute in 1892 when Dr. Andrew Taylor Still insisted on the different degree to be conferred upon those graduating as Doctors of Osteopathy. Osteopaths are unlimited in their practice of the medical profession in all states and in the District of Columbia. They fulfill the needs of the community in all of the accepted methods of treatment of disease and injury, including operative surgery and obstetrics, prescribing drugs, and administering physical therapy. It is in their use of manipulation therapy and in stressing its importance, however, that they differ from the Doctor of Medicine. This difference, however, is not always discernible. This is exemplified by a recent federal court case which awarded the title "M.D." to a Doctor of Osteopathy.[11]

The osteopath maintains that the early symptoms of a functional disease may be projected in the musculoskeletal system of the patient and that irregularities affecting the human being's total system may be corrected through diagnosis and corrective treatment. The two ideas basic to their modification in medical treatment stem from their assumption that all human functions are interrelated, and that man's body naturally possesses the ability to heal itself and to combat the stresses and strains which result in disease. It is therefore the duty of the osteopath to consider the whole man as sick, and to treat the man, and not so much the disease. This can be accomplished by doing all to maintain or to stimulate the normal, natural functions of the body. Manipulation can at times, they contend, be as necessary and effective as drugs or surgery. They place emphasis on the maintenance of health through prevention of disease by an unimpaired blood and nerve sturcture.

In the United States there are seven four-year colleges of osteopathic medicine training young men and women in their science. Entrance depends scholastically on a high average in at least three years of college, even though approximately 97 per cent of students have a bachelor's degree. The medical school entrants are rather evenly divided between those who have majored in the sciences and those who have humanities majors, but all students must have had a minimum of 28 credit hours distributed among the sciences. All applicants are required to take the Medical College Admissions Test. A broad academic background seems to be conducive to their large view of the function of medicine, but personal characteristics such as a pleasing personality, emotional stability, an inquiring mind, and keen senses are considerations to acceptance by the colleges of osteopathic medicine. An outstanding feature of the training at colleges of osteopathy is their emphasis on general practice. The college at Kirksville participates in a Rural Clinic Program which operates 11 clinics in communities which would otherwise go without any medical care. One hundred student doctors and 40,000 patients mutually benefit from the program each year.[12]

One year of internship is required following the four years of medical school and virtually all students fulfill this obligation in one of the approximately 250 osteopathic hospitals in the country. Residency is available to those who wish to specialize. As with all doctors, the osteopath must be licensed in each state in which he practices. He must first pass a written examination and the scrutiny of a state Board of Trustees, usually comprised of Doctors of Medicine as well as Doctors of Osteopathy.

Osteopaths serve as physicians in state and Federal Government agencies, the armed forces, and can provide treatment under Medicare, the Veterans Administration, and welfare agencies. They serve as coroners, medical examiners, school physicians, and county physicians, and they assist on boards of medical examiners— virtually the same posts open to medical doctors. Of the 14,000 osteopaths practicing, four-fifths are in private practice. Seventy-three per cent are in general practice, about 13 per cent of these having a specialty.[13] Less than 10 per cent limit their practice to manipulative therapy and clinical conditions amenable to such therapy. Osteopaths are widely distributed geographically, with about 50 per cent located in city areas while the other half practice in smaller communities.

This branch of medicine is united by the American Osteopathic Association. A high percentage of osteopaths support the Osteopathic Progress Fund which has provided physical help to their institutions and scholarships to their students. The total of U. S. Government grants made to D. O. research and training during a recent year was approximately 6.5 million dollars. Osteopathic colleges receive grants on essentially the same basis as those awarded to colleges conferring the M.D. degree.

## The Nurse

The nursing profession has come a long way since the great modernization of standards started by Florence Nightingale in the 1850's. No longer is it sufficient to give the patient prompt, pleasing, and interested attention in a neat, clean, and cheerful ward, although at one times these things were well-needed innovations. The functions, responsibilities, and roles of nurses and of nursing practice are undergoing change at an ever-accelerating rate. Forces responsible for this change are attributed to social legislation and governmental health care programs, and to the rapid advances in the medical, physical, and social sciences. Twenty-five years ago it would have been comparatively easy to define the scope and functions of the nurse. At the present time, it is almost impossible. Today, the nurse is more of an administrator who supervises the carrying out of many services by her assistants: practical nurses and nurses' aides. Rather than devoting her time to one or two patients, she has many under her care. The professional registered nurse plans, supervises, and gives bedside nursing care, administers medications, and carries out the treatments prescribed by the doctor. She observes, evaluates, and records the symptoms, reactions, and progress of each patient under her care. She co-ordinates all of the aspects of care for the patient directly or by supervising allied personnel. That is the duty of hospital nurses, comprising two-thirds of all registered nurses.

But the registered nurse may decide to join the 10 per cent assisting in private doctor's offices, or the 6 per cent employed in private duty. Another 5 per cent teach in schools of nursing. The newest and most rapidly growing field is that of the public health nurse, who carries her abilities and training into the home, industry, primary and secondary schools, military forces, and other public agencies. Approximately 10 per cent of the professional nurses are in this field. It is here that the growing pains of the profession are most acute.

A new role of responsibility for the nurse with initiative is emerging in the field of public health services. The Federal Government is endorsing the use of nurses with five to six years of education, superior clinical preparation, and practical experience to perform functions heretofore the prerogative of the physician. Some of their duties are the delivery of babies, the prescribing of medicines and drugs, the working out of treatment, taking case histories, making physical examinations, and even performing certain laboratory procedures. Such a program is designed to relieve the physician of house visits, especially in the rural areas of the South and West, and to give people living in outlying areas access to medical attention for perhaps the first time on a broader front.

As medical sciences advance, the physician tends to delegate more and more authority to the nurse, and the nurse in turn passes on some of her more routine functions to the practical nurse or nurse's aide or others. More educational preparation is demanded as well as keener initiative and judgment on all of the nursing levels. The registered nurse is now becoming less of a technician and more of a professional person entrusted with great responsibilities. The psychosocial needs of the patient are being assessed and satisfied by this new image of the nurse. Home care and self-care are being emphasized for the patient, the training supplied in great part by the nurse.

Giving help is the key to the nurse's professional life. She aids the patient, she aids the doctor to aid the patient, and she helps the patient and his family to help themselves. To assist her in her duties, most hospitals have found it convenient to group the patients according to the degree of illness and the needs of care. The nursing staff is then selected and trained in each group: intensive care, intermediate care, self-care, long-term care, and home care.

But in order to give help, the nurse must have certain personal and educational qualifications.

Because of her eventual role as supervisor, she must have the ability to make decisions based on common sense and knowledge. She must be able to organize and plan. She must be able to maintain emotional stability in the face of any situation. Sympathy and friendliness are important to her in carrying out her most important duty: to like, genuinely, people of all ages in their worst moments in order to help them get over their immediate crises.

The prospective registered nurse has three possibilities in achieving her education and degree. Each differs in time and in degree awarded and, naturally, in financial reimbursement. There are 1350 nursing schools. Of the graduates, 47 per cent completed the diploma program at a three-year nursing school. Twenty-one per cent were awarded a baccalaureate degree. Another 31 per cent attended the junior college level of two years of concentrated nursing courses culminating in the associate degree.[14] The basic nursing program consists generally of anatomy, physiology, microbiology, nutrition, psychology, medical and surgical nursing, nursing of babies and children, and community health nursing. The amount of work in the humanities, social, physical, and biological sciences depends upon the additional time spent to complete the degree. It is becoming more and more obvious that, as nursing duties broaden, the baccalaureate degree will become the minimum, as the ANA is already advocating. Already a bachelor's or a master's degree is customarily required for supervisory or admininistrative positions. Graduates of all schools of nursing must pass the state board examination and must be approved by the state board of nursing. Unlike most other medical professions, one state will generally endorse the licensure of a nurse by another state.

There are more than twice as many RN's as physicians according to the population ratio, with 748,000 nurses practicing in the United States. Although it is a field that has generally appealed to women, more and more men are entering the field. Some of the specialties include pediatric nursing, obstetrics, psychiatric, and orthopedic fields. Nursing is an excellent preparation to marriage and to raising a family. In fact, statistics show that two-thirds of the nurses employed are married, which upholds its qualifications as a rewarding job with security, and suitable hours and conditions. The rapid expansion in health care and the even more rapid expansion in nursing programs have led not only to dramatic challenges and opportunities but also have been the source of confusion, misunderstanding, and frustration within the nursing profession. Some leaders feel that nursing, as a field of endeavor, will be a casualty in the national battle to satisfy the public health care need.[15] Others are concerned about the controversy between diploma schools and baccalaureate degree programs, the proportion of time spent in direct patient care activities, and disagreement between educators and nurse administrators.[16] Although it is true that some nurses are reluctant to assume additional responsibilities, it is inevitable that the nursing profession will continue to assume a wider role in delivery of health care at an accelerated rate. Among other documents substantiating this development is the report of the committee created by the Secretary of HEW to study extended roles for nurses.[17] The degree of specialization as well as variations within specialized fields is multiplying. The nurse-midwife has already proven her value and effectiveness.[18] The primary care nurse has demonstrated her effectiveness as a generalist for family health care.[19] Demonstrations of the extension of nursing functions in clinical practice have grown and spread rapidly. The pediatric nurse practitioner is one example.[20] Another health worker who is prepared to assume some of the traditional patient-care responsibilities of the physician is the medical nurse practitioner.[21] One of the many functions performed by these well-trained people is the conducting of routine physical examinations for asymptomatic persons. A large segment of the American public regards an annual physical examination as a necessity but the available physician pool is inadequate to provide this service.[22] The extent and the degree of expanded roles for the visionary nurse seem to be limited only by the imagination. With the nursing colleges offering a multiplicity of graduate programs in specific areas of health care, the emerging student can rightfully take her place as a true colleague of the physician.

Adjunct to the profession of the registered nurse is the practical nurse, licensed in many cases after passing a qualifying state board examination. Although she must bear many of the same characteristics of the registered nurse, she requires less intensive education because of a less responsible role. For her, two years of high school are all that is required for entrance into training. Here again, it only takes 12 to 18 months of training in a hospital or a private community agency. Whereas most nursing schools will not take an applicant over 35, practical nursing students may begin their training as late as 50, which is very advantageous to older men and women. There are an estimated 427,000 LPN's in the United States. Financially, they make approximately 75 per cent of the professional nurse's pay. They are also in great demand as they take the burden of many routine chores off the registered nurse and the doctor, under whose supervision they work.

### The Dentist

Dentistry is one of the earliest of the medical professions. In crude forms, it dates back to prehistoric times. In early Egypt dentists as well as doctors took the Hippocratic oath. In fact, it is known that Hippocrates himself made a dentifrice and a mouthwash, perhaps the first of their kinds. Records of early attempts at false teeth are still being discovered in the skulls of Indians in both North and South America, and Etruscan findings show a surprising amount of skill in this dental area. The Middle Ages marked somewhat of a reversal, for barbers took on the duties of dentistry, which was limited largely to pulling teeth. This was also the early practice in America before physicians took on the extra duties of dentistry.

Pierre Fouchard of the early 1700's is considered the father of modern dentistry. It was not until 1840, however, that the most significant early dental landmarks were established. In that year the first dental school was opened in Europe and the first medical journal devoted to dentistry was founded. The discoveries of X ray and anesthesia were probably the most important single advancements affecting the progress of the profession.

Today dentistry has become a very sophisticated profession, using the latest drug discoveries and the most elaborate mechanical devices. More specifically, dentistry is that branch of the medical profession concerned with the diagnosis and treatment of the diseases of the teeth, the jaw, and all associated parts of the oral cavity, and the restoration of defective or missing tissue. The dentist in general practice

detects and fills cavities in the teeth, X-rays the mouth, straightens crooked teeth, removes deteriorated teeth and their nerves when necessary, and replaces them with bridges and plates designed for the individual. He also treats diseases of the gums.

It is estimated that 90 per cent of dentists are in general practice, while the remaining 10 per cent limit themselves to one of the eight specialty fields in dentistry. Public health dentistry emphasizes the prevention of tooth decay, and devotes itself to teaching the public the necessities of dental health and the available services, often on a local level. The oral pathologist treats diseases of the mouth and their systemic ramifications. The oral surgeon concerns himself with the surgery of the mouth and diseased gums, and extraction of teeth. The orthodontist specializes in straightening teeth and jaws. Pedodontists devote themselves to the special dental needs of children. The prosthodontist provides artificial replacements for missing teeth, a periodontologist treats gums and bone tissues supporting the teeth or dentures, and endodontists are concerned with the treatment of diseased tooth pulp and root canal therapy.[2][3]

Dentists are usually self-employed, but 10 per cent work in clinics, hospitals, and institutions, for public health agencies on a local and state level, in schools, and in the Armed Forces. (In the Army they are commissioned as captains, and in the Navy as lieutenants). The few that teach and conduct research often maintain a private practice in addition. Dentistry is generally recognized as one of the most financially rewarding of the allied medical professions.

The dentist often works with the physician, recognizing that tooth and gum troubles may be the cause or the effect of other physiological problems. According to the population ratio, there is only one dentist to every three doctors, and yet dentists, collectively, treat almost as many patients as are treated by physicians.

It is estimated that 98 per cent of the population in most areas have tooth decay (dental caries). Twenty per cent, however, never see a dentist. Once a child has reached the age of one year, soon after cutting his first teeth, he is susceptible to tooth decay, yet in some areas more than half of the children never see a dentist before five years of age. Half of the population at the age of 55 needs dentures. Forty million Americans never see a dentist and another 100 million do so only when in pain. The pain indicates, of course, that serious damage has already been done and complicated work often involving extraction or multisurface filling is necessary for repair. This very often could have been avoided by earlier and more regular treatment.

If a mouth discomfort is put off, it is often because of the sufferer's fear of pain, but too often it is because of the unavailability of a dentist. The need for dentists is urgent. The distribution of dentists by State varies widely. In general, States in the Northeast and Far West had dentist-population ratios higher than the national average, while the South and Southwest had ratios lower than the national average. It is estimated that it would take 250,000 dentists 10 years merely to catch up on the backlog of dental decay in America.

To fulfill this growing need, there are 51 dental schools to supply the necessary professionals. Admission is dependent upon a minimum of two years of predentistry in a liberal arts college, although over two-thirds of those students in dental schools have a baccalaureate degree. Admission is also contingent upon the score attained on the Dental Aptitude test taken by the predental student. This test, compiled under the surveillance of the American Dental Association, is designed to measure both scientific knowledge and practical manual dexterity. A prospective dental student must have not only a command of the biological and physical sciences but also must possess finger dexterity and enjoy detailed work.

In the dental schools the first two years are devoted to instruction and laboratory work in anatomy, bacteriology, and pharmacology. The last two years are spent chiefly in the school's dental clinic with practical experience in treating patients under the direct supervision of teaching and practicing dentists. Although the D.D.S. (Doctor of Dental Surgery) is the degree awarded by most of the schools, a few give the equally respected D.M.D. (Doctor of Dental Medicine).

Licensing within the state is universally required. After receiving the degree the applicant must pass the state boards of the individual state in which he wishes to practice, though 49 of the states recognize the ADA's National Board of Dental Examiners' exam as a substitute for the written portion of their state boards. There is little reciprocity between the states on licenses. Annual registration is required in some states. Since the initial cost of the dentist's office equipment is so high, far beyond the cost in most other medical professions, the beginning dentist will often join an established dentist, from whom he also gains the advantage of supervised experience.

Most of the dentists serve as general practitioners, working in the specialities as needed. In some states, however, an additional state examination is required to be a "specialist." This entails not only years of practice in the specialty, but two or three years of graduate education, available at most dental schools. The candidate may, instead, serve an internship or residency at one of the hospitals offering such a program. The dentist who desires to make a career of administration of dental public health must practice for at least a few years as a dentist. After such experience, a minimum of one year of additional study is necessary, culminating in the attainment of a Master of Public Health degree.

There are approximately 104 thousand active dentists in the United States. The large majority of these professionals have received training in the principles of "Four-handed dentistry," that is, the utilization of the chairside dental assistant in an efficient and effective manner. The actual number of dental assistants are in excess of the number of dentists since multiple helpers are frequently employed in one office practice.[24] Traditionally, dental assistants have been trained on the job by their dentist-employers. This training is now being assumed by educational institutions at an increasing rate, and presently there are 180 institutions offering accredited training programs for assistants. Dental hygienists, who are trained by courses at the college level and must be licensed, number 17,000. They often assist the dentist by doing such routine work as cleaning teeth and taking X rays. Although some dentists still do their own laboratory work, most of it is done by commercial laboratory firms who employ four-fifths of the 32,000 dental laboratory technicians. The solo practitioner working without assistance is least productive, most costly, and least effective. With the great need for expanded dental manpower, there have been strong recommendations and some pilot programs concerning extended utilization of non-licensed personnel. It has been recommended that both the dental hygienist and dental assistant be given assignments of greater responsibility and new job classifications created for additional helpers. These classifications are a dental associate, similar to a nurse practitioner or physician's assistant; dental therapist, assigned such functions as taking diagnostic impressions, and insertion of materials in prepared cavities; and the dental aide who would perform many of the routine tasks previously assigned to the dental assistant.[25]

The reaction of the dental profession to encroaching governmental programs has paralleled those of the physician. Some groups definitely oppose many of the changes, other groups appear to have assumed a "wait and see" attitude, while still others have accepted these changes as an inevitable progression toward more public involvement and accountability. The Association of American Dentists is a comparatively new group that appears to be taking an almost militant stand against further government involvement in dentistry.[26]

## The Podiatrist

Foot problems are probably the most common ailment of our older population and the doctors who specialize in their treatment are just beginning to receive their proper recognition. The podiatrist or chiropodist is an orthopedic specialist who diagnoses and treats diseases and deformities of the feet and attempts to prevent their occurrence. He increases personal comfort, lessens the possibility of additional medical and surgical complications, and minimizes confinement in or out of the hospital. Through the use of X rays, blood tests, and urinalyses as well as his personal patient contact, he is able to make his diagnosis. He treats corns, bunions, calluses, tumors, ulcers, shortened or strained tendons, ingrown toenails, skin and nail diseases, deformed toes, and arch conditions. Since foot problems often can be early warning signs of conditions such as arthritis, heart and kidney ailments, and diabetes, the podiatrist is alerted to this relation and is in a position to refer the patient to a physician before the disease fully develops.

The podiatrist treats his patients with drugs, physical therapy, and surgery, prescribes proper shoes, and makes and fits corrective prosthetic devices. Podiatry along with medicine, osteopathy, and dentistry is one of the four professions

having the training, legal qualifications, and license to diagnose and to treat patients from all aspects, and to make judgments as to their care.

The prospective podiatrist must exhibit the same qualities of intellectual acuteness, sound judgment, and ability to make correct decisions as all other health professionals. He must have the ability to coordinate eyes and hands or fingers rapidly and accurately in making precise movements. Mechanical aptitude is also very important as much of his work will be with machines, whirlpool or paraffin baths, plaster casts, short wave or low voltage currents, and prosthetic appliances, as well as the devices normally used by physicians.

Two years devoted primarily to sciences in a liberal arts college are the absolute minimum for entrance into a college of podiatry. Three-fourths of the total students in colleges of podiatric medicine have baccalaureate degrees. The first two of the four years spent in podiatry school are concentrated on classroom instruction and laboratory work in the basic sciences. Medically oriented courses plus a minimum of 2000 hr. of clinical experience occupy the student's last two years. At graduation from one of the five colleges of podiatry the successful candidate is awarded the degree of Doctor of Podiatric Medicine (D.P.M.). Licensure is necessary for practice in all states and is based upon graduation from an approved college, the passing of state board examinations, and, in three states, one year of internship in a hospital or clinic. Approximately one-half of the states accept the licenses issued by other states. Two professional associations are active in this field, the National Association of Chiropody and the American Podiatry Association. Membership in the latter group is available to those experienced podiatrists who prescribe to the Code of Ethics of that organization.

There are approximately 8000 podiatrists in the United States and about 90 per cent of them are in general practice.[28] Some, however, specialize in particular ailments, skin conditions, or children's podiatry. A few serve as consultants to shoe manufacturers, and others devote their lives to research or to teaching. Podiatrists are also employed in the armed forces, the Veterans Administration, and certain school districts.

As life expectancy is increased, and with it

the number of geriatric patients, podiatry promises to assume an even more prominent position. The physical and mental advantages of the aged remaining ambulatory are easily recognized, and the podiatrist will be called upon to a greater extent to exercise his skill. His training emphasizes the anatomical changes in the foot as a person ages, particularly changes in the musculoskeletal and nervous systems. Through his knowledge and help, greater numbers of older people can retain their walking ability for greater periods of time and thus maintain more independence.

Another of the great needs for podiatry in the future lies with the public health facilities. In 1964, the first full-time podiatry clinic was established in the municipal health department of Washington, D. C. The program now includes three full-time clinics, four part-time clinics, and a home care system. Since it seemed unreasonable for podiatrists to treat the results of neglect without trying to prevent the same problems in the next generation, a mass foot screening project for 20,000 children was established. The findings of this project revealed that 37 per cent of those screened had postural and orthopedic foot disorders, and 16 per cent had gait deviations.[29]

The chronic nature of the problems of the foot is entitled to more attention and care. For too long feet have been one of the most neglected parts of the anatomy. As more people learn of the help that they can receive for their feet, the need for podiatrists will rise at an even higher rate. As one of the partners on the health service team, today's podiatrists are intimately concerned with the dramatic changes and the need for improvement in the delivery of health care and have become firmly committed to public health.

## The Veterinarian

To think that with the appearance of the horseless carriage the veterinarian would become obsolete is pure contradiction of the fact, or to assume that with the movement from an agrarian to an urban society we would minimize the need for the veterinarian is exactly the opposite of what has occurred. Evidently the tribal medicine man who treated animals as well as human patients came closer to what history has demonstrated to be reality. We now recognize that human and animal well-being are irremediably linked, and that many animal diseases are transmitable to humans. Contrary to superficial expectations urban societies depend on veterinarians, serving unobtrusively in the background, to inspect the meat, poultry, fish, and dairy products which people consume in quantity. Even the imported animal foods must pass the rigorous tests of the veterinarians to meet our standards. It is veterinary research which has produced biologicals such as serums, toxoids, and antitoxins which are used in the prevention and treatment of so many human illnesses. Through the work of veterinarians, the danger of bovine tuberculosis, rabies, and brucellosis have all but been eliminated in this country. The veterinarian works with the physician, the dentist, the nurse, and other specialists to assure health and safety in the community.

Rural veterinarians work primarily with larger animals, while veterinarians in private practice in the cities treat mostly pets. A large portion of their work regardless of location is preventative, that is, the routine work of giving vaccinations, alerting through quarantines, and informing people how best to treat their pets and animals. For the farmer the veterinarian is a special aid in financial security, saving herds from epidemics, and advising and assisting in breeding of prize stock, as well as caring for the individual animals. He assures the farmer not only of increasing production of bigger and healthier stock but also, through his services as a health inspector, assures a continuing market at home and abroad. The consumer in the city, through the diligence of the veterinarian, is confident of abundant, uncontaminated, and cleanly prepared food.

To pet owners everywhere, the vet is the friend who can understand the complaints of a sick animal, who can relieve suffering, and who can help an injured, beloved companion. He not only increases the animals' chances for longevity, but he helps to eliminate any danger or trouble that they might be to their owners. Thanks to the veterinarian, a pet can become almost pure enjoyment.

Veterinarians have a key responsibility in special types of endeavors, such as the fur industry. By keeping the animals healthy and by developing nutritional supplements the quantity and the quality of furs have been greatly improved. Similar to the problems of the fur industry, where normally free animals are kept in captivity and thus become far more susceptible to disease, is the series of challenging situations presented by the zoo or circus. In these places the veterinarian not only serves the animal in an unusual capacity, but protects the zoo goer and circus watcher as well. Ancillary to this service has been the humane treatment of animals which has been far advanced by the veterinarian.

In the military departments the veterinarian performs still another type of special service. In such a closely confined community where effectiveness depends on health, it is his responsibility to see that servicemen receive only safe and nutritious foods, at home, and in foreign lands. He often has to develop more effective ways of preparing, producing, and serving foods from animal sources. Further, he has the obligation of giving medical care to animals used for guard duty and other special purposes.

In this atomic age with the threat of nuclear warfare, it will be the veterinarian's responsibility to check all animals and their food products to determine their safety for human consumption. Currently, he is studying the effect of modern day air pollution on animals and their subsequent effect on humans.

The training of the veterinarian has many similarities to the training required of other disciplines which award the professional doctor's degree. Although a baccalaureate degree is not mandatory for admission to a veterinary college, the majority of students have completed full college courses, usually with emphasis upon the physical and biological sciences. All but two of the 18 veterinary colleges in the United States are associated with state university systems. As such they are supported by state funds and must give preferential consideration to state residents. The four years of training in these colleges place emphasis upon both scientific theory and practical applications regarding cause, prevention, and treatment of animal diseases, as well as the zoonoses. Upon successful completion of this training the graduate is awarded the professional degree of Doctor of Veterinary Medicine (D.V.M.)

The practice of veterinary medicine is controlled through a licensing procedure in each state. Presently there is not a uniform licensing program among the various states. All states require a written examination, and some require one year's internship. Once licensed, the veterinarian is eligible for membership in the American Veterinary Medical Association.

There are approximately 27,500 veterinarians in the United States and approximately three-fourths are in private practice. The others are involved in regulatory veterinary medicine, veterinary public health, education, military veterinary practice, or laboratory services. There are a few employed by international organizations such as the World Health Organization and the Food and Agriculture Organization, primarily in research to alleviate indirectly the food shortages of the world.[30]

## THE PUBLIC HEALTH ROLE OF THE PRACTICING PHARMACIST

But if you are to be full members of the health care delivery system, then you must accept the responsibility for helping to improve that system—to restructure and reform it.

EDWARD M. KENNEDY*

If Pharmacy is to be a public health profession it too must better prepare pharmacists in their social role.

DON E. FRANCKE[31]

In recent years the pharmacy profession has been the recipient of overtures made from public health professionals, national voluntary health agencies, various segments of the Public Health Service and other Federal agencies, and from state and local health departments. Pharmacy leaders have been asked to testify before Federal and state legislative bodies concerning pending legislation, and pharmacy representatives have been welcomed to participate on health planning boards. In addition, public health agencies and state public health associations have sought the co-operation and active involvement of practicing pharmacists in programs designed to deliver more effective health care to needy segments of the population. These overtures, fortunately, are becoming more numerous and more pronounced. The reaction of pharmacists, at first hesitant and halting, is increasingly characterized by acceptance, willingness, and even an eagerness to participate in these co-operative ventures. Dialogues are established and strengthened be-

---

*From Keynote Address, American Pharmaceutical Association Annual Meeting, 1973.

tween pharmacy and other professions in the field of public health, and more pharmacists are appearing on committees and on programs of state public health associations. National leadership is exhibited by such active involvement as the Pharmacy Public Health Conference now held each year in conjunction with the annual convention of the American Public Health Association and cosponsored by the American Association of Colleges of Pharmacy and the American Pharmaceutical Association. In addition, a Public Affairs Committee has been functioning for a number of years within the American Pharmaceutical Association to keep pharmacists informed of developments within this very important area of activity and to enlist a continually greater degree of participation in public health endeavors.

Two questions may present themselves regarding this mutual courtship. In years past pharmacists in general were not closely associated with formalized community health agencies. Pharmacists customarily did not seek such association and their assistance was not openly sought by officials and administrators in the field of public health. Why, then, has there been this change in recent years? More specifically, the two questions that may be asked are (1) why are public health agencies now interested in the active involvement of pharmacists in their programs, and (2) why are knowledgeable, visionary pharmacists now urging their colleagues to participate in public health endeavors to an extent not previously anticipated?

The answer to the first question resides both in what the pharmacist knows and in his unique position as a readily available representative of the health professions. The pharmacist is either the most over-educated or the most underutilized member of the allied medical professions. His academic training cuts across a significant number of the social and scientific disciplines. He is schooled in the behavioral sciences, the physical sciences, and the biological sciences. He is health-oriented and thanks to recent changes in pharmacy college curricula and philosophies is becoming more patient-oriented.

As a knowledgeable health professional he is in a potentially ideal position to render a very valuable service in helping to improve the health of his community. It has been estimated conservatively that approximately 185 million persons enter our nation's pharmacies each week. The pharmacist is available to those who seek his counsel; he can be seen without prior appointment and, because most pharmacies are open from 9 to 13 hrs. each day, the services of a pharmacist can be utilized throughout the day or early evening. Many, many people, whether ill-advised or not, seek out their pharmacist for information in matters related to health.

A recent edition of the *Journal of the American Pharmaceutical Association* listed some of the specific health problems about which the public consults the pharmacist. Representatives from this list included such items as the following: gastrointestinal complaints, diarrhea, rectal ailments, contraceptives, genito-urinary problems, sleeping complaints, and menstrual problems. Also included in this list were burns, eye and ear ailments, muscular aches and pains, wounds and infections, problems of the oral cavity, respiratory ailments, and skin problems. Persons from all walks of life and all economic levels frequently consult their pharmacist about their health interests and problems. In low-income areas, however, the pharmacist is, in many instances, the health professional in closest contact with the people.[32]

The Federal Government, through its multiple programs of comprehensive health care and financing, is cooperating with state and local agencies to improve the health of all people in the nation's communities. Public health officials responsible for administration of these programs recognize the very valuable aid which the community pharmacist can render in assuring the success of these programs. People living in low income areas frequently are uninformed about healthful living and are in need of health education. The pharmacist in the community knows the language of his people. Many times he knows their problems, their fears, their superstitions, and their reservations. Often he is faced with finding solutions for persons supported by public welfare, and having rather complicated health problems. Thus, he is in an ideal position to explain the newer methods of health services delivery, to inform the patient how to make his way through the maze of organized health programs, and to enlist the cooperation of people in his community to utilize the neighborhood health centers more freely. The pharmacist is also a resource for epidemiological studies. He knows about the patterns of illness in his community and is a rich source of information regarding distribution, age groups involved, race, sex, and socio-economic factors in relation to particular diseases. It is small wonder, then, that public health agencies and public health associations have sought out the pharmacist as an ally in the campaign against disease and in the developing programs of preventive medicine.

But why should the pharmacist alter his historic role of filling prescriptions and assume a more active participation in the field of public health?

The answer to this question involves the changing roles which are being experienced in all of the allied medical professions. Nursing, pharmacy, medical technology, clinical medicine, and other related professions have found new avenues of service and have had to reappraise their customary practices in the light of their new obligations. These professions have a long and distinguished history in which each has developed a pattern of operation in order to cope with health problems within their area of interest and concern. Changing times, further development of technology, and newer methods of health delivery have, however, wrought changes in the historic patterns of the medical professions. Perhaps in no other profession has the rate of change been more profound than in pharmacy.

Prior to World War II the majority of medications prescribed by physicians were compounded in the pharmacy. It is true that most of the drugs were not very potent and some had questionable value but certainly the mortar and pestle, now observed mainly as pharmacy insignia, enjoyed far more prominence and use. In more recent years the vast bulk of all medications is mass produced under high quality specifications by large drug-manufacturing companies. The actual dispensing of prescriptions now consists largely of preparing appropriate quantities of the manufactured product for individual use, with individualized instructions for administering the drug. Although such dispensing is important and certainly requires supervision, much of the work is routine and involves non-decision-making activity. The increased use of unit dose packaging, particularly in hospitals, is another step toward wider utilization of technicians. Also, through mechanical innovation and the technological capacity of computers, it is possible to com-

pletely automate the counting, pouring, and labeling of prefabricated medications. Indeed, automated prescriptions systems presently are being marketed. In view of the extensive academic background required for registration of present-day pharmacists, questions are being raised in many circles about proper utilization of such highly trained personnel.

The nursing profession has taken the lead in assigning routine duties to those classes of nurses whose training is not so extensive and exacting, and have reserved for the professional registered nurse those decision-making responsibilities which utilize her preparation and background. Similarly, government agencies, medical institutions, and some pharmacy leaders are suggesting that much of the mechanical dispensing of prescriptions be delegated to trained technicians, under supervision, and the pharmacist be utilized for services and duties which are more commensurate with his rich training in the biological sciences. These suggestions have merit and may help significantly to promote the pharmacist into the much more realistic and effective roles of drug consultant for the medical professions and health consultant for the public. Certainly, the pharmacist is valued much more for what he knows that for what he does.

By relieving the pharmacist of much of his historic, routine duties it would be possible for this trained professional to assume responsibilities in health-related areas that need the services of an expert in drugs. A word of caution is indicated, however. In the enthusiasm of seeking extended roles for pharmacists, some leaders from both within and outside the pharmacy profession have advocated an almost total desertion of the historic dispensing function, leaving that important element almost completely to less qualified technicians. While we applaud the visionaries who project pharmacy into roles generally assumed by the clinical pharmacologist, we must also recognize that these new positions will not become immediately available in large quantities. There is a distinct danger, then, in abandoning one important role before being accepted into extended roles. In the rush toward rapid change there may well be the definite possibility of "throwing out the baby with the bath water."

Enlarged activities of the pharmacist as the resource person in all matters concerning drugs is the field of most practical expansion. This includes the management of all drug-related sources and drug distribution processes.[33] In a hospital setting the pharmacist has already demonstrated his capabilities as a clinical pharmacist, a drug information specialist, poison control consultant, and as a participant in continuing education for the other allied medical professions. Other duties that the pharmacist has discharged capably in clinical settings have been as a monitor of ongoing drug therapy, a prescriber of drugs, a participant in drug utilization review, a consultant in drug reactions and biological incompatibilities, and as an important team member in the discharge interview.[34]

It may be some time yet before the full potential of the pharmacist can be realized in the clinical environment. There are also indications that the drug-consulting role will be limited in future years since much of this type of information is being stored in computers. It is also true, however, that the drug consultant role of the pharmacist is extremely important at the present time. For the practicing physician to be expected to have a working knowledge of hundreds of drugs is unrealistic. The results obtained from a questionnaire mailed to a random sample of 1000 physicians demonstrates this problem. It was revealed that 54 per cent of the respondents felt their knowledge concerning drugs was inadequate, 62.5 per cent acknowledged difficulty in keeping up with drug information, and 75 per cent spent two hours or less per week in obtaining drug information.[35] The public health activities of practicing pharmacists, though, offer some of the greatest opportunities for service, both now and in years to come. Pharmaceutical practice for the community is essential and it will remain so, and it will be more intimately connected with community health problems and community health services.[36] Pharmacists are assuming a social responsibility in the realization that the health of one person is inextricably bound to the health of all the community in one way or another. Pharmacy in co-operation with the other medical professions has an equal stake in meeting and anticipating the health needs of society. Through dedicated, conscientious application of this social responsibility, traditional community pharmacy will be swept on to new professional horizons.

The public health role of practicing pharmacists can be exhibited both within their pharmacies and within their communities. Inside the store the pharmacist can serve as a health information specialist. Through greater involvement in the education of people in the community about acute and chronic diseases, and ways and means of developing healthful living, the pharmacist can demonstrate recognition of his social responsibility. Information is the first step to understanding, which leads to motivation and finally to action. These are the essential steps of effective health education. To help in this educative endeavor, many pharmacists maintain racks near their prescription counters containing folders and pamphlets on various aspects of health. The printed material is furnished by government health agencies, voluntary health associations, and insurance companies. The pamphlets are rotated periodically so that the contents of the rack remain a source of interest for the public. In order to be an additional source of information for further discussion, the pharmacist frequently reviews his knowledge concerning the health conditions described in his current pamphlets. In this regard the pharmacist may be called upon to lend his attention to a wide spectrum of illnesses, both, real and imaginary. Fortunately, the pharmacist is no longer charged with counter-prescribing when he discusses illnesses with his patients. If the patient is suffering from a visible injury such as wounds or sprains it is to be expected that the pharmacist would lend his expertise. The list continues to grow and also becomes more complicated. Whereas ready assistance can be given for injuries or nose bleeds, an additional amount of professional judgment is needed for ingrown toenails, earaches, prolonged fever or cough, and bleeding from the rectum or vagina.[37] The pharmacist appears to be in a key position as a health care middle man because of the decisions he makes on whether to prescribe medication or to refer the person to a physician.[38] Studies have shown that as the complaining symptoms become more severe the practicing pharmacists become more cautious in their help and guidance, commonly resulting in reference to a physician.[39] In addition to benefiting the public health, an improvement in public attitude toward pharmacy is enhanced through this pharmacist-patient communication regarding health matters.[40]

Another way that the pharmacist can serve

the public health is to become thoroughly familiar with government health programs, particularly those that directly affect some of his patients. Explaining the provisions to the elderly, the poor, and the uneducated can help these people obtain the medical services that they need. Although Federal and state health agencies have performed a mammoth task in publicizing the details and benefits of such legislation there remain significant numbers of potential recipients in our society who still do not understand the various provisions of the newer legislation. Terms such as "co-insurance" and "deductible" can be confusing to these people, particularly to those who understand that the government will pay for their total medical expenses. Continually expanding Federal legislation in the field of health will increasingly involve greater numbers of the health profession. This expansion can be viewed either as encroachment upon privileged domain or as an opportunity to participate on a co-operative basis with other health professionals and legislative intent. Two examples of this expansion are the HMO legislation and the 1972 Amendments to the Social Security Act, establishing Professional Service Review Organizations (PSRO's). HMO's may have either an in-house pharmacy or a vendor system with participating pharmacists in the community. Either one of these systems allows pharmacists to participate on governing boards, drug utilization review committees, and to lend their professional knowledge to upgrade and expand the pharmaceutical services. PSRO's provide the opportunity for subcontract review procedures for specialized services. Enterprising pharmacists can become involved in helping to establish accepted standards for pharmaceutical services in their geographical areas and can serve on the review committee for this specialty. In these ways, Federal legislation can help provide opportunities for expanded roles of the pharmacist.[41,42]

The pharmacist can render a public health service by familiarizing himself with the various voluntary health groups in his community. By determining the work performed by each agency, the organizational structure, and utilization of funds, he is in a better position to advise those who seek his counsel and those who need help. As discussed in Chapter 2, there are now so many voluntary health groups, each with its special appeal, that a need has

arisen for an unbiased evaluation of the agencies which are effective and worthy of support. Does an agency exist only for education, does it support research, does it furnish needed sickroom supplies, does it offer transportation to hospitals and clinics, and does it offer financial assistance to those patients in need? Information such as this, if available in pharmacies, further enhances the public health role of pharmacists.

Experience with diabetes screening and high blood pressure campaigns have demonstrated the value of the pharmacist in programs designed to encourage the co-operation and active involvement of the public. Through the use of his influence to persuade community support there is a much greater chance that these campaigns will be even more successful. Additional mass campaigns are planned to marketedly reduce certain diseases in a target population. Once again, the pharmacist will be present to show his concern for the public health.

Throughout this textbook we have discussed problems which pose a threat to the public health. The pharmacist, through conversations with his clientele, can assert a position and encourage community support in such areas as drug abuse, air and water pollution, venereal disease, mental health, civil defense, and planned parenthood. All of these problems are worthy of his support, and none of the programs designed to diminish such problems can succeed without community co-operation.

The pharmacist further fulfills his public health role by serving as a referral center for those in acute need. When the alcoholic or the narcotic addict finally recognizes the hopelessness of his situation, to whom can he turn for assistance? Where is the nearest suicide prevention center? What services are available for those who are in acute medical need but who are without funds? Information such as this, available in pharmacies, helps significantly to promote community health. While neighborhood health centers are still being established and some other health facilities are in the process of decentralization, neighborhood pharmacists are already geographically distributed throughout their communities and can provide accessible, walk-in facilities. Their presence is made visible in large letters and neon lights. Community pharmacists are ideally positioned to serve as a first point of planned contact between the patient and the health care enterprise. The responsibilities of the pharmacist can range from the operation of a simple screening service and primary health counseling to referral to an appropriate source of advanced service. In short, one of the very valuable public health services performed by pharmacists in a community setting is serving as an entry point into the health care system.[43]

A very effective public health service performed by the pharmacist is that of drug consultant to the self-medicating public. All of us recognize that many drug products are presold through extensive advertising. The alert and concerned pharmacist is aware that some of the ingredients found in over-the-counter medications can be potentially harmful to patients taking certain prescription drugs or to those suffering from particular chronic illnesses. Lists of biological incompatibilities grow almost daily and the pharmacist continues to be an increasingly important source of this type of drug information. If the pharmacist maintains a family prescription record, he is performing an even greater and more effective service. By cross-reference to such files he is in a better position to offer professional advice regarding which medications can be taken safely and which ones are contraindicated. For example, patients on prescription sedatives and tranquilizers may experience additional CNS depression and sedation if they drink alcohol or take over-the-counter (OTC) antihistamine cold and allergy preparations; aspirin can reduce blood sugar levels and thus complicate the therapy of diabetic patients, it can irritate the stomach and cause some blood loss, and is contraindicated in patients taking anticoagulant drugs; OTC nasal decongestants may cause hypertensive reactions in patients taking monoamine oxidase inhibitors; and sodium bicarbonate decreases the absorption of tetracycline an average of 50 per cent.[44] The pharmacist also can properly evaluate the relative merits of mouth washes, eye solutions, rubs, and inhalants. In his capacity as an expert on drugs he can render a great public health service. All too often patients take over-the-counter preparations which mask the symptoms of underlying, serious diseases. The alert and concerned pharmacist can detect some of these disease patterns and help the patient to seek medical assistance.

Along these same lines, the professional image of pharmacy also must be kept in focus if the public is to associate the community pharmacy as representative of the public health. It is paradoxical for a pharmacist to establish himself as a guardian of the community health and yet continue to sell products which are deleterious to health. Fortunately the incidence is decreasing, but there are still pharmacies which continue to sell intoxicating beverages on the premises. Also, the Surgeon General's Report along with literally dozens of other reports of scientific investigations have established a causal relationship between cigarette smoking, respiratory diseases, and lung cancer. In the face of this evidence many pharmacies continue to sell cigarettes as a convenience item for their customers. It is incumbent upon the professional pharmacist to deliberate this question and to determine whether he "practices what he preaches" regarding preventive medicine and public health.

The public health role of the practicing pharmacist is equally important outside the four walls of the pharmacy. The combination of scientific background, concern for the health of others, and involvement in community affairs highly recommend this trained professional as a key mover in Community Action Programs. As pharmacists become more knowledgeable in the total delivery of health services, they are being called upon more frequently to serve as advisors to government agencies. Planning and decision-making conferences on health programs and services certainly should include pharmacists as essential members. It must be kept in mind, however, that these community action councils are composed of volunteers; participation of the medical professions or of individuals within those professions is seldom solicited. It is usually necessary for the pharmacist and other interested health professionals to attend announced open meetings, to participate in discussions, to offer helpful suggestions, and to volunteer to serve where needed. By displaying both knowledge and concern, the value of the professional pharmacist will soon be recognized. Through such active involvement the pharmacist not only helps to ensure the success of community programs but also aids his profession. Pharmaceutical associations are seeking ways to be included in the newer Federal health programs. Also, the experience of pharmacists who are participating in co-operative community health ventures serves as a valuable resource in establishing guidelines. Certainly, the study of health delivery systems is an investment in the future. The health care system is being reconstructed in America. Although it will require adjustments, it will help provide the development of new public health opportunities for pharmacy.[45]

The public health role of the pharmacist also is exhibited in public speaking. Various service groups within the community and local PTA organizations are interested in health subjects, and the community-minded pharmacist is frequently called upon to discuss health problems of current interest. Topics such as poison control, drug abuse, family prescription records, and the pricing of prescriptions are among the popular subjects. Talks given in the public school systems related to career days and drug abuse are also of great importance. Such public speaking activities serve a 2-fold purpose. They not only enhance the public health of the community but also help public relations, which are sorely needed in pharmacy.

Still another public health contribution of the pharmacist is in the area of first aid. Accidents continue to plague our society with much needless suffering, disability, and loss of life. The pharmacy is a natural and historic repository for bandages, splints, and other supplies needed in such emergencies and the pharmacist frequently is called upon to render first aid when accidents occur in the neighborhood. In the case of a widespread disaster the first aid services of the pharmacist are utilized to an even greater extent. Since pharmacies are strategically located throughout the community both the needed supplies and a trained worker are readily available. Many pharmacists extend their first-aid services even further. In co-operation with the American Red Cross pharmacists qualify as first-aid instructors and conduct classes of instruction for various groups in their community. A growing number of pharmacy colleges are supporting this public health endeavor by incorporating first-aid instructor courses in their curricula so that the student is a qualified first-aid instructor when he graduates.

These, then, are but a few of the many ways that pharmacists can contribute to an effective public health program, in addition to their unfolding roles as therapeutic advisors and drug consultants to the medical profession. With the advent of newer government sponsored health

programs, emerging community mental health ventures, and the entire area of preventive medicine, which is only in its infancy, the possibilities for future roles of the pharmacist in public health programs appear to be limitless.

## NEW HEALTH PROFESSIONALS

Gross shortages of manpower plus a severe maldistribution of physicians and nurses have resulted in acute health problems in certain geographic areas of the United States. For example, there are 134 counties in the U.S. without physicians; and 55 million people live in rural communities of less than 2500 population where health care delivery is either inadequate or essentially non-existent.[46] Coupled with this is the skyrocketing costs of health care with relatively little in the way of increased productivity, although the allocation of ever-increasing amounts of money for health continues. Added to these issues is the inappropriate utilization and education of existing personnel. One study has shown that pediatricians spend 72 per cent of their time on well-child care and upper respiratory infections; these two areas definitely do not constitute the majority of training in their specialty.[47] At least one paper argues that since the physician's income is highly correlated with what he does, economic considerations influence him to retain these functions. In the same irreverent vein, obstetricians in the United States are described as the highest paid midwives in the world.[48] Certainly there can be no argument that there is a widespread misuse of medical expertise and a greater need for mid-level health workers. As we are moving more into a health care system instead of a medical cure system the demands for additional health manpower will continue. Since it is unreasonable to expect vast increases in the production of physicians, the next most logical procedure is to develop other types of health manpower to whom certain routine tasks can be delegated.

The process of delivering care is based on the same scientific knowledge for all the professions. The variations and differences in the combination and depth of knowledge of the basic sciences stems from a combination of role expectations and length of training. Due to legal sanctions and the wary guarding of professional territorial imperatives there has been relatively little utilization of task analyses or general acceptance of other than licensed practitioners. Furthermore, the high cost of training is creating a state of unrest and the public is starting to raise questions about whether a prolonged period is necessary to achieve professional skill. One author has referred to their process as the "great training robbery."[49]

Efforts to close this gap between available manpower and need have been attempted for many years. Other nations have helped to solve this problem through the development of mid-level professionals, usually working under medical supervision. The feldsher in Russia, the "barefoot doctor" in China, the "Medicatura Rurale" program in Venezuela,[50] and the extensive use of midwives in Western European countries demonstrate some of the notable successes Reports from China that the birth rate is dropping significantly; mass immunizations have been provided against polio, measles, and diphtheria; and health care is available to essentially all the rural population, have indicated that much of this progress can be attributed to the "barefoot doctor." Also, comparisons of maternal and perinatal mortality rates provide no evidence that the less intensive use of physicians for maternity care in Western Europe is associated with adverse effects upon the course and outcome of pregnancy.[51]

In the United States the need for additional health manpower has been increasingly stressed. It appears that each new clinical advance, each new generation of technological medicine, and each abrupt reawakening of the nation's conscience increases demand for health care services and for people trained to deliver these services.[52]

Some of the earlier programs were concerned with the efforts by the Office of Economic Opportunity to incorporate health aides and technicians into Neighborhood Health Center Extended Programs. The Allied Health Professions Personnel Training Act was another effort to supply additional help for the medical profession.[53] Reports in the literature reflect various degrees of success or failure with these programs. On the shadow side are reports that few paraprofessionals have moved beyond their entry positions, health services have not been significantly increased or improved, the main features of these service systems are unchanged, and the undisputed dictates of professionals are

largely undiminished. The teamwork between professionals and non-professionals has been described as being akin to the partnership of horse and rider. Also there has been the criticism that too many health workers have been encapsulated at the bottom to serve the angry, critical, poor who previously have not been well served. This arrangement has reduced the pressure on the professional but has been discouraging to the non-professional who feels that he is serving as a buffer.[54] On the brighter side have been numerous reports from well-satisfied administrators and professionals who have highly praised the work of their new helpers and have been able to extend health services to much greater areas. One report from a department of obstetrics and gynecology disclosed that workers with very little formal education background were competing in quality of workmanship with registered nurses.[55] Certainly, with increased government programs such as comprehensive health services, family planning, disease control, and health maintenance organizations the health manpower projections for the future are very high.[56] It is not only to be hoped, but anticipated that more effective use will be made of these trained personnel.

The spectrum of training programs for medical assistants is extremely wide and varied. Some of the programs have been developed in response to local need, some have been duplications of programs in other institutions, and others have been developed through the urging of lower-level workers who desired vertical mobility. For our discussion we will limit consideration to the "physician associate" and "physician assistant." In some cases these are new terms for personnel who have been working with the physicians on an informal basis for years.

## Physician Associates

Physician associates are health workers educated to the level where they can make some independent judgements as well as performing tasks in health counseling. Most of the workers in Physicians Associate Programs are registered nurses with baccalaureate degrees who have taken graduate work plus extended clinical experience. With such training and background, these people are frequently accepted as colleagues of physicians. A special need for such personnel exists in municipal hospitals that are often called on to provide primary care to a large population.[57] Other areas of demonstrated helpfulness are in rural populations and in the neighborhood health centers. The following list of physician associate titles reflects the extreme variation which presently exists and suggests a need for greater standardization[58]

Associate in Anesthesiology
Child Health Associate
Clinical Associate
Family Health Supervisor
Family Nurse Practitioner
Maternity Nurse
Clinical Specialist
Nurse Associate
Pediatric Nurse Associate
Pediatric Nurse Clinician
Pediatric Nurse Practitioner
Physician Associate
School Nurse Practitioner

The term "Physician Associate" is further confused by the former physicians assistant program at Duke University, presently called the Physicians Associate Program. Each student in this program is required to have at least 2000 hours of patient care experience before matriculation. The educational curriculum is divided into nine months of didactic work and the last 15 months to practical study in clinical settings.[59]

## Physician Assistants

Physician assistants are less educated and less independent than physician associates. They carry out tasks that are specifically delegated to them and usually reflect the specialty of the physician under whose direct supervision they work. They are usually employed directly by the physician and their independent action is legally limited. The topic of physician assistants has received so much publicity in medical literature that annotated bibliographies are being published.[60] With financial support from private foundations and the Bureau of Health Resources Development, programs to train physician assistants have mushroomed. Presently there are well over 1000 people already trained in the various programs and an additional 1900 trainees are currently enrolled in 24 states and the District of Columbia. Similar to the variation in titles of physician associates,

the titles of physician assistants are no less confusing.

Master Anesthesia Technologist
Clinical Corpsman
Community Health Medic
Marine Physician Assistant
MEDEX
Medical Emergency Technicians
Medical Service Assistant
Mental Health Technologist
Orthopedic Assistant
Pathologist Assistant
Pediatric Assistant
Physician Assistant
Surgeons Assistant
Urologist Assistant

The levels of training and competence of those now being prepared varies widely, so that any titles given to them tend only to confuse, not to enlighten. The situation is in a state of flux, with a definite possibility that a hierarchy of training and competence may emerge. It is expected that physician assistants can be deployed for practice in a variety of settings, but the possibility also exists that the distribution of these health workers may be determined more by the distribution of private practitioners then by the health needs of poor or rural people.[61]

The physician assistant program was first started at Duke University in 1965. This was followed shortly by the MEDEX Program in the state of Washington. These initial programs utilized returning servicemen with a considerable medical experience who had worked independently in their military assignments. Additional programs designed to bring medically trained servicemen into the health care system have been highly successful. Noteworthy among these are the MEDIHC Program (Military Experience Directed Into Health Careers), administered by the National Health Council,[62] and Project VEHTS (Versatile Employment of Health-Trained Servicemen), sponsored by the Manpower Administration of the U.S. Department of Labor.[63] The MEDEX program appears to have the greatest degree of standardization and is presently in the Universities of Washington, North Dakota, Alabama, Utah, South Carolina, and Hawaii; plus Dartmouth Medical School, Los Angeles, and Howard University. To start a MEDEX Program a medical association must initiate the process in conjunction with a medical school. The students are matched on a one-to-one basis with physicians before they finish their three-month intensive training at the university. They are then placed in nine-month on-the-job-training programs with the physicians who have previously agreed to hire the graduate MEDEX. The MEDEX is required to wear a blue coat instead of the white coat of physicians. The MEDEX Program has been proposed as a workable solution to health manpower shortage in many areas of the world.[64]

The increasing number of physician assistants has been viewed with mixed reaction. Generally, these new health workers have been a definite asset, particularly in rural areas.[65] Physicians are finding that these trained workers are reliable and dependable and thus feel justified in extending areas of work and responsibility. Some doctors are establishing protocols for their physician assistants to follow in treating patients with routine, chronic conditions.[66] In response to the growing need for standardization, the American College of Surgeons has adopted basic minimum requirements. The standards recommend that an assistant, prior to entering a training program, should have two years of college or its equivalent with courses in biological and physical sciences plus mathematics. The training program must have one year of preclinical work and one year of clinical training.[67] Also, the National Board of Medical Examiners has developed a national certification examination for physician assistants in primary care.[68]

Many questions are still left unanswered regarding physician assistants and their role in health care programs. The nursing profession is concerned that the nurse with her baccalaureate degree may have to be subservient to the physician assistant possessing only one or two years of academic training. Pharmacists are concerned that the physician assistants will be given the authority to write prescriptions, an authority not yet delegated to the pharmacist with his five or six years of intensive training in medical therapeutics. It is argued that the pharmacist should be given the legal right of prescribing long before this privilege is extended to those with far less training.

Certainly, there is a distinct need for standardized legislation regarding the role of physicians assistants. State legislation regarding at least some aspect of this classification of health workers has been enacted in approximately half of the individual states.[69] Some are granted legislative sanction through a general delegatory statute which amends the State Medical Practice Act and permits physician assistants to work under the supervision of physicians. Other states have enacted laws which authorize a State Board of Medical Examiners to establish rules and regulations with respect to the educational and employment qualifications of physician assistants. Under this latter regulatory authority statute, the physician who employs or supervises such an assistant is reported to be particularly vulnerable to malpractice claims.[70]

The National Academy of Sciences has defined three types of physician assistants. Type A is the preferred classification. This person is a generalist and is distinguished by his ability to integrate and interpret findings on the basis of general medical knowledge and to exercise a degree of independent judgement. Type B assistant possesses exceptional skill in one clinical specialty or, more commonly, in certain procedures within such a specialty. He is less qualified for independent action. Type C assistant performs a variety of routine tasks but his level of medical knowledge restricts his degree of independent synthesis and judgment.[71]

Considerable discussion, plus journal articles, has been generated regarding the certification or licensing of these new health professionals. Licensing laws were originally designed to specify minimum levels of professional competence necessary to protect the public. As the proliferation of health professions has increased, however, the stringent requirements have served to limit upward and lateral mobility, restrain movement of health professionals into other states, and confine personnel to limited functions as defined under statutory law. Several problems emerge in the licensing of new health professionals. Scope of functions for a given occupation are not easily delineated in such laws. It is difficult to filter out those duties that may be the sole responsibility of a given profession, those shared with other professions, and those not permissible for practice by a profession. Shortages of health personnel, particularly in rural areas or on late-night shifts have resulted in violation of rigid licensing laws.[72] Also the trend for each profession to establish its own set of license and educational requirements has limited the membership, and little planning has been done to establish cross-over points between licensed occupations.

Several alternatives have been proposed to modify these and other shortcomings. Most of these alternatives involve proposals to modify the State Medical Practice Act to allow broader delegatory powers in assigning tasks to allied health care personnel. It is proposed that broad delegatory powers should be given to health care institutions such as hospitals or health maintenance organizations.[73] Under this umbrella protection there could be considerable flexibility in assigning tasks throughout the wide range of health services. This broad delegation could also be extended to primary health care workers in remote areas where the person best qualified to render the needed health service would be the person legally permitted to deliver that service. In this consideration there could be a distinct difference between pharmaceutical service, physician service, or nursing service as compared to the services of a pharmacist, a physician, or a nurse. Another suggestion has been to encourage establishment of educational equivalency measures and job performance tests as alternative routes to licensing of health care personnel. Certainly, it obligates those who serve the public health to erase their preconceptions and orient themselves to the competencies of others whose skills supplement their own. New health professionals are needed in our expanded health care programs and should be encouraged to participate to the limits of their capabilities.

## REFERENCES

1. Rashkis, H. A. Urban health services of the future. *J.A.M.A., 217:* 6, 1971.
2. Berry, E. A., Jr., and Gordon, G. G. The Health Professions—A Paper Team? Bulletin Bureau of Pharmaceutical Services, School of Pharmacy, University of Mississippi, *6:* 7, 1970.
3. Atwell, R. J. Interdependence of medical and allied health education. *J.A.M.A., 213:* 2, 1970.
4. Mosow, S., Fifer, E. Z., and Guthman, J. Changing state laws regulating health manpower. *Amer. J. Public health, 63:* 1, 1973.
5. Christman, L. Education of the health team. *J.A.M.A., 213:* 2, 1970.
6. *Looking Into Health Care.* Health Manpower Conferences Project, Student American Pharmaceutical Association, 1973.
7. *Cost of Educating Medical Student May Reach $26,000.* News Front, Modern Medicine, Dec. 10, 1973.
8. *Educators Get Gloomy Financial Report.* American Medical News, Nov. 19, 1973.
9. *Percent Distribution of Non-Federal Physicians by Activity. Reference Data on the Profile of medical Practice.* American Medical Association, 1971.
10. *The Family Doctor.* American Academy of General Practice, 1973.
11. By any other name? *Time,* July 23, 1973.
12. *The Rural Clinic Program.* American Osteopathic Association.
13. *Fact Sheet.* American Osteopathic Association, 1973.
14. *Nursing and Related Services.* Health Resources Statistics, National Center for Health Statistics, DHEW Pub. (HSM) 73-1509, 1973.
15. Schaefer, M. J. The political and economic scene in the future of nursing. *Amer. J. Public Health, 63:* 10, 1973.
16. Lysaught, J. P. The house reunited: It must not fall. *Amer. J. Public Health, 62:* 7, 1972.
17. Extending the scope of nursing practice. A report of the Secretary's Committee to study extended roles for nurses. *J.A.M.A., 220:* 9, 1972.
18. Nurse-midwifery in the United States. *HSMA Health Rep., 86:* 5, 1971.
19. The primary care nurse: The generalist in a structured health care team. *Amer. J. Public Health, 62:* 6, 1972.
20. Standard, R. L., and Easley, H. D.C.'s new pediatric nurse practitioners. *Health Services Rep., 87:* 5, 1972.
21. Coulehan, J. L., and Sheedy, S. The role, training, and experience of a medical nurse practitioner. *Health Services Rep., 88:* 9, 1973.
22. Henriques, C. C., Virgadamo, V. C., and Kahane, M.D. Performance of adult health appraisal examinations utilizing nurse practitioners. *Amer. J. Public Health, 64:* 1, 1974.
23. *The Dentist and the Pharmacist.* American Dental Association, 1970.
24. *Dentistry and the Allied Services.* Health Resources Statistics, National Center for Health Statistics, DHEW Pub. (HSM) 73-1509, 1973.
25. Fisher, M. A. New directions for dentistry. *Amer. J. Public Health, 60:* 1970.
26. Waldman, H. B. The response of the dental profession to change in the organization of health care. *Amer. J. Public Health, 63:* 1, 1973.
28. Preliminary results of podiatry manpower survey. *Monthly Vital Statistics Rep., 19:* 11 Supplement, 1971.
29. Shapiro, J. Podiatry and public health: A 7-Year experience in the District of Columbia. *Amer. J. Public Health, 63:* 10, 1973.
30. *Veterinary Medicine.* Health Resources Statistics, National Center for Health Statistics, DHEW Pub. (HSM) 73-1509, 1973.
31. Francke, D. E. Career Opportunities for Students of Social Studies in Pharmacy. *Amer. J. Pharm. Ed.,* 1973.
32. Wilson, R. M. A Broader Range of Services for the Community Pharmacist. *J. Amer. Pharm. Assn., 14:* 1, 1974.
33. Froh, R. B. The Up and Coming Roles of the

Pharmacist. *J. Amer. Pharm. Assn., 12:* 8, 1972.

34. Brodie, D. C., Knoben, J. E., and Wertheimer, A. I. Expanded Roles for Pharmacists. *Amer. J. Pharm. Ed.,* 1973.

35. Hamm, M: N., Stanaszek, W. F., and Sommers, E. B. Survey of Physicians' drug information. *J. Amer. Pharm. Assn., 13:* 7, 1973.

36. Wilson, V. E. Medical care. *NARD J.,* March, 1971.

37. Waters, I. W. Understanding Your Patient: IV. Minor Ailments At *the Cash Register. School of Pharmacy,* University of Mississippi, Bulletin Bureau of Pharmaceutical Services, *9:* 12, 1973.

38. Lecca, P. J. Professional myopia in today's health crisis. *J. Amer. Pharm. Assn., 12:,* 8, 1972.

39. Linn, L. S., and Davis, M. S. Occupational orientation and overt behavior: The pharmacist as drug adviser to patients. *Amer. J. Public Health, 63:* 6, 1973.

40. Yellin, A. K., and Norwood, G. J. The public's attitude toward pharmacy. *J. Amer. Pharm. Assn., n.s., 14:* 2, 1974.

41. Davidson, S. M., Wacker, R. C., and Klein, D. H. Professional standards review organizations. *J.A.M.A., 26:* 9, 1973.

42. Rucker, T. D. PSRO's and Pharmacy. *J. Amer. Pharm. Assn. 13:* 10, 1973.

43. The pharmacist as a source for health information. *Action in Pharmacyy, 5:* 7, 1973.

44. Bicket, W. J. Autotherapy: The Future is Now. *J. Amer. Pharm. Assn., 12:,* 11, 1973.

45. Ladinsky, J. Research on pharmacy: Retrospect and prospect. *Amer. J. Pharm. Ed.,* 1973.

46. Henry, R. A. Use of physician's assistants in Gilchrist County, Florida. *Health Services Rep., 87:* 8, 1972.

47. Golden, A. S. Carlson, D. G., and Harris, B. Jr. Non-physician family health teams for Health Maintenance Organizations. *Amer. J. Public Health, 63:* 8, 1973.

48. Adamson, T. E. Critical issues in the use of physician associates and assistants. *Amer. J. Public Health, 62:* 9, 1971.

49. Kimmey, J. R. MEDEX-An operational and replicated manpower program: Increasing the delivery of health services Editorial. *Amer. J. Public Health, 62:* 12, 1972.

50. Drobny, A. Latin American experience related to the solution of rural health problems in the United States. *Amer. J. Public Health, 63:* 1, 1973.

51. Yankauer, A., *et al.* Performance and delegation of patient services by physicians in obstetrics-gynecology. *Amer. J. Public Health, 61:* 8, 1971.

52. Young, R. L. Apples and oranges and bananas. *Amer. J. Public Health, 64:* 2, 1974.

53. *The Allied Health Professions Personnel Training Act of 1966, as Amended.* Report to the President and the Congress. Washington, D. C.:

U. S. Gov't Printing Office, 1969.

54. Gartner, A., Health systems and new careers. *Health Service Rep., 88:* 2, 1973.

55. Ostergard, D. R., E. M., and Marshall, J. R. *Family Planning and Cancer Screening Services as Provided by Paramedical Personnel.* Paper Presented at Annual Meeting of American Association of Planned Parenthood Physicians, 1971.

56. *Health Manpower Source Book, Allied Health Manpower, 1950-80.* P.H.S. Pub. 263: 21, 1970.

57. Challenor, B., *et al.* A physician-associate program at a municipal hospital. *J.A.M.A., 225:* 1, 1973.

58. *Selected Training Programs for Physician Support Personnel,* DHEW Pub. No (NIH) 72-183, 1972.

59. Braun, J. A., Howard, D. R., and L. R. Pondy. The physician's Associate: A task analysis. *Amer. J. Public Health, 63:* 12, 1973.

60. *The Physician's Assistant: An Annotated Bibliography.* American Rehabilitation Foundation, 1970.

61. Kimmey, J. R. The physician's assistant and the provision of health care. Editorial. *Amer. J. Public Health, 63:* 1, 1973.

62. Operation MEDICH. *National Health Council, 3:* 1, 1973.

63. *Project VEHTS (Versatile Employment of Health-Trained Servicemen).* Preliminary Second Interim Report. Manpower Administration, U. S. Department of Labor, 1973.

64. Smith, R. A. MEDEX: A new approach to the global health manpower problem. *PAHO Bull., 7:* 3, 1973.

65. Litman, T. J., Public perceptions of the physician's assistant: A survey of the attitudes and opinions of rural Iowa and Minnesota residents. *Amer. J. Public Health,* March, 1972.

66. Komaroff, A. L., Protocols for physician's assistants. *N. Engl. J. Med., 290:* 6, 1974.

67. *ACS Lists Surgeon's Assistant Standards.* American Medical News, August 20, 1973.

68. 1900 expected to be enrolled in physician assistant trianing. *Health Resources News, 1:* 1, 1973.

69. Dean, W. J. State legislation for physician's assistants. *Health Services Rep., 88:* 1, 1973.

70. Curran, W. J. "Physician's assistants": The question of legal responsibility. *Amer. J. Public Health, 60:* 12, 1970.

71. Barkin, R. M., Need for statutory legitimation of the roles of physician's assistants. *Health Services Rep., 89:* 1, 1974.

72. Egelston, E. M. Licensure: Effects on career mobility. *Amer. J. Public Health,* Jan., 1972.

73. Shimberg, B., Esser, B. F., and Kruger, D. H. *Licensing in Health Occupations. Occupational Licensing and Public Policy.* Mapower Administration, U. S. Department of Labor, 1972.

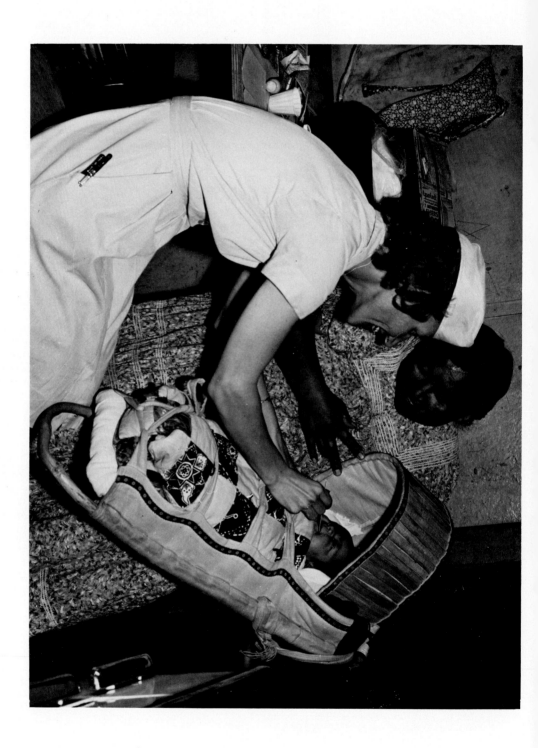

# 13

# Limitations to progress and opportunities for action

... the central plot of all social history—man's struggle to rearrange his social organization and institutions to keep pace with his accumulating knowledge, changing needs, and altered environment.
SOMERS, H. M., and SOMERS, A. R.,
*Doctors, Patients and Health Insurance*
Washington, D. C.: The Brookings Institution, 1961

Health cannot be simply given to the people; it demands their participation.
RENÉ SAND
So many worlds, so much to do,
So little done, such things to be.
ALFRED LORD TENNYSON

## LIMITATIONS TO PROGRESS

In a recent book, *The Biological Imperatives*,[1] Allan Chase points out that medical care and preventive medicine are only partial factors, albeit important ones, in the overall picture of the health of mankind. Adequacy of food supplies, proper housing conditions, freedom from occupational hazards and from stressful environments, and protection from pollution of air, food, and water are major determinants of human health. Man-made health hazards are not new, but actually began with the rise of industrialization in the 18th century. What is new about environmental disease factors is the rate at which they are now multiplying.

In a foreword to Chase's book, Doctor George Wald, noted biologist of Harvard University, states the matter clearly: "Lack of money decides one's chance to be born healthy, to survive infancy, to live out one's life span, to grow to one's genetic height, to have one physique rather than another, to be educated in the things one wants to learn. And so poverty is passed on from generation to generation, by social inheritance."

Much attention has been given in recent decades to the betterment of conditions in the impoverished segment of the American population. From Franklin Roosevelt on, each President has announced programs to alleviate the worst effects of poverty. Results to date have been fragmentary and only partially successful. It appears that the same determination and magnitude of effort must be devoted to social and human betterment as was concentrated on the Space program and other technological developments.

In a discussion before the Association of American Medical Colleges in 1969, Alan Pifer, President of the Carnegie Corporation, questioned whether piecemeal corrections of poverty situations can be successful. "Can any great social leap forward take place and be sustained in one sector of society without corresponding advances in others? Can we have good education in our inner cities without better housing, better job opportunities, better health facilities? Can we ever have good health without improved education, improved housing, and improved economic opportunity?"[2]

Although health and medical expenditures in the United States have risen from about $3.86 billion in 1940, to $12 billion in 1950, to $25.8 billion in 1960 to $68 billion in 1970, and to an estimated $94.1 billion in fiscal year 1973 and are likely to rise to at least $156 billion by 1980, all is not as it ought to be in respect to the health care of the American people. In Table 13.1, national health expenditures are summarized by source of funds and by types of expenditure. The health expenditures of 1973 are estimated to represent 7.7 per cent of the gross national product (see Fig. 13.1).

In spite of these large expenditures and in spite of the high level of medical competence that exists in the United States, progress in the organization of the system of delivery of medical care has lagged. According to Walter Reuther, former president of the United Auto-

523

Table 13.1

*Persons employed in the civilian labor force in Health services industry: 1950 and 1960 enumerations, 1966 estimates, and 1975 requirements*

| Industry and Occupation | 1950 | 1960 | 1966 | 1975 |
|---|---|---|---|---|
| Total, health services industry | 1,669,401 | 2,589,253 | 3,672,000 | 5,350,000 |
| Hospitals | 989,968 | 1,691,578 | 2,363,000 | 3,375,000 |
| Other health services | 679,433 | 897,675 | 1,309,000 | 1,975,000 |
| Selected health occupations within health services industry | | | | |
| *Other than "Allied Health"* | | | | |
| Dentists | 72,663 | 85,263 | 94,900 | 121,900 |
| Nurses, registered | 355,216 | 528,771 | 584,100 | 799,200 |
| Nurses, practical | 54,270 | 144,045 | 254,800 | 398,200 |
| Optometrists | 6,688 | 13,073 | 13,900 | 19,800 |
| Pharmacists | 3,510 | 6,504 | 10,600 | 11,300 |
| Physicians, including osteopaths | 186,525 | 222,162 | 254,500 | 371,900 |
| *"Allied Health"* | | | | |
| Attendants, hospital and office | 191,553 | 367,846 | 637,900 | 1,023,900 |
| Dietitians and nutritionists | 14,090 | 18,190 | 18,200 | 25,100 |
| Technicians, medical and dental | 69,208 | 127,947 | 203,600 | 376,400 |

Source: *Health Manpower Source Book* 21, M. Y. Pennell and D. B. Hoover, Public Health Service Publication, No. 263, Section 21, 1970.

mobile Workers,[3] approximately 2 million people in the United States currently receive no medical care; about 20 million people receive only a part of the care they require; and an additional 20 million who reside in urban ghettos receive less than adequate care. Reuther also points out that working people pay an increasingly large portion of their wages for prepaid health care benefits and see their hard-earned money purchase less care because of escalating costs.

### Restrictions of the Traditional System

Traditional public health agencies have been directed toward providing services to high risk groups in the population. On the whole there has been a low utilization of these services. Indeed, had there been a high utilization, the agencies would not have been prepared to provide the volume of services required. The agencies for the most part have been geared to a low demand for the services proffered.

The barriers to the full utilization of services by the poor are real. The health care offered is generally episodic, fragmented, and uncoordinated; it is not centered on the patient or the family unit, and is certainly not planned on a community-wide basis. The care is mostly symptomatic, and the patients are frequently sent back unchanged in their knowledge of, attitudes toward, and behavior within the same social environment that initially helped to produce their ill health.

An important barrier that separates the poor from health care is inaccessibility. This lack of accessibility is caused in part by the shortage of facilities and in part by a maldistribution of the available facilities. Clinics, health centers, and other facilities are frequently located to meet the convenience of the suppliers rather than that of the consumers of services. The service centers are often distant from the poverty areas which makes transportation difficult or expensive. In many situations, there is a failure to provide clinic hours that do not require the clients to miss employment or that accommodate the schedules of busy housewives.

In addition to inaccessibility, services provided for the poor often lack acceptability. Patients may spend long hours in uncomfortable and unattractive waiting rooms. Privacy and common human dignity are all too frequently ignored.

Another difficulty has been the failure of

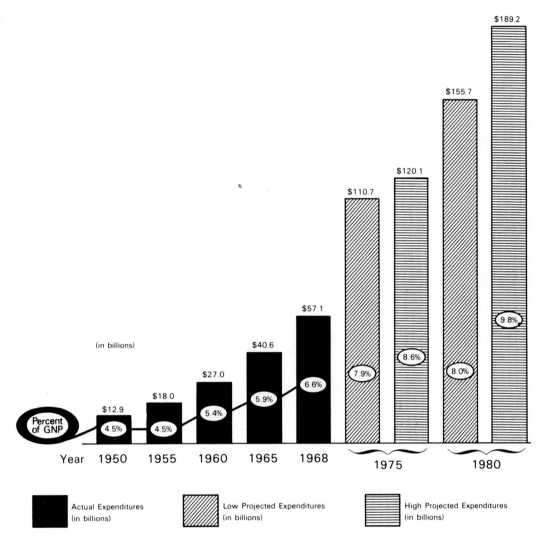

Fig. 13.1. Actual and projected national health expenditures and per cent of gross national product, selected years 1950-1980. Source: Research and Statistics Note, USDHEW, Social Security Administration, Office of Research and Statistics, Note No. 18, Oct. 30, 1970.

health departments and other public clinic services to recognize the total needs of the patient and the family. Programs have been developed for pregnant women, well babies, school children, and a number of specific disease problems. Routine preventive services have been separated from curative care which has resulted in a marked fragmentation of the health program.

In almost all communities, there are marked cultural differences between the poor and those charged with provision of health services. The cultural variations include language barriers, ethnic differences, and sharply divergent con-

cepts of sickness and health. These cultural gaps make it difficult for the poor to understand the value of the services being offered and to appreciate fully the necessity for preventive measures. Those who are in most need of health services frequently value them the least.

It is well known that those living at poverty levels and those belonging to certain ethnic groups experience illness more frequently than do more fortunate elements of the population. This aspect of health care in the United States is thoroughly explored in an excellent book sponsored by The Commonwealth Fund a few years ago.[4]

Other groups who suffer from a maldistribution of medical facilities are the populations of small towns and rural areas. Highly skilled professional workers in the health field tend to congregate in locations with large populations. In urban areas, there are 185 physicians per 1000 population, while rural areas have an average of 76 per 1000.

As pointed out in Chapter 3, the main complaint against current methods of medical practice, aside from the high cost, is its lack of continuity in the follow-up of patients over long periods. This is largely due to the scarcity of primary or family physicians. Patients frequently go directly to specialists who are restricted to narrow fields of medicine. Once the immediate complaint is relieved, the patient is seen no more.

Another criticism that has been leveled at American medicine is the excessive numbers of doctors who limit their practice to surgery. There are twice as many surgeons in proportion to the population in the United States as there are in the British Isles and they perform twice as many operations. In addition to those with specialist qualifications in surgery, large numbers of major operations are performed in the United States by general practitioners who lack proper surgical qualifications.

Failure of medical societies to discipline members who have become professionally incompetent for one reason or another or who have violated the code of medical ethics in their practices has drawn unfavorable comment from the public.

The public is also anxious to know that physicians and other professional health workers are keeping abreast with the tidal wave of new scientific and technical information that becomes available at an ever-increasing rate. Professional societies do urge members to take short courses and to attend scientific meetings to keep themselves informed. There is a movement toward requiring periodic examinations for the renewal of licensure for professional personnel to ensure that those allowed to practice have kept in touch with recent advances in their respective fields.

### Public Apathy and Ignorance

One characteristic of people living in poverty is that the level of education is far lower than the rest of the community. This signifies less interest in reading current publications; consequently, the poor are badly informed. Frequently language differences add to this difficulty. Unable to afford good housing, the poor tend to be segregated in low class residential areas. This creates a feeling of separateness from the other parts of the community and leads to increased difficulties in communication and a greater feeling of alienation. In dealing with such people, the public health officer must understand that their points of view may be so different from his own that what is reasonable in his terms may be quite unreasonable in theirs.

Some public health measures have, of course, been highly effective among the poor as well as the more fortunate. Public water supplies, which provide safe drinking water to all homes, and pasteurized milk, have greatly reduced some of the communicable diseases. More recently, the fluoridation of water has decreased dental caries. Smallpox vaccination was widely applied to children reaching school age; therefore, smallpox has virtually disappeared as a health problem in the United States. The contrary is true for other types of immunization such as measles, diphtheria, and poliomyelitis. These preventive measures are not nearly as well accepted by the poor as they are by other segments of the population. Partly, this lack of acceptance is caused by factors mentioned in the previous section.

It is apathy combined with ignorance that impedes the eradication of measles and poliomyelitis by immunization of the children of the United States. These human characteristics also account for the sharp rise in the prevalence of syphilis and gonorrhea among the youth of the nation.

Apathy is to some extent a characteristic of all people. There is a tendency for all humans to avoid or postpone experiences that are likely to prove unpleasant. Many individuals neglect going to a physician lest a diagnosis of heart disease or cancer be made. Among the poor, apathy is likely to be more of a problem. Often among the poor the cultural pressure to conform, which characterizes American society, is not as rigid as in other economic classes. A mother in a good residential area who neglects her child's teeth is almost surely to be reproved by her friends or neighbors. Because health standards are low in the poverty area, social pressures of that kind are unlikely to be expressed.

Another kind of apathy toward health hazards results from the human frailty of ignoring remote consequences. The public has been thoroughly warned by every imaginable means of the threat of cigarette smoking to health. The consequences of this injurious practice are distant in time, usually 10 to 20 years in the future. This very remoteness of the penalty makes people indifferent. The same applies to many other facets of personal behavior such as overeating, overindulgence in alcohol, and the sedentary life of ease so prized by many affluent individuals.

## Health Manpower Shortage

About 4.4 million persons were employed in the health professions and occupations in 1971, being listed under some 600 primary and alternate job titles. This total considerably exceeds the number that had been predicted for 1975 (see Table 13.1). Among professional workers, the greatest percentage increases were in the relatively newer occupational groups. Still with the growth of population in the United States (about 38 per cent increase between 1950 and 1973) and with the increased demand for personal health services, there are acute shortages in health manpower in almost every community.[5]

Over the past quarter of a century, there has been a substantial increase in the use of medical services. In 1930, Americans saw a physician on an average of two to three times each year; by 1964, the average had reached four and a half times; and in 1971, four and nine-tenths times. Hospital bed use has shown a similar increase. Annual admissions to general hospitals rose from 56 per 1000 population in 1930 to 145 per 1000 in 1964 to 160 per 1000 in 1972. Care of the sick in nursing homes has also risen substantially. Demands are expanding in two directions—toward intensification of care and toward a broader coverage.

Many social, economic, and technological factors influence the demands for health services. Population growth and increased numbers of elderly people are of prime importance. By 1980, it is expected that the population of the United States will increase another 14 million. Among these there will be one million more people over 65 years. The 65 and over age group requires twice as much service from physicians and uses over twice as many days of hospital care annually as do adults below that age.

The need for trained personnel in the health field is now so great and the demand so insistent that all sorts of persons trained and partially trained are being utilized. This shortage can become even more acute as health insurance expands. It is necessary to provide more health care personnel of the right kinds and to arrange a better geographical distribution of personnel and educational facilities to serve central urban and rural areas.

The Carnegie Commission on Higher Education in their 1970 report on "Higher Education and the Nation's Health"[6] sees the urgent need to expand the number of places for training doctors during this decade by 50 per cent and of dentists by 20 per cent. To achieve these goals, the Commission recommended that a number of new medical and dental schools be established; that the time required to become a practicing doctor be shortened from eight years after the B.A. to six years; reducing from four to three years the time required to get an M.D. degree; admitting two classes a year to medical and dental colleges; and reducing the time required for residency training. It was further recommended that the number of allied health personnel be greatly increased thereby raising the productivity of doctors, dentists, and nurses. To achieve these rather drastic changes in the training of medical and dental students, considerable outlays of money would be required. The Commission suggested that the major portion of these funds be provided by the Federal Government.

In addition to the new university health science centers and medical colleges, the Carnegie Commission recommended the development of the 126 new area health education centers located on the basis of careful regional planning. The objective would be to provide for enough area health centers so that no portion of a state or region would be remote from such facilities. These centers would be in essence satellites of university health science centers and would be visited regularly by the faculty of the university centers. The nucleus of the area health education centers would be a hospital. The functions of these centers would be to maintain high standard hospital facilities; to conduct educational programs under supervision of the university science centers; to provide clinical experience for medical and dental students and for students in allied health programs; to conduct continuing educational programs for health manpower of the area; to guide community colleges of the area in their development of training programs for allied health workers; and to cooperate with other hospitals and community agencies in the planning of more effective health care delivery systems.

*Physicians*

In 1971, the total number of active physicians (doctors of medicine and osteopathy) was 322,228. About 29,199 of these physicians were in Federal services. The ratio of physicians to the population has risen slightly for some years, but, because an increasing number are devoting their time to teaching, research, administration, and other activities, the ratio of physicians engaged in the delivery of personal services has declined. The situation would be much worse had it not been for the large scale migration of doctors from abroad to the United States. In 1972-73, 21,959 interns and residents in U. S. hospitals were graduates of foreign medical schools.

Based upon the estimate of several prepayment group practice plans, approximately 164 physicians are required per 100,000 population to provide present patterns of service. With the use of this ratio, it is estimated that by 1975 some 353,000 active physicians will be required, an addition of some 30,000 over the 1971 supply.

In the academic year of 1973-1974, there were 114 medical schools with students enrolled and seven osteopathic medical schools. First year enrollments in medical schools increased from 12,361 in 1971-1972 to 13,726 in 1972-1973. The number of graduates in 1973 increased by 842 over the previous year. Further increases are expected in each of the next five years. Entering students in the osteopathic schools are expected to increase from 580 in 1970 to 769 by 1976.

The Carnegie Commission of Higher Education recommends that entrants to medical schools be increased to 15,300 by 1976 and to 16,400 by 1978.

*Dentists*

In 1971, there were about 103,750 dentists in practice in the United States, a ratio of 47 per 100,000 population. It has been estimated that a doubling of output would be required to maintain that ratio of dentists to the population. In 1972 there were 52 dental schools (11 more than in 1950) graduating approximately 3775 dentists each year. By 1980, demands for dental care are expected to almost double as a result of rising incomes and education levels, increasing population, and dental insurance services.

It seems that there is little likelihood that the increase in practicing dentists will be sufficient to meet the needs. Probably there will have to be more use made of dental assistants to extend the quantity of services performed in dentist's offices.

*Nurses*

At the end of 1971, an estimated 748,000 registered nurses were practicing their profession in the United States. Approximately 30 per cent of these worked only on a part-time basis.

In 1910, there were 50,000 professional nurses employed in the United States or 55 for every 100,000 inhabitants. By 1930, the total rose to over 200,000 or 175 nurses per 100,000 population. Since that time, the growth has continued at a rate more than proportionate to the growth of population, and by 1970, there were 341 active nurses per 100,000 population. By 1980, it is estimated there will be between 379 and 406 nurses per 100,000 population. Of the nurses practicing in 1970, approximately 69 per cent were employed in hospitals or related institutions, 17 per cent as private duty or office nurses, 7 per cent as public health nurses, 4 per cent as nursing educators, and 3 per cent in occupational health fields (see Table 13.2).

In 1971, a total of 1350 schools offered 1363 programs in which 187,551 students were enrolled. The 1970-71 graduates totaled 47,001 of whom 48 per cent were graduated from diploma programs.

By 1975, the number of practicing registered nurses is expected to reach a level between 785,000 and 809,000. The prediction for 1980 is that between 864,000 and 924,000 registered nurses will be practicing their profession in the United States.

During the past 25 years, there has been a steady reduction in the number of nurses graduating from the old diploma schools usually operated by hospitals. At the same time,

Table 13.2

*Registered nurses in relation to population: selected years 1954–70;*
*projected 1975 and 1980*

| Year | Resident Population | Nurses in Practice | Nurses per 100,000 Population | Annual Change |
|------|-----|-----|-----|-----|
|  | *in thousands* | *in thousands* |  |  |
| 1954 | 159,825 | 402 | 252 |  |
|  |  |  |  | +3.5 |
| 1956 | 165,931 | 430 | 259 |  |
|  |  |  |  | +4.5 |
| 1958 | 171,922 | 460 | 268 |  |
|  |  |  |  | +7.0 |
| 1960 | 178,729 | 504 | 282 |  |
|  |  |  |  | +8.0 |
| 1962 | 184,598 | 550 | 298 |  |
|  |  |  |  | +4.0 |
| 1964 | 190,169 | 582 | 306 |  |
|  |  |  |  | +6.5 |
| 1966 | 194,899 | 621 | 319 |  |
|  |  |  |  | +6.0 |
| 1968 | 199,017 | 659 | 331 |  |
|  |  |  |  | +5.0 |
| 1970 | 205,395 | 700 | 341 |  |
|  |  |  |  | +4.6  +6.8 |
| 1975 | 215,588 | 785–809 | 364–375 |  |
|  |  |  |  | +3.0  +6.2 |
| 1980 | 227,510 | 863–924 | 379–406 |  |

Source:   Altman, S. H., *Present and Future Supply of Registered Nurses.* Public Health Service - National Institutes of Health, Bureau of Manpower Education, Division of Nursing, DHEW Publication (NIH) 73-134. Reprinted August, 1972.

the numbers of nurses receiving their education in two-year college courses (associate degree collegiate program) and in four-year collegiate courses leading to a degree has steadily risen.[7]

One point of interest in the nursing situation has been the increase in the numbers of foreign trained nurses becoming licensed in the United States. In 1950, such nurses averaged 1.7 per cent of the output of the United States nurse training programs; by 1960, this percentage had grown to 6.1, and by 1967 to 10 per cent. It is estimated that the foreign trained nurses will increase to 16.4 per cent of the number of nurses graduating from United States schools in 1980.[8]

The increase in the number of practical nurses has been rapid. By 1966, the number had reached 300,000. At least 50,000 more could have been used in hospitals and nursing homes. The requirements by 1975 may reach about 550,000, with the expected supply of 450,000.

To meet the expected needs, the annual number of graduates would have to be increased by an average of at least 7000 per year up to 1975.

About 700,000 nurse aides, orderlies, and attendants were employed in the United States in 1966, more than three times as many as had been employed in 1950. Shortages in each of the categories have been reported throughout the country. By 1975, the projected number of nurse aides, orderlies, and attendants will be about 1.1 million. Most of these individuals are trained in on-the-job programs.

*Pharmacists*

In 1972, approximately 130,750 pharmacists were practicing in the United States, about 18 per cent more than in 1955. Some 82 per cent of these worked in retail pharmacies, but most of the others were employed in hospitals, in manufacturing firms, or in Federal institutions.

In 1971-1972, there were 75 colleges of pharmacy in the United States and Puerto Rico which offered degrees in the profession–5,232 were graduated in the academic year 1971-72. The number of active pharmacists per 100,000 population has remained the same in recent years. Probably several new schools will be required to meet expected population growth.

*Clinical Laboratory Personnel*

As of 1971, an estimated 150,000 persons were engaged in full or part-time work in providing services in clinical laboratories in addition to physicians who specialize in clinical pathology. Some two-thirds of these are employed in hospitals. These persons include such specialties as bioanalysts, clinical chemists, microbiologists, clinical laboratory technologists, medical technologists, specialists in blood-bank technology, and cytotechnologists. In addition to these highly skilled persons, there are less well qualified people classified as clinical laboratory technicians, certified laboratory assistants, and medical laboratory technicians.

The number of those employed in clinical laboratory services has grown steadily. It is estimated that there were about 50,000 in 1955, 68,000 in 1960, about 85,000 in 1965, and some 150,000 in 1971. Automation and other technological advances may result in substantial savings of time for some skilled personnel. For example, the AutoAnalyzer in the clinical laboratory can perform in an 8-hr. day the equivalent of three weeks work of an average technician.

*Other Allied Health Professions*

Other members of the medical health team are in short supply, and future requirements will call for a stepping up in training and educational programs. To mention only a few of these allied medical professions points up the magnitude and complexity of the manpower problem. These professionals include dietitians; podiatrists; optometrists; occupational, physical, speech, and inhalation therapists; medical record librarians; dental hygienists; radiological technicians; and social workers.

In 1971, there were an estimated 16,800 dental hygienists in practice. These workers receive at least two years of education at the college level. The number of schools offering dental hygiene programs more than doubled between 1966 when there were only 58 such schools to 1971 when the number had grown to 133.

As for dental assistants, there were some 8000 maintaining their current registration in 1971. The two-year training period for these workers was offered by 46 institutions in 1971.

There were an estimated 31,150 dental technicians in 1971, mostly employed by commercial dental laboratories. Most of the dental technicians were trained on the job, but by 1971, 31 accredited institutions offered two-year academic programs.

One of the most hopeful developments in recent years for extending the professional skills of physicians and dentists is the employment of trained assistants. These are variously known as nurse clinicians, physician assistants or associates, and, in dentistry, as dental hygienists or dental assistants. Under the Comprehensive Health Manpower Training Act of 1971, more than 30 programs for training physician assistants have been supported. Prior to 1972, there was an accumulated total of 231 graduates; by the end of 1973, there were an additional 406; and by the end of 1974, an additional 793 will have been graduated. A national certification examination has been developed by the National Board of Medical Examiners and was administered for the first time in December, 1973.

Apart from the civilian sphere, each of the armed services and the Veteran's Administration has developed their own training programs for professional assistants.

The University of Colorado began training pediatric nurse practitioners in 1965. Since then, some 30 training programs for nurse practitioners and nurse midwives have been established. Up to the end of 1973, approximately 400 nurses have been trained in these programs.[9]

It must be understood that, in addition to providing for increased manpower needs, account must be taken of replacements necessitated by deaths, retirements, and other separations from the labor force and from transfers to other industries. Fortunately, many health workers who have left the labor force because of family responsibilities return to work at a later period.

*Public Health Personnel*

A task force at the University of North Carolina School of Public Health has recently completed a study of projected supplies of personnel to be trained by schools of public health, and an estimate of possible requirements for such trained personnel in community health programs in 1980 (see Table 13.3).

There are no reliable current data on the total supply of public health personnel, and certainly not according to specialty disciplines. The future of public health is uncertain with new specialties such as health planning, international health population studies, aerospace medicine, and family planning having either come into being or having been greatly expanded. A second difficulty has been to anticipate the outlines of the emerging health services delivery system. To complicate matters more, the Federal Government proposes policies that should increase the demand for health manpower while at the same time proposing drastic cuts in funds for training public health workers.[10]

*Aid for Educational Programs*

The Federal Government has supported health manpower education and training to meet its own needs for many years. Involvement in health manpower education and training to meet the needs of the civilian population originated in the mid-thirties with the inclusion in the Social Security Act of funds for the training of public health per-

Table 13.3

*Estimated supply of and requirements for selected categories of professional health manpower*

| Occupational Category | Base year supply (1970 unless specified) | Professionals with Masters Level Training or Higher[1] | | |
| | | 1980 Supply, assuming[2] | | |
| | | Constant school output | Reduced school output | Possible 1980 Requirements[3] |
|---|---|---|---|---|
| Environmental health | 2,200 | 4,300 | 3,800 | 5,000 |
| Epidemiology | 1,000 | 1,800 | 1,500 | 2,000 |
| Health education | 2,000 | 3,600 | 3,100 | 6,000 |
| Health services administration | 8,500 | 18,200 | 15,300 | 25,200 |
| Health statistics | 1,100 (1971) | 1,700 | 1,500 | 2,500 |
| Maternal health, family planning & child health | 800 | 1,800 | 1,500 | 2,000 |
| Mental health | 200 | 400 | 350 | 1,100 |
| Public health dentistry | 300 | 550 | 500 | 550 |
| Public health nursing | 2,457 (1968) | 5,200 | 4,500 | 5,700 |
| Public health nutrition | 1,000 | 1,800 | 1    0 | 2,600 |
| Public health veterinary medicine | 200 | 350 | 300 | 550 |

[1] Numbers over 1,000 are rounded to nearest 100, and below 1,000, to nearest 50.

[2] "Constant school output" is based on the size of the average graduating class in the early 1970's. "Reduced school output" assumes that the Administration's proposed FY 1974 budget was implemented according to plan, resulting in a 35 per cent reduction in the combined school output from the 1973–74 academic year on.

[3] The projected requirements *do not* take into consideration the continuing demands being made on American schools of public health to train foreign students in connection with the U. S. foreign assistance program and the requirements of the World Health Organization. Foreign student enrollments have averaged over 15 per cent in recent years.

Source: *Professional Health Manpower for Community Health Programs*, Task Force Report, Thomas L. Hall, Coordinator, Dept. of Health Administration, School of Public Health, U. of North Carolina, Chapel Hill, 1973.

sonnel. Since 1962, Federal assistance programs that foster the training of health manpower at all levels have increased in number and variety. Among the major enabling acts that have come into effect are the Manpower Development and Training Act of 1962, the Health Professions Educational Assistance Act of 1963, the Vocational Education Act of 1963, the Nurse Training Act of 1964, the Economic Opportunity Act of 1964, and a number of other acts leading up to the Comprehensive Health Manpower Training Act of 1971 and the Nurse Training Act of 1971. In an inventory taken, the Department of Health, Education, and Welfare lists 165 separate programs through which health personnel were being assisted under Federal agencies during fiscal year 1972. Nine Federal departments and five independent agencies administered programs. Two-thirds of these programs were supported or conducted by the Department of Health, Education, and Welfare.[11]

In his FY 1974 budget message to Congress, the President called for an abrupt termination of support to the schools of public health and a drastic reduction of traineeship funds for students in public health fields. This sharp cut in funds posed a critical situation for most schools. Congress acted to restore these funds to the 1974 budget, but the outlook for Federal aid in future years is most uncertain.

### Social and Economic Barriers

Man lives in a social as well as a physical environment. Health problems which arise among people are essentially social in character. In the past, public health agencies have too often attempted to avoid responsibility for the development of social policies for the solution of health problems.[12] This tendency is disappearing under the leadership of the Federal Government. In the words of former Secretary of Health, Education, and Welfare, John W. Gardner, "We have declared war on ignorance, disease, poverty, discrimination, mental or physical incapacity—in fact, on every condition that stunts human growth or diminishes human dignity."

These Federally sponsored programs—Medicare, Medicaid, War on Poverty, Housing and Urban Development, and others—have had a strong impact on every aspect of health and medical practice throughout the land. These social policies are the first steps toward abolition of the charity system of medicine, a system which has generally provided second class care.

It is well known that social conditions influence health markedly. The urban poor live in crowded surroundings where smog prevails, where refuse collects in the streets, where rats run, where plumbing fails, and where malnutrition is common. Such conditions invariably lead to high tuberculosis rates, to unnecessary infant mortality, to higher maternal death rates, and to increased occurrence of chronic diseases. For these people who need it the most, good medical care is least accessible. The same applies to many rural areas. Some 6 per cent of the American population live without the protection of local health services. In many rural areas, high quality medical care is inconveniently located and difficult for many families to finance.

On the other side of the coin, the pressures and anxieties resulting from business and professional competition, the complexities of society, overindulgence in food and drink, plus a sedentary existence, all of which characterizes a good proportion of affluent groups in Western society, lead to other forms of ill health—high blood pressure, coronary heart disease, duodenal ulcers, and nervous breakdowns.

In respect to financial barriers to health care, a great difficulty has been the steady rise in *per capita* personal health care costs. In 1960 personal health care costs were $147.20. By 1968, these expenditures had risen to $279.68 and by 1972 to $422.00 *per capita*. Estimates are that *per capita* costs will be over $500.00 by 1975 and between $669.94 and $814.25 by 1980 (see Table 13.4). The increase in expenditures has occurred primarily in the Federal sector. The government is now providing about 40 per cent of the total health expenditures.

In Chapter 3, Table 7, it is shown that the largest single item of expenditure—representing more than one-third of the total—was for hospital care, including both inpatient and outpatient services. Physician services are the next largest type of expenditure amounting to 21 per cent of the total. The remainder of the expenditures goes for a large number of health services including dentist's services, drugs, eyeglasses, appliances, nursing home care, and so on.

Over the past two decades, medical care costs have increased more rapidly than any other component of the consumer price index. The

Table 13.4

*Per capita national health expenditures, by type of service, selected years, 1960–80[1]*

| Type of Service | 1960 | 1968 | 1975 | | 1980 | |
|---|---|---|---|---|---|---|
| | | | Low | High | Low | High |
| Total | $147.20 | $279.68 | $508.91 | $551.81 | $669.94 | $814.25 |
| Health services and supplies | 137.86 | 259.97 | 481.85 | 521.61 | 640.74 | 777.07 |
| Hospital care | 49.35 | 101.63 | 221.54 | 240.97 | 328.70 | 398.45 |
| Short-term | 32.92 | 75.51 | 174.65 | 190.32 | 268.57 | 328.79 |
| Long-term | 16.44 | 26.12 | 46.88 | 50.65 | 60.12 | 69.66 |
| Physicians' services | 31.02 | 56.63 | 101.57 | 110.22 | 125.64 | 156.85 |
| Dentists' services | 10.79 | 17.69 | 30.30 | 32.76 | 36.10 | 45.57 |
| Other professional services | 4.70 | 6.57 | 10.23 | 11.11 | 11.98 | 15.09 |
| Drugs and drug sundries | 19.96 | 30.12 | 42.65 | 45.43 | 48.81 | 56.64 |
| Eyeglasses and appliances | 4.23 | 8.41 | 13.28 | 13.84 | 16.72 | 19.13 |
| Nursing-home care | 2.87 | 11.18 | 21.94 | 24.44 | 26.20 | 32.07 |
| Expenses for prepayment and administration | 4.71 | 9.05 | 12.27 | 12.76 | 14.15 | 15.99 |
| Government public health activities | 2.25 | 4.75 | 6.06 | 6.27 | 6.80 | 7.49 |
| Other health services | 7.98 | 13.94 | 21.99 | 23.80 | 25.66 | 29.81 |
| Research and medical-facilities construction | 9.33 | 19.71 | 27.06 | 30.20 | 29.20 | 37.18 |
| Research | 3.61 | 8.64 | 10.32 | 11.31 | 11.04 | 13.51 |
| Construction | 5.72 | 11.07 | 16.74 | 18.90 | 18.17 | 23.67 |

[1] Based on the following population estimates: 1960—183,246,000; 1968—204,173,000; 1975—217,557,000; 1980—232,412,000.

Source: *Projections of National Health Expenditures 1975 and 1980.* D. P. Rice and M. F. McGee, Research and Statistics Note, Social Security Administration, Note No. 18-1970, Oct. 30, 1970.

increase in average cost per patient day in community hospitals rose from $16 in 1950 to $103 in 1972. Probably the chief factor in this great increase in hospital costs is due to a rapid expansion of demand for such services. The growth of health insurance has promoted this increased public demand. The effect of prepaying for health care is to encourage hospitals to provide a product that is steadily more expensive.

In 1970, the national health care expenditures came to $61.8 billion. Of this total, 25.5 per cent was met by private health insurance; 38 per cent by direct out-of-pocket payments by consumers; 35 per cent by public funds; and 1.5 per cent by philanthropy. Four-fifths of the civilian population of the United States had some protection by private health insurance [13] (see Table 13.5).

Although insurance overall pays a substantial amount of medical bills and even a greater portion of hospital costs, individual coverage varies widely. Low-paid workers, those frequently unemployed, and those who are self-employed or work in small businesses, are not likely to be adequately insured. Families not eligible for group coverage can purchase insurance only on very disadvantageous terms. This lack of adequate coverage imposes a considerable residue of financial hardship on many families least able to meet it.

At the end of 1972, the Health Insurance Association of America estimated that a total of some 182 million individuals in the United States held some form of private health insurance policies, an increase of over 30 per cent over the 1962 total.

Every family (even those in the upper income brackets) is haunted by the possible occurrence of a catastrophic illness in its midst. Everyone

Table 13.5

*National health expenditures, by source of funds and per cent of gross national product, selected calendar years 1929-72*

| Year | Gross National Product | Total | | Private | | Public | |
|---|---|---|---|---|---|---|---|
| | | Amount | Per cent of gross national product | Amount | Per cent of total | Amount | Per cent of total |
| | *in billions* | *in millions* | | *in millions* | | *in millions* | |
| 1929 | $103.1 | $3,649 | 3.5 | $3,154 | 86.4 | $495 | 13.6 |
| 1935 | 72.2 | 2,936 | 4.0 | 2,372 | 80.8 | 563 | 19.2 |
| 1940 | 99.7 | 3,987 | 4.0 | 3,178 | 79.7 | 811 | 20.3 |
| 1950 | 284.8 | 12,662 | 4.5 | 9,222 | 72.8 | 3,440 | 27.2 |
| 1955 | 398.0 | 17,745 | 4.4 | 13,190 | 74.3 | 4,555 | 25.7 |
| 1960 | 503.7 | 26,895 | 5.3 | 20,259 | 75.3 | 6,637 | 24.7 |
| 1965 | 684.9 | 40,468 | 5.9 | 30,398 | 75.1 | 10,066 | 24.9 |
| 1966 | 749.9 | 44,974 | 6.0 | 32,153 | 71.5 | 12,821 | 28.5 |
| 1967 | 793.9 | 50,696 | 6.4 | 32,555 | 64.2 | 18,141 | 35.8 |
| 1968 | 864.2 | 56,587 | 6.5 | 34,999 | 61.8 | 21,588 | 38.2 |
| 1969 | 930.3 | 64,139 | 6.9 | 40,046 | 62.4 | 24,094 | 37.6 |
| 1970 | 977.1 | 71,619 | 7.3 | 44,729 | 62.5 | 26,889 | 37.5 |
| 1971 | 1,055.5 | 79,658 | 7.5 | 48,741 | 61.2 | 30,917 | 38.8 |
| 1972 | 1,155.2 | 89,516 | 7.7 | 54,075 | 60.4 | 35,441 | 39.6 |

Source: *National Health Expenditures Calendar Years* 1929-72, Cooper, B. S., N. L. Worthington, and P. A. Piro, Research and Statistics Note No. 3-1974, February 6, 1974, Social Security Administration, DHEW Publication No. (SSA) 74-11701.

knows of occasional unfortunate individuals whose medical and hospital expenses run into many thousands of dollars. The health insurance companies have attempted to meet this threat by the issuance of major medical policies. Beginning in 1951, this form of insurance has grown rapidly. By 1971, some 81 million persons were covered by major medical policies with maximum insurance coverage for medical expenses ranging up to $50,000 or more.[14]

The Social Security Amendments of 1965 opened a new era of health services. The health of the people has now been raised to the real of considered social policy. The first steps taken in Title 18A under the principle of compulsory social insurance are partial and timid. Benefits are limited to paying for hospital and certain types of hospital-related care, and the benefits are restricted to people 65 years of age and over. Under Title 18B coverage is voluntary and depends upon payment of monthly premiums. The benefits under Title 18B take the form of indemnification or reimbursement rather than service. This system involves no major departure from well-known private insurance plans.

Title 19 seems to open the door to an extension of free services to some groups other than welfare recipients. The limit of income of those eligible for Title 19 benefits is set by each state legislature and has varied rather widely among states.

In the past, the public medical care programs that have been enacted have been limited to special groups, such as veterans and workers under workmen's compensation, or to the indigent. All social classes come within the scope of Medicare. The public has been little concerned about the quality of the medical care that was supplied to the indigents. Now that the plan applies to all social classes, concern for setting good standards of care is embodied in the act.

The principal significance of Medicare and Medicaid is the deliberate use of social policy to remove partially the financial barriers to access to health services. It now seems inevitable that strong forces will demand an extension of the health benefits to other groups in the population.[15]

There is a saying that "the sick get poorer and the poor get sicker." Both poverty and ill health have multiple causes which are inter-

related. Poverty is neither a necessary nor a sufficient cause of ill health; well-to-do people also suffer from many diseases. Poverty denotes a wide variety of undesirable features of social life: unemployment, poor housing, loss of status, inadequacy, and social disruption. Whether it is a matter of poverty, insufficient education, or both, it is evident that the poor are likely to receive less health care than are more favored elements of the population. A few illustrations point up this situation. Among persons with annual family incomes of less than $2000 about 29 per cent have chronic conditions with limitation of activity, as contrasted with less than 7.5 per cent among persons with family incomes of $7000 or more. Children under age 15 average two physician visits per year in families with incomes under $2000 compared with four and four-tenths visits in families with incomes over $7000. In families with income under $4000, 22 per cent have never seen a dentist as compared with 7.2 per cent in families with incomes over $10,000.[16] (see Table 13.6).

Each year the Bureau of the Census updates the income figure separating the "poor" from the non-poor to reflect changes in the consumer price index. For 1972, the figure was $4275 for a non-farm family of four. According to the Bureau's survey early in 1973, there were about 24.5 million persons in the United States in families with incomes below the poverty level. This figure is 4.3 per cent lower than in 1971. Probably with the energy shortage, the low income families will increase again in 1973 to 1974. Table 13.7 shows the number and per cent of households by 1972 household income. It will be seen that 17.1 million households (24.9 per cent) had incomes under $5000.

In a paper entitled "The Pathology of Poverty", Doctor Ashley Weeks[17] states ". . . there are groups in the population that are especially likely to show a high incidence of poverty." Among these are the aged, persons over 65 years of age, especially women who are heads of families, and the non-whites. Those poorly educated are also likely to have a high incidence of poverty. Geographically there are differences in the distribution of the poverty group. In the north, poverty is more prevalent in the cities, while in the south, poverty is found more commonly in rural areas.

Paradoxically mortality rates may be higher among some high income groups than among

Table 13.6

*Number and per cent of households by 1972 household income*
*Households as of March 1973*

| Household Income | Households | |
|---|---|---|
| | Number | Per cent |
| Total | 68,251,000 | 100.0 |
| Under $1,000 | 1,523,000 | 2.2 |
| $1,000 to $1,999 | 3,605,000 | 5.3 |
| $2,000 to $2,999 | 4,276,000 | 6.2 |
| $3,000 to $3,999 | 3,894,000 | 5.7 |
| $4,000 to $4,999 | 3,777,000 | 5.5 |
| $5,000 to $5,999 | 3,652,000 | 5.4 |
| $6,000 to $6,999 | 3,558,000 | 5.2 |
| $7,000 to $7,999 | 3,752,000 | 5.5 |
| $8,000 to $9,999 | 7,178,000 | 10.5 |
| $10,000 to $11,999 | 7,025,000 | 10.3 |
| $12,000 to $14,999 | 8,647,000 | 12.7 |
| $15,000 to $24,999 | 13,139,000 | 19.3 |
| $25,000 and over | 4,227,000 | 6.2 |
| Median income | $9,698 | (X)[1] |

[1] Not applicable.

Source: Bureau of the Census, Current Population Reports, Series-P-60, No. 89, July 1973.

the poor. Millions of Americans who do not get enough to eat live in close proximity to more millions who eat too much. More Americans probably die of excess rather than of neglect and poverty.

The children of well-to-do parents who turn to drugs for everything from weight control, to control of acne, to birth control, to stay awake or to get to sleep, and for psychic stimulation are surely running risks with their health, as much as the middle-aged businessman who overeats, drinks to excess, smokes heavily, and takes no exercise.[18]

In the words of the former Prime Minister Harold Macmillan of Great Britain, "The winds of change are blowing." Now that health services have become a concern of social policy, many vested interests must yield some of their stubbornly held prerogatives. Voluntary hospitals must recognize that there is a public interest in their affairs, especially as an increasing portion of their funds will come from public sources. They can no longer be answerable only to their governing boards or to dominant professional groups. They are responsible to the public. It would be well that the public should have a broader representation on their governing councils.

The medical profession, which fought bitterly against the passage of Medicare, has a great responsibility in the years to come in helping to decide what course the distribution of health services may take. This is particularly true with regard to improving the quality of care for the average patient and, second, to controlling the rapidly growing costs of medical services. Constructive participation of the medical men in such important matters will do much to restore the partially lost confidence of the public in the high principles of the profession.

Health departments in general have confined their activities to preventive measures and ignored the gross inadequacies in community health services. All this is changing. Health departments are now administering home medical care programs and are becoming involved more frequently in administrative responsibility for publicly financed medical care programs. More and more public health agencies must become concerned with the quality of health services available to the public. The role of watchdog of the community in health matters

Table 13.7

*Trends in poverty: Number and per cent of persons poor, by age, 1959-71*

| Age | Total Civilian Noninstitutional Population[1] (in millions) | | | | Persons Poor (in millions) | | | | Per Cent Poor | | | |
|---|---|---|---|---|---|---|---|---|---|---|---|---|
| | 1959 | 1969 | 1970 | 1971 | 1959 | 1969 | 1970 | 1971 | 1959 | 1969 | 1970 | 1971 |
| All ages | 176.5 | 199.8 | 202.5 | 204.6 | 39.5 | 24.3 | 25.5 | 25.6 | 22.4 | 12.2 | 12.6 | 12.5 |
| Children under 18 | 64.0 | 69.8 | 69.9 | 68.5 | 17.2 | 9.8 | 10.5 | 10.3 | 26.9 | 14.1 | 15.0 | 15.1 |
| In families with male head | 58.3 | 61.7 | 60.8 | 59.3 | 13.1 | 5.4 | 5.7 | 5.5 | 22.4 | 8.8 | 9.3 | 9.3 |
| In families with female head | 5.7 | 8.0 | 9.0 | 9.1 | 4.1 | 4.4 | 4.8 | 4.8 | 72.2 | 54.4 | 53.4 | 53.1 |
| 18–54[2] | 81.0 | 93.0 | 94.9 | 97.5 | 13.4 | 7.7 | 8.2 | 8.8 | 16.5 | 8.2 | 8.6 | 9.0 |
| 55–64 | 15.5 | 18.2 | 18.4 | 18.8 | 3.3 | 2.0 | 2.1 | 2.2 | 21.5 | 11.1 | 11.4 | 11.4 |
| 65 and over | 15.9 | 18.9 | 19.3 | 19.8 | 5.6 | 4.8 | 4.7 | 4.3 | 37.7 | 25.3 | 24.4 | 21.6 |
| In families | 12.1 | 13.3 | 13.5 | 13.8 | 3.2 | 2.1 | 2.0 | 1.7 | 26.4 | 16.0 | 14.7 | 12.4 |
| Unrelated individuals | 3.8 | 5.6 | 5.8 | 6.1 | 2.4 | 2.7 | 2.7 | 2.6 | 66.0 | 47.3 | 47.1 | 42.3 |
| Men | 1.1 | 1.4 | 1.4 | 1.4 | .6 | .6 | .5 | .5 | 58.5 | 39.8 | 38.9 | 32.6 |
| Women | 2.6 | 4.2 | 4.4 | 4.7 | 1.8 | 2.1 | 2.2 | 2.1 | 69.1 | 49.9 | 49.7 | 45.1 |

[1] Includes Armed Forces in the United States living off post or with families on post.
[2] Includes some unrelated individuals and heads or wives under age 18.
Source: Annual Statistical Supplement, Social Security Bulletin 1971.

must be assumed even though it results in less comfortable relationships with medical practitioners.

## Man's Worst Enemy

As a leading cartoonist paraphrased Admiral Oliver Hazard Perry's message sent after the Battle of Lake Erie, "We have met the enemy and he is us." Man's worst enemy is himself. As recently stated by Burnet and White, "Civil war and rising incidence of crime, drug addiction, psychosomatic and mental disease are likely to be much more important results of overpopulation than any increase in infectious disease."[19]

In a similar vein, Denis Gabor in his book, *Inventing the Future,*[20] asserts that the future of man will be determined by three major requirements: (1) to prevent nuclear war on a global scale; (2) to keep population growth in reasonable step with planetary resources; and (3) to make socially acceptable use of the increasing leisure that comes with increasing affluence.

Whether man can manage these necessary accommodations with the future remains to be seen. Judging by his reckless misuse of the technological and scientific accomplishments of the past 100 years, one cannot help but have strong reservations. The greed of industrial corporations and the indifference and carelessness of the public has brought us to a situation of polluted air and water. The land is being progressively ravished and the oceans are rapidly becoming uninhabitable for marine life. All of these forms of pollution are potentially harmful to human health.

Unfortunately, the energy crisis has brought the Environmental Protection Agency in its efforts to improve air quality into conflict with efforts to deal with the shortage of energy. Automobile manufacturers are loudly calling for a postponement of the required reductions in emission standards.

Another quite different human characteristic that poses some health hazards is the desire of man to possess a pet. An article in the *U. S. News and World Report* states that in 1973 the American public possessed some 700 million domestic pets.[21] Of these, there were 40 million dogs, 40 million cats, 15 million birds, 10 million other mammals varying from rodents to monkeys, and 600 million fish. These pets pose various health threats such as rabies, psittacosis, salmonella infections, and others.

The cost of this prodigious pet industry runs around $4 billion per year.

In other sections of this textbook, man's intransigence in persisting in health-harmful habits has been referred to in connection with alcohol, drugs, tobacco, food excesses, and careless handling of cars on streets and highways. Perhaps the one beneficial result of gasoline shortage has been a marked reduction in highway deaths and accidents.

## Fallacious Advertising

Advertising occupies an ever increasing role in American life. Over 23 billion dollars are spent annually in the advertising industry. The techniques of popular appeal become ever more sophisticated. From the point of view of health, advertising makes valuable contributions. Probably advertising media have done more to promote personal hygiene than all other approaches added together. In immunization campaigns, notably that against poliomyelitis, the cooperation of advertising experts ensured that about every individual in the country understood the value and the availability of the procedures. In other fields of health education, the possibilities of advertising methods have scarcely begun to be fully explored. In general, it may be said that modern advertising has exerted many favorable influences toward better health. Unfortunately, advertising is expensive and health agencies are generally limited in their available funds.

In some directions advertising has had harmful effects on the health of the people. Almost certainly cigarette smoking has been popularized by intensive advertising campaigns. The same may be said for the consumption of beer and other alcoholic beverages. Americans have been turned into a pill-taking people. The Food and Drug Administration is responsible for regulation of the advertising of prescription drugs. A close watch is maintained on the public statements of pharmaceutical houses about their products, and frequently the FDA requires that some claims for commercial products be modified or withdrawn. There is a growing demand that the Federal Government take steps to control the advertising of cigarettes and other articles likely to be injurious to human health.

For many years, intensive advertising efforts have been directed to persuading the uninformed lay public of the wonderful healing powers of varied and numerous therapeutic agents, secret or patented. Great claims are made for the beneficent effects of these drugs on such common conditions as back pain, arthritis, or general lassitude. Inasmuch as many of these heavily advertised remedies are frequently ineffective, the public is defrauded of its money. Perhaps more important is that these carefully conceived sales campaigns persuade thousands of gullible people to engage in self-medication. Frequently, the self-medication leads to postponement of seeking medical advice until the underlying condition has advanced too far for remedial action that might have been effective earlier in the course of the disease.

One of the most inhuman facets of advertising in the health field is the advocacy of false cancer cures. Such fallacious advertising preys upon the victims of a chronic and highly fatal disease. Many of these patients have already spent a large proportion of their resources for medical expenses and can ill afford to invest in worthless remedies. The advertising of such valueless cancer cures is a public disservice.

## OPPORTUNITIES FOR ACTION

Interest in health, both personal and for the community, is at an all time high level among Americans. Programs for control of air and water pollution, improvement of housing, and relief of urban problems have been launched on an impressive scale. The construction of new health and medical facilities has proceeded at an unprecedented rate. New schools for the preparation of additional health personnel are coming into use and others are in the planning stage. Each year brings new vaccines, drugs, equipment, and apparatus at an increasing rate. Research in the basic sciences of biology and medicine provides more insight into the chemical and physical basis of life. Transplantation of organs offers possibilities for prolonging useful lives for many years. All of these and many other new measures developed in recent years have changed the prospects for improvement of human health. The challenge presented to this generation is to apply these beneficent measures to the widest possible degree.

### Remodeling the Health Service Structure

One of the most significant events in the restructuring of health services to meet current demands was the passage of Public Law 89-749, the Comprehensive Health Planning Act of 1966. This program is designed to bring all communities of the nation into a framework for comprehensive health planning. State governors were requested to designate a single state comprehensive health-planning agency which could be the existing state health department, an interdepartmental committee, or a new agency to administer the state's planning functions. A state health-planning council must be provided to advise the state agency in carrying out its functions. A majority of the membership of the advisory council must be representatives of consumers of health services.

In addition to state planning agencies, the act authorizes grants to governmental or voluntary non-profit agencies for developing comprehensive health plans for regional, metropolitan, or other local areas. These area-wide health planning groups must be concerned with the total health system. This signifies planning for the provision of the full spectrum of health services in the area.

Future grants to states from the Public Health Service must be spent in accordance with plans made by the state comprehensive health-planning agency.

There has not been enough time since the provisions of Public Law 89-749 went into effect to demonstrate what the impact of this act will be. It seems likely that over the years a better integrated, more efficient system for the distribution of health services will result. The large consumer representation on the Advisory Council will give the public a greater voice in the way that available funds will be apportioned for health facilities and services. Duplication of services and facilities should be avoided more readily and provision for the care of all segments of the population should be attained more quickly. Probably the broadly based planning agencies at both state and local levels can reduce the bickering and competitive struggles of health agencies that characterize so many local situations.

Another significant program under Federal auspices is the Comprehensive Health Services Programs administered by the Office of Economic Opportunity. The intent of this program is to provide personal health services, both preventive and curative, to low income families, readily accessible to them, with the greatest possible participation in each program of the poor themselves. This program is not based on the state or region or even the community as a whole, but on the neighborhood.

The dominant trend of primary health care for 25 years has been to draw closer to the hospital as the center of health services. The justification is that there is coordination with inpatient care, accessibility of consultants, and availability of specialized equipment. Unfortunately, there has been a steady withdrawal of the hospital and its staff from the community needing primary care. Differences in ethnic background, in education, and in economic status between health professionals and the poor seem to have increased in recent years.

In contrast, the comprehensive neighborhood health center stands in the middle of its community. Over 40 such health centers are functioning today serving neighborhood populations of from 6000 to 25,000. In a neighborhood center in Boston, Massachusetts, 87 per cent of the area population—5300 people—came to the center during the first 20 months of operation. A coordinated home care program is also an integral part of the service.

There is a growing interest on the part of medical colleges to participate in the organization and operation of comprehensive community health care programs. Academic institutions have come to regard such programs as an excellent facility for both teaching and research. Such a program is being undertaken in the Boston area by the Harvard University School of Medicine in cooperation with a number of teaching hospitals and health insurance companies. This plan will provide medical coverage for 30,000 persons.

The University of Rochester in 1968 has taken the lead in the organization of a neighborhood health center in the Baden-Ormond area of Rochester, New York. The Office of Economic Opportunity is financing a neighborhood health center in Atlanta, Georgia, established by the joint efforts of the county medical society and Emory University. The center is designed to serve about 28,000 people in a poverty stricken area of the city.

In Nashville, Tennessee, the Meharry neighborhood health center is also being financed by the Office of Economic Opportunity. In addition to Meharry Medical College, Vanderbilt University, Fish University, and the George Peabody College are cooperating agencies in providing care for some 37,000 low income families in Nashville.

Other medical colleges are in process of planning participation in similar neighborhood health programs. The experience gained in this type of experimental pattern for the delivery of health services will doubtless influence medical practice substantially throughout the country within a few years.

Obviously, there are difficulties in extending the neighborhood health center idea to all communities that badly need such a service—long-range financing is one, scarcity of properly motivated personnel is another, resistance of vested interests also poses severe problems. However, the experience already gained clearly points up the desirability of creating comprehensive service centers that are consumer-oriented. It is also clear that in the future such services must be more accessible to those who are to use them.

As has been discussed in Chapter 2, the Federal Government hopes through the provisions of the Health Maintenance Organization Act of 1973 to promote organization for a large number of prepaid group clinics across the nation which will provide comprehensive health care to citizens of all social and economic levels. The Administration has also proposed a National Health Insurance Bill based on a cooperative program between government and private health insurance companies. Possibly by the date this book appears, Congress may have enacted a national insurance program. The Congress also has before it for consideration bills to formulate a National Health Policy to provide guidelines for future developments in the health field. The decade of the 1970's indeed may be a memorable one in the history of American health progress. New legislation may very well abolish or markedly alter certain health programs now aided by Federal funds such as the Regional Medical Program (P. L. 89-239) and the Comprehensive Health Planning programs (P. L. 89-749).

Under Congressional mandate, the Department of Health, Education, and Welfare established a nationwide system of Professional Standards Review Organization (PSRO) to evaluate the necessity for and quality of medical care delivered in their area under Medicare, Medicaid, and the Maternal and Child Health programs. PSRO membership is limited to licensed practicing doctors of medicine or osteopathy. The primary emphasis of PSRO is on assuring the quality of medical care. PSRO will also determine whether services provided are medically necessary and are delivered in the proper setting (hospital, office, home, or nursing home) for the proper length of time.

PSRO will have to be multiple in all states except those that are small or sparsely populated. HEW will provide funding to the PSRO to cover all necessary expenses. A national council advises HEW on PSRO program matters.

PSRO is recognized as a program of potential significant benefit to the health professions and to health care institutions.

## Research in Community Health

Until quite recently health-related research was focussed mainly on specific diseases and on methods for their prevention or treatment. The heavily financed and intensive research program in poliomyelitis organized by the National Foundation is an excellent example of this type of program. Many health problems, especially in the chronic disease area, cannot be satisfactorily dealt with by such a limited approach. Lung cancer and coronary heart disease have been investigated most fruitfully by well-planned epidemiological studies in the community. Other such health problems are under intensive study on a community or population basis rather than solely in the individual patient or in the basic science laboratory.

The advent of the National Health Survey program in 1958 has strongly indicated the value of the information that can be obtained by sampling methods. Now reliable data are available on dozens of health problems whereas only guesses or crude estimates were formerly available. One can only hope that these valuable surveys will be continued and expanded in the years to come.

Perhaps the most urgent need for research on community health is in the area of distribution of health services. There has been during the past 30 years a number of significant efforts in this direction. Early attempts to develop group practice, hospital-based home care programs, and prepaid comprehensive medical care plans are only a few such projects. In the latter field, the Health Insurance Plan for Greater New York has provided a continuous flow of valuable research data.

In the field of public health, research is needed to define objectives better, to evaluate old programs, to find more efficient methods to distribute services, and to coordinate services with the activities of other agencies. Health manpower will continue to be scarce. Studies to determine how to use professional personnel to best advantage by employment of less well-trained staff are now being undertaken.

Plans to use less well-trained, less expensive personnel to supplement and extend the services of the physician are gaining momentum.

As already mentioned, medical colleges are now developing departments of community medicine designed to bridge the gaps between teaching hospitals and the public at home. Numerous investigations are being undertaken to learn more about the motivations that impel people to act as they do in seeking health care. Other studies on the barriers that deter people from making use of available health facilities are of particular significance.

It is already clear from what has been learned in recent years that the dispensers of health services have acted all too often blindly upon outmoded conceptions of what the consumer will accept. This will not serve the future. Research is demanded to clarify the best courses for action.

## Health Education and Motivation

Advances in medical technology and the gradual disappearance of economic barriers are making effective health care much more accessible to the general public. There still remain social and behavioral factors associated with causation and distribution of disease, health practices, and the utilization of health services. It is in this area that health education is most important. To be effective the health educator requires a knowledge of relevant social and behavioral factors that lead people to act as they do. The needs, the expectations, and the priorities of the consumer should be carefully considered in planning every health program. The task of the health educator is to bridge the communication gap that frequently exists between the consumer and the health professionals. Health educators through their special knowledge and training can also assist in the making of plans well adapted to the needs and desires of the consumer. Such carefully tailored health programs should be more readily accepted by the public.

In a recent book[22] Knutson, Professor of

Behavioral Sciences, at the School of Public Health, University of California, Berkeley, presents a full discussion of the basic factors that determine the reaction of the individual and of society to health. The comments of this perceptive author point up the difficulties of changing basic human concepts as related to health. Fortunately, progress in discovering better methods of communication with people as a result of current research in psychology is continuing at an accelerated rate.

In 1973, the President's Special Committee on Health Education recommended a National Center for Health Education to oversee efforts to provide better health information to the public. The proposed center would be a private, non-profit organization authorized by Congress and financed by public and private funds. A 25-member board of directors appointed by the President would oversee the affairs of the Center. The functions of the Center would be to conduct research, coordinate national, state, and local public health education programs, and serve as an information clearinghouse.

The need for consumer protection is one form of health education that appeals to the public. The greatest advocate of the public against predaceous corporations is Ralph Nader who almost single-handedly challenged the automobile manufacturers on the lack of safety devices in the cars they produce each year. Making a career of defending the public's interest, Nader has been able to secure sufficient funds and to attract able, eager young research colleagues. His "Study Group" has produced informative reports on water and air pollution, the dangers of pesticides, and food additives such as hormones and antibiotics in meat and poultry. These reports are well documented and clearly point out the "public be damned" attitude of many large industrial companies. Nader's group has strongly emphasized the health hazards of many of the industrial processes and the reluctance of corporations and responsible government agencies to provide the necessary corrective measures.[23,24]

The reaction of people to health programs is only one aspect of all human behavior, but the complexities and multiple motivation of all human actions are reflected in attitudes toward health. There are no easy explanations or simple ways of producing change. This has been demonstrated by the unsatisfactory results of the campaign against smoking cigarettes. The threat of lung cancer or of chronic lung disease is remote; the satisfaction of smoking is immediate. Few will change their fixed habit patterns because of the roll of distant drums. The same applies to dietary changes. To change such time-honored customs in favor of simplified less appealing diets is difficult for most people to accept.

It appears then that there are two basic functions of health education. One is generally understood and can be effectively applied—that is, to assist health agencies in making their activities more popular and acceptable to the population groups to which they are directed. This is largely a matter of learning to communicate with the clientele and minimizing objectionable features of the programs. There is a strong movement to employ people from the ethnic groups being served to be used to explain and persuade their fellows of the value of the programs being provided. The skills required by the health educator are largely directed toward interpretation and popularization of specific preventive health measures. One can expect wider and more successful application of such methods.

A second and more difficult role for health education is to convince the public to alter its accustomed ways of living, its personal hygiene, and its behavioral patterns with the view to the promotion of better health over the years. All of the techniques of human psychology and of the behavioral sciences are required to develop methods that promise positive results in this area. Much research is being undertaken currently to discover new and more effective approaches to influence personal motivation.[25,26] The need is great—the opportunities limitless.

## Public Relations

All too often health workers have failed to take the public into their confidence in launching programs of far-reaching implications with unfortunate results. The failure of many communities to provide for fluoridation of the public water supplies is an illustration of this lack of confidence in their health agencies. Good public relations require the exercise of tact, skill, and constant attention to human attributes.

The rather steady decline of the public image

of the medical profession over the past 30 years illustrates the sad consequence of poor public relations. The American Medical Association carries on many valuable functions in the way of raising educational and professional standards and protecting the public from false therapies and unethical practices, but the general public's knowledge of the Association is limited to the narrow bigoted opposition to constructive legislation to assist in the provision of medical care to the needy. All too often now one hears sour comments on the emphasis of physicians on income rather than service. For these and other reasons, the hospital is assuming an ever increasing part as a provider of medical care.

Physicians, nurses, voluntary agencies, public health agencies, and others involved in health work are dependent to a large degree on public good will. Rivalries, jealousies, duplication of services, and petty bickering do not inspire public confidence.

It is particularly important for hospitals to create a favorable image for the public. Almost all community hospitals depend to a considerable extent upon public contributions to finance renovations and new construction. Most of them are acutely aware of this need for public interest and confidence. Some employ public relations experts to control their news releases and to solicit the support of influential groups in their communities.

Possibly the greater participation of consumer representatives in the councils of the comprehensive health-planning agencies at both state and local levels will bring a better awareness of the importance of informing the public of what is to come and of securing its acceptance of the plans. Public health agencies have long been used to depending on legislative bodies for their financial support. One could learn useful lessons by studying the varying success that such appeals have met in one state or another. Probably the competence and astute personal attributes of the local health leaders are the important factors in obtaining legislative support. In every state with first class health services, one finds a continuous and carefully planned campaign to keep the public informed of what the health services have done and are doing. The public cannot be fooled all the time.

The social problems presented by an affluent, permissive society are calling for sophisticated techniques to get the health education program across to those most in need of it. Not only must the concerns for individual health such as nutrition, dental care and conservation of sight and hearing be emphasized, but sociological health problems relating to abuse of tobacco, alcohol, and drugs must be made clear. In this period of sex experimentation, young people must be made to understand such matters as family planning, avoidance of venereal infection, and personality development. If civilization, as we know it, is to survive, people must be taught to have concern for the care of their environment and to take an interest in the health and welfare of their fellow human beings in the world. These and a myriad of other important aspects of human health are to a large degree dependent upon educating and motivating the people of our country.

## Legislation

The constitution of the United States does not mention the word health. Federal authority for concerning itself with health matters stems from the clauses relating to general welfare, from the provisions to regulate interstate commerce, and from the power to levy taxes. The powers not granted to the Federal Government in the constitution reside in the states, each of which may delegate some powers to local governmental units. The legal basis for action by states in the health field is the exercise of police power, which gives states the authority to regulate its internal affairs to protect and promote the health, safety, morals, welfare, and general convenience of its citizens.

During recent years, the Federal Government has become far more active than formerly in initiating legislation in the health field. Brief accounts of some of the recent health-related legislative acts have already been given. Amendments to these acts and additional new legislation are sure to come. Indeed the trend these days is to believe that legislation is the surest and best method of obtaining health objectives. Probably this reliance upon legislation is justified if the new regulations are based on adequate information and study, and if the legislative action is timely. Another consideration that has a bearing on the advisability of legislation is the choice of suitable subjects for action. It has been demonstrated in numerous instances that ill-considered, untimely, and unsuitable legislative acts are impossible to enforce and frequently do more harm than good. The Liquor Prohibition Amendment and the Volstead Prohibition Enforcement Act of 1919 probably set back the cause of rational control of the use of alcoholic drinks for many decades. Nearly all hotly disputed legislation represents a series of compromises that often turn a reasonably good bill into a weak or bad one.

With all these admonitions concerning the limitations of the legislative process, it must be admitted that health agencies and other interested parties will seek such measures frequently in the years ahead. This is an age of planning. Those who plan want to have their concepts preserved in a legalistic framework. Perhaps this eagerness on the part of many to rush to legislatures for support of their schemes should stimulate to action those who would prefer to see problems handled whenever possible by other means.[27]

The Medicare and Medicaid Acts with their amendments have profoundly influenced the distribution and quality of standards of medical care. Many difficulties remain to be solved before full effectiveness of these and other measures can be achieved. Changes in forms of medical and hospital practice will have to be made. These adaptations could be accomplished by private actions, but, if not, some legislative intervention is almost sure to be enacted.

Analysts of Washington affairs predict that Congress will pass some form of National Health Insurance before the next presidential election year in 1976. What form this legislation may take is as yet uncertain. Probably there will be a mixture of private and public funds to provide health care for those unable to bear the whole financial burden.

## FUTURE PROSPECTS

What can be said about the prospects for public health and community medicine in the future? René Dubos has vigorously warned us not to be beguiled by utopian ideas of life without disease in which every individual may live to a great old age. It is true that life expectancy at birth has been growing steadily during recent decades, but this increase has resulted almost entirely from the great decrease in deaths in infancy and early childhood. Longevity for individuals over 45 years of age has changed slowly. The ultimate human span still remains for most individuals close to the biblical estimate of "three score and 10 years."

As old problems disappear, such as bacterial pollution of water, new ones arise, as is the case with air pollution. New and effective drugs are available in increasing numbers, but there has been a sharp rise in ill health caused by drug reactions. Nutritional deficiencies are replaced by the excessively rich diets consumed by physically inactive people. The uncertainties and stresses of modern society bring frustrations, fear, and tensions to a good proportion of the population which aggravates the compulsion to eat and drink.

Be that as it may, the public is aware of the exciting advances in medicine and wish to have for their families and for themselves an opportunity to share whatever benefits that can be provided. As more sophisticated diagnostic and therapeutic procedures are developed, their use can no longer be restricted to those able to meet the costs. Indeed, future prospects point toward a better distribution of all health services without the intervention of financial barriers.

Computer technology is being developed and applied to the health field at an increasingly rapid pace. Computer systems are being applied in biomedical research and in direct patient care such as monitoring of patients in operating rooms and in intensive care units. In diagnosis, computers assist physicians in identifying a broad range of diseases and in automated laboratory systems one is able to perform dozens of tests in less time than it took to do one test by former methods. Hospitals and clinics find computers useful in their accounting and billing procedures. It is certain that automation and computer systems will be employed far more widely in medicine in future years.[28,29]

Experience of other countries with publicly financed medical care points out the dangers of soaring costs and increasing demands for services. The short experience in the United States with Medicare has demonstrated that rising costs will be difficult to control.

As pointed out earlier in this chapter, a greater degree of community planning is essential to meet future health requirements. The laissez-faire methods of the past have resulted in the duplication of facilities and in the construction of unneeded hospital beds which have left large segments of the community with unmet needs. Even in an affluent nation, these wasteful policies cannot be long continued. Under the guidance of Federal, state, and local planning agencies in which all community interests must be represented, progress will·be made toward the goal of comprehensive health services for all the people. Possibly hospitals will serve as the primary centers of health service,[18] with neighborhood centers, group clinics, and private physicians integrated to provide service and to carry on teaching and research. Colleges of medicine and nursing and other centers for the training of allied medical personnel will be the nerve centers for setting standards of quality and for the education of health manpower. Required changes may proceed slowly, and a considerable amount of experimentation is needed to determine the best patterns for distribution of service in different regions. Change appears to be the hallmark of this generation.

## REFERENCES

1. Chase, A. *The Biological Imperatives.* New York: Holt, Rinehart and Winston, 1971.
2. Pifer, A. (President, Carnegie Corporation of New York). Bulletin Association of American Medical Colleges, Vol. IV, 80th Annual Meeting AAMC, Cincinnati, Ohio, October 30-November 3, 1969.
3. Reuther, W. P. The need for comprehensive national health insurance and the health service corps. In *Medicine in a Changing Society,* edited by L. Corey, S. E. Saltman, and M. F. Epstein, St. Louis: C. V. Mosby Co., 1972.
4. *Poverty and Health: A Sociological Analysis,* edited by J. Kosa, A. Antonovsky and I. K. Zola. Cambridge: Harvard University Press, 1969.
5. *Health Resources Statistics 1972-73,* National Center for Health Statistics, DHEW Publication No. (HSM) 73-1509.
6. *Higher Education and the Nation's Health.* The Carnegie Commission on Higher Education. New York: McGraw-Hill Book Co., 1970.
7. *Health Manpower 1966-1975: a study of requirements and supply.* United States Department of Labor Report 323. Washington, D. C.: Bureau of Labor Statistics, 1967.
8. Altman, S. H. *Present and Future Supply of Registered Nurses.* Public Health Service, Division of Nursing. DHEW Publication No. (NIH) 73-134. Reprinted August, 1972.
9. Sadler, A. M., Jr., Sadler, B. L. and Bliss, A. A. *The Physician's Assistant—Today and Tomorrow,* New Haven: Yale University Press, 1972.
10. Hall, T. L. (Coordinator). *Task Force Report.* Professional Health Manpower for Community Health Programs. Department of Health Administration, School of Public Health, University of North Carolina, Chapel Hill, 1973.
11. *Inventory of Federal Programs Supporting Health Manpower Training.* Public Health Service, Bureau of Health Manpower Education. DHEW Publication No. (NIH) 73-146, 1973.
12. Terris, M. A social policy for health. *Amer. J. Public Health, 58:* 5-12, 1968.
13. Mueller, M. S. Private health insurance in 1970: population coverage, enrollment and financial experience. *Soc. Sec. Bull., 35:* 3-19, Feb. 1972.
14. *Source Book of Health Insurance Data 1973-74,* Ed. 15. Health Insurance Institute, New York.
15. Burns, E. M. Social policy and the health services: the choices ahead. *Amer. J. Public Health, 57:* 199-212, 1967.
16. *Delivery of Health Services for the Poor.* U. S. DHEW Office of the Assistant Secretary (Planning and Evaluation), U. S. Government Printing Office, 1968.
17. Weeks, A. The pathology of poverty. In *Medicine in a Changing Society,* edited by L. Corey, S. E. Saltman, and M. F. Epstein. St. Louis: C. V. Mosby Co., 1972.
18. Somers, A. R. *Health Care in Transition: Directions for the Future.* Hospital Research and Educational Trust, Chicago, 1971.
19. Burnet, F. M., and White, D. O. *Natural History of Infectious Disease,* Ed. 4. Cambridge: Cambridge University Press, 1972.
20. Gabor, D. *Inventing the Future.* London: Secker and Warburg, 1963.
21. Overlooked boom: The pet industry. *U.S. News and World Report,* January 1, 1973, pages 54-55.
22. Knutson, A. L. *The Individual, Society and Health Behavior.* New York: Russell Sage Foundation, 1965.
23. Esposito, J. C., and Silverman, L. J. *Vanishing Air,* The Ralph Nader Study Group Report on Air Pollution. New York: Grossman Publishers, 1970.
24. Wellford, H., *Sowing the Wind—a Nader Report.* New York: Grossman Publishers, 1972.
25. *New Directions in Health Education,* edited by D. A. Read. New York: MacMillan Co., 1971.
26. Read, D. A., and Greene, W. H. *Creative Teaching in Health.* New York: MacMillan Co., 1971.
27. Conant, R. W. *The Politics of Community Health: Report of the Community Action Studies Project,* National Commission on Community Health Services. Washington, D. C.: Public Affairs Press, 1968.
28. *Computer Techniques in Biomedicine and Medicine,* Edited by E. Haga *et al.* Philadelphia: Auerbach Publishers, Inc., 1973.
29. Kernodle, J. R., and Ryan, G. A. *Computers in Medicine—a Look Ahead. J.A.M.A., 220:* 1489-1491, June 12, 1972.

# 14
# National health organizations

ADDICTS ANONYMOUS
Box 2000
Lexington, Kentucky 40501

ALCOHOLICS ANONYMOUS
P.O. Box 459
Grand Central Annex
New York, New York 10017

ALLERGY FOUNDATION OF AMERICA
801 2nd Avenue
New York, New York 100117

ALLIED YOUTH, INC.
Suite 1011
1901 Fort Meyer Drive
Arlington, Virginia 22209

AMERICAN ACADEMY OF FAMILY PHYSI-
CIANS
Volker Boulevard and Brookside
Kansas City, Missouri 64112

AMERICAN ACADEMY OF PEDIATRICS
1801 Hinman Avenue
Evanston, Illinois, 60204

AMERICAN ASSOCIATION FOR GIFTED
CHILDREN
15 Gramercy Park
New York, New York 10003

AMERICAN ASSOCIATION FOR HEALTH,
PHYSICAL EDUCATION, AND RECREA-
TION
1201 16th Street, N.W.
Washington, D.C. 20036

AMERICAN ASSOCIATION FOR MATER-
NAL AND CHILD HEALTH, INC.
116 South Michigan Avenue
Chicago, Illinois 60603

AMERICAN ASSOCIATION OF FOUNDA-
TIONS FOR MEDICAL CARE
1255 New Hampshire Avenue, N.W.
Washington, D.C. 20036

AMERICAN ASSOCIATION OF OPHTHALM-
OLOGY
1100 17th Street, N.W.
Washington, D.C. 20036

AMERICAN ASSOCIATION OF PHYSICIANS
ASSISTANTS
Duke University Medical Center
P.O. Box 2914 (CHS)
Durham, North Carolina 27706

AMERICAN CANCER SOCIETY
219 East 42nd Street
New York, New York 10017

AMERICAN DENTAL ASSOCIATION
211 East Chicago Avenue
Chicago Illinois 60611

AMERICAN DIABETES ASSOCIATION, INC.
18 East 48th Street
New York, New York 10017

AMERICAN DIETETIC ASSOCIATION
620 North Michigan Avenue
Chicago, Illinois 60611

AMERICAN EUGENICS SOCIETY
230 Park Avenue
New York, New York 10017

AMERICAN FOUNDATION FOR THE BLIND
15 West 16th Street
New York, New York 10011

AMERICAN GENETIC ASSOCIATION
1028 Connecticut Avenue, N.W.
Washington, D.C. 20036

AMERICAN HEART ASSOCIATION, INC.
44 East 23rd street
New York, New York 10010

AMERICAN LUNG ASSOCIATION
1740 Broadway
New York, New York 10019

AMERICAN MEDICAL ASSOCIATION: EDU-
CATION AND RESEARCH FOUNDATION
535 North Dearborn Street
Chicago, Illinois 60610

AMERICAN NATIONAL RED CROSS
17th and D Streets, N.W.
Washington, D.C. 20006

AMERICAN NURSES' ASSOCIATION
2420 Pershing Road
Kansas City, Missouri 64108
[

AMERICAN OSTEOPATHIC ASSOCIATION
212 East Ohio Street
Chicago, Illinois 60611

AMERICAN PHARMACEUTICAL ASSOCIA-
TION
2215 Constitution Avenue, N.W.
Washington, D.C. 20037

AMERICAN PHYSICAL THERAPY ASSOCIA-
TION
1156 15th Street, N.W.
Washington, D.C. 20005

AMERICAN PODIATRY ASSOCIATION
20 Chevy Chase Circle, N.W.
Washington, D.C. 20015

AMERICAN PSYCHIATRIC ASSOCIATION
1700 18th Street, N.W.
Washington, D.C. 20009

AMERICAN PUBLIC HEALTH ASSOCIATION
1015 18th Street, N.W.
Washington, D.C. 20036

AMERICAN    REHABILITATION    COM-
MITTEE, INC.
28 East 21st Street
New York, New York 10010

AMERICAN    REHABILITATION    FOUNDA-
TION, INC.
Keany Rehabilitation Institute
1800 Chicago Avenue
Minneapolis, Minnesota 55404

AMERICAN SCHOOL HEALTH ASSOCIA-
TION 107 South DePeyster Street
Kent, Ohio 44240

AMERICAN SOCIAL HEALTH ASSOCIA-
TION
1790 Broadway
New York, New York 10019

AMERICAN SPEECH AND HEARING AS-
SOCIATION
9030 Old Georgetown Road
Washington, D.C. 20014

ARTHRITIS FOUNDATION
1212 Avenue of the Americas
New York, New York 10036

ASSOCIATION FOR VOLUNTARY STERILI-
ZATION
14 West 40th Street
New York, New York 10018

BRAIN RESEARCH FOUNDATIONS, INC.
An Affiliate of The University of Chicago
343 South Dearborn Street
Chicago, Illinois 60604

CHILD STUDY ASSOCIATION OF AMERICA
9 East 89th Street
New York, New York 10028

CHILD WELFARE LEAGUE OF AMERICA,
INC.
67 Irving Place
New York, New York 10003

CLEVELAND HEALTH MUSEUM
8911 Euclid Avenue
Cleveland, Ohio 44106

DAMON RUNYON MEMORIAL FUND FOR
CANCER RESEARCH, INC.
33 West 56th Street
New York, New York 10017

DEAFNESS RESEARCH FOUNDATION
366 Madison Avenue
New York, New York 10017

EPILEPSY FOUNDATION OF AMERICA
1828 L Street, N.W., Suite 406
Washington, D.C. 20036

FIGHT FOR SIGHT, INC.
National Council to Combat Blindness, Inc.
41 West 57th Street
New York, New York 10019

LEONARD WOOD MEMORIAL FOR THE
ERADICATION OF LEPROSY
American Leprosy Foundation
79 Madison Avenue
New York, New York 10016

MARGARET SANGER RESEARCH BUREAU
17 West 16th Street
New York, New York 10011

MATERNITY CENTER ASSOCIATION
48 East 92nd Street
New York, New York 10028

MEDIC-ALERT  FOUNDATION  INTERNA-
TIONAL
1000 North Palm Street
Turlock, California 95380

MUSCULAR DYSTROPHY ASSOCIATIONS
OF AMERICA, INC.
1790 Broadway
New York, New York 10019

MYASTHENIA GRAVIS FOUNDATION, INC.
2 East 103rd Street
New York, New York 10029

NATIONAL ASSOCIATION FOR VISUALLY
HANDICAPPED
3201 Balboa Street
San Francisco, California 98121

NATIONAL ASSOCIATION OF HEARING
AND SPEECH AGENCIES
919 18th Street, N.W.
Washington, D.C. 20006

NATIONAL ASSOCIATION FOR MENTAL
HEALTH
1800 North Kent Street
Rosslyn, Virginia 22209

NATIONAL ASSOCIATION FOR RE-
TARDED CHILDREN
2709 Avenue E East
Arlington, Texas 76010

NATIONAL COUNCIL ON ALCOHOLISM
2 Park Avenue
New York, New York 10016

NATIONAL CYSTIC FIBROSIS RESEARCH
FOUNDATION
3379 Peachtree Road, N.E.
Atlanta, Georgia 30326

NATIONAL FOUNDATION
800 Second Avenue
New York, New YOrk 10017

NATIONAL HEALTH COUNCIL
1790 Broadway
New York, New York 10019

NATIONAL GENETICS FOUNDATION, INC.
250 West 57th Street
New York, New York 10019

NATIONAL HEMOPHILIA FOUNDATION
25 West 39th Street
New York, New York 10018

NATIONAL KIDNEY FOUNDATION
116 East 27th Street
New York, New York 10016

NATIONAL MULTIPLE SCLEROSIS SOC-
IETY
257 Park Avenue South
New York, New York 10010

NATIONAL PARAPLEGIA FOUNDATION
333 North Michigan Avenue
Chicago, Illinois 60601

NATIONAL PITUITARY AGENCY
210 West Fayette Street
Baltimore, Maryland 21201

NATIONAL SAFETY COUNCIL
425 North Michigan Avenue
Chicago, Illinois 60611

NATIONAL EASTER SEAL SOCIETY FOR
CHIPPLED CHILDREN AND ADULTS, INC.
2023 West Ogden Avenue
Chicago, Illinois 60612

NATIONAL SOCIETY FOR MEDICAL RE-
SEARCH
1330 Massachusetts Avenue, N.W.
Suite 103
   Washington, D.C. 20005

NATIONAL SOCIETY FOR THE PRE-
VENTION OF BLINDNESS
79 Madison Avenue
New York, New York 10016

PAN AMERICAN HEALTH ORGANIZATION
525 23rd Street, N.W.
Washington, D.C. 20037

PARKINSON's DISEASE FOUNDATION
William Black Medical Research Building
640 West 168th Street
New York, New York 10032

PEOPLE TO PEOPLE HEALTH FOUNDA-
TION, INC.
2233 Wisconsin Avenue, N.W.
Washington, D.C. 20007

PLANNED PARENTHOOD-WORLD POPULA-
TION
810 Seventh Avenue
New York, New York 10019

RESEARCH TO PREVENT BLINDNESS, INC.
598 Madison Avenue
New York, New York 10022

SEX INFORMATION AND EDUCATION
  COUNCIL OF THE UNITED STATES
1855 Broadway
New York, New York 10010

SOCIETY FOR PUBLIC HEALTH EDU-
  CATORS

655 Sutter Street
San Francisco, California 94102

UNITED CEREBRAL PALSY ASSOCIATION
66 East 34th Street
New York, New York 10016

# 15

# Glossary

**Acetylate**—to introduce one or more acetyl radicals into a compound.

**Acidosis**—a condition of reduced alkaline reserve of the blood and other body fluids, with or without an actual decrease in pH.

**Adipose**—fatty, relating to fat.

**Adrenals**—endocrine glands near or upon the kidney.

**Age adjusted**—a method used to make valid statistical comparisons by assuming the same age distribution among different groups being compared.

**Alkylate**—to substitute a side chain radical into an aromatic compound.

**Allantois**—a fetal membrane; in the fowl, it lies close beneath the porous shell and serves as an organ of respiration.

**Amino acids**—an organic acid in which one of the hydrogen atoms has been replaced by $NH_2$; included among the products of the hydrolysis of protein.

**Amnion**—the innermost of the membranes enveloping the developing embryo.

**Anaphylaxis**—an exaggerated or extreme hypersensitivity that may be induced in various animals as the result of the injection of even a small dose of foreign material.

**Aneuploid**—having an abnormal number of chromosomes.

**Aneurysm**—circumscribed dilation of an artery.

**Angina pectoris**—a severe constricting pain in the chest due to failure of blood supply to the heart muscle.

**Angiography**—X ray of vessels after the injection of a radiopaque material into an artery.

**Antibody**—a modified protein in the serum of an animal, usually formed in response to an injection of antigen.

**Antigen**—any of various sorts of material, mostly protein in nature, that as a result of coming in contact with appropriate tissues of an animal stimulate an immune response.

**Antimetabolites**—cytotoxic drugs that substitute for normal components in enzymatic reactions in the body.

**Aplasia**—defective development of a tissue or an organ or a cessation of the usual regenerative process.

**Aplastic anemia**—failure in the production of blood cells by the bone marrow.

**Arachnoid**—a membrane, or middle layer of membranes, covering the brain and spinal cord.

**Arteriosclerosis**—hardening of the arteries.

**Arthus phenomenon**—the hypersensitive inflammatory reaction in rabbits resulting from repeated injections of antigen.

**Atheroma**—an accumulation of lipid-containing material in deposits in the intima or subintima of arteries.

**Atherosclerosis**—sclerosis or hardening of the inner lining or intima of the arteries.

**Atopic**—relating to a form of allergy characterized by immediate reaction of sensitive tissue to a specific exciting agent.

**Autosomal**—relating to chromosomes other than sex chromosomes.

**Axillary**—relating to the axilla or the armpit.

**Bioanalysts**—usually non-M.D. directors of clinical laboratories.

**Biopsy**—examination of tissue taken from a living patient.

**Bronchopneumonia**—an inflammation of the walls of the smaller bronchial tubes with areas of inflamed and consolidated lung tissue usually corresponding to the affected tubes.

**Calcified**—hardened tissue as the result of precipitates or larger deposits of insoluble salts of calcium.

**Caseous**—the appearance of tissue affected by coagulative necrosis, a cheese-like consistency.

**Cell-mediated immunity**—immunity provided by cells that can detect a microbial invasion and can provide a mechanism for resisting it without secretion of antibody.

**Cellulitis**—inflammation of cellular or connective tissue.

**Census tract**—small areas into which large cities are divided. Data collected by the Bureau of the Census are tabulated by these small areas.

**Cerebrovascular**—relating to the blood supply to the brain.

**Cerebrum**—the principal part of the brain, including most parts within the skull, except the medulla, pons, and cerebellum.

**Chemotherapy**—treatment of disease by means of chemical substances or drugs.

**Cholera**—an acute epidemic infectious disease caused by a specific agent (*Spirillum cholerae asiaticae*) marked by diarrhea, muscular cramps, vomiting and collapse.

**Cholesterol**—a fat-like monatomic alcohol

found in all animal fats, in bile, blood, brain tissue, milk, yolk of egg, and other foods; occurs in atheroma of the arteries.

**Chorea**—a disorder, usually of childhood, characterized by irregular, spasmodic, involuntary movements of the limbs or facial muscles.

**Chromatin**—portion of a cell nucleus that is readily stained by dyes.

**Chromosome**—a body in the cell nucleus that is the bearer of genes and is capable of reproducing through successive cell divisions.

**Cilia**—minute hair-like processes attached to free cell surfaces, as epithelial lining of bronchi.

**Clinic**—a medical institution where ambulatory patients are cared for.

**Clinical**—relating to the symptoms and course of a disease.

**Clinician**—a physician engaged in medical practice caring for patients.

**Coliform**—resembling the colon bacillus or belonging to the coli group of bacilli.

**Collagen**—whitish fibers in the skin, tendons, and connective tissue; the fibers are composed of fibrils bound together by a cementing material.

**Conjunctiva**—the mucous membrane covering the anterior surface of the eyeball and lining the lids.

**Conjunctivitis**—inflammation of the mucous membrane covering the anterior surface of the eyeball and lining the lids.

**Cytomegalovirus**—salivary gland disease virus. Invasion of tissue causes giant cell formation.

**Desquamation**—the shedding of the epithelial elements, chiefly of the skin, in scales.

**Diabetes mellitus** (literally, siphoning honey )—a metabolic disease in which sugar is excreted in the urine.

**Dimorphic**—existing in two forms.

**Dominant**—ruling or controlling, referring to genetic factors.

**Droplet nuclei**—sneezing or coughing produces infected droplets which evaporate in the air leaving nuclei of a few millimicrons in diameter frequently containing one microorganism or more.

**Dyscrasia**—a diseased state of the blood due to the action of toxic materials.

**Dysphasia**—lack of coordination in speech.

**Eczema**—an inflammation of the skin presenting moist or dry lesions and often accompanied by itching and burning.

**Edema**—excessive accumulation of clear watery fluid in the tissues.

**Edentulous**—toothless. Without teeth.

**Electrocardiograph**—an instrument for recording the potential of the electrical currents that traverse the heart and initiate its contraction.

**Electroencephalograph**—an apparatus which records the alternating currents of the brain.

**Embolus**—a plug, composed of a detached clot, mass of bacteria, or other foreign body occluding a blood vessel.

**Endemic**—the presence of a disease in a community on a continuous basis.

**Enzyme**—a protein, secreted by the body cells, that acts as a catalyst, inducing chemical changes in other substances, itself remaining apparently unchanged in the process.

**Epidemic**—extensive prevalence, in a community, of a disease brought from without, or a temporary increase in the number of cases of an endemic disease.

**Epithelioid**—resembling epithelium.

**Epithelium**—cellular, avascular layer covering all the free surfaces, cutaneous, mucous, and serous, including the glands.

**Erythema**—redness of the skin.

**Erythrogenic Toxin**—an exotoxin which causes the red skin eruption in scarlet fever.

**Etiology**—the study of causes, usually causes of disease.

**Exchange Transfusion**—substitution transfer of blood from one person to another.

**Exudative**—relating to the process of exuding or oozing.

**Fetus**—the unborn young of a viviparous animal after it has taken form in the uterus.

**Fibril**—a minute fiber.

**Fibrin**—an elastic, filamentous protein derived from fibrinogen by the action of thrombin in coagulation of the blood.

**Fibrinogen**—a globulin of the blood plasma that is converted into the coagulated protein, fibrin, by the action of thrombin in the presence of ionized calcium.

**Fibroblast**—an elongated, flattened cell present in connective tissue and thought to produce fibrous tissues.

**Fibrocystic disease of the pancreas**—a congenital metabolic disorder in which glands of external secretion function abnormally.

**Gamma globulin (immune serum globulin (ISG)**—an antibody-rich fraction of pooled plasma from normal donors.

**Gene**—the functional unit of heredity.

**Gestation period**—the length of time of pregnancy.

**Giant cell**—a large-sized cell with many nuclei.

**Glaucoma**—a disease characterized by high pressure in the eyeball.

**Glomerulonephritis**—renal disease characterized by bilateral inflammatory changes in glomeruli which are not the result of infection of the kidneys.

**Glomerulus**—a tuft formed of capillary loops at the beginning of each uriniferous tubule in the kidney.

**Gross National Product (GNP)**—the total national output of goods and services valued at market prices.

**Harelip**—a congenital fissure in the upper lip, often combined with cleft palate.

**Hashimoto's thyroiditis**—chronic inflammation of the thyroid gland thought to be an autoimmune disease.

**Hemolysis**—breaking up of red blood cells in such a manner that hemoglobin is liberated in the surrounding medium.

**Hemolytic**—destructive to blood cells, resulting in the liberation of hemoglobin.

**Heterozygotes**—individuals produced by the union of two germ cells of dissimilar genetic composition for certain characteristics.

**Histamine**—a powerful chemical derived in the body from histidine. It is liberated in the skin as a result of injury.

**Histidine**—an amino acid produced by the hydrolysis of protein.

**Hives (urticaria)**—an eruption of itching wheals usually of systemic origin due to hypersensitivity to foods or drugs, foci of infection, or psychic stimuli.

**Homozygotes**—individuals produced by the union of two germ cells genetically identical for certain genes.

**Hypercholesterolemia**—an abnormally large quantity of cholesterol in the cells and plasma of the circulating blood.

**Hypercoagulability**—tendency of the blood to clot too readily.

**Hyperlipemia**—an abnormally large quantity of total lipids in the blood.

**Hypersensitivity**—abnormal and excessive susceptibility of the body to certain agents, for example, pollens in hay fever.

**Hypoglycemia**—an abnormally low concentration of glucose in the circulating blood.

**Hypoxia**—decreased amount of oxygen in organs and tissues.

**Iatrogenic**—relating to abnormal states or conditions produced by the physician in a patient as a result of a therapeutic or diagnostic procedure.

**Incidence**—the number of cases of a disease reported during a stated period of time.

**Idiopathic**—referring to a disease that arises without apparent external cause.

**Immunotherapy**—treatment directed at the production of immunity.

**Incipient**—beginning to exist, coming into existence.

**Infarct**—death of tissue resulting from obstruction of the artery supplying the part.

**Infiltration**—the accumulation in a tissue of substances not normal to it.

**Insecticide**—a chemical that kills insects.

**Intracranial**—within the skull.

**Ischemic**—relating to a local anemia due to mechanical obstruction to the blood supply.

**Isotope**—substances chemically identical but whose nuclei contain different numbers of neutrons; many are radioactive.

**Ketosis**—a condition of acidosis in the body in which acetone substances or ketone bodies are found.

**Lesion**—a wound or injury, a more or less circumscribed pathological change in the tissues.

**Leukemia**—a disease characterized by an uncontrolled multiplication of one of the types of white blood cells.

**Leukocyte**—one of the several kinds of white blood cells.

**Lumen**—the space in the interior of a tubular structure, such as an artery or the intestine.

**Lupus erythematosis**—a disease of the skin and mucuous membranes of unknown etiology characterized by lesions frequently presenting a butterfly formation on the face. Disease may become disseminated.

**Lymphocyte**—a white blood cell formed in lymphoid tissue throughout the body.

**Lymphoma**—a general term that includes various tumors of the lymphoid tissue.

**Lymphosarcoma**—a form of malignant lymphoma

**Macrophage**—large mononuclear cells found in various tissues and organs of the body, sometimes called "wandering cells"; their function is to engulf foreign particles, bacteria, or other invading microorganisms.

**Macula**—a small discolored spot on the skin, not elevated.

**Mediastinum**—the dividing area between the left and right lungs in the thorax, containing the heart, large blood vessels, and other important organs.

**Meninges**—the membranous envelope covering the brain and spinal cord.

**Metastasis**—the spread of a disease, or its local manifestations, from one part of the body to another, generally applied to neoplasms.

**Miliary**—resembling a millet seed in size (about 2 mm.); marked by the presence of nodules of millet seed size on any surface.

**Millimicron**—one thousandth of a micron, or one millionth of a millimeter.

**Monocyte**—a large mononuclear white blood cell.

**Morbidity**—the ratio of sick to well in a community.

**Morphology**—the science which treats of the configuration or the structure of animals and plants.

**Mortality**—death rate, the ratio of the number of deaths to a given population.

**Mosaicism**—relating to the juxtaposition in an

organism of genetically different tissues resulting from somatic mutation.

**Mucinase**—an enzyme which hydrolyzes mucin, the chief constituent of mucus.

**Mucoprotein**—a protein containing a carbohydrate group; does not coagulate upon heating, but otherwise acts chemically as a protein.

**Mutation**—a change in the character of a gene that is perpetuated in subsequent divisions of the cell in which it occurs.

**Myocardium**—the muscular substance of the heart.

**Myosthenia gravis**—a disease characterized by a chronic progressive muscular weakness.

**Necrosis**—the pathological death of one cell or more or of a portion of tissue or organ.

**Neoplasm**—new growth of cells or tissues usually applied to malignant tumors.

**Nephritis**—inflammation of the kidneys.

**Nephritogenic**—capable of initiating inflammation of the kidney, or nephritis.

**Niacin**—nicotinic acid; vitamin B group.

**Nocturia**—urinating at night.

**Nosocomial**—relating to a hospital.

**Organ of Corti**—a structure in the internal ear.

**Oropharynx**—central portion of the pharynx.

**Palpitation**—forceful beats of the heart perceptible to the patient.

**Pandemic**—widely epidemic, involving many regions of the world.

**Pathogen**—any microorganism or other substance causing disease.

**Pathogenesis**—the mode of origin or development of any disease or morbid process.

**Pathogenic**—possessing ability to cause infection.

**Pathology**—the medical science that deals with all aspects of disease especially the essential nature and functional changes resulting from the disease processes.

**Pesticide**—a chemical product that destroys fungi, insects, rodents or any other pest.

**Phagocyte**—a cell possessing the property of ingesting bacteria, or any foreign particles that enter the tissues.

**Phenylalaninemia**—an abnormal increase in quantity of phenylalanine, an essential amino acid, in the blood.

**Photochromagen**—a microorganism capable of producing pigment in culture if exposed to light.

**Pinta**—a disease caused by a spirochete, endemic in Mexico and Central America, marked by an eruption of patches of varying color on the skin that finally become white.

**Placenta**—the organ of metabolic interchange between fetus and mother.

**Plasma**—the fluid portion of the circulating blood.

**Pleurisy**—inflammation of the serous membrane enveloping the lungs and lining the walls of the thoracic cavity.

**Polymorphonuclear**—a leukocyte having nuclei of varied forms.

**Polypeptide**—a peptide formed by the union of an indefinite (usually large) number of amino acids.

**Polyploid**—pertaining to the state of a cell nucleus containing three or a higher multiple of the haploid number of chromosomes.

**Polysaccharide**—a carbohydrate containing a large number of saccharide groups.

**Precipitin**—an antibody formed in the blood serum of an animal that has received intravenously a series of gradually increasing doses of a foreign protein.

**Precordial**—relating to the surface of the lower thorax over the heart.

**Prevalence**—number of cases of an illness occurring at a point of time.

**Prognosis**—the foretelling of the probable course of a disease.

**Proliferative**—relating to the growth in numbers of similar cells.

**Properdin**—a high-molecular-weight antigenic fraction of human euglobulin with marked antimicrobial activity against some pathogenic organisms.

**Protamine**—a group of proteins, highly basic and rich in arginine, found in fish spermatozoa in combination with nucleic acid.

**Puerperal fever**—an illness characterized by high fever in a woman who has just given birth to a baby.

**Punctate**—marked with points or dots.

**Pyloric stenosis, congenital**—an hereditary narrowing of the outlet of the stomach.

**Recessive**—not dominant, referring to genetic factors.

**Retina**—the inner nervous tunic of the eyeball which comprises an optic portion which receives the visual rays.

**Rheumatoid arthritis**—a disease affecting the joints and other organs whose etiology is unknown; a severe disabling disease.

**Rodenticide**—an agent lethal to rats, rabbits, guinea pigs, or other rodents.

**Saccharide**—a sugar compound.

**Salpingectomy**—removal of the Fallopian tubes.

**Scleredema**—hardening and swelling of the skin and subcutaneous tissue.

**Sequelae**—pathological conditions following an attack of a disease.

**Serological surveys**—collection of blood specimens for immunity tests to determine previous distribution of a specific infectious disease.

**Serology**—the study of sera and their reactions.

**Sickle cell anemia**—an hereditary and familial hemolytic anemia peculiar to Negroes and people of the Mediterranean area characterized by crescent-shaped red blood cells.

**Somatic**—relating to the body, including the head and neck, without the limbs.

**Sporadic**—occurring singly, not grouped; neither epidemic nor endemic.

**Stabilized population**—a population is stablized when the number of births has come into balance with the number of deaths, with the result that, the effects of immigration aside, the size of the population remains relatively constant.

**Sternum**—the breast bone.

**Subarachnoid**—beneath the arachnoid membrane that covers the brain and spinal cord.

**Subclinical**—causing no symptoms, inapparent.

**Suppurative**—forming pus.

**Teratogenic**—relating to the origin or production of an abnormal fetus.

**Thrombus**—a clot that more or less occludes a blood vessel or may form in a cavity of the heart.

**Thymus**—a lymphoid organ located in the lower part of the neck of babies which through gradual change decreases to small size in adults.

**Toxoplasmosis**—a systemic protozoan disease; early prenatal infections may cause death of fetus; infections in adults may be mild and go undetected.

**Trachea**—air tube extending from the larynx to the bronchi.

**Trisomy**—state of an individual having 47 chromosomes instead of the normal 46.

**Tubercle**—a characteristic nodular reaction in the tissues caused by tuberculosis infection.

**Tuberculin**—a preparation made from cultures of the tubercle bacillus used as a skin test for the study of tuberculosis.

**Typhoid**—an acute infectious disease with high fever caused by a bacillus, *Salmonella typhi*.

**Uterine cervix**— the neck of the uterus; the lower part of the uterus extending from the isthmus of the uterus into the vagina.

**Vasectomy**—excision of a segment of the vas deferens.

**Vasodilator**—an agent that causes dilation of the blood vessels.

**Ventricle**—a small cavity, especially one in the brain or the heart.

**Waldeyer's ring**— lymphoid ring formed by tonsils and other lymphoid tissue in the throat.

**Yaws**—an infectious disease of the tropics, marked by ulcerations of the skin and destructive changes in bones.

# Index